Pharmacokinetics: Advanced Principles and Applications

Pharmacokinetics: Advanced Principles and Applications

Edited by **Sean Boyd**

FOSTER ACADEMICS

New Jersey

Published by Foster Academics,
61 Van Reypen Street,
Jersey City, NJ 07306, USA
www.fosteracademics.com

Pharmacokinetics: Advanced Principles and Applications
Edited by Sean Boyd

International Standard Book Number: 978-1-63242-319-1 (Hardback)

Printed in China.

Contents

Preface

Every book is a source of knowledge and this one is no exception. The idea that led to the conceptualization of this book was the fact that the world is advancing rapidly; which makes it crucial to document the progress in every field. I am aware that a lot of data is already available, yet, there is a lot more to learn. Hence, I accepted the responsibility of editing this book and contributing my knowledge to the community.

The advanced principles and applications of pharmacokinetics have been discussed in this book. It contains updated information and practical analyses regarding the study of drug pharmacokinetics in animals as well as humans. The aim of this book is to serve as a source of reference for scientists, researchers and clinicians and help them to logically develop their knowledge regarding this field from basics to advanced applications. The book consists of analyses of advanced theories which cover topics like bioequivalence studies, simulation theories on the basis of computers, pharmacogenomics in association with pharmacokinetics, drug interactions of herbal medicines and veterinary pharmacokinetics. It also covers practical aspects providing numerous examples of procedures and applications in advanced pharmacokinetics.

While editing this book, I had multiple visions for it. Then I finally narrowed down to make every chapter a sole standing text explaining a particular topic, so that they can be used independently. However, the umbrella subject sinews them into a common theme. This makes the book a unique platform of knowledge.

I would like to give the major credit of this book to the experts from every corner of the world, who took the time to share their expertise with us. Also, I owe the completion of this book to the never-ending support of my family, who supported me throughout the project.

Editor

Section 1

Advanced Concepts

1

Bioequivalence Studies

Aisha Qayyum
National University of Sciences and Technology
Pakistan

1. Introduction

During last four decades there is an increased use of generic drug products in order to lower the healthcare cost. With increased availability and use of generic drug products, healthcare professionals are encountered with a large number of multisource products from which they have to select therapeutically equivalent products. Generic substitution is of concern not only for healthcare professionals but also for pharmaceutical industries, consumers and government officials. Many research papers have pointed out the concern regarding standards for approval of generic products which may not always ensure therapeutic equivalence (Boix-Montanes, 2011; Skelly, 2010; Tothfalusi et al., 2009; Midha et al., 2005; Chen & Lesko, 2001; Chen et al., 2000; Strom, 1987; Lamy, 1986). To alleviate this fear many guidelines/guidance and regulations covering the licensing of generic products have been introduced to ensure that the medicinal products reaching the market have well-established efficacy and safety profile (FDA, 1992, 1996, 2001a, 2001b, 2003, 2011; CDSCO, 2005; SFDA, 2005; Health Canada, 2004; CPMP, 2000; WHO, 1986).

Generally, demonstration of bioequivalence (BE) is the most appropriate method of ensuring therapeutic equivalence between two medicinal products. Bioequivalence studies should be conducted for comparison of medicinal products containing same active substance. Such studies need to be carefully designed to take into account biopharmaceutical, ethical, medical, pharmacokinetic, analytical and statistical considerations. The studies should be aimed to critically assess the possibility of alternate use of these products. In the 2003 United States Food and Drug Administration (FDA) guidance, bioequivalence is defined as:

> "the absence of a significant difference in the rate and extent to which the active ingredient or active moiety in pharmaceutical equivalents or pharmaceutical alternatives becomes available at the site of drug action when administered at the same molar dose under similar conditions in an appropriately designed study" (FDA, 2003).

Bioequivalence is actually the comparison of the bioavailability of two drug products. In the 2003 United States Food and Drug Administration (FDA) guidance, bioavailability is defined as:

> "the rate and extent to which the active ingredient or active moiety is absorbed from a drug product and becomes available at the site of action. For drug products that are not

intended to be absorbed into the blood stream, bioavailability may be assessed by measurements intended to reflect the rate and extent to which the active ingredient or active moiety becomes available at the site of action" (FDA, 2003).

According to World Health Organization (WHO) guidelines, bioavailability is defined as:

"the rate and extent to which the active drug ingredient or therapeutic moiety is absorbed from a drug product and becomes available at the site of drug action" (WHO, 1986).

According to the United States Food and Drug Administration (FDA) "pharmaceutical equivalents" are drug products that contain identical active ingredients and are identical in strength or concentration, dosage form, and route of administration (FDA, 2011).

The CPMP (Committee for Proprietary Medicinal Products) guidance on bioavailability and bioequivalence confers the concept of therapeutic equivalence as:

"A medicinal product is therapeutically equivalent with another product if it contains the same active substance or therapeutic moiety and, clinically, shows the same efficacy and safety as that product, whose efficacy and safety has been established. In practice, demonstration of bioequivalence is generally the most appropriate method of substantiating therapeutic equivalence between medicinal products, which are pharmaceutically equivalent or pharmaceutical alternatives, provided they contain excipients generally recognized as not having an influence on safety and efficacy and comply with labeling requirements with respect to excipients. However in some cases where similar extent of absorption but different rates of absorption are observed, the products can still be judged therapeutically equivalent if those differences are not of therapeutic relevance. A clinical study to prove that differences in absorption rate are not therapeutically relevant, will probably be necessary"(CPMP, 2000).

In early 1960's extensive work in pharmacokinetics offered substantial evidence that composition and dosage form of a drug product can affect *in vivo* properties as well as therapeutic effects. These differences have been attributed to the effect of different drug excipients used, variations in manufacturing procedures and the properties of final dosage form on the rate and extent of the drug absorption from its site of administration. The importance of bioavailability came into lime-light after an incidence in Australia where a change in an inactive excipient of phenytoin formulation by the manufacturer resulted in low plasma levels of active drug leading to therapeutic failure and seizures in epileptic patients who were previously well-controlled with the same dose of same drug. Similarly in Europe marked variations in the plasma levels of digoxin were observed with different preparations of the drug resulting in either toxicity or therapeutic failure (Crawford et al., 2006; Welage et al., 2001; Soryal & Richens, 1992; Lindenbaum et al., 1971; Tyrer et al., 1970).

Bioequivalence and bioavailability studies are important during drug development of both new drug products and their generic equivalents. Provision of bioavailability and/or bioequivalence study data is an important element in support of Investigational New Drug Applications (INDs), New Drug Applications (NDAs), Abbreviated New Drug Applications (ANDAs) and their supplements. The term generic drug product has been defined as "interchangeable multi-source pharmaceutical product". Generic products are the copies of brand-name drugs with same dosage form, strength, route of administration, intended use and toxicity profile as the original innovator drug. Concern about lowering healthcare costs has resulted in an increase in the use of cheaper generic drug products instead of branded products. The innovator drugs are protected from copying by patents that last for 20 years from the first filing of the new chemical entity. Many people are concerned why generic drugs are often cheaper than the brand-name versions. It is because all the development work and clinical trials on new chemical entity are carried out by innovator to get initial drug approval which is later on reflected in its high price whereas the generic manufacturers only need to submit the bioequivalence data of the generic product to get a product license. The new products need to undergo bioequivalence testing before they are marketed. The difference may exist in absorption reflected in differing bioavailability profile of various brands, production batches or dosage forms of a drug. This can lead to either over- or under-medication if one entity is substituted for the other. The under-medication can lead to therapeutic failure and on the other hand over-medication can lead to toxicity. To avoid such risk it is best to study the bioavailability of all products but practically it is not possible. So each drug and any change in formulation must be considered individually while keeping in mind the real medical need for such studies in order to ensure efficacy and safety of these drugs. Many clinicians while switching or interchanging the different products are concerned with the safety and effectiveness of the new product. This concern is because of the fact that small changes in bioavailability can lead to significant changes in the efficacy or safety of the drug. Bioequivalence studies are designed with this concern in mind and to devise the strategies that minimize the risk to the patient. So when the generic product is pharmaceutically equivalent as well as bioequivalent to the innovator drug, then it is expected to be therapeutically equivalent (Kowalski et al., 2006; Crawford et al., 2006; FDA, 2003; Welage et al., 2001; Vasquez & Min, 1999; Banahan & Kolassa, 1997; Benet & Goyan, 1995; Marzo and Balant, 1995; WHO, 1986).

2. Design and conduct of bioequivalence studies

The basis of a bioequivalence study is the comparison of the drug product to be tested with an appropriate reference product (branded innovator drug). In bioequivalence studies an applicant compares the systemic exposure profile of a test drug to that of a reference drug product. Bioequivalence of two products can be assessed using *in vitro* standards, pharmacokinetic profile, clinical or pharmacodynamic end points. Different approaches for determination of bioequivalence of a drug product are:

- An *in vivo* test in humans in which the concentration of the active ingredient and when appropriate, its active metabolites, in blood, plasma, serum or other suitable biological fluid is measured as a function of time.
- An *in vivo* test in humans in which the urinary excretion of the active ingredient and when appropriate, its active metabolites are measured as a function of time.
- An *in vitro* test that has been correlated with and is predictive of human bioavailability profile or the one acceptable to FDA (e.g. dissolution rate test) that ensures human *in vivo* bioavailability.
- An *in vivo* test in humans in which an appropriate pharmacological effect of the active ingredient and when appropriate, its active metabolites are measured as a function of time if this effect can be measured with adequate accuracy, sensitivity and reproducibility.

- Well-controlled clinical trials that establish the efficacy and safety of the drug product, for purpose of determining bioavailability, or comparative clinical trials, for purpose of demonstrating bioequivalence.
- Any other approach considered adequate by the FDA to measure bioavailability or ascertain bioequivalence.

Bioequivalence for most of oral tablets or capsules is demonstrated *in vivo* by comparing the rate and extent of absorption that is bioavailability of the generic product with that of the innovator product. This is done by measuring the active ingredient concentration in blood, plasma, serum or other biological fluids over a certain period of time for both the generic and innovator products, also called test and reference drugs respectively. By doing so the bioequivalence studies frequently rely on pharmacokinetic measures such as area under the concentration-time curve (AUC) and peak drug concentration (Cmax) (Niazi, 2007; FDA, 2001a, 2003; Pidgen, 1996; Nation & Sanson, 1994).

2.1 Study design

Many authors have debated whether multi-dose or single-dose studies should be used to assess bioequivalence. Generally single-dose pharmacokinetic studies are recommended for both immediate- and modified-release drug products as they are more sensitive in assessing the active ingredient released from drug into circulation. For assessing bioequivalence of two formulations of a drug, two-sequence, two-period, crossover study is conducted after administration of single dose under fasted conditions. In crossover design the subjects serve as their own controls and they crossover from one treatment to the other. A large variability in drug clearance often exists among the individuals. However the intrasubject variation is usually smaller relative to inter-subjects variability. Parallel studies are appropriate if the drug has extremely long half life, repeated pharmacokinetic profile is difficult to obtain, or residual pharmacodynamic effects are relevant. Furthermore, if carry over effects from one treatment period to another are of concern or if intrasubject variability is high, then replicated design is used. Nonreplicate study designs are usually recommended for bioequivalence studies of most of the orally administered, modified-release and immediate-release dosage forms. Replicate study designs are often recommended for bioequivalence studies of highly variable drug products (intra-subject coefficient of variation $\geq 30\%$), including those that are modified-release, immediate release, and other orally administered drug products. Replicate study designs have several scientific advantages compared to nonreplicate designs. (SFDA, 2005; FDA, 2001a, 2003; Welage et al., 2001; Nation & Sanson, 1994; Steinijans et al., 1992; Metzler, 1989).

2.2 Study subjects

The subjects should be selected with the objective of minimizing variability and permitting detection of difference between the drug products. Therefore, the study is normally carried out with healthy subjects. The study is performed in accordance with the Declaration of Helsinki for biomedical research involving human subjects (WMA Declaration of Helsinki, 2008) and the Guideline for Good Clinical Practice (FDA, 1996). The subjects recruited for bioequivalence studies should be 18 years of age or older and capable of giving informed consent. Generally adults between 20-40 years should be selected. According to FDA guidance and Canadian and European guidelines a minimum of 12 subjects are recruited for bioequivalence studies. For logistic reasons the total number normally does not exceed 24 subjects. The subjects should be in good health. The subject's health is assessed by medical examination including medical history and laboratory tests. They should be screened for the history of use of medications or drugs of abuse, alcohol intake and smoking. The subjects should not take any medication one week before start of study (CDSCO, 2005; FDA, 2001a, 2003; Marzo & Balant, 1995; Nation & Sanson, 1994; WHO, 1986).

2.3 Drug administration and sampling

A bioequivalence study should be a single dose comparison of test drug with appropriate reference drug product carried out in healthy adults. The drug is administered to the subjects in fasting state, unless some other approach is more suitable for valid scientific reasons. Co-administration of food with oral drugs may either enhance or interfere with drug absorption. Thus, feeding increases the inter- and intra-subject variations in rate and extent of absorption. The sponsor should provide the rationale for conducting bioequivalence study under fed or fasting conditions. The subjects are randomly selected for each group in the study and the sequence of drug administration is randomly assigned to the individuals. In a typical situation of comparing a test formulation (T) with a reference formulation (R), the two-period, two-sequence crossover design is the RT/TR design as shown in table 1. Subjects are randomly allocated to two treatment sequences; in sequence 1, subjects receive the reference drug and test drug in periods 1 and 2 respectively, on the other hand in sequence 2, subjects receive the drug products in reverse order. The administration of each product is followed by a sufficiently long wash out period of time to ensure complete elimination of drug before next administration. A time period of more than 5 half-lives of the drug is considered adequate washout period. In selected cases, it may be necessary for the test and reference products to be compared after multiple-dose administration to determine steady-state levels of the active drug moiety. A multiple-dose study should be crossover in design, unless a parallel or other design is more suitable for valid scientific reasons (Hauschke et al., 2007; Niazi, 2007; FDA, 2003; Makoid et al., 1999).

In fasted state studies an overnight fast of at least 10 hours is recommended. Generally in single dose studies the highest marketed strength is administered. The doses of the test and reference products should be same. The test or reference products are administered with 240 ml of water. Liquids are allowed after one hour and standard meal after 4 hours of drug administration. In all the studies the standardization of study environment, diet, fluid intake and exercise is important (CDSCO, 2005; FDA, 2003; WHO, 1986).

Sequence	Period 1	Washout	Period 2
1	R		T
2	T		R

Table 1. RT/TR Design

Under most of the conditions blood or plasma is collected rather than urine or tissue. Blood samples are drawn at appropriate times to assess the absorption, distribution and elimination phases of the drug. For most of the drugs 12-18 samples are recommended including pre-dose sample from each subject. Generally sampling for a period equal to at least 3 times the terminal half life of the drug is recommended. Other approach is that the duration of sampling should be sufficient to define at least 80% of the total area under the concentration–time curve (AUC). The exact timings for sampling depend on nature and pharmacokinetic profile of individual drug and its dosage form (FDA, 2001a, 2003; Nation & Sanson, 1994; WHO, 1986).

2.4 Bioanalytical methodology

The measurement of drug concentration in collected samples is done through bioanalytical methods. Prior to sample analysis, the selected analytical method is validated in accordance with the recommended guidelines (Niazi, 2007; ICH, 2005; FDA, 2001b). Assay validation involves different steps:

- Quality control samples
- Identification and specificity
- Sensitivity and limit of detection
- Range, linearity and limit of quantitation
- Precision and accuracy
- Analyte and system stability
- Reproducibility

A properly validated assay method is crucial for the acceptance of any pharmacokinetic study. During validation, quality control samples are run in replicates to assess the intra- and inter-day variability during sample analysis.

2.5 Data analysis

Data analysis is carried out:

- By direct observation and measurement
- By simple mathematical calculations
- By use of different softwares

2.5.1 Pharmacokinetic analysis

Pharmacokinetic analysis is done using the blood or plasma concentration-time profile. The pharmacokinetic parameters to be measured depend on the type of study whether single-dose or multiple-dose study (FDA, 1992).

For single dose bioequivalence study the parameters are:

- Area under the plasma / blood concentration-time curve from time zero to time t (AUC_{0-t}), calculated by trapezoidal rule, where t is the last measurable time point.

- Area under the plasma / blood concentration-time curve from time zero to time infinity ($AUC_{0-\infty}$) where

$$AUC_{0-\infty} = AUCt + Ct / \lambda z$$

  Ct is the last measurable drug concentration and λz is the terminal elimination rate constant calculated according to an appropriate method. The terminal or elimination half life of the drug should also be documented.
- Peak drug concentration (Cmax) and the time to peak drug concentration (Tmax), obtained directly from the data without interpolation.

For multiple-dose studies, the parameters measured are:

- Area under the plasma / blood concentration-time curve from time zero to time τ over a dosing interval at steady state ($AUC_{0-\tau}$), where τ is the dosing interval.
- Peak drug concentration (Cmax) and the time to peak drug concentration (Tmax), obtained directly from the data without interpolation, after the last dose is administered.
- Drug concentrations at the end of each dosing interval during steady state (C_{min}).
- Average drug concentration at steady state (C_{av}), where $C_{av} = AUC_{0-\tau} / \tau$.
- Degree of fluctuation (DF) at steady state, where $DF = 100\% \times (C_{max} - C_{min}) / C_{av}$.

2.5.2 Statistical analysis

The pharmacokinetic parameters AUC and Cmax are analyzed statistically to determine if the test and reference products produce comparable values. The FDA's statistical criteria for approval of test or generic drugs requires calculation of a confidence interval (CI) for the ratio between the means of test and reference product's pharmacokinetic variables. The two products are said to be bioequivalent if the 90% CI for the ratio of test to reference formulation falls within the bioequivalence acceptance range of 80-120% for data in original scale and 80-125% for log-transformed data of AUC and Cmax. This method is equivalent to a testing procedure called two one-sided tests (TOST) procedure, where one test verifies that the bioavailability of the test product is not too low and the other to show that it is not too high as compared to standard reference product. The current practice is to carry out two one-sided tests (TOST) procedure with the null hypothesis (H_0) of non-bioequivalence at 5% level of significance (α=0.05). Traditional statistical approach is often designed to test the null hypothesis of equality. If data is sufficiently strong, null hypothesis is rejected and alternate hypothesis (H_1) is accepted. Before 1980s, most of the bioequivalence studies were conducted in this way; researchers tested for differences between drug formulations and if they found none, they concluded them to be bioequivalent (i.e. H_0 = bioequivalence, H_1 = non-bioequivalence). During further studies, many flaws were recognized in this approach. If sample size was large enough, minor differences even not important clinically, were found to be significant, whereas if sample size was small, the potential important differences were neglected. The purpose of bioequivalence (BE) study is generally not to demonstrate a difference but to assess the equivalence of test product to that of reference standard. So the method of difference statistics with null hypothesis of no difference is not applicable to BE studies.

Instead, the equivalence testing with the null hypothesis of a difference or non-bioequivalence is used. According to the FDA this difference is set at -20 / +25 percent. In order to verify that -20 / +25 percent rule is satisfied, the two one-sided tests are carried out. The rejection of the two one-sided tests null hypotheses at 5% level of significance (α=0.05) is equivalent to the inclusion of the 90 percent CI in the acceptance range (Hauschke et al., 2007; Riffenburgh, 2006; Welage et al., 2001; FDA, 1992, 2001a; Pidgen, 1996; Hauck & Anderson, 1992; Schuirmann, 1987).

The statistical analysis ANOVA (analysis of variance) is used to calculate estimates of the error variance. ANOVA should be performed on AUC and Cmax accounting for the sources of variation which are:

- Sequence (group)
- Subjects in a sequence
- Period (phase)
- Treatment (drug formulation).

The results of ANOVA are calculated at 5% level of significance (α=0.05). The sponsor may use untransformed or log-transformed data. The choice should be made with concurrence by the FDA prior to conducting the study. The validity of statistical analysis is improved by log-transforming the raw data prior to analysis (FDA, 1992).

2.6 Presentation and documentation of data

The drug concentration in the biological fluid at each sampling time point for all the subjects should be presented in original form. Pharmacokinetic parameters like C_{max}, C_{min}, T_{max}, are directly observed from original data. Pharmacokinetic parameters like AUC_{0-t}, $AUC_{0-\infty}$, $AUC_{0-\tau}$, λz, $t_{1/2}$ are derived from original data by mathematical calculations or by using different softwares like APO MWPHARM, PK Solutions, PK-fit and WinNonlin PK software. The pharmacokinetic data recommended for submission is:

- Plasma concentrations and time points
- Subject, period, sequence, treatment
- AUC_{0-t}, $AUC_{0-\infty}$, λz, $t_{1/2}$, C_{max} and T_{max}
- $AUC_{0-\tau}$, C_{min}, C_{av} and degree of fluctuation are also submitted for multiple-dose studies
- Intersubject, intrasubject, and/or total variability

The mean values and standard deviation (SD) can be calculated by computer programs like Microsoft Excel, SAS, SPSS. The statistical analysis for bioequivalence testing is carried out by using different computer softwares like EquivTest 2.0, Minitab Release 13.1, BioEquiv and DAS 2.0 software. The statistical information recommended to be provided for pharmacokinetic parameters are:

- Geometric mean
- Arithmetic mean
- Ratio of means
- Confidence interval

Bioequivalence parameters can be presented in tabulated form as shown in table 2.

Parameters	Test mean ± SD	Reference mean ± SD	Ratio of Geometric means	90 percent confidence interval
$AUC_{(0\text{-}t)}$ (hr.mg/l)				
$AUC_{(0\text{-}\infty)}$ (hr.mg/l)				
Cmax (mg/l)				
Tmax (hrs)				

Table 2. Bioequivalence Parameters

3. Waivers of *in vivo* bioequivalence studies

Under certain circumstances, FDA may waive the requirement for *in vivo* bioequivalence studies if drug product meets one of the following criteria:

- When the drug product is a parentral solution intended solely for administration by injection, and contains the active drug ingredient in the same solvent and concentration as a solution that is subject of an approved full New Drug Application (NDA).
- The drug product is a topically applied preparation intended for local therapeutic effect e.g. ophthalmic/otic solutions or it is administered by inhalation and contains the active drug ingredient in the same dosage form as a drug product that is the subject of an approved full NDA and ANDA.
- The drug product is a solution for application to the skin, an oral solution, elixir, syrup, tincture, a solution for nebulization, a nasal solution, or similar other solubilized form, and contains an active drug ingredient in the same concentration and dosage form as a drug product that is the subject of an approved full NDA or ANDA, and contains no inactive ingredient or other change in formulation from the drug product that is the subject of an approved full NDA and ANDA that may significantly affect absorption of the active drug ingredient or moiety for products that are systemically absorbed, or that may significantly affect systemic or local availability for products intended to act locally.
- The drug product is a solid oral dosage form (other than controlled release or enteric-coated) that has been determined to be effective for at least one indication in a Drug Efficacy Study Implementation (DESI) notice and is not included in the FDA list of drugs for which *in vivo* bioequivalence testing is required.
- The *in vivo* bioavailability or bioequivalence may be self-evident for certain drug products. The FDA may waive the requirement for the submission of evidence obtained by *in vivo* measuring the bioavailability or demonstrating the bioequivalence of these drug products. A drug product's *in vivo* bioavailability or bioequivalence may be considered self-evident based on other data in the application.
- For certain drug products, bioavailability or bioequivalence may be demonstrated by evidence obtained *in vitro* in lieu of *in vivo* data. The FDA may waive the requirement of the submission of *in vivo* data if a drug product meets the following criteria:

- The drug product is in the same dosage form, but in the different strength, and is proportionally similar in its active and inactive ingredients to another drug product for which the same manufacturer has got the approval and certain conditions are met, that the bioavailability of this other drug product has been measured and both meet an appropriate *in vitro* test approved by the FDA; and the applicant submits evidence showing that both products are proportionally similar in their active and inactive ingredients.
- The drug product is shown to meet an *in vitro* test that assures bioavailability, that *in vitro* test has been correlated with *in vivo* data.
- The drug product, for which only an *in vitro* bioequivalence data has been required by FDA for approval.
- The drug product is a reformulated product that is identical, except for a different color, flavor, or preservative, to another drug product for which the same manufacturer has obtained approval and the following conditions are met: the bioavailability of the other product has been measured; and both the drug products meet an appropriate *in vitro* test approved by the FDA.

In above circumstances bioequivalence studies may be waived by the drug regulatory authorities (FDA, 2011, 2000, 2003; Niazi, 2007; CDSCO, 2005; Makoid et al., 1999).

4. Conclusion

Keeping in view the health-care cost, the pharmaceutical companies are manufacturing and marketing cheaper generic drug products. It is vital for the regulatory authorities of every country to ensure the efficacy and safety of these generic formulations. Carefully planned and designed bioequivalence studies are the only way to ensure uniformity in standards of quality, efficacy and safety of pharmaceutical products.

5. Acknowledgement

The author thanks Prof M. H. Najmi (Professor of Pharmacology and Therapeutics Foundation Medical University) and Prof Muhammad Nawaz (Vice Chancellor of University of Veterinary and Animal Sciences) for their guidance and inspiration. The author appreciates the financial assistance provided by National University of Sciences and Technology (NUST) for producing this piece of work.

6. References

Banahan, B. F. & Kolassa, E. M. (1997). A physician survey on generic drugs and substitution of critical dose medications, *Archive of Internal Medicine*, 157, 2080-2088.

Benet, L. Z. & Goyan, J. E. (1995). Bioequivalence and narrow therapeutic index drugs, *Pharmacotherapy*, 15, 433-440.

Boix-Montanes A. (2011). Relevance of equivalence assessment of topical products based on the dermatopharmacokinetics approach, *European Journal of Pharmaceutical Sciences*, 42 (3), 173-9.

Central Drugs Standard Control Organization (CDSCO) (2005). Guidelines for bioavailability and bioequivalence studies. Directorate General of Health Services,

Ministry of Health and Family Welfare, Government of India, New Delhi. Available from:
http://cdsco.nic.in/html/BE%20Guidelines%20Draft%20Ver10%20March%2016,%2005.pdf

Chen, M. L. & Lesko, L. J. (2001). Individual bioequivalence revisited, *Clinical Pharmacokinetics*, 40 (10), 701-6.

Chen, M. L. ; Patnaik, R. ; Hauck, W. W. ; Schuirmann, D.J. ; Hyslop, T. & Williams, R. (2000). An individual bioequivalence criterion: regulatory considerations. Stat Med, 19 (20), 2821-42.

Committee for Proprietary Medicinal Products (CPMP) (2000). Note for guidance on the investigation of bioavailability and bioequivalence, The European Agency for the Evaluation of Medicinal Products (EMEA) - Evaluation of medicines for human use. London, 14 Dec 2000 CPMP/EWP/QWP/1401/98. Available from:
http://www.eme.europa.eu/docs/en_GB/ducument_library/Scientific_guideline/2009/09/WC500003519.pdf

Crawford, P. ; Feely, M. ; Guberman, A. & Kramer, G. (2006). Are there potential problems with generic substitution of antiepileptic drugs? A review of issue, *Seizure*, 15, 165-176.

FDA (1992). Guidance for industry, Statistical procedures for bioequivalence studies using a standard two-treatment crossover design. U.S. Department of Health and Human Services. Food and Drug Administration, Center for Drug Evaluation and Research (CDER), July 1992. Available from:
http://www.fda.gov/downloads/Drugs/GuidanceComplianceRegulatoryInformation/Guidances/ucm072878.pdf

FDA (1996). Guidance for industry, E6 Good Clinical Practice: Consolidated Guidance. U.S. Department of Health and Human Services. Food and Drug Administration, Center for Drug Evaluation and Research (CDER), April 1996. Available from: http://www.fda.gov/downloads/Drugs/GuidanceComplianceRegulatoryInformation/Guidances/ucm073122.pdf

FDA (2000). Guidance for industry, Waiver of *In vivo* Bioavailability and Bioequivalence Studies for Immediate-Release Solid Oral Dosage Forms Based on a Biopharmaceutics Classification System. U.S. Department of Health and Human Services. Food and Drug Administration, Center for Drug Evaluation and Research (CDER) August 2000. Available from:
http://www.fda.gov/downloads/Drugs/GuidanceComplianceRegulatoryInformation/Guidances/ucm070246.pdf

FDA (2001a). Guidance for industry, Statistical approaches to establishing bioequivalence. U.S. Department of Health and Human Services. Food and Drug Administration, Center for Drug Evaluation and Research (CDER), January 2001. Available from: http://www.fda.gov/downloads/Drugs/GuidanceComplianceRegulatoryInformation/Guidances/ucm070244.pdf

FDA (2001b). Guidance for industry, Bioanalytical Method Validation. U.S. Department of Health and Human Services. Food and Drug Administration, Center for Drug

Evaluation and Research (CDER), Center for Veterinary Medicine (CVM), May 2001. Available from:
http://www.fda.gov/downloads/Drugs/GuidanceComplianceRegulatoryInformation/Guidances/ucm070107.pdf

FDA (2003). Guidance for industry, Bioavailability and bioequivalence studies for orally administered drug products - General considerations. U.S. Department of Health and Human Services. Food and Drug Administration, Center for Drug Evaluation and Research (CDER) March 2003. Available from:
http://www.fda.gov/downloads/Drugs/GuidanceComplianceRegulatoryInformation/Guidances/ucm070124.pdf

FDA (2011). CFR - Code of Federal Regulations Title 21 - Part 320 Bioavailability and bioequivalence requirement. U.S. Department of Health and Human Services. Food and Drug Administration, Center for Drug Evaluation and Research (CDER). Available from:
http://www.accessdata.fda.gov/scripts/cdrh/cfdocs/cfcfr/cfrsearch.cfm?cfrpart=320

Hauck, W. W. & Andersos, S. (1992). Types of bioequivalence and related statistical considerations, *International Journal of Clinical Pharmacology, Therapy and Toxicology*, 28, 105-10.

Hauschke, D. ; Steinijans, V. & Pigeot, I. (2007). *Bioequivalence studies in drug development.* John Wiley and Sons Ltd, The Atrium, Southern Gate, Chichester, West Sussex PO19 8SQ, England. ISBN-13: 978-0-470-09475-4 (HB).

Health Canada (2004). Draft Guidance for Industry, Preparation of comparative bioavailability information for drug submissions in the CTD format - Minister of Public Works and Government Services Canada 2004. Available from: http://dsp-psd.pwgsc.gc.ca/Collection/H42-2-97-4-2004E.pdf

ICH Harmonized Tripartite Guideline. (2005). International conference on harmonization of technical requirements for registration of pharmaceuticals for human use. Validation of analytical procedures: Text and methodology. Available from: http://www.ich.org/fileadmin/Public_Web_Site/ICH_Products/Guidelines/Efficacy/E9/Step4/E9_Guideline.pdf

Kowalski, P. & Bieniecki, M. (2006). Pharmacokinetics and bioavailability study of l-ornithine–l-aspartate in healthy volunteers—A comparative study of two oral formulations, *Journal of Pharmaceutical and Biomedical Analysis*, 41 (3), 1061-1064.

Lindenbaum, J. ; Mellow, M. H. ; Blackstone, M. O. & Butler, V. P. Jr. (1971). Variation in biologic availability of digoxin from four preparations, *The New England Journal of Medicine*, 285 (24), 1344-7.

Lamy, P. P. (1986). Generic equivalents: issues and concerns. *Journal of Clinical Pharmacology*, 26 (5), 309-16.

Makoid, M. C. ; Vuchetich, P. J. & Banakar, U. V. (1999). *Basic Pharmacokinetics.* The Virtual University Press. *REV.* 99.4.25 http://kiwi.creighton.edu/pkinbook/ Available from:
http://www.nova-transnet.com/zonanova/downloads/documentos/Basic%20Pharmacokinetics.pdf

Marzo, A. & Balant, L. P. (1995). Bioequivalence. An updated reappraisal addressed to applications of interchangeable multi-source pharmaceutical products, *Arzneimettel-Forschung*, 45, 109-115.

Metzler, C. M. (1989). Bioavailability / bioequivalence: study design and statistical issues, *Journal of Clinical Pharmacology*, 29, 289-292.

Midha, K. K. ; Rawson, M. J. & Hubbard, J. W. (2005). The bioequivalence of highly variable drugs and drug products, *International Journal of Clinical Pharmacology and Therapeutics*, 43 (10), 485-98.

Nation, R. L. & Sanson, L. N. (1994). Bioequivalence requirements for generic products, *Pharmacology and Therapeutics*, 62, 41-55.

Niazi, S. A. (2007). *Handbook of Bioequivalence Testing*. Informa Healthcare USA, Inc. 52 Vanderbilt Avenue, New York, NY 10017. ISBN-13: 978-0-8493-0395-1.

Pidgen, A. (1996). Bioequivalence and generic prescribing: an industrial view, *Journal of Pharmacy and Pharmacology*, 48, 11-16.

Riffenburgh, R. H. (2006). *Statistics in Medicine* (2nd Ed.). Elsevier Academic Press, 30 Corporate Drive, Suite 400, Burlington, MA 01803, USA.

Saudi Food and Drug Authority (SFDA) (2005). Bioequivalence requirements guidelines. Drug Sector, Kingdom of Saudi Arabia, Draft May 2005. Available from: http://www.sfda.gov.sa/NR/rdonlyres/6A114B70-4201-46EF-B4C7-127FD66D3314/0/BioequivalenceRequirementGuidelines.pdf

Schuirmann, D. J. (1987). A comparison of the two one-sided tests procedure and the power approach for assessing the equivalence of average bioavailability, *Journal of Pharmacokinetics and Biopharmaceutics*, 15, 657-680.

Skelly, J. P. (2010). A history of biopharmaceutics in the food and drug administration 1968–1993, *The American Association of Pharmaceutical Scientists Journal*, 12 (1), 44-50.

Soryal, I. & Richens, A. (1992). Bioavailability and dissolution of proprietary and generic formulations of phenytoin, *Journal of Neurology, Neurosurgery and Psychiatry*, 55 (8), 688–691.

Steinijans, V. W. ; Hauschke, D. & Jonkman, J. H. G. (1992). Controversies in bioequivalence studies, *Clinical Pharmacokinetics*, 22, 247-253.

Strom, B. L. (1987). Generic drug substitution revisited, *The New England Journal of Medicine*, 316 (23), 1456-62.

Tothfalusi, L. ; Endrenyi, L. & Arieta, A. G. (2009). Evaluation of bioequivalence for highly variable drugs with scaled average bioequivalence, *Clinical Pharmacokinetics*, 48 (11), 725-43.

Tyrer, J. H. ; Eadie, M. J. ; Sutherland, J. M. & Hooper, W. D. (1970). Outbreak of Anticonvulsant Intoxication in an Australian City, *British Medical Journal*, 4 (5730), 271–273.

Vasquez, E. M. & Min, D. I. (1999). Transplant pharmacist's opinions on generic product selection of critical dose drugs, *American Journal of Health-System Pharmacy*, 56, 615-621.

Welage, L. S. ; Kirking, D. M. ; Ascione, F. J. & Gaither, C. A. (2001). Understanding the scientific issues embedded in the generic drug approval process, *Journal of the American Pharmacists Association*, 41 (6), 856-867.

World Health organization (1986). Guidelines for the investigation of bioavailability. World Health organization Regional Office for Europe, Copenhagen.

World Medical Association Declaration of Helsinki – Ethical Principles for Medical Research Involving Human Subjects. Adopted by the 18th WMA General Assembly Helsinki, Finland, June 1964 and amended by the 59th WMA General Assembly, Seoul, October 2008, Available from: http://www.wma.net/en/30publications/10policies/b3/17c.pdf

2

Genetic Variation in Drug Disposition

Balmukunda Regmi and Laxman Bharati
Tribhuvan University Institute of Medicine,
Maharajgunj, Kathmandu,
Nepal

1. Introduction

Genetic variation is an important source of pharmacokinetic variability and leads to modification of drug response. It is one of the several factors contributing to variability in drug disposition. Any alteration in drug disposition, influences circulating drug concentrations, as well as the concentrations at the sites of action. Drug disposition is mainly affected by drug metabolizing enzymes, drug transport proteins, plasma protein binding and transcription factors. The knowledge about the factors influencing drug disposition is useful in predicting potential drug interactions and pharmacokinetic variations. Among the above factors the most important mechanism by which genetic variation modifies drug response is by altering drug metabolizing enzymes that in turn alter drug metabolism. These enzymes are proteins that catalyse the chemical alteration of drugs and other molecules inside the body. Metabolism converts most of the drug to inactive product but few others to more toxic product. The main organ for drug metabolism is liver; kidney, GI mucosa and lungs play smaller role. The drug metabolizing enzymes can either be functionalizing (oxidation, reduction, and hydrolysis) or conjugating (glutathione, glucuronide). Genetic variation in drug metabolizing enzymes can either increase or decrease drug metabolism. For example some individuals have genetically determined insufficiency to metabolise succinylcholine, a short-acting neuromuscular-blocking drug, widely used as muscle relaxant and in anaesthesia. It is normally rapidly hydrolysed by plasma cholinesterase. If succinylcholine is administered to such individual, he/she fails to inactivate succinylcholine rapidly and experiences prolonged neuromuscular block. This is because a recessive gene gives rise to an abnormal type of plasma cholinesterase and this abnormal enzyme has a modified pattern of substrate and inhibitor specificity.

Plasma binding proteins often bind a large fraction of a drug in circulation Binding varies from drug to drug. Sometimes drug bind more than 99%. Albumin is main plasma protein to which drug bind and mostly acidic drug bind with plasma albumin. Other drug binding plasma proteins are globulin, alpha acid glycoprotein etc. Protein binding affects pharmacology of drug. It alters unbound drug concentration in circulation and only unbound (free) drug can enter tissues. So any genetic variation in plasma protein brings about variation in drug response. Similarly, transcription factors are proteins that regulate gene expression. When bound to exogenous chemicals, certain transcription factors induce the expression of drug metabolizing enzymes and modify drug response. Some genetically determined drug response based on factor other than pharmacokinetic variation. Consider an example of the individuals having red blood cells deficient in an enzyme called glucose-6- phosphate dehydrogenase. Deficiency of this enzyme increases the risk of hemolysis, if certain drugs such as aspirin and sulfonamides are administered.

Differences in metabolism, transportation, plasma protein binding of drugs are significant factors affecting drug disposition and results modification of drug action. This chapter summarizes the reviews of the findings on genetic variation related with drug disposition.

Genetic variation is an important source of pharmacokinetic as well as pharmacodynamic variability and leads to modification of drug response. It is one of several factors contributing to variability in drug disposition. The branch of science that deals with individual variation in drug response is termed pharmacogenetics. It deals with the genetic basis of variability of drug response in an individual and is a useful parameter for individualization of drug therapy. It is a rapidly emerging branch in which thousands of studies are carried out annually. Besides, it has important role in clinical practice and on drug development.

Recently, pharmacogenetic deals with the study of drug response in unrelated individuals. The difference in drug response is due to the variation of genotype, that encodes for drug-metabolizing enzymes, receptors for the drug, drug transport proteins, transcription factors and various ion channels. A change in genotype or a mutation in gene sequence may increase quantity and/ or activity of a protein or an essential enzyme. In some cases, such a change results in an exaggerated or reduced therapeutic response to a drug. In general, variation in genotype account for15%-30% of inter-individual differences in drug metabolism and response, but for some drugs, genetic factors are of most common and account for up to 95% of inter-individual variability in drug disposition and effects.

The important drugs under different therapeutic categories are shown in Table 1.

The knowledge about the factor influencing drug disposition is useful in predicting potential drug interaction and pharmacokinetic variation.

The genetic mechanisms for variation of drug response are variation in gene sequence. It includes changes in the primary nucleotide sequence of coding, regulatory, and splice regions of a gene. Less common forms are variability in the structure and function of the genome. Among these are sequence variation in microRNA (miRNA) binding sites, which affects the ability of miRNA to regulate translation; pharmacoepigenetics, which examines heritable chromatin modifications; and copy number variation.

2. Pharmacokinetic variability

The effectiveness of the medication is determined by how much of the drug is present at its site of action and how long sufficient concentrations of the drug remain at the site. Pharmacokinetics is the quantitative study of the time course of drug concentration in the body. It is the term used to describe the disposition of a drug throughout the body – that is, the drug's absorption, distribution, metabolism, and excretion (ADME). Pharmacokinetic variability is the variation in drug movement throughout the body. Drugs produce an effect

CYP2D6		CYP2C9	CYP2C19
Analgesica, Antitussives	**Antiemetics**	**Angiotensin II blockers**	**Anticonvulsants, hypnosedatives, muscle relaxants**
Codeine	Ondansetron	Irbesartan	Diazepam
Dextromethorphan	Tropisetron	Losartan	Phenytoin
Ethylmorphine			
Tramadol	**Antiestrogen**	**Anticonvulsant**	**Antidepressants**
	Tamoxifen	Phenytoin	Amitriptyline
Antiarrhythmics			Citalopram
Flecainide	**Antipsychotics**	**Antidiabetics**	Clomipramine
Mexiletine	Haloperidol	Glibenclamide	Imipramine
Propafenone	Perphenazine	Glimepiride	Moclobemide
	Risperidone	Glipizide	
Antidepressants	Thioridazine	Nateglinide	**Anti infectives**
Amitriptyline	Zuclopenthixol		Proguanil
Doxepin		**Anti-inflammatories**	Voriconazole
Fluoxetine	**β-blockers**	Celecoxib	
Fluvoxamine	Metoprolol	Diclofenac	**Proton pump inhibitors**
Imipramine	Propranolol	Ibuprofen	Omeprazole
Maprotiline	Timolol	Piroxicam	Lansoprazole
Mianserin		Tenoxicam	Pantoprazole
Nortriptyline			Rabeprazole
Paroxetine		**HMG-CoA reductase inhibitor**	
Venlafaxine		Fluvastatin	**β-blocker**
			Propranolol
		Oral anticoagulant	
		(*S*)-Warfarin	

Sistonen J.Pharmacogenetic variation at *CYP2D6, CYP2C9,* AND *CYP2C19*. Population Genetic and Forensic Aspects Department of Forensic Medicine University of Helsinki Finland 2008

Table 1. Common drug substrates of *CYP2D6, CYP2C9,* and *CYP2C19* according to therapeutic Categories

only if they can reach its physiological target(s) in sufficient concentration. These processes determine the fate of a drug in the body. A combination of metabolism and excretion constitutes drug elimination. Following factors are the sources of individual variation in drug disposition.

1. Drug-metabolizing enzymes,
2. Drug transport proteins,
3. Receptors for the drug,
4. Various ion channels

2.1 Drug-metabolizing enzymes

Metabolism is biochemical reaction that takes place inside body. Almost all tissues are capable to metabolize drugs but the liver is the major site of metabolism. Besides liver, GI tract, kidney and lungs also metabolize certain fraction of drug. The main objective of metabolism is to convert lipophilic to hydrophilic so that drug is easily excreted from the body. In general, metabolites lack pharmacological activity and are more water soluble than the parent substance. But in few conditions, active metabolites are formed from inactive parent drugs; such parent drugs are termed as *prodrug*. The chemical reactions that involve in drug metabolism are categories into two types - Phase 1 reactions and - Phase 2 or *conjugation* reactions.

Phase 1 reactions occur in the cytosol, mitochondria, microsomes of cells of the liver and other organs. It includes oxidation, reduction, hydrolysis, cyclization and decyclization reactions. Much phase I drug metabolism is performed by polymorphic enzymes, particularly various forms of cytochrome P450 (CYP). The influence of genetic polymorphisms of drugs metabolized by *CYP2C9, CYP2C19,* and *CYP2D6* indicates polymorphisms and affects the metabolism of 20%–30% drugs.

In Phase 2 reaction drugs or metabolites combine with other substances and results in increased water solubility of the substance, which decreases the amount that is reabsorbed through renal tubules and thereby increases the fraction that is excreted in the urine. It is also known as conjugation. The most common conjugation reaction is glucuronide, glycine, glutathione, glutamate and sulfate conjugation.

The cytochrome P450s are a multigene family of enzymes found predominantly in the liver, that are responsible for metabolism. Genetically determined variability in the level of expression or function of these enzymes has a profound effect on drug efficacy. Genetic polymorphisms for many drug-metabolizing enzymes and drug targets have been identified. Polymorphisms refer to sequence variations with an allele frequency of greater than or equal to 1%. Polymorphism in any one of many genes—including those encoding drug receptors, drug transporter are important determinants of clinical response. Polymorphisms have now been identified in more than 20 human drug metabolizing enzymes. Important examples are polymorphisms in the cytochrome P450 enzymes and in thiopurine methyltransferase. Polymorphism not only affects drug disposition but can also be important in the conversion of prodrugs into their active form. For example, codeine is metabolized into the analgesic morphine by CYP2D6, and the desired analgesic effect is not achieved in CYP2D6 poor metabolizers.

Cytochrome P450 system refers to a family of enzymes (usually hepatic) which are located on the endoplasmic reticulum, which performs oxidative metabolism of broad array of substances. Cytochrome P450 comprises the most important group of phase I enzymes. The most important CYP 450 enzymes are:

CYP3A4 (50% of P450 metabolism) followed by
CYP2D6 (20%),
CYP2C9 and CYP2C19 (together 15%)
Others: CYP2E1, CYP2A6, and CYP1A2.

2.1.1 Some common drug metabolizing enzymes and genetic polymorphisms

CYP2D6 – The notable substrates for this enzyme include the tricyclic antidepressants amitriptyline, clomipramine, desipramine, amphetamines, ß-blockers, imipramine, and nortriptyline. Metabolism of these drugs is influenced by the polymorphism in gene that code CYP2D6. Polymorphism in gene that code CYP2D6 may either reduce the rate of the metabolism and increased plasma concentrations of above mentioned drugs when given in recommended doses, or it may enhance the rate of metabolism and results into therapeutic failure because the drug concentrations at normal doses are far too low.

CYP 3A4- The notable substrates for this enzyme include alprazolam, triazolam, carbamazepine, methadone, pimozide, quetiapine, risperidone, zolpidem.

Isoform	Examples of drug substrates	Nature of polymorphism	Effect on activity
CYP1A2	Clozapine, olanzapine theophylline and caffeine	Polymorphisms in non-coding sequences may affect expression or induction.	No absence of activity reported. Some effects on expression or induction.
CYP2A6	Coumarin and nicotine	Non-synonymous mutations, large deletion and upstream polymorphisms.	Absence of activity seen at low frequency. Ultrarapid metabolizers may also occur.
CYP2B6	Cyclophosphamide and efavirenz	Non-synonymous and upstream polymorphisms.	No absence of activity reported. Variation in activity common.
CYP2C8	Paclitaxel, retinoic acid, rosiglitazone and repaglinide	Non-synonymous and upstream polymorphisms.	No absence of activity reported. Variation in activity common.
CYP2C9	Warfarin, ibuprofen, diclofenac, tolbutamide and phenytoin	Non-synonymous polymorphisms common. Also upstream polymorphisms.	Very low activity in some individuals.
CYP2C19	Omeprazole, diazepam, clobazam and clopidogrel	Splice site, initiation codon, non-synonymous and upstream polymorphisms.	Absence of activity common. Some ultrarapid metabolizers.
CYP2D6	Codeine, amitriptyline, nortriptyline, tamoxifen, metoprolol, timolol, tropisetron, dextromethorphan, atomoxetine, venlafaxine thioridazine, zuclopenthixol, perphenazine, risperidone and haloperidol.	Splice site, small and large deletions and non-synonymous polymorphisms. Duplication and other amplifications.	Absence of activity common. Some ultrarapid metabolizers.
CYP2E1	Ethanol and isoniazid	Non-synonymous polymorphisms rare. Upstream polymorphisms common.	No absence of activity reported. Some variation in activity.
CYP3A4	Midazolam, cyclosporine, tacrolimus, erythromycin, nifedipine, simvastatin atovastatin, diltiazem verapamil, vincristine and dapsone	Non-synonymous polymorphisms rare. Upstream polymorphisms common.	No absence of activity reported. Some variation in activity.
CYP3A5	Broadly similar to *CYP3A4* above	Non-synonymous polymorphisms rare. Splice site polymorphisms common.	Absence of activity common.

Daly AK. Pharmacogenetics and human genetic polymorphisms (2010). Biochem. J. 429: 435–449

Table 2. CYP genes and polymorphic drug metabolism

CYP2C9 – The notable substrates for this enzyme include warfarin. tolbutamide, glipizide, and phenytoin.

The CYP genes (See Table 2) have well characterized roles in pharmacogenetic studies on drug metabolism. Other CYP genes also contribute to drug and xenobiotic metabolism or have physiological roles, but pharmacogenetic data is more limited.

2.2 Drug transport protein

In addition to metabolizing enzymes, drug transport proteins also contribute to alteration in drug disposition. Many drugs are transferred by active transporter systems, membrane proteins that maintain both inward and outward transport of drugs and their metabolites in cells. Variation in a drug transporter producing a clinical impact is less common than is observed for other pharmacokinetic mechanisms. However, there are examples of variation in drug transport that can be attributed to adverse drug effects. One such example is the *SLCO1B1* gene that encodes a polypeptide, OATP1B1, which mediates hepatic uptake of anionic drugs, including most HMG-CoA (3-hydroxy-3-methylglutaryl-coenzyme A) inhibitors (statins). Although statins are the safest drugs, they sometimes develop myopathy in relatively small percentage of treated individuals. Variability in drug transporters also contributes to resistance to a variety of medicines, most commonly observed in the treatment of a variety of cancers.

Transport proteins are embedded in a the cell membrane and responsible for transport of endogenous compounds or drugs into the cell or outside of the cell i.e. across the biological membranes. They are classified into either efflux or uptake proteins, depending on the direction of transport. The extent of expression of genes coding for transport proteins can have a profound effect on the bioavailability and pharmacokinetics of various drugs. Additionally, genetic variation such as single-nucleotide polymorphisms (SNPs) of the transport proteins can cause differences in the uptake or efflux of drugs. Genetic variants of transport proteins can cause or contribute to a number of diseases, such as anemia.

There are two superfamilies of transport proteins that have important effects on the absorption, distribution, and excretion of drugs. These are the ATP-binding cassette (ABC) and the solute-carrier (SLC) superfamilies.

ATP-binding cassette (ABC) transporters are present in cellular and intracellular membranes and can be responsible for either importing (influx) or removing (efflux) of substances from cells and tissues. They often transport substances against a concentration gradient by using the hydrolysis of ATP to drive the transport.

2.2.1 ABC transporters

There are at least 49 ABC transporter genes. These genes are particularly important for drug transport. Genetic polymorphisms affecting ABC transporter genes expression or changing their affinity for substrates and alter the absorption and elimination of drugs. It also alters drug concentrations at the site of action despite similar blood concentrate. The majority of ABC transporters move compounds from the cytoplasm to the outside of a cell, although some of them move compounds into an intercellular compartment such as the endoplasmic reticulum, mitochondria, or peroxisome. ATP-binding transporters are responsible for the efflux of drugs and substrates, including bilirubin, several anticancer drugs, cardiac glycosides, immunosuppressive agents and glucocorticoids.

2.2.2 Solute Carrier Proteins

Solute carrier proteins (SLCs) are important in the transport of ions and organic substances across biological membranes in the maintenance of homeostasis. Members of the SLC superfamily consist of membrane channels, facilitative transporters, and secondary active transporters. Examples of some of the endogenous solutes that are transported include steroid hormones, thyroid hormones, and prostaglandins. Additionally, SLCs are important in the transport of a large number of drugs. In all, more than 40 families of transporters make up the SLC superfamily. Genetic variants of solute carrier proteins, such as *SLC6A3* gene encodes for the dopamine transporter DAT1, the *SLC6A4* gene codes for the serotonin transporter (SERT) that has been associated with variation in drug response.

2.3 Receptors for the drug

Receptors are the macromolecules that are located in cell membrane or inside cell or in organism to which drugs bind to initiate the series of biochemical reaction that leads to biological response. Most receptors are regulatory proteins (hormones, neurotransmitter), enzymes (dihydrofolate reductase), transport proteins (Na+/K+ ATPase) and structural proteins (tubulin). Sequential variations in the receptor protein can affect target molecules or the structural integrity of the receptor and change ligand binding.

Genetic variation not only varies towards drug response by altering metabolism but also have important role in drug receptors. A growing number of drug targets (e.g., receptors) are known to exhibit genetic polymorphisms and alter drug response in humans. Many researches have been conducted to show polymorphisms in the gene encoding receptor/effectors contribute variation in drug response e.g. β2-adrenergic receptor, is encoded by the gene ADRB2. This receptor interacts with endogenous catecholamines and various medications altering the effects of medications. Polymorphisms in the gene encoding this receptor have been associated with altered expression, down-regulation, and altered cell signaling and finally on clinical responses to endogenous and exogenous agonists.

2.4 Various ion channels

Ion channels are multimeric protein complexes and exert functionally overlapping control over excitability and signaling in both the plasma membrane and intracellular organelles. These channels control the electrical activity of muscles and nerves. There are various genes encoding the ion channels that have been identified.

Ion channel genes constitute about 1.2% of known protein coding genes. Mutations of these genes alter the functioning of ion channel resulting into a diverse array of clinical disorders in the body, especially in brain, nerve, muscle and heart. Predisposition of some common disorders like migraine and epilepsy might be mediated by genetic variation in ion-channel genes. Genetic variation in cellular ion transporter can also have a role in the alteration of drug response.

The most important ionic pores for generation and control of the action potential are voltage-dependent sodium and potassium channels. Specific genes coding for these channels are expressed in the central nervous system. So, it could be expected that a mutation in these genes may be at the origin of unbalance between excitation and inhibition and thus could cause epilepsy. Three types of epilepsies have been linked to mutations in human genes encoding subunits of:

- The neuronal nicotinic acetyl choline receptor (nAChR) (α4, *CHRNA*4, and β2, *CHRNB*2, subunits),
- The voltage-gated potassium (*KCNQ*2, *KCNQ*3) channels and
- The voltage-gated sodium (*SCN*1*A*, *SCN*1*B*) channels.

Mutations in *CHRNA*4 and *CHRNB*2 are associated with some cases of familial epilepsies classified as autosomal dominant nocturnal frontal lobe epilepsies with an important intra and interfamilial clinical heterogeneity. Mutations in voltage-gated potassium channels *KCNQ*2 and *KCNQ*3 have been identified in benign familial neonatal convulsions.

The sodium channel is composed of four homologous domains that contain well-characterized voltage-sensing and pore regions. The four domains form a sodium-permeable pore within the membrane that is remarkably selective for the individual ion that it conducts. Each domain comprises six membrane-spanning segments, each of which has an α-helical structure. And each sodium channel α subunit associates with one or more different β subunits. This association of α and β auxiliary subunits has an important influence on the voltage dependence, kinetics and cell-surface expression of most voltage-gated ion channels. Most neurological channelopathies associated with dysfunction of voltage-gated ion channels are caused by mutations in the gene encoding the pore-forming subunit.

Myotonia is a clinical disorder in which patients experience muscle stiffness because of a failure of normal electrical inactivation of activated muscle. Myotonia can result from mutations in either the *CLCN1* gene, that encodes the muscle voltage-gated chloride channel, or *SCN4A* encoding the voltage-gated sodium channel.

3. Pharmacogenetics and adverse drug reactions

Drug is any substance or product that is used or intended to be used to modify or explore the physiological system or pathological state for the benefit of the recipients. Interacting with receptors drugs not only produce desire effect but also produce undesired effect. Most undesirable effect associated with drugs is overdose/ poisoning, development of resistance, and adverse drug reaction (ADR). Amongst these effects ADR are important and leads to morbidity and mortality. Fortunately, when drugs are used properly, many ADR can be avoided or at least kept to a minimum. According to WHO 'ADR is any noxious, unintended and undesirable effect that occur at doses normally used in men for prophylaxis, diagnosis or therapy of the disease or modification of physiological function'. Adverse effect to drug may develop promptly or only after prolonged medication or even after stoppage of medications. Type B ADRs, which are not directly predictable from drug pharmacology and are unrelated to pharmacological actions of the drugs and often caused by immunological and pharmacogenetic mechanism, these effects are rare, but they are potentially very serious consequences for the patient. Type A (Predictable), can be predictable from drug pharmacology and is dose dependent. It is common and found to occur in 80%. It includes side effects, toxic effect, withdrawal symptoms.

Polymorphisms in the genes that code for drug-metabolizing enzymes, drug transporters, drug receptors, and ion channels can alter drugs pharmacokinetics as well as pharmacodynamics. Polymorphism results in individual's risk of having adverse drug reactions

Some pharmacogenetically determined adverse drug reactions include prolonged muscle relaxation after succinylcholine injection due to inherited deficiency of a plasma cholinesterase, resulting alteration of metabolism. Haemolysis is caused by antimalarials and sulfonamides due to glucose-6-phosphate dehydrogenase deficiency.

It was found that the genetic polymorphism of the drug-metabolising enzyme CYP2D6 due to the antiarrhythmic drug, sparteine, is responsible for adverse drug reactions such as nausea, diplopia, and blurred vision. Similarly, orthostatic hypotension after the antihypertensive agent debrisoquine is also due to genetic polymorphism. It was found that ticlopidine induced hepatotoxicity. The incidence of hepatotoxicity is more common among Japanese patients than Europeans because hepatotoxicity is associated with *HLA* (human leucocyte antigen) genes. HLA gene is predominantly presented in Japanese. Carbamazepine, a widely used anticonvulsant, can cause hypersensitivity reactions but rarely showed Stevens–Johnson syndrome. Various study showed that Taiwanese have high incidence of CBZ-induced Stevens–Johnson syndrome because they have very strong association between the *HLA gene* and CBZ-induced SJS.

4. Clinical applications

The importance of genetic variation has been best illustrated by the approval of BiDil, a cardiovascular combination product of isosorbide dinitrate and hydralazine, by FDA for the Afro-American population in 2005. Similar race- or gene-specific drugs are likely to be marketed in near future as a response to need for safer and more effective drugs.

4.1 Cancer treatment

Genetic variation at *CYP2D6* has important therapeutic implications in cancer treatment. Tamoxifen are used to treat breast cancer. It is a pro-drug, requiring metabolic activation to active metabolites endoxifen and 4 hydroxytamoxifen. These reactions are catalyzed by CYP2D6. Variation in gene coding CYP2D6 enzyme activity has been shown to affect tamoxifen treatment outcomes. Besides, CYP2D6 polymorphism can also affect the efficacy of antiemetic drugs, which are often used for nausea and vomiting induced by cancer chemotherapy. Serotonin type receptor antagonist ondansetron, is metabolized by enzyme CYP2D6. CYP2D6-related rapid metabolism decrease therapeutic effect (severe emesis) and dose adjustment is necessary.

4.2 Oral anticoagulation therapy

Warfarin, as the most commonly used anticoagulation therapy, is indicated for the prophylaxis and/or treatment of thromboembolism. It is also indicated for treatment and prophylaxis of deep vein thrombosis, acute myocardial infarction, and stroke. Warfarine act as vitamin K antagonists by inhibiting the liver microsomal enzyme, vitamin K epoxide reductase, which is essential in the vitamin K cycle and formation of clotting factors.

Warfarin is administered as a racemic mixture of *R*- and *S*-enantiomers, the latter of which is predominantly responsible for the anticoagulant effect and metabolized by CYP2C9. Similar doses of warfarin given to different individuals can result in varied drug responses. Patients with a two genetic variants have a significantly increased occurrence of a serious or life-threatening bleeding incident. This is due genetic polymorphism of drug metabolizing enzyme *CYP2C9*.

4.3 Proton Pump Inhibitor (PPI) therapy

PPIs, such as omeprazole, lanzoprazole, are widely used for the treatment of acid-related diseases, including gastroesophageal reflux disease and peptic ulcer, as well as for the eradication of *Helicobacter pylori* in combination with antibiotics. PPIs are mainly metabolized by CYP2C19 in the liver, and the clinical outcome of drug therapy depends on genetic variation at the encoding gene CYP2C19. Ultra-rapid CYP2C19-related metabolism is an important factor contributing to therapeutic failures in drug treatment with PPIs, especially in European populations.

4.4 Psychiatric drug therapy

Genetic variation is an important factor for the variation in psychiatric drug response. The meta-analysis conducted by Kirchheiner *et al.* showed that of 36 commonly used antidepressants, for 20 of those, data on polymorphic CYP2D6 or CYP2C19 were found and that in 14 drugs such genetic variation would require at least doubling of the dose in extensive metabolizers in comparison to poor metabolizers. They also showed that out of 38 antipsychotics, CYP2D6 and CYP2C19 genotype was of relevant in 13 drugs. Amitriptyline has relatively narrow therapeutic range and high toxicity at increased concentrations, leading to severe adverse effects. The main CYPs involved in amitriptyline metabolism are CYP2C19. Genetic variation of these enzymes has been shown to correlate with the serum concentrations of amitriptyline, as well as with the occurrence of side-effects related to amitriptyline therapy.

5. References

Classsen T et al. Exome Sequencing of Ion Channel Genes Reveals Complex Profiles Confounding Personal Risk Assessment in Epilepsy (2011). *Cell* 145: 1036–1048,

Daly AK. Pharmacogenetics and human genetic polymorphisms (2010). Biochem. J. 429: 435–449

Evans WE and McLeod HL. Pharmacogenomics — Drug Disposition,Drug Targets, and Side Effects (2003) N Engl J Med 348: 553-549.

Kirchheiner J et al. Pharmacogenetics of antidepressants and antipsychotics: the contribution of allelic variations to the phenotype of drug response (2004). *Mol Psychiatry.* 9 (5):442-73.

Konig J, Seithel A, Gradhand U, Fromm MF. Pharmacogenomics of human OATP transporters. *Naunyn Schmiedebergs Arch Pharmacol* (2006). 372(6):432-443.

Meyer UA. Pharmacogenetics and adverse drug reactions (2000). *The Lancet* 356: 1671-1675

Sistonen J. Pharmacogenetic variation at *CYP2D6, CYP2C9,* AND *CYP2C19*: Population Genetic and Forensic Aspects Department of Forensic Medicine University of Helsinki Finland 2008

Wikinson GR. Drug Metabolism and Variability among Patients in Drug Response (2005). N Engl J Med ;352:2211-21.

3

Evaluation of Percutaneous Drug Permeation Using a Lateral Sectioning Approach

Nobuhiro Goi, Katsunori Morishita,
Akihito Taniguchi and Takayuki Ishii
Mikasa Seiyaku Company Limited
Japan

1. Introduction

Local enhanced tissue delivery (LETD) of non-steroidal anti-inflammatory drugs (NSAIDs) provides a means to avoid adverse effects, such as gastrointestinal disorders (Hawkey & Truelove, 1983; Taha et al., 1994). Regarding the skin dispositions of drugs, it is considered to be more important to evaluate the drug LETD from the formulation than the drug uptake into the body from the cutaneous microvascular network (Morgan et al., 2003). Assessment of drug concentrations in the skin is crucial for the development of topical products, such as patches, and other transdermal formulations. Several studies have demonstrated the skin permeabilities and local tissue concentrations of NSAIDs after topical administration (Singh & Rogerts, 1994; Grupta et al., 1995). However, the drug concentrations in those *in vitro* studies were calculated as accumulated volumes across the skin, and the drug contents within the skin consequently remain unclear. It has also been suggested that the diffusion length of the viable epidermis and dermis is longer *in vitro* than *in vivo* (Scheuplein, 1976), thereby leading to possible discrepancies in the permeation data between *in vitro* and *in vivo* studies. Almost all previous *in vivo* studies have evaluated drug concentrations within the whole skin layer after topical application. In addition, only one or two points of the skin were sampled and measured for their drug concentrations, and it therefore remains unclear how drugs permeate the skin layer from the surface to the deep regions over time.

To solve such problems, we developed a new evaluation method involving transdermal pharmacokinetics (Goi et al., 2010). In this chapter, we first explain the details of the dermal lateral sectioning approach and clearly summarize the results. Next, we apply this evaluation method to a more realistic model. Finally, we analyze the correlation between the time course changes of the drug concentration at the deepest layer of skin and the expression rate of drug efficacy, and suggest that our lateral sectioning approach is an ideal method for predicting therapeutic expression.

2. Evaluation method of transdermal drug permeability

The aim of this study was to establish a new method for clearly analyzing the flow of drugs in the skin layers and evaluating the drug levels in the target area of the skin tissue.

2.1 Animals

All experiments were carried out in accordance with the Institutional Animal Care and Use Committee of Mikasa Seiyaku Co. Ltd. (Tokyo, Japan). Male hairless rats (8 weeks of age, weighing 190–250 g; Japan SLC Inc., Shizuoka, Japan) were used in all experiments. The rats were housed in an animal room with a room temperature of 23±2°C, relative humidity of 55±15% and 12-h/12-h light/dark cycle (lights on at 07:00). The animals had free access to a mouse/rat diet (#5002, pellet form; PMI Nutrition International Inc., Richmond, IN) and tap water throughout the experiments.

2.2 Drugs

Flurbiprofen and ketoprofen are racemic propionic acid-derived NSAIDs with proven efficacy and safety in the treatment of osteoarthritis, rheumatoid arthritis and acute musculoskeletal disorders (Brogden et., 1979; Buchanan & Kassam, 1986; Waikakul et al., 1997). As a matter of course, tape-type patches of flurbiprofen (FP-T) and ketoprofen (KP-T) have been used and investigated for their anti-inflammatory and analgesic effects on local tissues (Martens, 1997; Mazieres, 2005).

The FP-T tape-type patches (ZEPOLAS® TAPE; Mikasa Seiyaku Co. Ltd., Tokyo, Japan) contained 2.2% flurbiprofen (1.1 mg/4 cm^2) in a hydrophobic adhesive-like styrene/isoprene/styrene copolymer without water. The KP-T tape-type patches (MOHRUS® TAPE; Hisamitsu Pharmaceutical Co. Ltd., Tosu, Japan) contained 2% ketoprofen (1.1 mg/4 cm^2). Both patches are widely used clinically. Other chemical agents used were flurbiprofen and ketoprofen (purity, >99.7%; Daito Pharmaceutical Co. Ltd., Toyama, Japan).

2.3 *In vivo* evaluation of the transdermal permeability of drugs

Rats were anesthetized with ether and 2.0×2.0 cm flurbiprofen or ketoprofen patches were individually applied to the center of their abdomen. The region with the applied patch was covered with a bonded-fiber fabric bandage and the body was wrapped with an adhesive elasticized bandage (Elastopore® No. 50; Nichiban Co. Ltd., Tokyo, Japan) to prevent the patch from becoming dislodged. The rats were then housed individually in blanket cages (240 mm width × 380 mm length × 200 mm height) and supplied with food and water *ad libitum*. Both types of patches were removed at 2, 4, 8, 12, 14, 16 and 24 h after application, including an extra time point of 1 h after application for FP-T, and the rats were euthanized by collection of whole blood from the abdominal aorta under ether anesthesia. The area of skin tissue where each patch was applied was removed and the harvested skin tissues were embedded in OCT compound (Sakura Finetechnical Co. Ltd., Tokyo, Japan) and frozen at –80°C.

The most important part of the technique was the procedure for freezing skin tissues in a flat manner. As shown in Fig. 1, the embedding agent was poured into a case to about half-full and frozen in advance. The case was then left for about 15 min at room temperature and 1) the surface of the embedding agent was lightly rubbed with the flat part of a finger to make the surface parallel. 2) Subsequently, the harvested skin tissues were placed on the flat surface and 3) pins were placed at the corners of the skin tissues to clarify the outline (because the place where the skin existed became unknown after the OCT compound was frozen). 4) Finally, the embedding agent was gently poured into the rest of the case and frozen at –80°C.

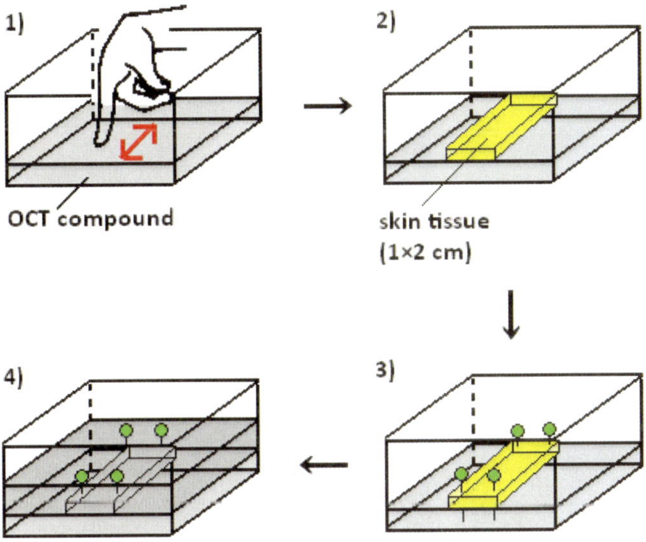

Fig. 1. Procedure for freezing skin tissues in a flat manner.

One-half of each frozen skin tissue sample (1.0×2.0 cm) was cut with a microtome (Cryotome CR-502; Nakagawa Co. Ltd., Tokyo, Japan) into 20 μm-thick slices parallel to the surface. The drug concentrations in the individual slices were measured after the slices were weighed. At this point in the slicing, the most crucial part of the handling was how the initial slice of frozen skin was cut parallel to the plane surface of the skin. When continued slicing became able to catch the embedded skin surface along the way, the angle of the cutting plane was adjusted and the slicing was operated several more times. This procedure was repeated until the cut plane became parallel to the surface of the skin tissue. Once the slicing of the skin was initiated, the operation was carried through without any further adjustments. The drug concentrations were obtained by dividing the measured amount of the drug in each skin slice by the weight of the slice. The microtome was not able to slice frozen samples thicker than 20 μm. The other half of each frozen skin tissue sample was sliced perpendicular to the skin surface and stained with hematoxylin and eosin (HE) for measurements of the skin thickness. Images were obtained using a fluorescence microscope (IX81-ZDC; Olympus, Tokyo, Japan). For measurement of the thickness of each layer, 10 points of the layer in a microscopic field were randomly picked up and the thickness was calculated using the software Lumina Vision LV-WIN TM-SOFT (Mitani Co. Ltd., Fukui, Japan). The average value from each image was taken as the individual thickness of each layer.

The thicknesses of the stratum corneum, epidermis and other tissues (dermal and subcutaneous tissues) were measured (Table 1) when the rats were 8 weeks of age (n=4). The whole skin thickness was approximately 700 μm and 35 pieces of skin tissue were theoretically obtained when the frozen tissues were sliced laterally every 20 μm. However, it was necessary to take account of individual differences and surface irregularities. Therefore, the skin tissue was sliced an extra five times (=100 μm thickness) and weighed, and the drug concentrations in the skin layers from 0 to 800 μm were measured. Images of the slicing and measuring protocol are shown in Fig. 2.

stratum corneum	epidermis	dermal and subcutaneous tissues
15.9 ± 0.9	38.4 ± 2.0	659.8 ± 32.6

(μm)

Table 1. Skin layer thicknesses of hairless rats

2.4 Analytical methods

The frozen skin tissue samples were dissolved in a solution at room temperature. Briefly, a piece of skin sample (about 3 mg) was added to 250 μL of 1 mol/L KOH and incubated at 60°C for 15 min. Next, 750 μL of 5% (v/v) H_3PO_4 was added, and 500 μL of the resulting solution was subjected to solid-phase extraction (Oasis® MAX 96-Well Plate 30 μm; Waters, Milford, MA) after the cartridge had been successively prewashed with 1 mL of methanol and 1 mL of water. The cartridge was consecutively rinsed with 1 mL of 50 mM sodium acetate (pH 7.0) and 1 mL of methanol, and eluted with a mixed solution (isopropanol/acetonitrile/formic acid = 58:40:2). A 5-μL aliquot of each eluate was analyzed by HPLC and LC/MS.

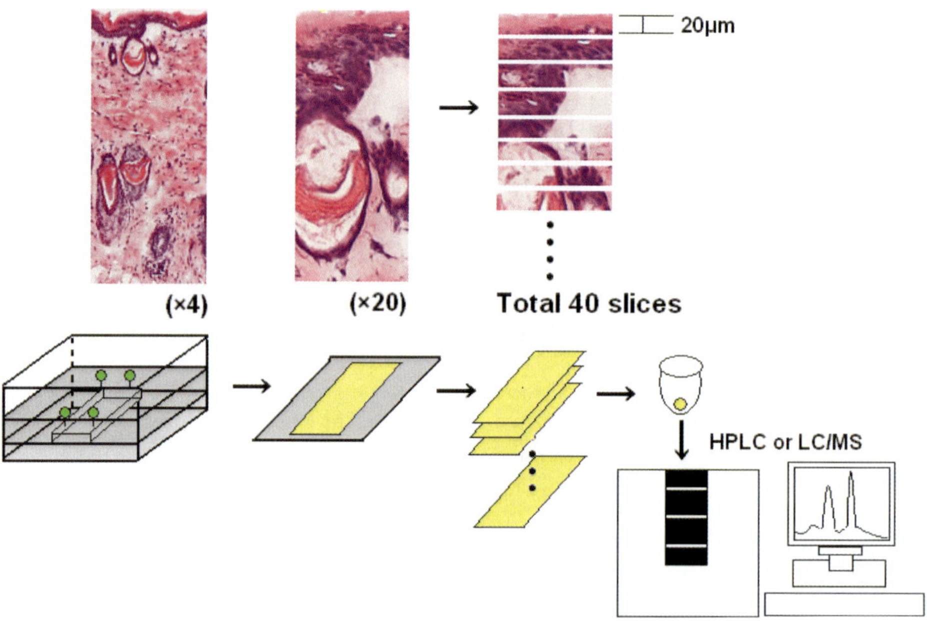

Fig. 2. Images of skin slicing and analysis of the drug contents of individual slices.

The concentrations of flurbiprofen in the dissolution media were determined by HPLC. The HPLC conditions were as follows: pump, LC-20AD; detector, RF-10A$_{XL}$; system controller, CBM-20A; auto-injector, SIL-20AC$_{HT}$; column oven, CTO-20AC (Shimadzu Co. Ltd., Kyoto, Japan); column, ZORBAX SB-C18 (150×4.6 mm, 1.8-μm particles; Agilent Technologies Inc.,

Wilmington, DE); column temperature, 60°C. The mobile phase consisted of acetonitrile and 0.1% (v/v) formic acid at a ratio of 60:40, delivered at a flow rate of 1 mL/min. The fluorescence was determined at 310 nm (emission) and 260 nm (excitation). The retention time of flurbiprofen was approximately 5.5 min.

The concentrations of ketoprofen were measured by LC/MS. Mass spectrometry was used to confirm the chromatographic profile obtained by a diode-array detector. The Shimadzu LCMS-2010A system used was equipped with a column (ZORBAX SB-C18, 150×2.1 mm, 3.5-μm particles; Agilent Technologies Inc.), a photodiode array detector (SPD-M20A) and a single quadrupole analyzer (LCMSF-2010EV). The other pieces of equipment were the same as those used for the HPLC analyses. Identification was achieved using the full-scan mode at a mass range of *m/z* 100-500. The mobile phase consisted of acetonitrile and 0.1% (v/v) formic acid at a ratio of 60:40, delivered at a flow rate of 0.2 mL/min.

The accuracy values of blank skin samples with added flurbiprofen and ketoprofen (2.5, 10 and 80 ng/mL) were in the ranges of 102.7–111.5% and 98.1–107.1%, respectively, within 24 h for the sample preparation and measurements by HPLC and LC/MS described above. The recovery rates of the individual drugs from the skin tissue samples were both >93.0%.

The flurbiprofen and ketoprofen contents of the FP-T and KP-T patches were also measured by HPLC. The residual ratios were calculated as follows:

$$\text{Residual ratio (\%)} = \frac{\text{Drug contents in patches after application}}{\text{Drug contents in patches before application}} \times 100 \quad (1)$$

The HPLC conditions were as follows: column, Mightysil RP-18 GP (150×4.6 mm, 5.0-μm particles; Kanto Chemical Co. Inc., Tokyo, Japan); column temperature, 40°C. The mobile phase consisted of acetonitrile and 0.1% (v/v) formic acid at a ratio of 60:40. The retention times of flurbiprofen and ketoprofen were both approximately 4.0 min. The other conditions were the same as those used for the skin tissues.

2.5 Statistical analysis

The results were expressed as means ± SD. The significance of differences between measurements for the FP-T-applied and KP-T-applied groups was evaluated using the Mann–Whitney *U* test. The criterion for statistical significance was a value of $P<0.05$ for all statistical evaluations.

3. Estimation of the percutaneous permeation of flurbiprofen and ketoprofen from the surface to the deep layer

To examine the drug permeation in the skin tissue, the skin areas where the tapes were applied were cut into 20 μm-thick horizontal slices from the surface, and the drug concentrations in the slices were measured individually. Later, we calculated each drug concentration in the skin tissue per 100 μm thickness, corresponding to five pieces of skin tissue, to clearly indicate the drug distributions, because we considered that it was not easy to evaluate the drug disposition in the finely-divided state (every 20 μm).

3.1 Single application of FP-T and KP-T

The drug levels in the skin tissues after application of FP-T and KP-T are shown in Fig. 3. Initially, the flurbiprofen concentrations in the skin layers from 0 to 400 μm were highest at 2 h after FP-T application and then decreased gradually, although the concentrations in the skin layers from 0 to 300 μm increased transiently after 12 h (Fig. 3A). The flurbiprofen concentrations at 2 h after application of FP-T were 2270±770, 1410±260, 1110±200 and 650±160 ng/mg of skin layer from 0 to 100 μm, 100 to 200 μm, 200 to 300 μm and 300 to 400 μm, respectively. Subsequently, the flurbiprofen concentrations in the skin layers from 400 to 800 μm, except for 500 to 600 μm, were highest at 4 h after FP-T application and then decreased until 24 h after FP-T application (Fig. 3C). On the other hand, the ketoprofen concentrations in the skin layers from 0 to 500 μm reached their peaks after 4 h of tape application (Fig. 3B and D).

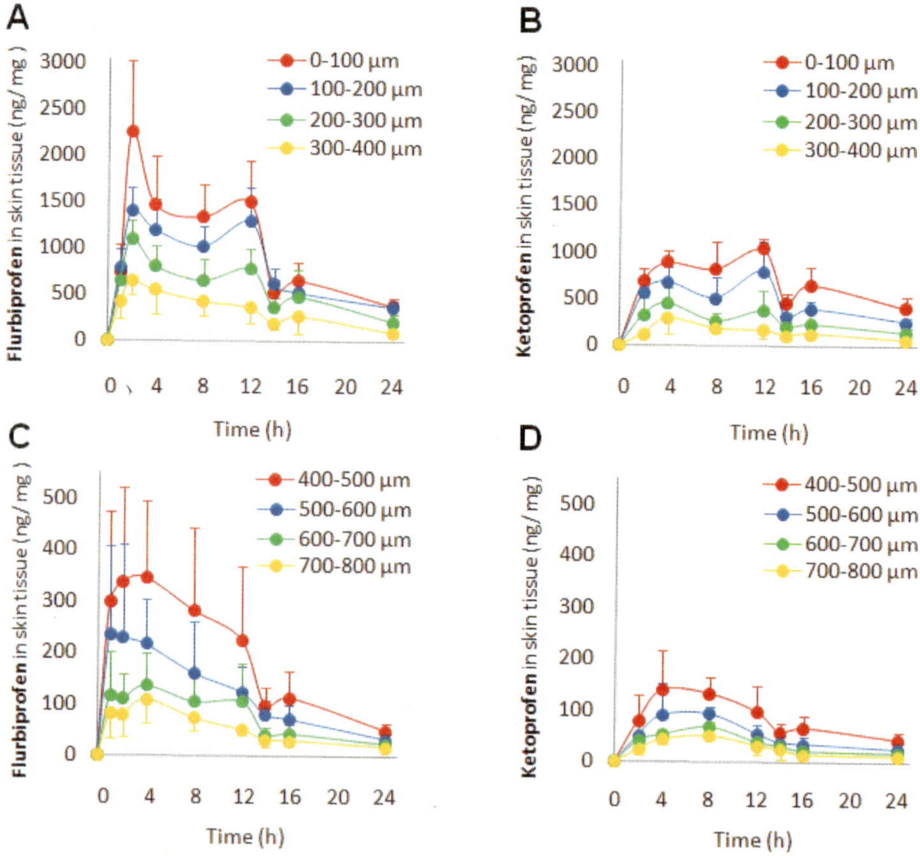

Fig. 3. Time-course profiles of the skin tissue concentrations of flurbiprofen and ketoprofen after FP-T and KP-T application. (A) Flurbiprofen concentrations in the layers from 0 to 400 μm. (B) Ketoprofen concentrations in the layers from 0 to 400 μm. (C) Flurbiprofen concentrations in the layers from 400 to 800 μm. (D) Ketoprofen concentrations in the layers from 400 to 800 μm. Each point represents the mean ± SD (n=5).

The ketoprofen concentrations at 4 h after application of KP-T were 900±130, 680±170, 460±160 and 300±160 ng/mg of skin layer from 0 to 100 μm, 100 to 200 μm, 200 to 300 μm and 300 to 400 μm, respectively. Similar to the case for flurbiprofen, the ketoprofen concentrations in the skin layers from 0 to 300 μm increased transiently after 12 h. The ketoprofen concentrations in the skin layers from 500 to 800 μm were highest at 8 h after KP-T application and decreased until 24 h (Fig. 3D).

Traditionally, information on percutaneous absorption has been obtained using *in vitro* skin diffusion chambers, mathematical models (Potts & Guy, 1992; Singh & Roberts, 1996) and indirect methods such as radiolabeled drug absorption techniques *in vivo* (Schaefer et al., 1978). However, percutaneous absorption depends on various multiple components, and consequently the series of equations is complicated. Autoradiography has the advantage that the drug levels are represented visually, but is not considered to be a quantitative method. Our technique of lateral sectioning of frozen skin tissues and measurement of the drug concentration in each slice may be primitive, but allowed us to clearly understand the diffusion of drugs in the skin layers.

Table 2 shows the time courses of the changes in the residual ratios of flurbiprofen and ketoprofen after topical application of FP-T and KP-T. No significant differences between flurbiprofen and ketoprofen were observed with respect to the residual ratios until 12 h after patch application, suggesting that the drug release rates of FP-T and KP-T were nearly equal and that the higher skin concentrations of flurbiprofen shown in Fig. 3 followed another mechanism that was separate from the drug release rate. From 12 to 16 h, a high volume of flurbiprofen was released compared with ketoprofen. Therefore, flurbiprofen seemed to be released from FP-T to the greatest possible extent until 16 h and no more flurbiprofen was subsequently released until 24 h, whereas ketoprofen was continuously released from KP-T until 24 h after application.

	Time after tape application (h)					
	2	4	8	12	16	24
Flurbiprofen	73.7 ± 2.6	65.1 ± 2.6	45.3 ± 6.2	37.3 ± 2.0	22.7 ± 1.2*	22.0 ± 2.6
Ketoprofen	76.8 ± 4.0	60.0 ± 2.9	48.7 ± 3.8	40.8 ± 6.2	34.7 ± 5.7	22.3 ± 2.8

(%)

Table 2. Residual ratios of flurbiprofen and ketoprofen after tape application. Each value represents the mean ± SD (n=4). *$P<0.05$ *vs.* ketoprofen.

3.2 Second application of FP-T

Since the FP-T patch is removed and replaced with a new patch every 12 h, we also investigated the flurbiprofen concentrations in the skin tissues after a second application of FP-T. The second FP-T was applied to the same skin site as the first patch under the assumption that patches are applied to the same affected area more than once. The time courses of the changes in the concentrations of flurbiprofen in the whole skin layer (0 to 800 μm) after tape application are shown in Fig. 4. It was clearly demonstrated that flurbiprofen rapidly reached the deepest layer of the whole skin within a short time, but there was a low content of flurbiprofen in the area deeper than 600 μm from 16 to 24 h after administration with only a single application. This was because a very low amount of flurbiprofen was released from FP-T from 16 to 24 h, as shown in Table 2. On the other hand, the flurbiprofen concentration in all regions of the whole skin increased promptly after 14 h and a high concentration of flurbiprofen was maintained until 24 h after application, even in the deepest layer in cases where a second application was carried out.

The time courses of the changes in the concentrations of flurbiprofen and ketoprofen in the deepest skin layer (700 to 800 μm) after FP-T application are shown in Fig. 5. This layer is adjacent to the intramuscular tissue and plays a major role in the evaluation of drug permeability and pharmacodynamics. The concentration of flurbiprofen (109.4±44.8 ng/mg) was significantly higher than that of ketoprofen (44.4±9.8 ng/mg) at 4 h after tape application, but there were no significant differences in the concentrations of the two drugs at 12 h and thereafter, except for 16 h. However, the flurbiprofen concentration in the deepest skin tissue layer increased again at 2 h (total exposure, 14 h) after the second application of FP-T (115.3±44.6 ng/mg) and was maintained at a significantly higher level than ketoprofen for the next 10 h (total exposure, 24 h).

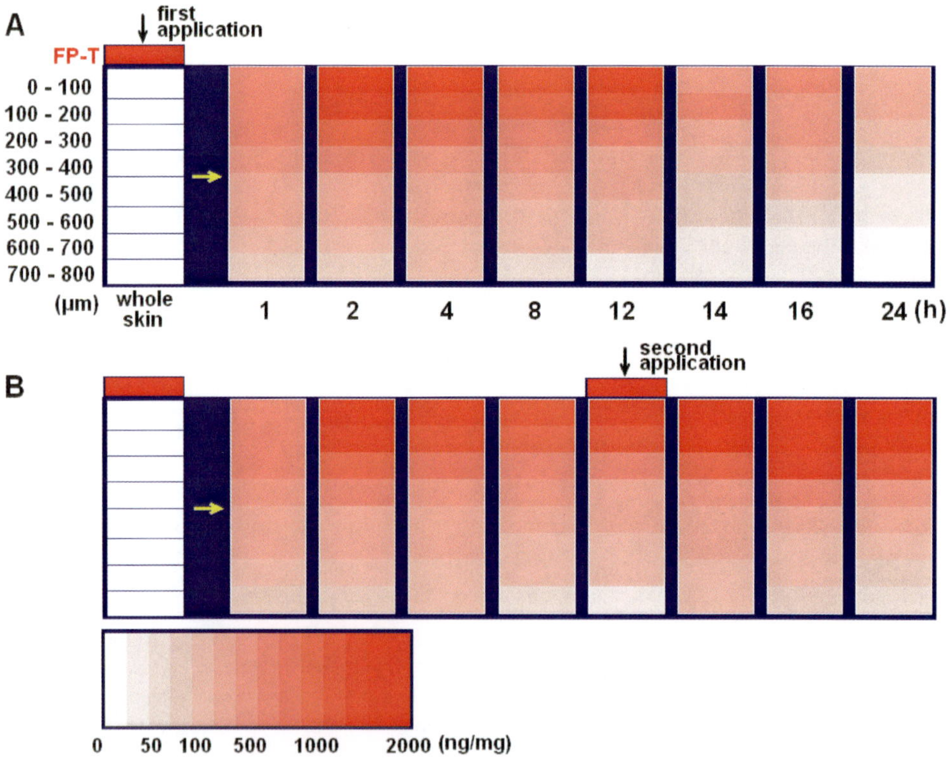

Fig. 4. Time-course profiles of the skin tissue concentrations of flurbiprofen after FP-T application. (A) Single application. (B) First and second applications. The color density is dependent on the drug concentration in the skin tissues.

A second application of FP-T reduced the time required to reach the maximal concentration in the deepest skin layer (700 to 800 μm) from 4 h to 2 h after administration (Fig. 5). The skin permeation of a drug is generally enhanced by occlusive application (Schaefer & Redelmeier, 1996). Hydration of corneocytes and weakening of the stratum corneum barrier function induced by 12 h of continuous FP-T application appeared to comprise the main mechanisms for how the permeability rate of flurbiprofen released from the new FP-T patch was increased. In addition, the flurbiprofen contents in the superficial layer (0 to 300 μm) increased slightly at 12 h after administration compared with the contents at 8 h (Fig. 3A). This observation means that enormous proportions of the flurbiprofen were stored in the superficial layer, and that this layer acted as a drug reservoir. Fundamentally, stored flurbiprofen is slowly released to the deeper tissues (Sugawara et al., 1987). However, it should be considered that the powerful driving force produced by the application of a second FP-T extruded the deposited flurbiprofen and a greater amount of flurbiprofen was able to permeate quickly into the deepest layer of the skin as a result. These findings are consistent with a previous study in which T_{max} was decreased by successive patch applications (Taburet et al., 1995).

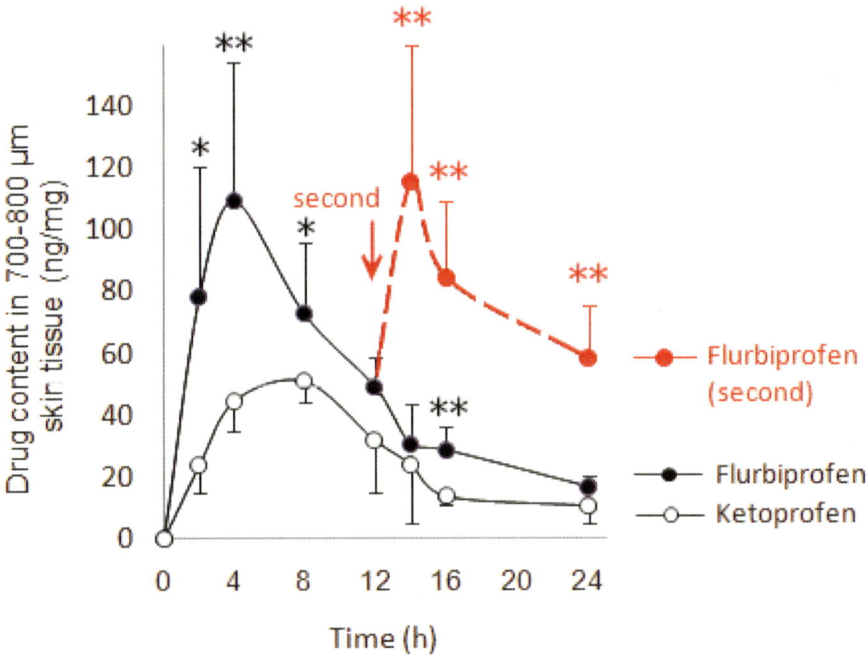

Fig. 5. Time-course profiles of the skin tissue concentrations of flurbiprofen and ketoprofen in the layer from 700 to 800 μm after FP-T and KP-T application. The unbroken lines for flurbiprofen and ketoprofen show data for continuous FP-T and KP-T administration for 24 h. The broken line for flurbiprofen shows data after a second administration of FP-T from 12 to 24 h (the previous FP-T was removed and the new patch was applied at 12 h). Each point represents the mean ± SD (n=5). *P<0.05 and **P<0.01 *vs.* ketoprofen.

3.3 Effect of stratum corneum stripping on the transcutaneous permeability of flurbiprofen

What factors would affect the LETD of NSAIDs in practical usage? The FP-T patch is removed and replaced with a new patch every 12 h as mentioned above. We observed that the stratum corneum was hardly stripped when FP-T was removed after 4 h of adhesion, but was slightly stripped to about 1.5-μm thickness after removal of the first FP-T patch at 12 h (Table 3). To investigate the effect of this decrease in the thickness of the stratum corneum on the transcutaneous penetration of flurbiprofen, we measured the concentrations of flurbiprofen in skin layers of 100-μm thickness with and without tape-stripping.

Normal	Time after FP-T administration (h)			
	2	4	8	12
15.9 ± 0.9	15.1 ± 1.0	15.2 ± 1.6	14.5 ± 0.6	14.5 ± 0.9

(μm)

Table 3. Stratum corneum thicknesses after removal of adherent FP-T at a fixed time. Each value represents the mean ± SD (n=4).

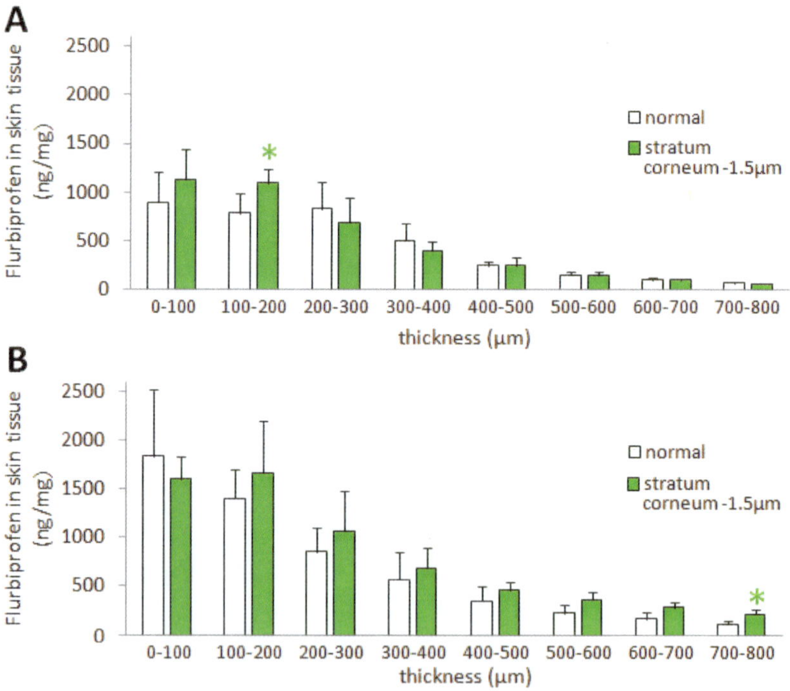

Fig. 6. Effect of stratum corneum stripping on the transcutaneous permeability of flurbiprofen. The skin tissue concentrations of flurbiprofen per 100-μm thickness are expressed after FP-T application for 2 h (A) and 4 h (B). The data represent means ± SD (n=4). *P<0.05 *vs.* the non-stripped group (=normal).

Tape-stripping is used to measure drug uptake into the skin (Touitou et al., 1998; Bashir et al., 2001). The tapes have different propensities to cause barrier disruption. Some individuals do not exhibit increased TEWL despite an equivalent mass of stratum corneum being removed compared with those who do show a response (Bashier et al., 2001). In our situation, the abdominal skin of some rats was tape-stripped using two strokes of adhesive tape (Transpore® Surgical Tape; Sumitomo 3M Co. Ltd., Tokyo, Japan) before placing FP-T patches. The score of TEWL was 9.3±0.4 g/m^2h before stripping and increased slightly to 11.6±0.5 g/m^2h after two strokes of tape-stripping. Therefore, it seemed that two strokes of tape-stripping replicated the decrease in thickness of the stratum corneum when FP-T was removed after 12 h of adhesion without disrupting the horny layer formation. We compared the drug concentrations in the skin tissues between the stripping and non-stripping models to evaluate the effect of stratum corneum stripping on the transcutaneous permeability of flurbiprofen.

At the time when the skin tissue was previously stripped and FP-T had been administered for 2 h, the skin tissue concentrations of flurbiprofen were higher than those without stripping in the layers from 0 to 200 μm, and a significant difference was observed in the layer from 100 to 200 μm (Fig. 6A). In the deeper layers beyond 200 μm, there were no significant differences in the flurbiprofen concentrations between the two groups. Likewise, at the time when the skin tissue was previously stripped and FP-T had been administered for 4 h, the skin tissue concentrations of flurbiprofen were higher than those without stripping in the layers from 100 to 800 μm, and a significant increase was observed in the deepest layer (Fig. 6B). Therefore, the transcutaneous permeability of flurbiprofen into the deepest layer of the skin tissue was not affected by stratum corneum stripping when FP-T had been applied for 2 h, but was affected by stripping after FP-T had been administered for 4 h. Our evaluation method revealed that only a small 10% decrease in the thickness of the stratum corneum could change the drug LETD to the deepest layer.

4. Pharmacokinetics

4.1 Pharmacokinetic parameters

Blood samples (0.2 mL) were collected from the jugular vein of the rats at 2, 4, 8, 12, 14, 16 and 24 h after both types of patches were applied. The analytical methods were slightly modified compared with those for the skin tissues. Briefly, 50 μL of plasma sample was applied to measure the drug contents. The mobile phase of HPLC consisted of acetonitrile and 0.1% (v/v) formic acid at a ratio of 55:45, delivered at a flow rate of 1 mL/min, and the mobile phase of LC/MS consisted of acetonitrile and 0.1% (v/v) formic acid at a ratio of 50:50, delivered at a flow rate of 0.2 mL/min.

The pharmacokinetic parameters following topical administration of flurbiprofen and ketoprofen are summarized in Table 4. These pharmacokinetic values are based on the plasma concentration/time profiles of the drugs after administration of one patch. FP-T exhibited higher and more rapid flurbiprofen permeation compared with ketoprofen permeation from KP-T. As shown in Table 4, FP-T exhibited a higher C_{max} value (4.6±0.7 μg/mL) and shorter T_{max} value (6.3±2.1 h) than KP-T. Moreover, FP-T administration produced a high $AUC_{0\text{-}12h}$ value of 44.5±7.3 μg•h/mL, which was five times higher than that of KP-T (8.6±1.8 μg•h/mL). The plasma concentration of flurbiprofen peaked at 6.3±2.1 h after the first FP-T application, although this peak was shortened to 3.2±1.1 h after the second FP-T application. The C_{max} and $AUC_{0\text{-}12h}$ values for the second FP-T application were slightly increased, and the $T_{1/2}$ value after the successive applications was longer than that after the first FP-T application. The drug delivery during the second patch application indicated relatively good permeability as mentioned previously, and this is probably the reason why the shorter T_{max} value and higher C_{max} and AUC values were observed.

	Flurbiprofen		Ketoprofen
	first	second	
Dose (mg/kg)	4.5	4.5	4.5
C_{max} (μg/ml)	4.6 ± 0.7	5.9 ± 0.4	1.5 ± 0.2
T_{max} (h)	6.3 ± 2.1	3.2 ± 1.1	19.2 ± 3.4
$T_{1/2}$ (h)	7.3 ± 1.1	10.3 ± 1.3	—
$AUC_{0\text{-}12h}$ (μg•h/ml)	44.5 ± 7.3	55.2 ± 2.6	8.6 ± 1.8
A.B. (%)	43.0	53.4	14.8

Table 4. Pharmacokinetic parameters following topical administration of flurbiprofen and ketoprofen. Each value represents the mean ± SD (n=3–5). C_{max}: maximum plasma concentration; T_{max}: time to reach C_{max}; $T_{1/2}$: terminal half-life; $AUC_{0\text{-}12h}$: area under the plasma concentration-time curve from time 0 to 12 h; A.B.: absolute bioavailability in an intravenous group.

4.2 Differences in the time-course changes in the skin and plasma concentrations between flurbiprofen and ketoprofen

The time-course changes in the flurbiprofen concentrations in the skin layer from 700 to 800 μm were very similar to the plasma concentrations of flurbiprofen after both single and repeated applications (Fig. 7A). In contrast, the transcutaneous absorption of ketoprofen into the systemic circulation was relatively slow, and the plasma concentration of ketoprofen peaked about 8 h later than the peak in the skin layer from 700 to 800 μm (Fig. 7B).

The two formulations of NSAIDs examined have their own characteristic features. FP-T with a twice-daily application frequency induced a quick increase in the skin concentration of flurbiprofen and maintained a high level in the deepest layer via LETD (Fig. 7A). This shows the potential for prompt onset and prolonged duration of NSAID activity in intramuscular tissues. However, the systemic concentrations of the drug increased at the same rate as the concentrations in the deepest layer of the skin, which may increase the risk of adverse effects. On the other hand, the diffusion of ketoprofen from KP-T to the maximal depth of the skin by LETD was relatively slow (Fig. 7B), suggesting the possibility that several hours are required to realize its efficacy as an anti-inflammatory drug. However, the plasma concentrations of ketoprofen absorbed by the systemic circulation route were relatively low, which may lower the risk of adverse effects. These observations are consistent with previous reports indicating that ketoprofen is an effective and safe therapeutic option for the treatment of local painful inflammation (Mazieres, 2005; Flouvat et al., 1989). In many studies, including the present study, pharmacokinetics parameters have been evaluated using the time courses of the total plasma or serum concentrations. However, the theory of practical pharmacokinetics emphasizes the importance of the unbound fraction of a drug in understanding concepts such as clearance, apparent volume of distribution and pharmacodynamic action (Wright et al., 1996). Borgå & Borgå (1997) reported that the lowest dissociation constant (highest affinity) was found with flurbiprofen, which exhibited an 80-fold difference compared with the highest affinity for ketoprofen. This high affinity of flurbiprofen for albumin may contribute to a reduction in the incidence of gastrointestinal disorders, although its plasma concentration was still much higher than that of ketoprofen.

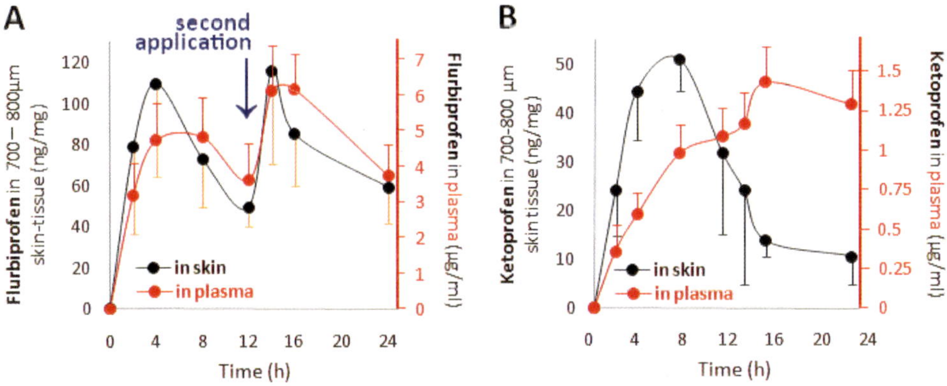

Fig. 7. Time-course profiles of the skin tissue and plasma concentrations of flurbiprofen and ketoprofen after FP-T and KP-T application. (A) The skin tissue concentrations of flurbiprofen in the layer from 700 to 800 µm are expressed on the left axis and the plasma concentrations of flurbiprofen are expressed on the right axis. (B) The skin tissue and plasma concentrations of ketoprofen are expressed in the same way as described for (A). Each point represents the mean ± SD (n=3–5).

Skin concentrations result from the balance of permeation into the tissue and clearance from the tissue, combined with partitioning into the various skin components (Kretsos et al., 2008). Percutaneous absorption depends on the physicochemical properties of the compound, and small moderately lipophilic molecules are generally the most readily absorbed. The log Ko/w values for flurbiprofen and ketoprofen are 3.75 and 2.76, respectively (Valko et al., 2003). The binding affinity of flurbiprofen for albumin is superior to that of ketoprofen, as mentioned above, and the binding ratios of the two drugs are 99.9% and 98.7%, respectively (Valko et al., 2003). It is notable that both the viable epidermis and dermis contain, on average, about 2% extravascular albumin, to which both flurbiprofen and ketoprofen can bind (Bert et al., 1986). The high lipophilicity and an effect of the superior protein-binding activity on the clearance mechanism are likely to be the major reasons why the skin concentration of flurbiprofen was higher than that of ketoprofen. Besides, other important factors may affect the transdermal absorptions of the two drugs. In general, LETD-mediated drug permeation has been explained in terms of passive diffusion of non-ionized compounds (Potts, 1992). However, several studies have focused on the possible involvement of transporters expressed in the skin, similar to the case for other tissues (Schiffer et al., 2003; Bonen et al., 2006; Li, 2006). Organic anion transporter 2 (OAT2) is thought to be a candidate for an exchanger involved in the uptake and/or efflux of flurbiprofen in the skin, and the flurbiprofen permeability in the absorptive direction was higher than that in the secretory direction (Ito et al., 2007). The superior permeability of flurbiprofen in the skin may be attributable to a more predominant exchange capacity with several transporters compared with other NSAIDs.

5. Pharmacodynamics

From our lateral sectioning approach, it was predicted that FP-T had the potential for prompt onset and prolonged duration of NSAID activity, while KP-T needed several hours to demonstrate its efficacy as an anti-inflammatory drug in intramuscular tissues. Therefore, we investigated whether the results for the percutaneous drug permeation using lateral slicing were in accordance with the drug efficacies.

5.1 Topical anti-inflammatory efficacy in carrageenin-induced rat paw edema

The topical anti-inflammatory efficacy was evaluated for carrageenin-induced inflammation edema in Wistar rats weighing 124±11 g. The activities of the drugs were evaluated by measuring the changes in paw volume with a plethysmometer (TK-101CMP; Muromachi Co. Ltd., Tokyo, Japan). FP-T or KP-T (0.5×3.5 cm) was applied to the right paw for 3 h with the help of adhesive tape, at 0.5 h prior to the carrageenin injection. Acute inflammation was produced by injecting 0.1 mL of 1% (w/v) carrageenin solution into the subplantar region of the right hind paw. The paw volume was measured at 0, 3, 4 and 5 h after the injection.

The percentage of swelling in the paw was calculated by the following formula.

$$\text{Swelling } (\%) = \frac{b-a}{a} \times 100 \qquad (2)$$

where a is the paw volume before producing the edema and b is the paw volume measured after producing the edema.

In this acute model, the percentage swelling was promptly suppressed by flurbiprofen released from FP-T, whereas it required some time to be suppressed by ketoprofen from KP-T (Fig. 8). In addition, the FP-T efficacy was much stronger than that of KP-T. These findings support the accuracy of the evaluation method of percutaneous drug permeation using a lateral sectioning approach.

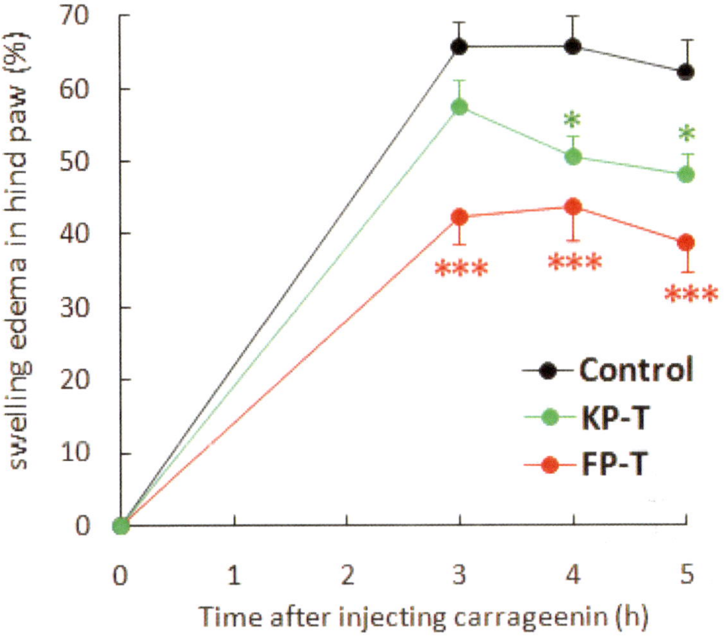

Fig. 8. Effects of FP-T and KP-T on edema produced by carrageenin in the hindpaw of rats. Each point represents the mean ± SE (n=7). *$P<0.05$ and ***$P<0.001$ *vs.* Control by Dunnett's test.

5.2 Antinociceptive efficacy in the inflamed paw pressure test

This experiment was performed according to the method of Randall & Selitto (1957) using Wistar rats weighing 114±19 g. FP-T or KP-T (0.5×3.5 or 1.0×3.5 cm) was applied to the right paw for 3 h with the help of adhesive tape, at 0.5 h prior to an injection of baker's yeast. Briefly, 0.1 mL of a 10% (w/v) solution of baker's yeast in saline was given by subplantar injection into the hind paw. Nociception was measured by applying an increased weight to the paw with a pressure meter (Ugo Basile, Varese, Italy) until the rats vocalized or drew their feet back. The algesic threshold was measured at 2, 3 and 4 h after the injection and the level of the algesic threshold was expressed as the sum of the algesic thresholds between 2 and 4 h.

As shown in Fig. 9, FP-T significantly increased the paw pressure threshold required for the nociceptive response, indicating a probable analgesic action. Besides, the drug efficacy depended on the applied area of FP-T. However, KP-T had no effect on the nociceptive response, even when its applied area was expanded.

From these pharmacodynamics studies, our predictions derived from the lateral sectioning approach were consistent with the facts that FP-T had the potential for prompt onset and prolonged duration of NSAID activity and that KP-T required a reasonable time to demonstrate its efficacy.

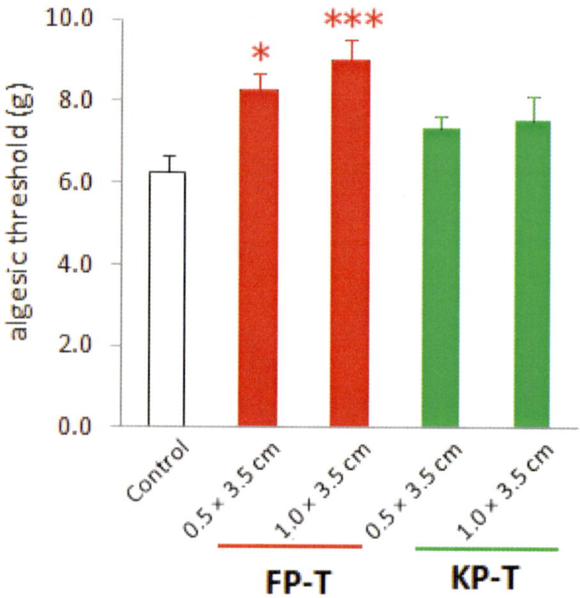

Fig. 9. Effects of FP-T and KP-T on nociception produced by baker's yeast in the hindpaw of rats. Each column represents the mean ± SE (n=10). *P<0.05 and ***P<0.001 *vs.* Control by Dunnett's test.

6. Evaluation of the technique

There are several limitations to our technique for evaluating transdermal permeability. First, information on the percutaneous absorption is obtained from invasive skin biopsies and this method cannot be applied to humans. Next, this technique is limited by the location. As previously mentioned, this technique depends on the procedure for freezing and slicing samples in a flat manner. Therefore, the abdominal skin is a suitable area for removal and preparation as samples. However, there are many sites in the body other than the abdominal area that are not flat, such as the circumferences of joints, and we ought to measure the drug concentrations at these sites. Our pharmacodynamic studies focused on the hindpaw and not on the abdominal area, although our predictions were derived using the abdominal region. Nevertheless, the therapeutic expressions were accordance with the efficacy predictions. This means that the lateral sectioning approach at the abdominal area could be applied to understand drug flow in other places of the body. Furthermore, it is well known that rodent skin is generally more permeable than human skin (Poet et al., 2000). Therefore, another method is required to precisely calculate the drug permeability in human skin. However, our lateral sectioning approach can simply and clearly indicate the time courses of the flow of drugs in skin tissues and the obtained data should facilitate the prediction and estimation of the pharmacodynamics of patches with other transdermal formulations. Recently, a hydrogel patch has been applied as a transcutaneous vaccination system against viral and bacterial infections (Ishii et al., 2008; Matsuo et al., 2011). In this case, the drug levels in the epidermal layer where Langerhans cells reside are crucial, and there is no point in measuring the total amounts of drugs that permeate the whole skin. Furthermore, we can check the conformational changes of the protein in the process of passing through the stratum corneum to judge whether the activity of the protein is maintained at that site.

As a matter of course, the sites in the skin where different drugs have efficacy tend to differ. However, our slicing method makes it possible to evaluate the drug levels at the skin sites where individual drugs exert their beneficial effects. These studies focused on the skin region for the present data, and clarification of the musculocutaneous pharmacokinetics is an issue for future studies. In addition, we would like to concentrate on the surrounding environments of the drugs in the skin tissues.

7. Conclusions

The present experimental data suggest that our approach involving lateral sectioning of frozen skin tissues and measurement of the drug concentration in each slice makes it possible to easily and clearly determine the tissue concentrations of drugs in skin layers adjacent to the target area, albeit in a rodent model. This technique has the advantage of simplicity and therefore has the potential to be applied to evaluations of the pharmacokinetics of other transdermal formulations.

8. References

Bashir, S. J.; Chew, A. L.; Aniqboqu, A.; Dreher, F. & Maibach, H. I. (2001). Physical and physiological effects of stratum corneum tape stripping. Skin Research and Technology, Vol.7, No.1, (February 2001), pp. 40-48, ISSN 0909-752X

Bert, J. L. (1986). Pearce RH, Mathieson JM. Concentration of plasma albumin in its accessible space in postmortem human dermis. *Microvascular Research*, Vol.32, No.2, (September 1986), pp. 211-223, ISSN 0026-2862

Bert, J. L.; Mathieson, J. M. & Pearce, R. H. (1982). The exclusion of human serum albumin by human dermal collagenous fibres and within human dermis. Biochemical Journal, Vol.201, No.2, (February 1982), pp. 395-403, ISSN 0264-6021

Bonen, A.; Heynen, M. & Hatta, H. (2006). Distribution of monocarboxylate transporters MCT1-MCT8 in rat tissues and human skeletal muscle. *Applied Physiology and metabolism*, Vol.31, No.1, (February 2006), pp. 31-39, ISSN 1715-5312

Borgå, O. & Borgå, B. (1997). Serum protein binding of nonsteroidal antiinflammatory drugs: A comparative study. *Journal of Pharmacokinetics and Biopharmaceutics*, Vol.25, No.1, (February 1997), pp. 63-77, ISSN 0090-466X

Brogden, R.N.; Heel, R. C.; Speight, T. M. & Avery, G. S. (1979). Flurbiprofen: a review of its pharmacological properties and therapeutic use in rheumatic diseases. *Drugs*, Vol.18, (December 1979), pp. 417-438, ISSN 0012-6667

Buchanan, W. W. & Kassam, Y. B. (1986). European experience with flurbiprofen. A new analgesic/anti-inflammatory agent. *American Journal of Medicine*, Vol.80, No.3A, (March 1986), pp. 145-152, ISSN 0002-9343

Flouvat, B.; Roux, A. & Delhotal-Landes, B. (1989). Pharmacokinetics of ketoprofen in man after repeated percutaneous administration. *Arzneimittelforschung*, Vol.39, No.7, (July 1989), pp. 812-815, ISSN 0004-4172

Goi, N.; Morishita, K.; Taniguchi, A. & Ishii, T. (2010). Evaluation of percutaneous permeation of flurbiprofen and ketoprofen after application of transdermal patches using a lateral sectioning approach in hairless rats. *Pharmaceutical Development and Technology*, Vol.15, No.6, (December 2010), pp. 658-665, ISSN 1083-7450

Gupta, E.; Wientjes, M. G. & Au, J. L. (1995). Penetration kinetics of 2′, 3′-dideoxyinosine in dermis is described by the distributed model. *Pharmaceutical Research*, Vol.12, No.1, (January 1995), pp. 108-112, ISSN 0724-8741

Hawkey, C. J. & Truelove, S. C. (1983). Inhibition of prostaglandin synthetase in human rectal mucosa. *Gut*, Vol.24, (March 1983), pp. 213-217, ISSN 0017-5749

Ishii, Y.; Nakae, T.; Sakamoto, F.; Matsuo, K.; Quan, Y. S.; Kamiyama, F.; Fujita, T.; Yamamoto, A.; Nakagawa, S. & Okada, N. A transcutaneous vaccination system using a hydrogel patch for viral and bacterial infection. *Journal of Controlled Release*, Vol.131, No.2, (October 2008), pp. 113-120, ISSN 0168-3659

Ito, K.; Kato, Y.; Tsuji, H.; Nguyen, H. T.; Kubo, Y. & Tsuji, A. (2007). Involvement of organic anion transport system in transdermal absorption of flurbiprofen. *Journal of Controlled Release*, Vol.124, (August 2007), pp. 60-68, ISSN 0168-3659

Kretsos, K.; Miller, M. A.; Zamora-Estrada, G. & Kasting, B. (2008). Partitioning, diffusivity and clearance of skin permeants in mammalian dermis. *International Journal of Pharmaceutics*, Vol.346, (January 2008), pp. 64-79, ISSN 0378-5173

Li, Q.; Tsuji, H.; Kato, Y.; Sai, Y.; Kubo, Y. & Tsuji, A. (2006).Characterization of the transdermal transport of flurbiprofen and indomethacin. *Journal of Controlled Release*, Vol.110, No.3, (February 2006), pp. 542-556, ISSN 0168-3659

Martens, M. (1997). Efficacy and tolerability of a topical NSAID patch (local action transcutaneous flurbiprofen) and oral diclofenac in the treatment of soft-tissue rheumatism. *Clinical Rheumatology*, Vol.16, (January 1997), pp. 25-31, ISSN 0770-3198

Matsuo, K.; Ishii, Y.; Quan, Y. S.; Kamiyama, F.; Mukai, Y., Okada, N. & Nakagawa, S. (2011). Characterization of transcutaneous protein delivery by a hydrogel patch in animal, human, and tissue-engineered skin models. Biological and Pharmaceutical Bulletin, Vol.34, No.4, (2011), pp. 586-589, ISSN 0918-6158.

Mazieres B. (2005). Topical ketoprofen patch. *Drugs in Research and Development*, Vol.6, No.6, (2005), pp. 337-344, ISSN 1174-5886

Morgan, C.J.; Renwick, A. G. & Friedmann, P. S. (2003). The role of stratum corneum and dermal microvascular perfusion in penetration and tissue levels of water-soluble drugs investigated by microdialysis. *British Journal of Dermatology*, Vol. 148, (March 2003), pp. 434-443, ISSN 0007-6963

Poet, T. S.; Corley, R. A.; Thrall, K. D.; Edwards, J. A.; Tanojo, H.; Weitz, K. K.; Hui, X.; Maibach, H. I. & Wester, R. C. (2000). Assessment of the percutaneous absorption of trichloroethylene in rats and humans using MS/MS real-time breath analysis and physiologically based pharmacokinetic modeling. *Toxicological Sciences*, Vol.56, No.1, (July 2000), pp. 61-72, ISSN 1096-6080

Potts, R. O. & Guy, R. H. Predicting skin permeability. *Pharmaceutical Research*, Vol.9, No.5, (May 1992), pp. 663-669, ISSN 0724-8741

Randall, L. O. & Selitto, J. J. (1957). A method for measurement of analgesic activity on inflamed tissue. *Archives internationals de pharmacodynamie et de therapie*, Vol.111, No.4, (September 1957), pp. 409-419, ISSN 0301-4533

Schaefer, H & Redelmeier, T. E. (1996). Skin Barrier, S Karger Pub, ISBN 978-3805563260, Basel, Switzerland

Schaefer, H.; Stüttgen, G.; Zesch, A.; Schalla, W. & Gazith, J. (1978). Quantitative determination of percutaneous absorption of radiolabeled drugs in vitro and in vivo by human skin. *Current Problems in Dermatology*, Vol.7, (1978), pp. 80-94, ISSN 1421-5721

Scheuplein, R. J. (1976). Percutaneous absorption after twenty-five years: or "old wine in new wineskins". *Journal of Ivestigative Dermatology*, Vol.67, (July 1976), pp. 31-38, ISSN 0022-202X

Schiffer, R.; Neis, M.; Höller, D.; Rodríguez, F.; Geier, A.; Gartung, C.; Lammert, F.; Dreuw, A.; Zwadlo-Klarwasser, G.; Merk, H.; Jugert, F. & Baron, J. M. (2003). Active influx transport is mediated by members of the organic anion transporting polypeptide family in human epidermal keratinocytes. *Journal of Investigative Dermatology*, Vol.120, No.2, (February 2003), pp. 285-291, ISSN 0022-202X

Singh, P. & Roberts, M. S. (1994). Skin permeability and local tissue concentrations of nonsteroidal anti-inflammatory drugs after topical application. *Journal of Pharmacology and Experimental Therapeutics*, Vol.268, No.1, (January, 1994), pp. 144-151, ISSN 0022-3565

Singh, P. & Roberts, M. S. (1996) Local deep tissue penetration of compounds after dermal application: structure-tissue penetration relationships. *American Society for Pharmacology and Experimental Therapeutics*, Vol.279, No.2, (November 1996), pp. 908-917, ISSN 0022-3565

Sugawara, S.; Ohno, H.; Ueda, R.; Ishigami, M.; Fujiwara, H.; Hashimoto, S.; Satoh, Y. & Yamazaki, K. (1987). A study of the concentration in the synovial fluid and tissues of patients treated with the transdermal topical application of flurbiprofen (FP-A). *Therapeutic Research*, Vol.6, No.1, (January 1987), pp. 289-294, ISSN 0289-8020

Taburet, A. M.; Singlas, E.; Glass, R. C.; Thomas, F. & Leutenegger, E. (1995). Pharmacokinetic comparison of oral and local action transcutaneous flurbiprofen in healthy volunteers. *Journal of Clinical Pharmacy and Therapeutics*, Vol.20, No.2, (April 1995), pp. 101-107, ISSN 0269-4727

Taha, A. S.; Dahill, S.; Sturrock, R. D.; Lee, F. D. & Russell, R. I. (1994). Predicting NSAID related ulcers - assessment of clinical and pathological risk factors and importance of differences in NSAID. *Gut*, Vol.35, (July 1994), pp. 891-895, ISSN 0017-5749

Touitou, E. Meidan, V. M. & Horwitz, E.(1998). Methods for quantitative determination of drug localized in the skin. *Journal of Controlled Release*, Vol.56, (December 1998), pp. 7-21, ISSN 0168-3659

Valko, K.; Nunhuck, S.; Bevan, C.; Abraham, M. H. & Reynolds, D. P. (2003). Fast gradient HPLC method to determine compounds binding to human serum albumin. Relationships with octanol/water and immobilized artificial membrane lipophilicity. Journal of Pharmaceutical Sciences, Vol.92, Vol.92, (November 2003), pp. 2236-2248, ISSN 0022-3549

Waikakul, S.; Penkitti, P.; Soparat, K. & Boonsanong, W. (1997). Topical analgesics for knee arthrosis: a parallel study of ketoprofen gel and diclofenac emulgel. *Journal of the*

Medical Association of Thailand, Vol.80, No.9, (September 1997), pp. 593-596, ISSN 0125-2208

Wright, J. D.; Boudinot, F. D. & Ujhelyi, M. R. (1996). Measurement and analysis of unbound drug concentrations. Clinical Pharmacokinetics, Vol.30, No.6, (June 1996), pp. 445-462, ISSN 0312-5963

4

Computer Simulations as a Tool for Optimizing Bioequivalence Trials

Carmen Navarro-Fontestad[1], Victor Mangas-Sanjuán[2], Isabel González-Álvarez[2], Alfredo García-Arieta[3,*], Carlos Fernández-Teruel[1], Vicente G. Casabó-Alós[1] and Marival Bermejo[2]

[1]*Universidad de Valencia,*
[2]*Universidad Miguel Hernández de Elche,*
[3]*Agencia Española de Medicamentos y Productos Sanitarios (AEMPS),*
Spain

1. Introduction

The analyte to be measured in a Bioequivalence study when an oral drug undergoes a metabolic step in intestine or liver is still today a controversial issue with different recommendations in European Medicines Agency (EMEA/EMA) and Food and Drug Administration (FDA) guidance documents (EMA, 2010; EMEA, 2001; FDA, 2002).

In the current EMA guidance it is stated that in principle, evaluation of bioequivalence should be based upon measured concentrations of the parent compound (also for inactive pro-drugs) as the Cmax of the parent compound is usually more sensitive to detect differences in absorption rate than the Cmax of the metabolite. Only for some pro-drugs with very low plasma concentrations and quickly eliminated it is acceptable to demonstrate bioequivalence for the main active metabolite without measurement of parent compound. Nevertheless in these exceptional cases the applicant should adequately justify that it is not possible to reliably measure the parent compound after single dose administration (even with supra-therapeutic doses) and moreover the applicant should present any available data supporting the view that the metabolite exposure will reflect parent drug and that the metabolite formation is not saturated at therapeutic doses (EMA, 2010)

FDA guidance recommends metabolite measurement if it is formed as a result of gut-wall or other pre-systemic metabolism and if the metabolite contributes meaningfully to safety and/or efficacy. In this case parent drug data is used to confidence interval approach whereas metabolite data is used as supportive evidence of comparable therapeutic outcome (FDA, 2002).

The extent of pre-systemic metabolism and the non-linearity of the metabolic processes are the controversial aspects that require harmonization with regards to analyte selection. The lack of agreement in FDA and EMEA/EMA recommendations and the changes in the new

* This article reflects the author's personal opinion and not necessarily the policy or recommendations of the AEMPS.

EMA guideline makes evident that the simulations on which those recommendations were based, if any, were performed in different set of scenarios under a different set of assumptions leading to different answers to the same question.

2. Simulation models of bioequivalence scenarios

The critical issues that have been considered in the literature to create the simulated scenarios, apart from the true differences in extent and/or rate of absorption are

a. the extent of pre-systemic metabolism, intestinal or hepatic
b. the non-linearity of the metabolic processes
c. the intrinsic clearance magnitude (high or low) and
d. the intra-subject variability (high or low)

For instance Chen and Jackson (Chen & Jackson, 1991,1995) and Jackson (Jackson, 2000) constructed models of two compartments with and without a linear metabolic step. They considered the difference in absorption rate with Cmax as target parameter and the final criterion to select the best analyte was intra-individual variability.

The factor of parent drug or metabolite variability, nevertheless, is an arguable aspect to make a decision about the analyte. Once a study design is selected, the larger the intra-subject (inter-occasion) variability of the analyte, the lower the percentage of successful bioequivalent studies for a given real difference. In another words, the lack of power can be solved by increasing the number of patients in the study but the lack of sensitivity cannot be improved once the insensitive analyte has been selected. The ability to reflect the formulations differences in the estimations (accuracy) should not be confounded with the variability of the estimations (precision). The analyte selection should be based on the accuracy of the estimations. Statistically, the consumer and producer risk offered by each analyte (with the adequate sample size) should be the main determinants for this decision (Fernandez-Teruel et al., 2009b).

The issue of parent drug and metabolite variability has been addressed in other papers based on simulations with controversial conclusions (Blume & Midha, 1993; Jackson, 2000; Rosenbaum, 1998). Many of these simulation works have employed the percentage of failed studies as end-point to select the analyte to be measured. This depends not only on the difference between formulations but also, and in a higher extent, on the variability of the analytes. In spite of the interest of sponsors in decreasing the percentage of failed studies, to select the analyte based on its rate of failures should never be the regulatory criterion. On the contrary, the study design and analyte should be defined according to their ability to detect differences between formulations (i.e reducing the consumer risk of accepting bioinequivalent formulations)(Fernandez-Teruel et al., 2009a; 2009c)

Brady and Jackson (Braddy & Jackson, 2010) used a model similar to Chen and Jackson models but with non linear metabolism. As in the previous papers the main conclusion was that the parent drug (either AUC or Cmax data) was more sensitive to formulation differences than the metabolite. Apart from their simplicity the main objection of these models was the over parameterization as the first-pass metabolic clearance was modelled as a different and independent parameter than the metabolic systemic clearance.

A second group of papers present simulations based on semi-physiological models (Rosenbaum, 1998; Rosenbaum & Lam, 1997; Tucker et al., 1993) that solved the over-parameterization issue but they do not included in the simulations the problem of non-linear metabolism. In all the cases, their simulations showed that parent drug and metabolite have the same sensitivity to detect differences in extent of absorption (AUC) when the system is linear, but the Cmax of parent drug is more sensitive to differences in rate of absorption.

The study design (single dose versus steady state studies) has also been addressed by simulation approaches (el-Tahtawy et al., 1994, 1995; 1998; Jackson, 1987, 1989, 2000; Zha & Endrenyi, 1997) with the conclusion that single dose studies are more sensitive to detect differences in absorption rate.

3. BCS-based simulations

The Biopharmaceutic classification system (BCS) has changed the focus of bioequivalence demonstration from plasma levels to the absorption site, as permeability of the intestinal membrane (P), solubility (S) in luminal fluids and in vivo dissolution rate are recognized as the main determinants of rate and extent of absorption. The combination of the two levels of the permeability and solubility factors (High (H) or Low (L) permeability and High or Low solubility) defines the 4 BCS classes (Class 1: HP, HS ; Class 2: HP, LS; Class 3: LP, HS; Class 4: LP, LS) (Amidon et al., 1995; FDA, 2000)

It is generally accepted, and it has been shown through gastrointestinal simulation technology (computer simulations) that for class 1 and 3 formulation impact on extent of absorption is minimal, and regarding absorption rate, the formulation influence is also minimal for class 3 drugs while it could be reflected in Cmax differences for class 1 drugs (Kuentz, 2008). Class 2 drugs having good permeability but low solubility are the candidates showing a great dependence on formulation factors as for these drugs solubility and in vivo dissolution rate are the limiting factors. As BCS classification is relevant for the probabilities of bioequivalence problems related to the formulation, this classification system has been taken into account recently for the simulation approach to the analyte selection discussion (Fernandez-Teruel et al., 2009a; 2009b; 2009c; Navarro-Fontestad et al., 2010)

The authors addressed all the issues mentioned in the previous section that have been discussed in the literature i.e. the intrinsic clearance magnitude, the variability of the analyte, the linearity of the metabolic step and single dose versus steady state designs. In top of that, the four drug BCS classes were simulated in formulations of decreasing quality compared to the reference one. Results were analyzed from the point of view of the analyte giving the right answer to the BE criteria. As BE scenarios were simulated for each drug, it was possible to calculate which analyte detects better the lack of pharmaceutical quality.

The authors explored semi-physiological models of increasing complexity starting with a model considering hepatic first pass effect under linear and non linear conditions, then, adding the intestinal metabolic step and finally considering the existence of two metabolic pathways of different magnitude. The latest addition to those models is the involvement of intestinal transporters that could eventually lead to a non linearity in the absorption process.

In all the models the scheme for generating the scenarios is depicted in Figure 1 and briefly explained in the next section.

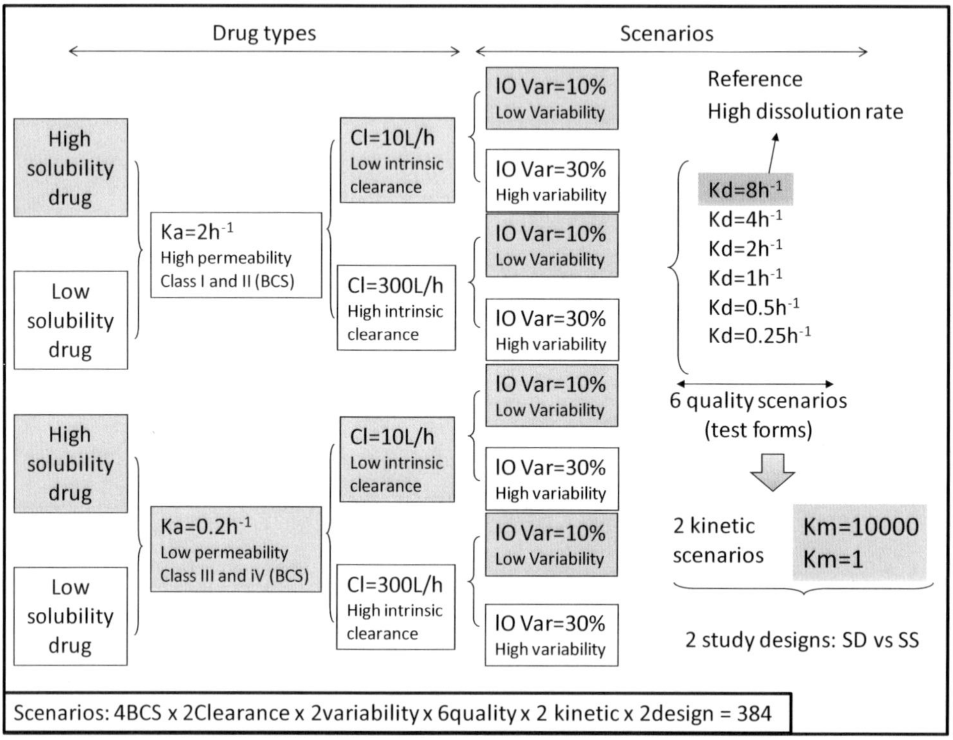

Ka: absorption rate constant; Kd: in vivo dissolution rate constant; IO Var: inter-occasion variability expressed as %; SD: single dose; SS: steady state

Fig. 1. Scenarios and drug types generation scheme for performing the BCS-based simulations. The semiphysiological models of increasing complexity were tested under these assumptions for a given set of pharmacokinetic parameters. (Fernandez-Teruel et al., 2009b, with permission from the authors).

3.1 Description of drug types, study designs and explored scenarios

The aim of these simulations was to define the most sensitive analyte, parent drug or metabolite, for in vivo bioequivalence studies. In this way, several drug types, study design and scenarios are used:

- *Drug types*: simulations can be made for different class of drugs by varying the kinetic parameter values as clearance, permeability, solubility. Simulations have been performed for:

    - Four drug classes corresponding to Biopharmaceutical Classification System by combining high and low permeability (Ka) and solubility (S).
    - High and low intrinsic hepatic clearance ($Cl_{int,0H}$).
    - High and low inter-individual variability in intrinsic hepatic clearance (this point will be explained in detail in the model).
    - High and low Michaelis-Menten constant (Km_H): differences between this parameter and liver drug concentrations defines the metabolic pathway saturation so when KmH is small (it takes values around liver drug concentrations) the metabolism becomes non-linear (saturated), but when Km_H is large (it takes values so much greater than liver drug concentrations) the metabolic system remains linear (non-saturated).
- *Study design*: it refers to perform the bioequivalence study after dosing the drug in single dose or in multiple doses. In the case of multiple doses, drug is administered every 8 hours (or a dosing scheme considered) and the bioequivalence study should be performed when steady state is reached.
- *Scenarios*: defining the most sensitive analyte to detect differences in pharmaceutical quality performance requires comparing a reference product with different test products of varying quality. This pharmaceutical quality has been defined in these simulations as similar dissolution rate constant, so good quality has been considered when reference and test products have similar dissolution rate constant value (in vivo in lumen), and six different scenarios were explored by decreasing the value of this parameter from 100% to 3% of reference value.

The combination of all these different factors and levels correspond to a total of 384 bioequivalence scenarios: 32 drug types explored at single dose and steady state, by using 6 different formulations of decreasing quality compared to the reference one. The pharmacokinetic parameters used in Table 1.

3.2 The model implementation

A detailed explanation of the mathematical description of this semi-physiological approach is presented here as well as some examples of the outcomes that could be obtained in order to illustrate how this tool can be applied to particular drugs with known pharmacokinetics parameters in order to not only select the best analyte and study design but also to explore the impact of the quality of the formulation on the outcome of the Bioequivalence trial thus allowing to risk-analysis based decisions. A basic scheme of the model is shown in Figure 2.

The model is a semi-physiological one which includes six compartments: intestinal lumen (C1), liver (C2), systemic compartment (C3), metabolite compartment (C4), solid dosage form (C5) and kidney (C6). Each compartment is represented by Cn, and the processes involved in drug pharmacokinetics are represented by En.

The solid dosage form is administered by oral route, and it dissolves in lumen (E1). Then, the dissolved fraction can be degraded in lumen (E2) or absorbed (E3), but the absorption process duration depends on the intestinal transit time. Once absorbed, the drug is partially metabolized in the liver (E4) and it reaches the systemic plasma compartment, where the drug is rapidly distributed. Finally, the drug is eliminated by both routes: hepatic metabolism (E4) and renal excretion (E5), while the metabolite formed is eliminated by renal excretion (E6).

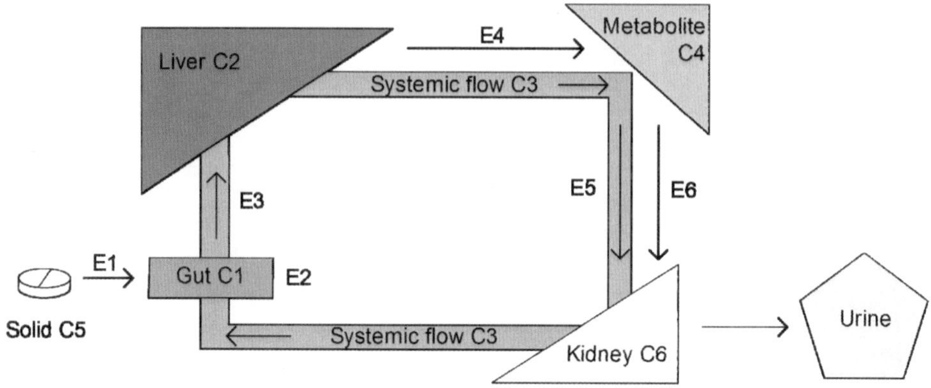

Fig. 2. The basic semi-physiological model used to perform simulations of BE trials for all BCS drugs. These model can be updated with more processes (as intestinal metabolism, or different metabolic routes).

Parameter	Value
Operative absorption time (OAT) (h)	7
Degradation rate in lumen (h−1)	0
Dissolution rate for reference form (h−1 mg−1)	4
Maximum soluble amount (mg)	10
	1000
Intrinsic absorption rate constant of the drug(h−1)	0.2
	2
Intrinsic clearance (L/h)	10
	300
Km intrinsic clearance (mg/L)	1
	10000
Renal clearance of parent drug (L/h)	0.05
Clearance of metabolite (L/h)	20
Hepatic flow (QH) (L/h)	90
Central compartment volume (L)	40
Hepatic volume (L)	1
Metabolite compartment volume (L)	40

Table 1. Pharmacokinetic parameters used in the simulations of Bioequivalence trials

1. Dissolution in lumen (E1) is considered limited by the solubility:

$$E1 = Kd \cdot A5 \cdot (S - A1) \tag{1}$$

Where E1 is the dissolution rate, A1and A5 represent the amount of drug in lumen and in solid dosage form respectively and S is the maximum soluble amount. The term Kd should not be interpreted as the first order dissolution rate as it has units of $h^{-1} \bullet mg^{-1}$. This parameterization is equivalent to this second one:

$$E1 = Kdis \cdot A5 \cdot \left(1 - \frac{A1}{S}\right) \tag{2}$$

where Kdis would represent the typical first order intrinsic dissolution rate constant and its units would be h^{-1}.

2. The drug dissolved can be degraded in lumen (E2) or absorbed (E3):

$$E2 = K\deg \cdot A1 \tag{3}$$

Where E2 is the degradation rate, Kdeg is the first order degradation rate constant and A1 the amount of drug in lumen. The luminal degradation was fixed to zero in the simulations, but both the degradation kinetic model and the value of the corresponding parameters can be easily changed to accommodate a degradation step in lumen.

Drug absorption can be implemented as a first order process:

$$E3 = (Ka \cdot A1) \cdot \alpha \tag{4}$$

Where E3 is the absorption rate, Ka the first order absorption rate constant and A1 the amount of drug in lumen and α is the operator to account for the intestinal transit time. α takes value "1" when the time is less than the intestinal transit time (or operative absorption time OAT in the model) and is set to "0" when time is higher than OAT.

After the OAT the compartment dose C5 was reset to zero, simulating the effect of the intestinal transit and therefore the drug in solid form was not accumulated in the gut for the scenarios of multiple dosage administrations.

Other absorption kinetics can be easily implemented, as an active absorption transport or an efflux mechanism, by adding the corresponding term to the equation.

For example in order to account for an efflux transport mechanism, a new compartment (C_{gut}) should be added, and the equation describing the rate of absorption would be:

$$E3 = (Ka \cdot A1)\alpha - \frac{Vm_E \cdot C_{gut}}{Km_E + C_{gut}} \tag{5}$$

where Vm_E and Km_E are the Michaelis-Menten parameters and C_{gut} is the concentration in gut wall.

3. The drug is partially metabolized in the liver (E4) after its absorption:

$$E4 = \phi H \cdot EH \cdot C2 \tag{6}$$

The hepatic metabolic rate E4 depends on the hepatic blood flow (ΦH), the drug concentration in the liver (C2) and the hepatic extraction ratio (EH).

EH is a parameter dependent on the hepatic blood flow (ΦH), and the intrinsic clearance at concentration C($Cl_{int, CH}$).

$$EH = \frac{Cl_{int,CH}}{Cl_{int,CH} + \phi H} \tag{7}$$

in which $Cl_{int, CH}$ is

$$Cl_{int,CH} = \frac{Cl_{int,0H} \cdot Km_H}{Km_H + C2} \tag{8}$$

Thus $Cl_{int, CH}$ is a non-linear function of three parameters: clearance at infinite blood flow and zero hepatic concentration ($Cl_{int, 0H}$), the Michaelis-Menten value (Km_H) and liver drug concentration (C2).

Thanks to this modeling of the hepatic metabolism a wide range of drug types and scenarios can be explored by changing the value of the intrinsic clearance or by changing the value of Km_H. that would lead to linear or non linear conditions depending on the liver concentrations compared to Km_H. In another words first-pass effect was managed as linear using a high value of Km_H and as non linear using a Km_H value around the drug concentration found in liver.

4. Drug is eliminated by hepatic metabolism (E4) and renal excretion (E5):

$$E5 = Clrenal \cdot C3 \tag{9}$$

Where E5 represents the renal excretion rate. Clrenal is the renal clearance of drug and C3 is the drug concentration in systemic compartment (so it is assumed that systemic concentration equals the concentration in kidney).

As in the other kinetic processes, different excretion mechanism or kinetics (linear-non linear) can be considered and easily implemented.

a. Gut metabolism:(Navarro-Fontestad et al., 2010) In order to describe a first pass metabolic step in small intestinal tissue, similar equations as the ones used for describing hepatic metabolism can be implemented:

$$E = \phi G \cdot EG \cdot C_{gut} \tag{10}$$

$$EG = \frac{Cl_{int,CG}}{Cl_{int,CG} + \phi G} \tag{11}$$

$$Cl_{int,CG} = \frac{Cl_{int,0G} \cdot Km_G}{Km_G + C_{gut}} \tag{12}$$

where 'G' corresponds to 'GUT' parameters, and C_{gut} is the drug concentration in gut compartment. The other parameters having the same meaning than previously explained i.e

E metabolism rate, EG extraction ratio in gut and Cl_{int} intrinsic clearance (in the examples presented in this chapter gut metabolim was not included.)

b. Several metabolic pathways:(Navarro-Fontestad et al., 2010) it can be considered that drug is metabolized by two different routes, leading to different metabolites. The way to implement this model is equivalent to the present one, but it is important to estimate in a good way the extraction ratio, because EH (or 'EG') is different for each metabolite:

$$Cl_{int,0H}^{M1} = \frac{Cl_{int,CH}^{M1} \cdot Km_H^{M1}}{Km_H^{M1} + C2} \tag{13}$$

$$Cl_{int,0H}^{M2} = \frac{Cl_{int,CH}^{M2} \cdot Km_H^{M2}}{Km_H^{M2} + C2} \tag{14}$$

$$EH^{M1} = \frac{Cl_{int,CH}^{M1}}{Cl_{int,CH}^{M1} + Cl_{int,CH}^{M2} + \phi H} \tag{15}$$

$$EH^{M2} = \frac{Cl_{int,CH}^{M2}}{Cl_{int,CH}^{M1} + Cl_{int,CH}^{M2} + \varphi H} \tag{16}$$

where M1 and M2 correspond to parameters (intrinsic clearance, Michaelis-Menten constant or extraction ratio) for metabolite 1 and 2 respectively and the other terms have been already defined.

5. Metabolite formed is eliminated by renal excretion (E6):

$$E6 = Clmet \cdot C4 \tag{17}$$

where E6 represents the excretion rate of the metabolite, Clmet is the renal clearance of metabolite and C4 is the plasma concentration of metabolite.

Metabolite elimination could be also described a sequential phase where the first generation of metabolites is also eliminated by metabolism so a second generation of metabolite(s) is formed.

Once the individual kinetic processes have been described, the next step is to build the equations describing the time-concentration profile in each compartment:

- *Intestinal lumen*: drug is dissolved in lumen (E1) and then it can be degraded in lumen (E2) or absorbed (E3).

$$\frac{dA1}{dt} = Kd \cdot A5 \cdot (S - A1) - K\deg \cdot A1 - (Ka \cdot A1) \cdot \alpha \tag{18}$$

where dA1/dt represents the drug amount change over time in lumen.

- *Liver compartment:* after absorption (E3), drug is partially metabolized in the liver (E4), and it is distributed to systemic compartment.

$$\frac{dA2}{dt} = (Ka \cdot A1) \cdot \alpha - \phi H \cdot EH \cdot C2 + \phi H \cdot C3 \tag{19}$$

where dA2/dt represents the drug amount change over time in liver and ΦH•C3 represents distribution from systemic compartment to the liver.

- *Systemic compartment*: Drug is rapidly distributed in systemic compartment, and the elimination of parent drug is renal (E5) and hepatic (E4).

$$\frac{dA3}{dt} = \phi H \cdot FH \cdot C2 - \phi H \cdot C3 - Clrenal \cdot C3 \tag{20}$$

where dA3/dt represents the drug amount change over time in plasma and ΦH•FH•C2 corresponds to the fraction of drug escaping metabolism in liver (FH=1-EH)

- *Metabolite compartment*: finally, the metabolite formed (E4) is eliminated by renal excretion (E6)

$$\frac{dA4}{dt} = \phi H \cdot EH \cdot C2 - Clmet \cdot C4 \tag{21}$$

- *Solid dosage form compartment*: Dosage solid form has to be dissolved in lumen (E1) in order to release the drug for absorption. This compartment was added at the end of model, although dissolution form solid form is the first kinetic process, because of model development reasons as in first place the behaviour of the model was checked for a drug solution and then the dissolution from different dosage forms (or formulations) was implemented.

$$\frac{dA5}{dt} = -Kd \cdot A5 \cdot (S - A1) \tag{22}$$

dA5/dt represents the dissolution from the dosage form and the other terms have been previously defined.

3.3 Description of bioequivalence studies

All bioequivalence studies were evaluated with 2400 simulations per study. The number of healthy volunteers per study was 24, and they were distributed into two groups of 12 volunteers receiving the formulations in a cross-over design. Each volunteer received an oral dose of 100mg of drug products, reference and test in solid dosage form, with a period of a washout between the doses.

A total of 17 samples of both analytes, parent drug and metabolite, were collected for each individual at 0.1, 0.2, 0.4, 0.8,1, 2, 4, 6, 8, 10, 12, 14, 16, 18, 20, 24, 48h after the administration of the drug at single dose. In the case of multiple doses, drug was administered every 8 h until steady state was attained (160 hours) and a total of 10 samples of parent drug and metabolite were collected at 0.1, 0.2, 0.4, 0.8, 1, 2, 4, 6, 8h after the administration of reference or test product.

For the bioequivalence analysis, AUC0-t (calculated by trapezoidal rule) and Cmax were considered: differences between dissolution rates from test and reference products are transformed into AUC and Cmax ratios of both analytes for each drug type and scenario:

$$AUC\ ratio=(AUC\ test)/(AUC\ reference) \tag{23}$$

$$Cmax\ ratio=(Cmax\ test)/(Cmax\ reference) \tag{24}$$

These results are then presented as bar graphs where each color and group bars represents a different analyte and scenario, respectively.

For the bioequivalence analysis, 90% confidence intervals (90%CI) were calculated for the ratio of AUC0-t and Cmax values for the test and reference dosage forms, using logarithmic transformed data. ANOVA was used to assess the formulation, subject and period effects. Finally, reference and test dosage forms were considered bioequivalent if the 90%CI ofAUC0-t and Cmax ratios lay inside 80–125% limits.

On the other hand, the percentage of studies which would conclude bioequivalence using each analyte separately (with this particular study design of 24 subjects) can be estimated and compared to the nominal percentage of failure of 5%. (Type I error: failure is considered when a bioequivalence study states bioequivalence when the products were actually non-equivalent.)

3.4 Individual parameters and data simulation

Parameter values presented in Table 1 correspond to the population parameters values. The individual parameters were generated from these population parameters using an exponential model. Moreover, an inter-occasion variability was added to the individual parameters due to reference and test products are administered in different times:

$$Pi = Pp \cdot e^{\eta IID} \cdot e^{\eta IO1 \cdot O1} \cdot e^{\eta IO2 \cdot O2} \tag{25}$$

where Pp is the population parameter; Pi is the individual parameter; ηIID is the inter-individual variability; ηIO1 is the inter-occasion variability corresponding to first administration (O1) and ηIO2 is the inter-occasion variability corresponding to second administration (O2). O1 and O2 are the identifier variables for occasion 1 and 2

In these simulations, inter-individual variability of 20% was added to all parameters, while an inter-occasion of 10% was fixed in all parameters with the exception of intrinsic hepatic clearance for which a high (30%) or low (10%) level of inter-occasion (or intra-individual) variability was considered.

Finally, the individual plasma concentrations were simulated with the structural model, the individual parameters and a proportional residual error:

$$Cp_i = f\left(Pi, Dose, Time\right) \cdot \left(1+\varepsilon\right) \tag{26}$$

where Cpi is the individual concentration and ε is the residual error.

Other different approach can be used in order to generate population and individual parameters: if it is necessary to add different effects to the parameters, as sequence, period or formulation effects, the population parameters could be generated by using a multiplicative model as:

$$Pp = Pt \cdot Eseq^{seq} \cdot Eper^{per} \cdot Eform^{form} \tag{27}$$

where Pt is the typical parameter; "Eseq", "Eper" and "Eform" are the effects corresponding to the sequence, period and formulation respectively; and "seq", "per" and "form" are the identifiers of sequence, period and formulation respectively.

All these effects can be coded in the model and fixed to zero, in order to be easily modified.

All simulations were performed in NONMEM VI. The control files were edited under Microsoft Excel worksheet and the lines containing the parameters which defined the scenarios were identified. These lines were modified to produce all the scenarios using a Visual Basic (VB) code for Excel. The code included specific commands under 6 layers which were treated as loops for: solubility, absorption, clearance of parent drug, Km, inter-occasion variability in intrinsic hepatic clearance and dissolution rate for test. The VB code created 192 scenarios which were executed under batch processing. The same control file was used for single and multiple dosage simulations as the databases defined this additional layer to simulate the 384 scenarios above declared.

The control file managed the differential equations to simulate the plasma concentrations for test and reference drugs following the conditions defined in Table 1. Additionally the control file calculated the individual AUC and Cmax which were updated for each time. Therefore, the last time contained the final value of AUC and Cmax of each volunteer. All this information was reported in tables after run execution.

The tables generated in each simulation had hundreds of thousands of records and were filtered with SPSS syntax to select the last record of each volunteer which contained the individual Cmax and AUC.

The final step was to capture the 192 filtered tables under MS Excel and calculate using VB programming the AUC and Cmax ratios and ANOVA test for each simulated trial in each scenario. The results were reported into a worksheet of the Excel file with the mean AUC and Cmax ratios for each scenario and the percentage of bioequivalence achieved between test and reference.

4. Results and discussion

Modelling and simulation approaches are useful tools to assess the potential outcome of different scenarios in bioequivalence studies. The aim of these studies was to propose a new semi-physiological model for bioequivalence trial simulations and apply it for different drug classes by considering a basic structural model that can be easily modified to accommodate other kinetic processes or non-linearities in any of them.

In order to present the results in a way easy to understand and useful for regulatory decisions or for optimization of the trial design, the AUC or Cmax ratios were plotted versus the pharmaceutical quality (decreased dissolution rate in vivo in lumen) and relative absorbed fraction. An example of this kind of plots is shown in Figures 2 and 3. These type of figures allow assessing how the decrease of biopharmaceutical quality of test product in each scenario is reflected in the average AUC or Cmax ratios of parent drug or metabolite so it is easily observed which one is more sensitive to the changes in quality.

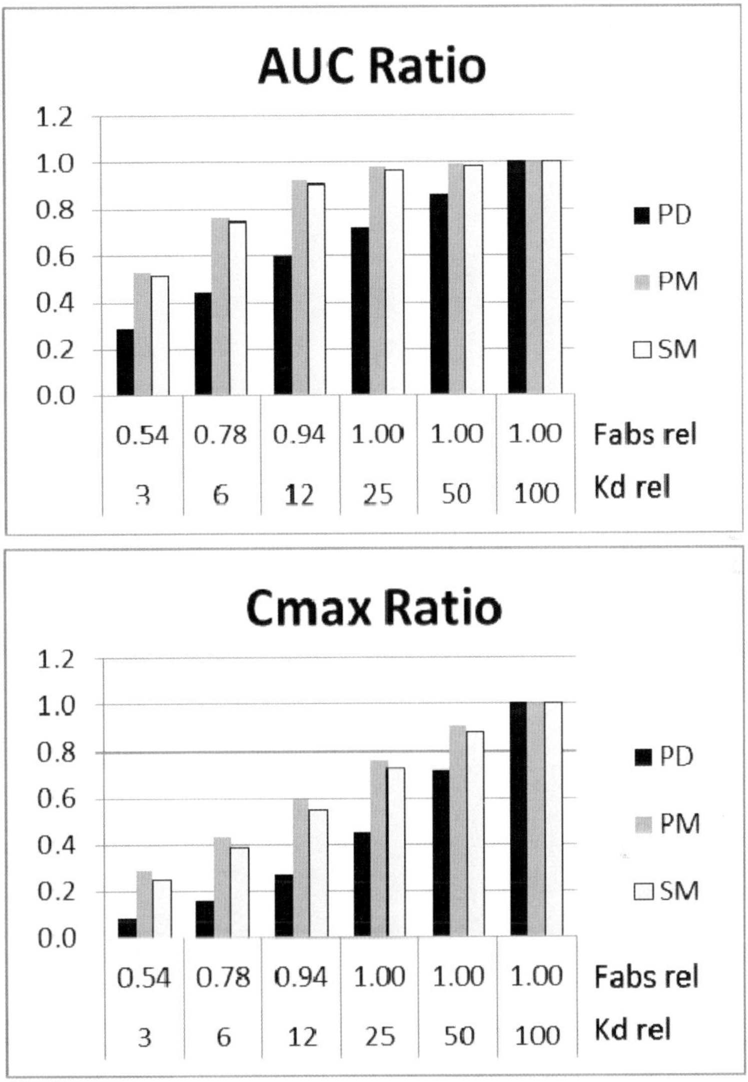

PD: Parent drug; PM: Principal metabolite; SM: Secondary metabolite

Fig. 3. True AUC and Cmax ratios (y axis) versus the relative absorbed fraction (Fabs rel) and the relative dissolution rate constant (Kd rel expressed as %) (x axis) obtained for each scenario. This model corresponds to a class III drug, administered at low dose scheme in single dose, when both metabolic pathways become saturated

In all the simulations performed with these models parent drug is the most sensitive analyte to detect the differences of in vivo dissolution. Some exceptions to this rule have been detected but it would be desirable to check these results with real examples of pharmacokinetic parameters. i.e. with known parameters from particular drugs.

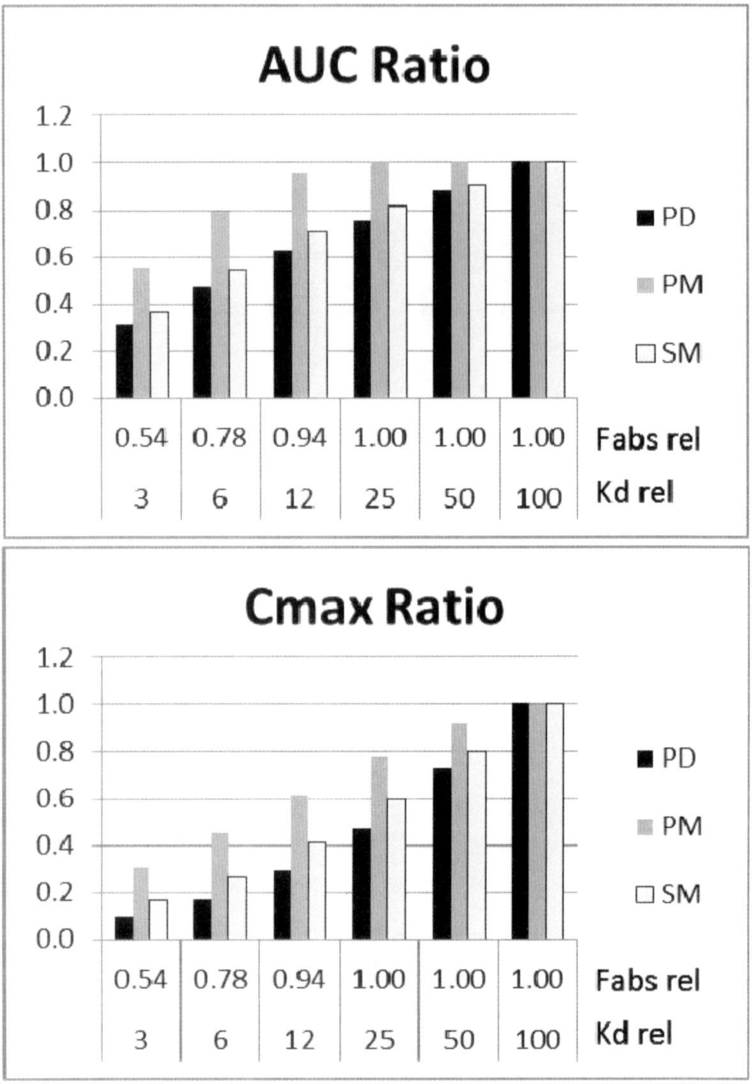

PD: Parent drug; PM: Principal metabolite; SM: Secondary metabolite

Fig. 4. True AUC and Cmax ratios (y axis) versus the relative absorbed fraction (Fabs rel) and the relative dissolution rate constant (Kd rel expressed as %) (x axis) obtained for each scenario. This model corresponds to a class III drug, administered at low dose scheme in single dose, when the principal metabolic pathway becomes saturated.

For instance when a model with pre-systemic metabolism (intestinal and hepatic) was checked (Navarro-Fontestad et al., 2010) it was concluded that, the metabolites (either principal or secondary metabolite) do not show higher sensitivity than the parent drug to detect changes in the pharmaceutical performance, even when pharmacokinetics of the parent drug is non-linear. In case of non-linear metabolism, higher parent drug sensitivity can be found, as compared with non-linear metabolites. Same conclusion was achieved in the case of linear hepatic metabolism despite of FDA requirements (Fernandez-Teruel et al., 2009c).

In the case of BCS classes with hepatic metabolism under linear conditions the differences in Cmax are detected more sensitively with the parent drug in the single dose study, except in the case of class III drugs with low intrinsic clearance (Fernandez-Teruel et al., 2009c)

In the particular examples represented in Figures 3 and 4 where the participation of an efflux transporter at intestinal level has been included, the parent drug is the most sensitive analyte to detect the lack of pharmaceutical quality in the problem formulation versus the reference one. The presence of an efflux carrier in the structural part o of the model even if it is non-saturated does not change the outcome in relation to previous scenarios.

Regarding the study design (single dose versus steady state) this aspect has been investigated in a model with hepatic metabolism under linear or non linear conditions and considering that a low percent of the dose is eliminated by renal clearance. With these assumptions interestingly, for class III drugs with non-linear pharmacokinetics the steady state design is necessary in addition to the single dose study, as required by EMEA and in contrast to FDA requirements, to compare with the highest sensitivity the Cmax of the **parent drug** not only in case of low intrinsic clearance but also in case of high intrinsic clearance and a small worsening of the in vivo dissolution (relative kd= 0.5). In the case of AUC (class III drugs) the steady state design is more sensitive in case of drugs with low intrinsic clearance but as sensitive as the single dose study when the intrinsic clearance is high (Fernandez-Teruel et al., 2009a)

A particular concern about this result is that following the Biopharmaceutic and Drug Disposition Classification System, BDDCS (Benet et al., 2008; Chen et al., 2010; Wu & Benet, 2005) it would be arguably that such a drug with high solubility, low permeability and highly metabolized (even if at slow rate) is an exception or does not exists. Further simulations with a higher renal clearance of parent drug to allow for a lower percent of the dose being metabolized should be done to clarify if the behavior is the same.

5. Conclusions

A simulation model of Bioequivalence trials have been developed taking into account the biopharmaceutical properties that determine rate and extent of absorption i.e. permeability, solubility and dissolution rate in relation with the human intestinal transit time. This BCS approximation have not been included in the previous simulation exercises found in the literature.

This work illustrates a methodology that could be implemented by the applicant of a marketing authorization of a generic product in order to justify the selected study design and analyte. Once the pharmacokinetic behaviour of the drug under investigation in known it is possible to identify the sensitivity of the different active species in the different study designs. Some structural models have been explored but as it has been explained the model could be adapted to incorporate other kinetic processes and non linear components on them as well as it could be possible to perform the simulations in saturating or non saturating conditions for each particular non linear step.

The final objective would be to develop customized models for each particular drug in order to justify the selection of the bioequivalence study design and analyte or, when the most sensitive scenario cannot be performed due to analytical or tolerability/safety limitations, to estimate the loss of sensitivity of an alternative design that has to be used pragmatically. In summary, virtual bioequivalence studies may serve as a tool to guide regulatory decisions both for sponsors and Regulatory Agencies.

6. Acknowledgements

This work is part of work-package nº 2 of BIOSIM project, funded by EU (NOE LSMB-CT-005137). The work has received funds also from Plan Nacional de I+D+I del Ministerio de Ciencia e Innovación de España (SAF2009-12768) , Consolider Ingenio 2010, CSD2007–00063 (Fun-C-Food) and from Programa alfa iii of the EC: Red Biofarma Project: DCI-ALA/19.09.01/10/21526/245-297.

7. References

Amidon, G. L., et al. (1995). A theoretical basis for a biopharmaceutic drug classification: the correlation of in vitro drug product dissolution and in vivo bioavailability. *Pharm Res*, Vol.12, No.3, (Mar-1995), pp. (413-420), ISSN 0724-8741

Benet, L. Z., et al. (2008). The use of BDDCS in classifying the permeability of marketed drugs. *Pharm Res*, Vol.25, No.3, (Mar-2008), pp. (483-488), ISSN 0724-8741

Blume, H. H. & Midha, K. K. (1993). Bio-International 92, conference on bioavailability, bioequivalence, and pharmacokinetic studies. *J Pharm Sci*, Vol.82, No.11, (Nov-1993), pp. (1186-1189), ISSN 0022-3549

Braddy, A. C. & Jackson, A. J. (2010). Role of metabolites for drugs that undergo nonlinear first-pass effect: impact on bioequivalency assessment using single-dose simulations. *J Pharm Sci*, Vol.99, No.1, (Jan-2010), pp. (515-523), ISSN 1520-6017

Chen, M. L., et al. (2010). The BCS, BDDCS, and regulatory guidances. *Pharm Res*, Vol.28, No.7, (Jul-2010), pp. (1774-1778), ISSN 1573-904X

Chen, M. L. & Jackson, A. J. (1991). The role of metabolites in bioequivalency assessment. I. Linear pharmacokinetics without first-pass effect. *Pharm Res*, Vol.8, No.1, (Jan-1991), pp. (25-32), ISSN 0724-8741

Chen, M. L. & Jackson, A. J. (1995). The role of metabolites in bioequivalency assessment. II. Drugs with linear pharmacokinetics and first-pass effect. *Pharm Res*, Vol.12, No.5, (May-1995), pp. (700-708), ISSN 0724-8741

el-Tahtawy, A. A., et al. (1994). Comparison of single and multiple dose pharmacokinetics using clinical bioequivalence data and Monte Carlo simulations. *Pharm Res*, Vol.11, No.9, (Sep-1994), pp. (1330-1336), ISSN 0724-8741

el-Tahtawy, A. A., et al. (1995). Evaluation of bioequivalence of highly variable drugs using Monte Carlo simulations. I. Estimation of rate of absorption for single and multiple dose trials using Cmax. *Pharm Res*, Vol.12, No.11, (Nov-1995), pp. (1634-1641), ISSN 0724-8741 el-Tahtawy, A. A., et al. (1998). Evaluation of bioequivalence of highly variable drugs using clinical trial simulations. II: Comparison of single and multiple-dose trials using AUC and Cmax. *Pharm Res*, Vol.15, No.1, (Jan-1998), pp. (98-104), ISSN 0724-8741

EMA, 2010. Guideline on the investigation of bioequivalence Committee for Medicinal Products for Human Use (CHMP)

EMEA, 2001. CPMP/EWP/QWP/1401/98 Note For Guidance On Investigation Of Bioavailability & Bioequivalence. Committee for Medicinal Products for Human Use (CHMP)

FDA, 2000. Waiver of In Vivo Bioavailability and Bioequivalence Studies for Immediate Release Solid Oral Dosage Forms Based on a Biopharmaceutics Classification System.

FDA, 2002. Guidance for Industry Bioavailability and Bioequivalence Studies for Orally Administered Drug Products-General Considerations.

Fernandez-Teruel, C., et al. (2009a). Computer simulations of bioequivalence trials: selection of design and analyte in BCS drugs with first-pass hepatic metabolism: Part II. Non-linear kinetics. *Eur J Pharm Sci*, Vol.36, No.1, (Jan 31-2009a), pp. (147-156), ISSN 1879-0720

Fernandez-Teruel, C., et al. (2009b).6 Virtual Bioequivalence trials as a tool for regulatory decisions., In:*Clustering Algorithms and Mathematical Modeling*, Wilson, C.L. (Ed.), pp. (1-14), Nova Science Publishers, Inc.,

Fernandez-Teruel, C., et al. (2009c). Computer simulations of bioequivalence trials: selection of design and analyte in BCS drugs with first-pass hepatic metabolism: linear kinetics (I). *Eur J Pharm Sci*, Vol.36, No.1, (Jan 31-2009c), pp. (137-146), ISSN 1879-0720

Jackson, A. J. (1987). Prediction of steady-state bioequivalence relationships using single dose data I-linear kinetics. *Biopharm Drug Dispos*, Vol.8, No.5, (Sep-Oct-1987), pp. (483-496), ISSN 0142-2782

Jackson, A. J. (1989). Prediction of steady state bioequivalence relationships using single dose data II-nonlinear kinetics. *Biopharm Drug Dispos*, Vol.10, No.5, (Sep-Oct-1989), pp. (489-503), ISSN 0142-2782

Jackson, A. J. (2000). The role of metabolites in bioequivalency assessment. III. Highly variable drugs with linear kinetics and first-pass effect. *Pharm Res*, Vol.17, No.11, (Nov-2000), pp. (1432-1436), ISSN 0724-8741

Kuentz, M. (2008). Drug absorption modeling as a tool to define the strategy in clinical formulation development. *AAPS J*, Vol.10, No.3, (Sep-2008), pp. (473-479), ISSN 1550-7416

Navarro-Fontestad, C., et al. (2010). Computer simulations for bioequivalence trials: selection of analyte in BCS drugs with first-pass metabolism and two metabolic pathways. *Eur J Pharm Sci*, Vol.41, No.5, (Dec 23-2010), pp. (716-728), ISSN 1879-0720

Rosenbaum, S. E. (1998). Effects of variability in hepatic clearance on the bioequivalence parameters of a drug and its metabolite: simulations using a pharmacostatistical model. *Pharm Acta Helv*, Vol.73, No.3, (Aug-1998), pp. (135-144), ISSN 0031-6865

Rosenbaum, S. E. & Lam, J. (1997). Bioequivalence Parameters of Parent Drug and Its First-Pass Metabolite: Comparative Sensitivity to Sources of Pharmacokinetic Variability. *Drug Development and Industrial Pharmacy*, Vol.23, No.3, 1997), pp. (337-344)

Tucker, G.T., et al. (1993).Bioequivalence—a measure of therapeutic equivalence?, In:*Bio-International: Bioavailability, Bioequivalence and Pharmacokinetics,* Midha, K.K., Blume, H.H. (Eds.), pp. (35-43), Medpharm Scientific Publishers, Stuttgart

Wu, C. Y. & Benet, L. Z. (2005). Predicting drug disposition via application of BCS: transport/absorption/ elimination interplay and development of a biopharmaceutics drug disposition classification system. *Pharm Res,* Vol.22, No.1, (Jan-2005), pp. (11-23), ISSN 0724-8741

Zha, J. & Endrenyi, L. (1997). Variation of the peak concentration following single and repeated drug administrations in investigations of bioavailability and bioequivalence. *J Biopharm Stat,* Vol.7, No.1, (Mar-1997), pp. (191-204), ISSN 1054-3406

5

Pharmacogenomics Dictate Pharmacokinetics: Polymorphisms in Drug-Metabolizing Enzymes and Drug-Transporters

Debasis Mondal*, Samantha L. Gerlach,
Amrita Datta, Geetika Chakravarty and Asim B. Abdel-Mageed
Tulane University School of Medicine
Department of Pharmacology, New Orleans, LA
USA

1. Introduction

1.1 Drug discovery and clinical evaluation

The discovery of a drug is focused on the goal of producing a useful therapeutic agent through a process utilizing the multiple skills and expertise of basic scientists, pharmaceutical chemists, toxicologists, clinical investigators, governmental regulators and clinicians (Mager DE, 2009; Michel MC, 2009; Nagase H, 2011). Drug development and its clinical evaluation is thus a very lengthy and expensive endeavor. One has to first come up with a novel mechanism, identifying relevant target(s) and pathway(s) towards formulation of a new chemical entity (NCE) to treat a disease. Both *in vitro* and *in vivo* models that are relevant to the disease form the basis of preclinical testing and identification of lead compounds, and the development of an Investigational New Drug (IND), and ultimately the entry of only a select few into human clinical trials. Therefore, initial studies in drug developments involve the synthesis and extraction of new compounds, their biological screening and pharmacological testing, followed by small animal model testing of toxicology and safety profiles. These early pharmacokinetic (PK) measurements guide researchers to formulate effective pharmaceutical dosage, *in vivo* stability, elimination and eventually the therapeutic index of lead compound(s). In pre-clinical studies, a favorable PK outcome can lead to the FDA approval for the phase-I, -II and -III clinical evaluation process (Fasolo A, 2009). However, even after clinical approval, drugs have to be continuously monitored towards improvements in their bioavailability, therapeutic, and toxicologic differences especially in a large patient population with patient-specific variability. For example, the azathioprine and mercaptopurine intolerance in patients were found to be linked to the deficiency of a metabolic enzyme, thiopurine S-methyltransferase, and formed the genetic basis for a molecular diagnostic test to designate specific population (Yates CR, et al. 1997). Thus, before testing in humans can start, a significant body of pre-clinical data on PK must be compiled and an appropriate dose should be established to ensure human safety. Toxicology, pharmacology and pharmaceutical sciences all represent the core of pre-

* Corresponding Author

clinical drug development which is repeatedly addressed in the clinical trials and post-clinical approval phases. Each phase of drug development has to be designed to accrue the necessary information to assess the probability of success of an NCE which remains the fundamental pathway to successful clinical approval (DiazGranados N, 2008). The continually expanding knowledge base on the development of new agents and novel delivery and formulation strategies are enabling a favorable *in vivo* PK and a more efficacious drug discovery process. Advances in the understanding of multiple factors that regulate drug disposition and response in individuals are elucidating the molecular basis of ethnic and inter-individual variability in drug action (Xie HG, et al. 2001; Soldin OP, et al. 2009). Furthermore, due to their *in vivo* safety and efficacy profiles, a number of natural products have recently entered clinical trials as potent anti-inflammatory agents (Basnet P, 2011; Abdel-Tawab M, 2011), however, their role in drug-drug interaction issues is not being addressed in specific patient populations.

1.2 Importance of preclinical *in vivo* models

The use of *in vivo* models to obtain vast quantities of PK/PD data is a well-established pre-clinical approach. Before any clinical testing can be initiated in humans, it is important to compare the PK and PD properties of candidate molecules; model potential relationships among dose, concentration, efficacy, and/or toxicity in appropriate animal model systems (Sausville EA, 2006; Kennedy AJ, 2010; Miyagawa F, 2010). For a more thorough and comprehensive understanding of the experimental approaches in mouse models, please refer to 'The handbook of experimental animals' by Elsevier Academic Press (Hans H, 2004). Numerous inbred mouse models are available to delineate the efficacy of drugs in specific disease models, such as the WKY and SHR strains which are optimal for studying antihypertensive and antidiabetic agents (Kennedy AJ, 2010) and the leptin knockout mice (ob/ob) as models for obesity and insulin resistance (Lijnen HR. 2011). Several disease specific knockout and transgenic mouse models are also used, for instance, to study cardiovascular drugs (Avila MD, 2011; Xiangdong L, 2011; Zaragoza C, 2011) and autoimmune disease targeting agents (Gulinello M, 2011; Schroeder MA, 2011). Immunodeficient animals, such as nude, SCID and SCID/NOD tumor xenograft mouse models, are also important for testing and development of new chemotherapeutic drugs (Sausville EA, 2006; Khan N, 2009; Umar A, 2010; Baiocchi M, 2010). The utility of these animal models to study cancer-initiating cells which are responsible for tumor recurrence and resistance, is showing great promise towards development of more potent anti-cancer agents (Wee B, 2011).

Studies completed in laboratory animals give useful indications for drug development, and many lead compounds that show compromised potency *in vitro* can turn out to be more effective *in vivo* because of their favorable pharmacokinetics, e.g. greater absorption, better distribution and stability, etc. Studies are first initiated in small animal models, e.g. mouse, rats, rabbits, to test for acute, sub-chronic and then chronic toxicity. In acute toxicity tests, one administration of the drug or chemical is given to each animal in order to generate a safe and effective dose–response curve. Appropriate pharmacological testing in disease models are carried out to determine 50% effective dose (ED_{50}). For some anti-tumor and anti-viral agents, even IC_{90} (90% inhibitory concentration) is incorporated in these initial studies in order to demonstrate the potency (Cummins CL, et al, 2003). Following acute administration, analytical methods are developed for determination of absorption, distribution, metabolism and excretion (ADME) of the drug. The subchronic toxicity tests usually involve animals exposed to the drug for 60–90 days duration. Both multiple administrations and/or continuous exposure via food or water to one dose level of a chemical per animal, is carried out to measure drug accumulation and possible toxicities. Depending on the animal species being used, the chronic toxicity tests usually takes 2 to 5 years to complete and may include both multiple administrations per day or continuous exposure measures via subcutaneous or intramuscular depot. Indeed, alterations in drug elimination rates and toxic outcomes are particularly important when drugs are given repeatedly. Certain therapeutic agents tend to accumulate toxic concentrations in tissues and organs when eliminated slowly or their metabolism is compromised, drug accumulation may occur with toxic concentrations reached in important tissues and organs. Alternately, faster elimination than expected due to increased breakdown of the agent may cause sub therapeutic concentrations to be reached, thus enabling the rapid selection of drug resistance, often observed with antibiotics and antimicrobials. Therefore, a commonly employed formula for ascertaining therapeutic dose levels in both pre-clinical and clinical models is, "*Maintenance dose = Dosing amount X Dosing interval*". Both *in vitro* and *in vivo* uptake experiments in rats have been able to predict the hepatic and renal clearance of a number of drugs, and were able to delineate drugs which are substrates for drug-metabolizing enzymes and drug-transporters (Watanabe T, et al. 2009). Several transgenic and knockout mouse models have also been used to understand the role of drug-metabolizing enzymes and drug-transporters, and in the discovery of novel inhibitors of these factors in order to increase drug efficacy *in vivo* (Salphati L. et al., 1998; Shitara Y. et al., 2002; van Waterschoot RA, 2011). Because the drug levels in plasma or tissues are often more predictive of a safe dose which can be extrapolated to humans, preclinical toxicology in animals underscores the importance of PK studies. The choice of endpoints and correct surrogate markers are very important and careful consideration must be given to the definition of therapeutic efficacy. Safety is the most important concern in clinical trials and then the emphasis is directed towards drug efficacy. In addition to examining safety and effectiveness, studies in animal models also emphasize critical aspects of drug kinetics, including proper dose determination, biotransformation, drug binding to plasma proteins, induction or inhibition of enzymes and potential interaction with other drugs (Evans W, et al. 1989; Evans W, et al. 1992). The choice of representative controls is also an essential component in PK studies in both preclinical and clinical settings. Indeed, most concurrently controlled trials are double-blind and randomized studies where both objective evidence and subjective complaints are taken into account towards a clearer representation of therapeutic value of the drugs being tested for a specific disease indication.

2. Pharmacokinetics

Cell membranes are biologic barriers that selectively inhibit passage of drug molecules. Drugs may cross cell membranes by passive diffusion, facilitated passive diffusion, active transport, or pinocytosis. Thus, drug PK is critically affected by body mass, obesity as well as age and health status of the subject. Since numerous currently used drugs may manifest toxic effects and may have long-term teratogenic effects, therapeutic drug monitoring in children has become an essential component of clinical testing as emphasized by pediatric pharmacokinetics (McLeod HL, et al. 1992). In general, drug elimination may occur through biotransformation and by the passage of molecules from the blood to the outside of the body through urines, bile or other routes. Therefore, the PK study relies on measurements of levels of the test drug in blood and urine at various times after administration. If a drug is ineffective at the given dose, the above measurements resolve issues of efficacy vs. poor absorption or rapid elimination. All the organs except the lungs are in parallel because they are perfused by a fraction of the whole blood in each passage. Drug levels in blood achieve equilibrium with drug entry into subvascular tissues and drug levels which are excreted or metabolized. PK studies investigate the parameters which regulate therapeutic concentrations of drugs and/or its metabolites, and their movement in different parts of the body (Ritschel WA & Kearns GL. 1999). Initial studies of *in vivo* PK measurements required complex mathematical modeling of absorption (A) and distribution (D). Absorption indicates the passage of drug molecules from the administration site to the blood, and distribution indicates the passage of drug molecules from blood to the tissues. As the roles of liver and kidney in drug disposition become clearer, essential components, such as the rate of drug metabolism (M) and drug excretion (E) from the body are increasingly examined. The choice of best route of drug administration establishes the best dose regimen and determines whether dose individualization would be necessary based on patient and disease characteristics, e.g. drug elimination rates (Ritschel WA & Kearns GL. 1999). Recent findings clearly indicate that these two later parameters in ADME are also critically regulated by intracellular drug metabolizing enzymes and membrane bound drug-transporters (Wikinski, S. 2005). Flexibility in the design of studies is very desirable at this stage. Furthermore, extremely slow metabolism of certain drugs may result in their accumulation and toxicity, thus mandating changes in subsequent doses. All drugs are eventually excreted from the body, and many require bio-activation to form the active compound [Figure-1].

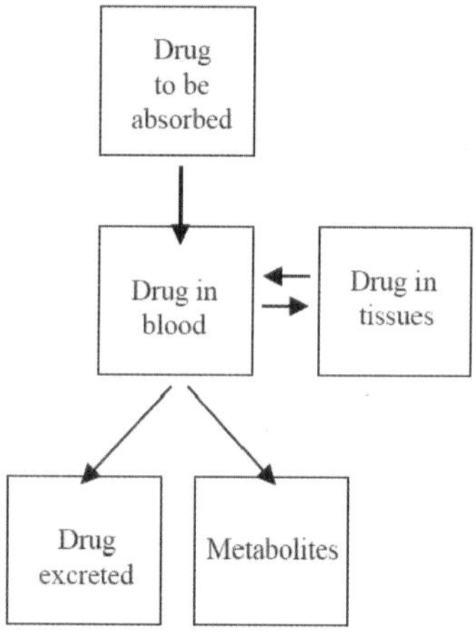

Fig. 1. *Drug absorption and disposition.* A graphic representation of drug disposition is shown where drug entry first occurs in the blood circulation and then drugs pass through tissues and organs. Blocks designate the equilibrium seen between drug absorption, distribution, metabolism and elimination (ADME) parameters.

2.1 Routes of administration

To gain a proper understanding of drug PK, first of all, it is essential to understand, compare and contrast different routes of drug administration, and acknowledge their advantages and disadvantages. Drug absorption is determined by the drug's physicochemical properties, formulation and route of administration. Depending on the preclinical findings on ADME in animal models, administration could be either Enteral (oral, buccal/sublingual) or Parenteral [subcutaneous (SC), intramuscular (IM) or intravenous (IV)] (Evans W, et al. 1992; Ritschel WA. 1999; Hans H. 2004). Dosage forms (e.g., tablets, capsules, solutions) are formulated to be given by various routes. Regardless of the route of administration, drugs must be in solution to be absorbed. Unless given IV, a drug must cross several semipermeable cell membranes before it reaches the systemic circulation. Oral drug delivery is highly advantageous since it is convenient and cheap and patient compliance is good. Different formulations such as fast release tablets, capsules, enteric coated pills, suspensions and mixtures can be used to enhance drug uptake by intestinal epithelial lining and to facilitate drug stability in the stomach and small intestine. However, there are several disadvantages related to oral delivery, especially its inefficiency in reaching therapeutic plasma levels. Low oral bioavailability can be due to decreased stability and solubility of the drug in the gastrointestinal (GI) tract. In addition, the GI lining expresses a number of Cytochrome P450 (CYP450) enzymes and drug-efflux transporters which can suppress drug uptake and enhance metabolism.

Presystemic metabolism is a significant challenge even after intestinal uptake due to the transport of drugs to the liver via the hepatic portal vein. Examples of drugs that experience a significant 'first-pass effect' are imipramine, morphine, propranolol, buprenorphine, diazepam, midazolam, demerol, cimetidine, and lidocaine. The first pass effect and liver metabolism can be bypassed via buccal or sublingual administration which significantly increases bioavailability (Brockmeier D. 1988; Haber PS, 1996; Brown AS, 1998). In recent years, the first pass effect has also been exploited in converting an inactive form of a drug (e.g. 3-methylmorphine or Codeine) to the pharmacologically active form (morphine) by first pass metabolism (KuKanich B. 2010; Nieminen TH, 2010). However, under most circumstances, the oral drug delivery approach is inconvenient and only small doses can be accommodated. Hence, several strategies to directly infuse drugs, so that rapid plasma levels can be achieved, are SC, IM and IV delivery methods. One advantage of SC delivery is that drugs can be self-administered. Although absorption is slow via this route, it can be improved by local massage or heat. Unfortunately, this method can be painful and irritant drugs can cause local tissue damage. In contrast, IM injections can accomodate a larger volume of drug delivery, and now a number of drugs are using IM strategies to facilitate depot formation for sustained release effects. The trained personnel are required for IM injections, however, the site of injection can significantly influence systemic absorption of the drug. A quicker response is possible with IV drug delivery and large doses may be given into a peripheral vein over 1 to 2 minutes or longer by infusion. In most of the pre-clinical PK studies, this is the route of choice for drug infusion and monitoring of toxicity, especially of chemotherapeutic agents (Wong J, 2008; Serwer LP, 2011). The IV method however requires trained personnel to maintain sterility, and pyrogen testing, while the cost of preparation, transport and storage of such preparations can be expensive.

2.2 Fick's law of diffusion

Drugs diffuse across a cell membrane from a region of high concentration to one of low concentration. Diffusion rate is directly proportional to the gradient but also depends on the molecule's lipid solubility, size, degree of ionization, and the area of absorptive surface. Lipid-soluble drugs diffuse most rapidly and small molecules tend to penetrate membranes more rapidly than larger ones. Drug effectiveness using any of the above delivery approaches ultimately requires transport across membrane barriers. In addition, membrane transporters play active roles in both drug influx and efflux and therapeutic levels in sequestered tissues. Oral drugs need efficient transport across intestinal epithelial lining and subsequently through the endothelial lining of blood capillaries. Drugs diffuse across a membrane in an attempt to equalize the drug concentration on both sides of the membrane. Fick's law was the driving force that represented a tendency for molecules to move from levels of higher concentration to lower concentration in accordance with random molecular motion. This has been attributed to the fact that the rate of diffusion across a membrane is directly proportional to the concentration gradient of a substance on either side of the membrane and is inversely related to the thickness of the membrane. Therefore, the rate of drug transport across the membrane has been described by the Fick's law of diffusion [Figure-2].

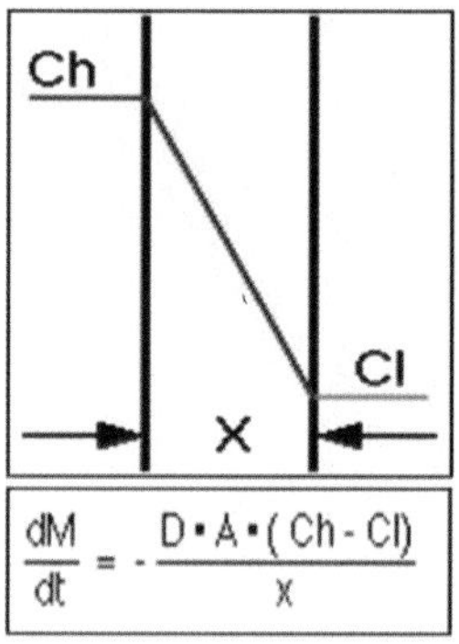

Fig. 2. *Fick's law of diffusion.* Molecules tend to move from a higher concentration to a lower concentration where the rate of diffusion across a membrane is directly proportional to the concentration gradient and inversely related to the thickness of the membrane. Rate of movement of Molecules per unit time = (Area)x(Permeability coefficient)x(Ch - Cl)/ Thickness.

Previously, most drugs were thought to cross biologic membranes by passive diffusion which occurs when the drug concentration on one side of the membrane is higher than on the other side. Therefore, in the past, the absorption principles for a drug molecule were primarily dependent on its aqueous diffusion, especially within large aqueous components (e.g. interstitial space, intracellular cytosol). This view of drug movement is dictated by their ability to transport drugs across epithelial and endothelial membrane tight junctions (Matsuhisa K, 2009; Furuse M. 2010). Both physiological conditions and disease status, especially inflammatory cytokines, are known to regulate drug transport from the blood to the tissues via these tight junctions (Tarbell JM. 2010; Srinivas SP. 2011). This drug absorption into tissues is also facilitated via transport through aqueous pores which allows diffusion of molecules with molecular weights up to 30 kDa. Lipid diffusibility of drugs is also an essential component in a drug's ability to be transported from one compartment to another since many lipid barriers separate tissue compartments and drug partition coefficients between aqueous and lipid environments. In addition, the ionization states of drugs have been studied to determine their PK efficacy and bioavailability. However, rapid dissolution and absorption is not always the objective. Sometimes a slower release is required, e.g. for Tolbutamide (used to lower blood sugar): a more sustained release is better, causing a more gradual reduction in blood sugar (Tassaneeyakul W, 1992; Lee CR,

2003). In addition, as mentioned earlier, the rate at which a drug dissolves is also dependent on its solubility and acid-base dissociation constants, according to the 'Henderson Hasselbalch equation, e.g. free acid or base forms of Penicillin achieve different serum levels. Also, absorption of antimicrobials can be extended by using IM injection of their less insoluble salt forms (e.g. Penicillin G). For other drugs, suspensions or solutions in nonaqueous vehicles (e.g., crystalline suspensions for insulin) are designed to delay absorption. Most drugs are weak organic acids or bases, existing in un-ionized and ionized forms in an aqueous environment. The un-ionized form is usually lipid soluble (lipophilic) and diffuses readily across cell membranes. The ionized form has low lipid solubility (hydrophilic) and high electrical resistance and thus cannot penetrate cell membranes easily. The proportion of the un-ionized form present (and thus the drug's ability to cross a membrane) is determined by the pH and the drug's pK_a (acid dissociation constant). However, whether a drug is acidic or basic, most absorption occurs in the small intestine because the surface area is larger and membranes are more permeable.

Although the surface area of the epithelial lining allows for high rate of absorption, the endothelial lining of blood vessels is relatively non-porous. For numerous diseases of the central nervous system (CNS), e.g. gliomas, AIDS dementia, epilepsy, etc., drug absorption into the brain has been a significant problem (Aragon-Ching JB, 2007; Reichel A. 2009). This is especially due to the presence of blood-brain barrier (BBB) and blood-cerebrospinal fluid (CSF) barrier (Mehdipour AR, 2009; Johanson CE, 2011). The membranes between the blood and brain have effectively no pores and prevent many polar materials (often toxic materials) from entering the brain. However, smaller lipid materials or lipid soluble materials, such as diethyl ether, halothane, can easily enter the brain. Several *in vitro* models have been developed to overcome drug inefficacies in the brain (Wilhelm I, 2011; Tóth A, 2011; Potschka H. 2010). The absorption of a drug and/or its metabolites into the kidney is also very crucial in dictating drug elimination and in suppressing accumulation of toxic levels of the drug. This is especially important since the membranes of the renal tubules and renal glomerulus are quite porous allowing non-polar and polar molecules (~ M.W. 70 kDa) to pass through and allows for rapid excretion of polar substances (drug and waste compounds) (Verbeeck RK, 2009; Hartmann B, 2010). However, lipophilic compounds or non-ionized species are reabsorbed dependent on the pH and pKa of the drug which dictates the elimination rate and is measured in patients via creatinine clearance rates (CCR) (Kooman JP. 2009; Bogard KN, 2011; Fesler P, 2011), a parameter which will be emphasized later in this chapter in relation to drug-transporter expression in the liver and the kidney.

In contrast to passive diffusion, active transport is selective, requires energy expenditure and may involve transport against a concentration gradient. Active transport seems to be limited to drugs structurally similar to endogenous substances (e.g. ions, vitamins, sugars, amino acids). These drugs are usually absorbed from specific sites in the small intestine. As will be discussed in more detail in this chapter, we have discovered that complex mathematical modeling is necessary to determine the volume of distribution and therapeutic window for drug action. Furthermore, we now appreciate the role of special carriers present on lipid membranes that regulate drug transport into various compartments.

2.3 Compartmental models and important PK parameters

Compartmental analysis uses kinetic models to describe and predict the concentration-time curve. PK compartmental models are often similar to kinetic models used in other scientific disciplines such as chemical kinetics and thermodynamics. At different times after drug administration, much information can be obtained on the passage of drug molecules between blood and tissues and on the rate of drug elimination in the urine or feces by measuring the concentrations of drugs in different body fluids or within tissues [Figure-3]. The advantage of compartmental over some non-compartmental analyses is the ability to predict the concentration at any time post drug infusion; however, the disadvantage of this complex system is the difficulty in developing the proper model and validating the proper rate constants for the ADME principles.

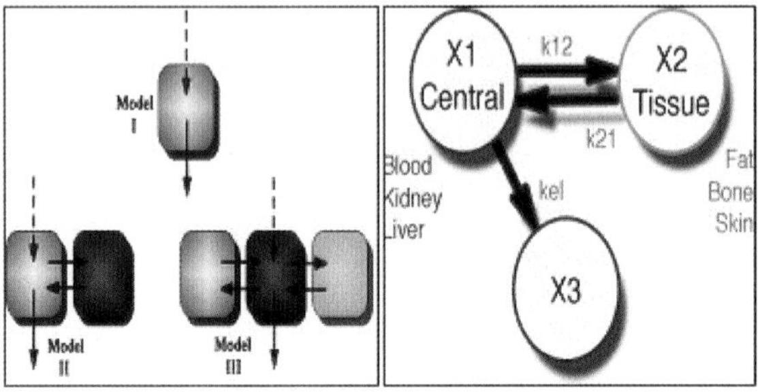

Fig. 3. *Compartment models used in drug disposition measurements.* The simplest PK compartmental model (Model-I) is the one-compartmental PK model with IV bolus administration and first-order elimination. In multicompartmental modeling, the rate constants for drug transport to-and-from the central reservoir (blood) to tissues such as fat, bone or skin (k_{12} and k_{21}) and the rate of elimination by the kidney and liver (k_{el}), are needed to be determined.

The planning, execution and analysis of the results of a PK study depends closely on the purpose of the experiment. For example some studies may be planned to get accurate estimates of drug absorption or to obtain information on the drug elimination kinetics (Evans W, et al. 1989; Evans W, et al. 1992; Ritschel WA & Kearns GL. 1999). Consequently the experimental protocols may vary considerably. Hence, to effectively plan a pharmacokinetic experiment, the following conditions should be well defined: the route of drug administration, dose regimen, which tissues to sample, sample times, analytical method, and the animal species. In clinical settings, the inclusion and exclusion criteria of subjects for observation and the population kinetics of the drug are taken into account.

Mathematical models are essential tools in PK measurements because these models aid in defining a set of parameters that describe drug disposition and the relationship of underlying biological processes. In model building, the linear compartmental models, the clearance models, and the multiexponential functions, constitute various passages of drugs through different compartments. Starting from a simple description of the drug profile in the plasma, the experimenter may gain better insight and reasonable approximations of the biological and physiological aspect of the system. The analysis of the assumptions, approximations of the model, and a comparison of the performance of different models may thus be very useful in identifying new aspects of the system and to design experiments able to deliver continuous and increasingly relevant knowledge. This chapter will only touch briefly on each of these important PK parameters to familiarize the reader with the concepts, but for detailed descriptions of these mathematical models the reader is requested to consult the following more comprehensive reviews on PK (Evans W, et al. 1992; Ritschel WA & Kearns GL. 1999).

During mathematical calculations estimate drug disposition rates, to compartmental models have been beneficial tools to understand the effects of the overall system under study. Both single and multicompartmental modeling is needed to obtain accurate measures of drug levels in tissues and possible efficacies at site of action. This is carried out following oral or IV infusion of the drug and sampling of plasma concentrations at different time points. The following parameters are determined simultaneously which include peak plasma concentrations (C_{max}), peak time to attain C_{max} (T_{max}), half-life ($t_{1/2}$), and area under the plasma concentration curve (AUC). It should be noted that each parameter of this model which deals with the rate constants, do not represent a single physical variable, but a set of variables which may not be distinguished at a given time point. The kinetic profile of a single drug in the plasma may be well summarized by the above parameters, and is depicted in the plasma concentration vs. time curves [Figure-4].

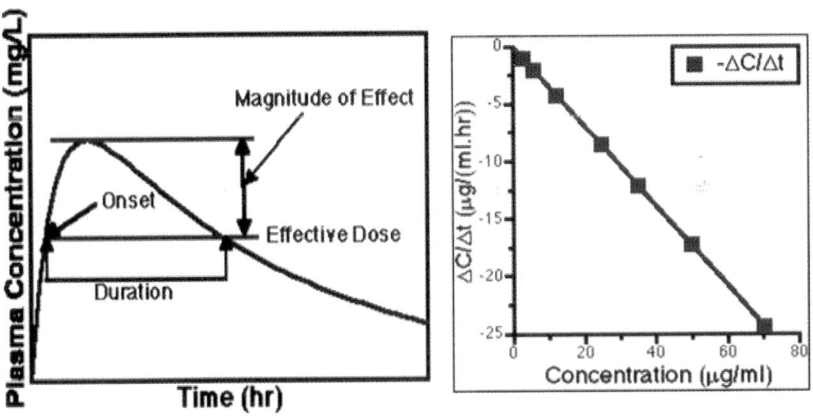

Fig. 4. *The plasma concentration vs. time curve.* The curve on the left illustrates plasma concentration of the drug at different times following IV introduction. The onset of drug effect, magnitude and duration of drug effect, as well as the therapeutic window for the drug can be determined from these *in vivo* measurements. The line graph on the right illustrates the rate of change in plasma concentration ($\Delta C/\Delta t$) of the drug which is dependent on the initial drug concentrations. This type of rate change analysis is helpful in determining the rates of elimination and metabolism, as well as the half-life of the drug.

The C_{max} and T_{max} may be directly obtained from experimental observations of each subject and these two parameters are closely dependent on the experimental protocol because the concentrations are always decreasing after the initial dose. The peak time corresponds to the time of infusion if the drug is infused by IV at a constant rate. However, after oral administration C_{max} and T_{max} are dependent on the extent and the rate of drug absorption, and on the disposition profile of the drug. Consequently these two parameters can characterize the properties of different formulations of the drug in the same subject. All of the initial information on C_{max} and T_{max} should be generated when presenting the design of a pharmacokinetic study.

The half life of a drug has a significant relevance in the determination of dosage of a drug. Half-life ($t_{1/2}$) is derived from a mathematical property of the monoexponential function curve which results in elimination of half of the drug after a fixed time interval [Figure-5]. This means that the kinetic profile of many drugs is well approximated by a monoexponential function in the terminal phase and consequently it makes sense to define the half-life, or terminal half-life, in order to characterize the slope of the curve in this phase. Therefore, the drug elimination rate (K_{el}) is the sum of the rate constants due to the rate of metabolism (K_m) and the rate of excretion (K_{ex}), and it can be defined as Kel = Km + Kex. Since drug elimination is an exponential process, the time required for a twofold decrease is proportional to ln(2) or 0.693 which equals the natural logarithm of two, and $t_{1/2} = (0.693)/Kel$. Therefore, if Co is the drug concentration at time 0 and λ is dependent on the half-life of the curve, then the following relationship can be extrapolated as: $t_{1/2} = 0.693 / \lambda$. With a single compartmental model, a monoexponential function can thus be used to calculate plasma concentration at a specific time after administration. This can be written as:- $c(t) = C_0 \times e^{-\lambda . t}$ where $c(t)$ is the drug concentration at time t. Indeed, the terminal half-life is often used to describe decay of the drug concentration during the terminal phase.

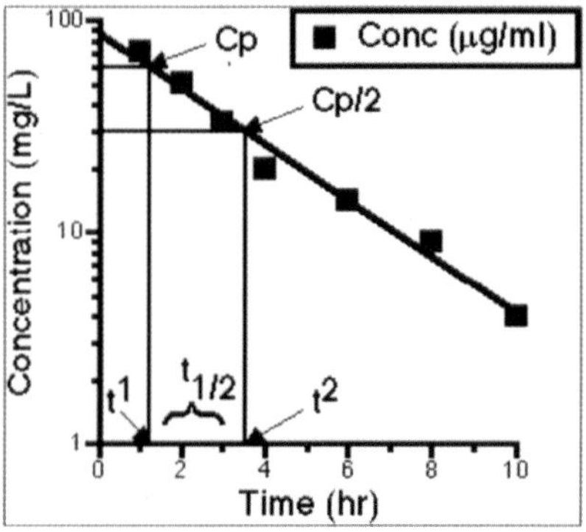

Fig. 5. *The half life of drugs in vivo.* Half life of a drug is dependent on Rate of Elimination of the drug. The semi-log plot shows plasma levels of drugs (Cp) and different time post infusion (e.g. t_1, t_2, etc.). It is a constant rate of decline which is independent of the starting time of drug administration.

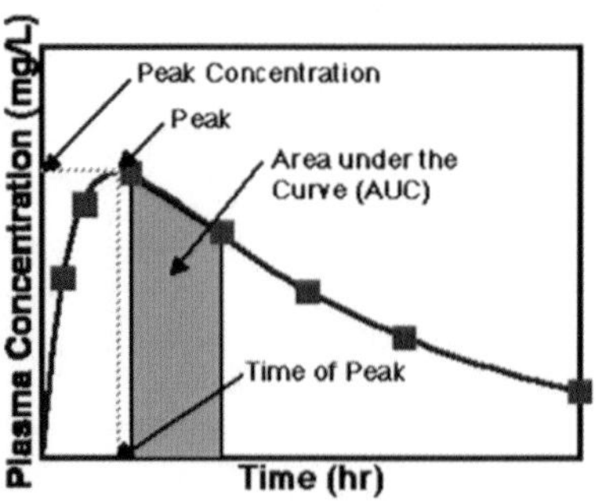

$$AUC = \int_{t=0}^{t=\infty} Cp^t \cdot dt \quad \text{Equation 1}$$

$$AUC = \frac{DOSE}{V \cdot kel} = \frac{Cp^0}{kel} \quad \text{Equation 2}$$

Fig. 6. *The AUC analysis.* The AUC is calculated by adding the different AUC-segments together. Each very narrow segment has an area of Cp.dt. The AUC depends on the volume of distribution (V) and the rate of elimination (Kel). It is calculated from time 0 (administration time, Cp0) to infinity as shown in equations 1 and 2.

The extent and rate of drug absorption and distribution thus play important roles in pharmacokinetics. These parameters are usually referred to as the drug bioavailability (BA). The area under the plasma concentration curve (AUC) value is very useful for calculating the relative efficiency and BA of different drugs and possibly their metabolic products, e.g. the metabolic products of the anti-cancer agent irinotecan (Mathijssen RH, et al. 2001). The AUC is calculated by adding the AUC-segments together under the plasma concentration vs. time curve. Each very narrow segment of the cure has an area equal to plasma concentration at different time intervals (i.e. Cp x dt) [Figure-6]. The AUC is calculated from time 0 (administration time) to infinity after single drug administration, and within the dose interval after multiple dose treatment. By integrating this equation that $t_{1/2} = 0.693 / \lambda$ between 0 and infinity, we can obtain the values for AUC = Co/λ. This suggests that the area under the curve can also be computed easily from the Co, e and λ values. The Co and λ can be estimated by a non-linear regression technique or by linearizing the data using the log-transformation.

The AUC can also be used to measure both the volume of distribution (Vd) and the drug elimination process. Under very general assumptions, the AUC is closely dependent on the drug amount that enters into the systemic circulation and on the ability that the system has to eliminate the drug (clearance). Therefore, AUC can be used to measure the drug amount absorbed or the efficiency of physiological processes that characterize drug elimination. Clearance (CL), on the other hand, depends on the functionality of the eliminating organs, i.e. the kidney or the liver, therefore possible inefficiencies of these organs can have consequences on clearance, AUC and drug levels. For example, a fraction of a dose may be metabolized during the early passage through the gastrointestinal (GI) tract or through the liver after an oral dose and part of the dose may not even reach the blood due to drug malabsorption. The consequences are incomplete absorption of the drug into the systemic circulation and incomplete drug availability which may result in an ineffective treatment. Evidence that drug PK may drastically be changed due to either IV or oral administration of the anti-diabetic agent metformin, were also clearly shown in these early studies (Pentikainen PJ, 1979). From the plasma AUC and the CL, it is possible to compute the drug amount which enters into the systemic circulation in a particular subject. The following very general definitions can be given: $CL = D/AUC \times V_d$ where CL = drug amount eliminated per unit of time/drug concentration in plasma, and the volume of distribution (V_d) = drug amount in the body/drug concentration in plasma [Figure-7].

For drugs with narrow therapeutic index and significant side-effect profiles, it is common that multiple exponential terms are needed to fit the plasma concentrations after an IV bolus, and more complex mathematical modeling is carried out to more accurately determine the PK parameters. In order to get a good interpolation of the data after oral or extravascular administration, multiple exponential terms should be added to the above simple equations of PK. Although plasma drug concentrations are increasing just after oral administration and decreasing after the peak time, the predicted data may be biased when fitted by a monoexponential function, and interpolation of oral or IV profile may be obtained by adding new exponential terms with the following equation: $C_{(t)} = A_1 \times e^{-\lambda_1 \cdot t} + A_2 \times e^{-\lambda_2 \cdot t}$, which is called a biexponential function. In order to get the best fit of the experimental data and the best accuracy in the estimated parameters, a number of these exponential terms should be chosen. By taking into account the numerous compartments that the drug can be distributed to, as well as the number of rate constants necessary to ultimately determine the drug concentration remaining at a certain time, the above equation is frequently changed to represent an integration function: $C_{(t)} = \Sigma A_i \times e^{-\lambda_i \cdot t}$. Following these calculations, the initial drug level and the AUC can be computed by the integrated parameters of the curve as represented by the equation: $Co = \Sigma A_i \times e \times AUC = \Sigma_i A_i / \lambda_i$ where Co is equal to 0 after oral or extravascular administration. This literally means that the terminal half-life is always represented by $0.693/\lambda_n$, where the λ_n is the lowest exponent.

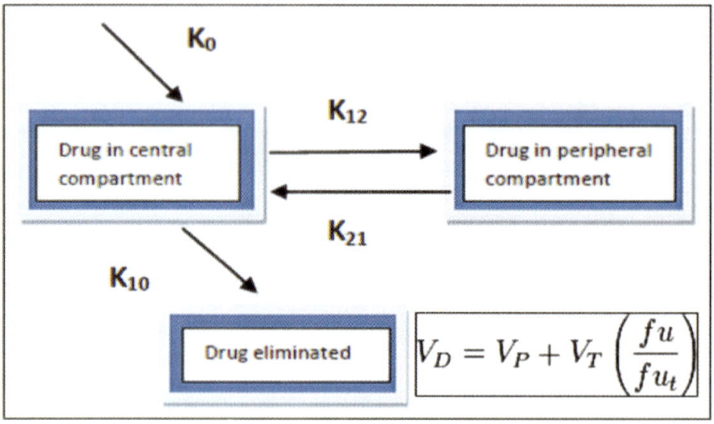

Fig. 7. *Multicompartmental Models.* Frequently, a multicompartmental model and equation are implemented where the rate constants for drug absorption and distribution are calculated. In this model, the k_0 represents initial absorption process and the processes of tissue absorption, distribution and excretion are denoted by using multiple rate constants such as k_{12}, k_{21}, and k_{10}. In this multicompartmental system, a drug appears to be dissolved in total body volume which is also referred to as the 'apparent' volume of distribution (V_D). The V_D can be used to determine how readily a drug will displace into the body tissue compartments relative to the blood, where: V_P = plasma volume; V_T = apparent tissue volume; fu = fraction unbound in plasma and fu_T = fraction unbound in tissue.

Although these multiexponential functions require complex calculations, they are needed to determine drug disposition in both preclinical and clinical settings. The importance of such rigorous calculations was recently underscored by findings that Clopidogrel, an anti-platelet drug used to treat heart attack and stroke, which had a very narrow therapeutic index and caused significant side effects in the elderly (Roden, DM. & Stein, CM. 2009), needed careful dose adjustments depending on the patient's renal clearance rates (Goteti K, 2008).

The majority of drugs currently used have approximately a biexponential profile in plasma after an intravenous bolus, but there are exceptions especially after oral administration. Indeed, very often the drug profile is not monoexponential, and the concentrations of many drugs in plasma and tissues may not decay in a linear fashion (Evan W., 1989). Highly comprehensive data on drug profiles, not only in the plasma, but also in all other tissues or fluids, and especially addressing the differences due to the routes of administration are needed. Therefore, for a given drug, a single kinetic profile may be well summarized by Cmax, Tmax, $t_{1/2}$ and AUC, however, with drugs having more than one profile, the mean and standard deviation of these individual parameters, may be needed to summarize the drug kinetics especially in multiple animals or in the whole population (Dreisbach AW, 2008 & 2009).

3. Drug metabolizing enzymes and drug-transporters

Until recently, when a drug exhibited poor oral bioavailability, it was generally assumed that this was due to either physicochemical problems associated with poor solubility in the GI fluids or inability to diffuse through the intestinal membrane, or alternatively, due to significant first-pass hepatic metabolism. Based on a series of cellular, animal and human studies, we now realize that both intestinal metabolic enzymes and efflux transporters, working together as a protective mechanism, may be responsible for the poor bioavailability of a number of drugs (Furuta T, 1998; Schellens JH, 2000; Luo FR, 2002). Drug metabolizing enzymes and drug-transporters critically regulate the extent of drug distribution throughout the body and the rate of drug clearance from the body (Volm M, 1991; Wacher VJ, 1995). The CYP450 enzymes are the major enzymes involved in drug metabolism and bio-activation, accounting for ~75% of the total metabolism. The CYP enzymes catalyze the oxidation of organic substances such as lipids, steroidal hormones, and xenobiotics, and they are the primary enzymes involved in drug metabolism and bioactivation (Guengerich, 2008). The first evidence of the Cyp450 system in regulating drug-interactions was observed when the effects of ketoconazole, a potent inhibitor of multiple drug-metabolizing enzymes, were shown to increase digoxin absorption and disposition in a rat model (Salphati, L. 1998). The ATP-binding cassette (ABC) transporters are a family of transmembrane proteins that harness the energy of adenosine triphosphate (ATP) hydrolysis to translocate a variety of substrates including lipids, sterols, metabolic products and drugs across extra- and intracellular membranes (Davidson et al., 2008).

PROCESS	ENZYMES	TRANSPORTERS
ABSORPTION	-	++
DISTRIBUTION	-	+++
METABOLISM	+++	+
EXCRETION	-	+++

Table 1. Both drug metabolizing enzymes and drug-transporters regulate ADME.

Over the past several decades, considerable efforts to delineate the characteristics influencing activation and regulation of these enzymes and proteins have provided a valuable foundation of data illustrating their different effects on the distribution, metabolism and clearance of drugs. Increasing evidence suggests that CYP450 enzymes and ABC transporters significantly impact drug bioavailability, and a variety of factors including age, sex, health and genetics influence their activity (Sai K, 2003; Allabi AC, 2004). The following section summarizes how the aforementioned factors may impact PK and PD to ultimately guide health care providers in making informed decisions about the type of drug, dosage and dosage scheduling for safe administration. Since all drugs are eventually excreted from the body, and many require bio-activation to form the active compound, the field of PK has begun to focus not only on drug metabolism by the CYPs, but also on the full spectrum of drug disposition, including a growing list of transporters that influence absorption, distribution and excretion [Table-1].

3.1 The CYP450 system

CYP450 enzymes are present in most tissues of the body and play important roles in hormone synthesis and breakdown (including estrogen and testosterone synthesis and metabolism), cholesterol synthesis and vitamin D metabolism (Salphati, L. 1998; Guengerich, 2008; Bjorkman S. 2005). CYP450 enzymes also function to metabolize potentially toxic compounds, including drugs and products of endogenous metabolism such as bilirubin, principally in the liver. A subset of CYP450 enzymes play important roles in the synthesis of steroid hormones (steroidogenesis) by the adrenals, gonads, and peripheral tissue: CYP11A1 (steroid 20α-hydroxylase), CYP11B1, CYP17A1, CYP21A1 (in the adrenal cortex conducts 21-hydroxylase activity) and CYP19A all catalyze aromatization of androgens to estrogens. These enzymes belong to the superfamily of proteins containing a heme cofactor and, therefore, are hemoproteins which have been named on the basis of their cellular (cyto) location and spectrophotometric characteristics (chrome). When the reduced heme iron forms an adduct with carbon monoxide (CO), the P450 enzymes absorb light at wavelengths near 450 nm, identifiable as a characteristic Soret peak, thus the name CYP450.

These drug metabolizing enzymes are primarily membrane-associated proteins, located either in the inner membrane of mitochondria or in the endoplasmic reticulum of cells. Often, they form part of multi-component electron transfer chains, called P450-containing systems. Each enzyme is termed an isoform since each derives from a different gene. It should be noted, however, that structural similarity of enzymes cannot be used to predict which isoforms will be responsible for a drug's metabolism. Because of the vast variety of reactions catalyzed by CYPs, the activities and properties of the many isoenzymes differ in many respects. Each CYP450 enzyme and their isozymes can metabolize multiple drugs and recognize molecules with disparate structures as their substrates. Drug interactions involving the CYP450 isoforms generally result from one of two processes, enzyme inhibition or enzyme induction. Enzyme inhibition usually involves competition with another drug for the enzyme binding site. This process usually begins with the first dose of the inhibitor and onset and offset of inhibition correlate with the half-lives of the drugs involved (Dossing M, 1983; Murray M, 1990). Enzyme induction occurs when a drug stimulates the synthesis of more enzyme protein, enhancing the enzyme's metabolizing capacity. It is somewhat difficult to predict the time course of enzyme induction because several factors, including drug half-lives and enzyme turnover, determine the time course of induction. Broadly, the CYPs are divided into two categories, i.e. Phase-I enzymes that introduce or remove functional groups in a substrate through oxidation, reduction or hydrolysis; and Phase-II enzymes that transfer moieties from a cofactor to a substrate via conjugation. According to a standardized nomenclature system adapted in 1996, the CYPs are divided into 18 families and 43 subfamilies on the basis of amino acid sequence homology (Ingelman-Sundberg M. 2004 & 2009; Nelson, DR. 2009). A schematic of recent guidelines for the nomenclature of CYP450 isoenzyme families, is provided [Figure-8].

The Phase-I CYP450 is a gene superfamily consisting of more than 57 genes coding for functional proteins, and 58 pseudogenes. The most common reaction catalyzed by the Phase-I enzymes is a monooxygenase reaction, e.g. insertion of one atom of oxygen into an organic substrate (RH) while the other oxygen atom is reduced to water: $RH + O_2 + 2H^+ + 2e^- \rightarrow ROH + H_2O$. The majority of these genes are polymorphic. Current information on genetic variants can be found at the human CYP allele home page (http://www.imm.ki.se/CYPalleles/ and http://www.cypalleles.ki.se/). More than 434 different alleles of the genes encoding xenobiotic metabolizing P450 enzymes are presented on this site. Among these, three subfamilies of CYPs, including CYP1, CYP2, and CYP3, contribute to the oxidative metabolism of more than 90% of clinically used drugs. Overall, approximately 10 of the CYP450 enzymes are responsible for the metabolism of a large number of pharmacologic agents in human beings, and six of them are considered most important: CYP3A4, CYP2D6, CYP2C19, CYP2C9, CYP1A2 and CYP2E1. CYP3A4 is the most abundantly expressed cytochrome and composes 30 to 40% of the CYP in the liver and in the small intestine. CYP2D6 is implied (at 20%) in the metabolism of active compounds and CYP2C9 coupled with CYP2C19 can metabolize at least 15% of commonly prescribed drugs (Desta Z, 2006).

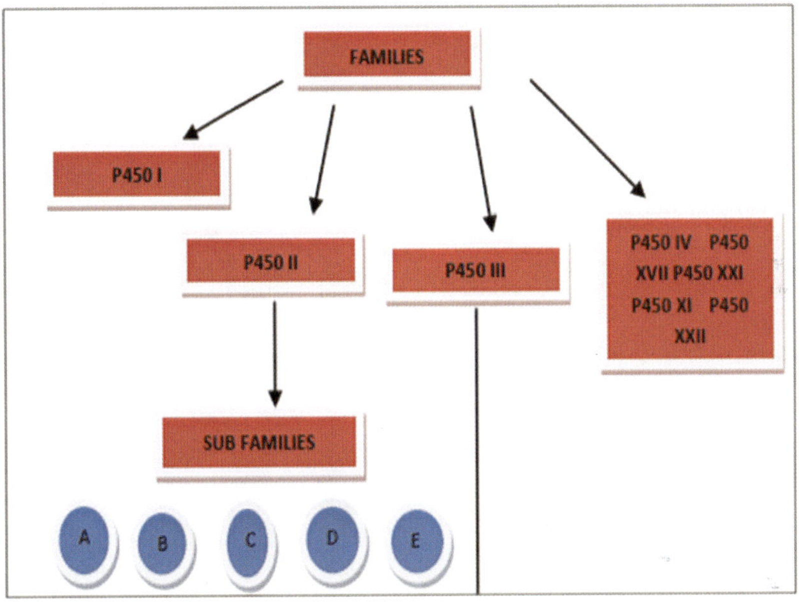

Fig. 8. *CYP450 gene nomenclature.* Enzymes that share at least 40% sequence homology are assigned to a family designated by an Arabic numeral, whereas those sharing at least 55% homology makeup a particular subfamily designated by a letter (A, B, C, etc.). Single members of a subfamily represent a particular enzyme and are designated by the number following the subfamily description (e.g. CYP2D6, CYP3A4). For each enzyme, the most common or "wild-type" allele is denoted as -1, and allelic variants are sequentially numbered as they are identified (i.e. -2, -3, etc.).

The most clinically important Phase-II enzymes are uridine diphosphate glucuronosyltransferase (UGT), sulfotransferase (SULT), glutathione S-transferases (GST), N-acetyltransferase (NAT) and thiopurine methyltransferase (TPMT). The human UGT superfamily is a group of conjugating enzymes that catalyze the transfer of the glucuronic acid group of uridine diphosphoglucuronic acid to the functional group (e.g. hydroxyl, carboxyl, amino, and sulfur) of a specific substrate. Glucuronidation increases the polarity of the substrates and facilitates their excretion in bile or urine. Seventeen human UGT genes have been identified thus far and are classified into two subfamilies (i.e. UGT1 and UGT2) (Nagar S, 2006). The super family of human GST catalyzes the conjugation of glutathione

(GSH) to a wide range of endogenous metabolites and xenobiotics including alkylating and free radical generating anticancer drugs (Townsend DM, 2005; Board PG. 2007). NAT2 plays an important role in the activation and/or deactivation of a large and diverse number of aromatic amine and hydrazine drugs used in the clinic, and therefore the NAT2 genotype is particularly relevant to the response to these drugs (Hein DW. 2002). TPMT is best known for its key role in the metabolism of the thiopurine drugs (e.g., 6-mercaptopurine, azathiopurine and 6-thioguanine) which are clinically used to treat cancers or as immunosuppressants (Booth RA, 2011).

3.2 The ABC and SLC transporters

Our knowledge of membrane expressed drug transporters has increased considerably in the past decade. Several transporters have been cloned and advances have been made in understanding their structure- function and characteristics (Davidson AL, 2008; Borst P, 2000; Shitara Y, 2002). Many tissues express these drug transporters such as the brain, liver, kidney and intestine; and they play an important role in defining characteristics of drug absorption, distribution and excretion of drugs. Thus, they are pivotal in affecting absorption and tissue distribution, hepatic uptake and export, as well as renal and biliary elimination of a variety of drugs. Conversely, the active transporters dictate the entry of drugs into different compartments and actively efflux drugs from intracellular compartments. Thus, drug transport via these membrane pumps could be classified as passive or active [Figure-9].

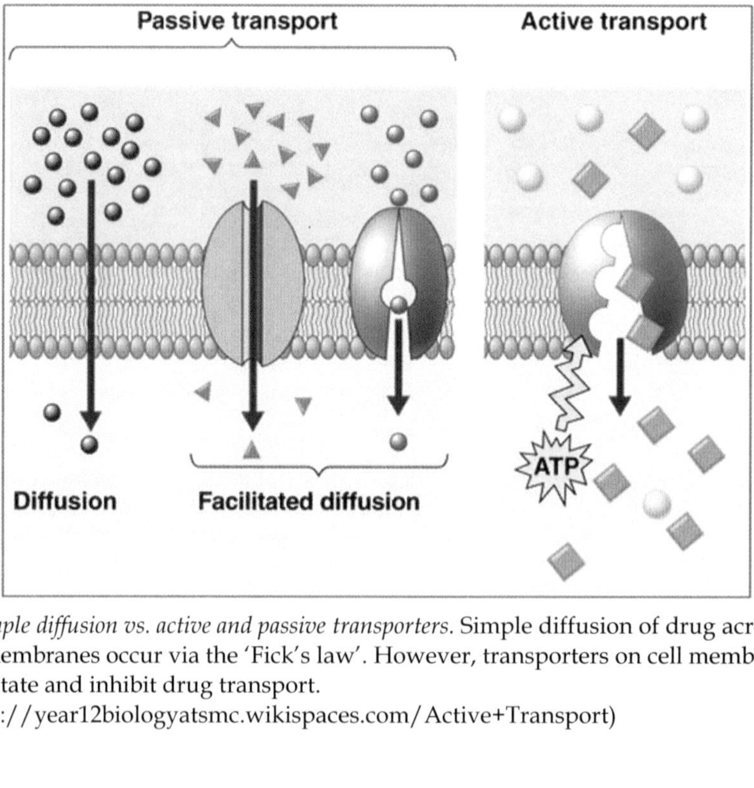

Fig. 9. *Simple diffusion vs. active and passive transporters.* Simple diffusion of drug across cellular membranes occur via the 'Fick's law'. However, transporters on cell membranes can both facilitate and inhibit drug transport.
URL: http://year12biologyatsmc.wikispaces.com/Active+Transport)

A drug that moves across a membrane along its concentration gradient without expending metabolic energy is said to be transported passively. The intestinal uptake of glucose in the human body serves as a good example of passive transport (Awad WA, 2007; Durán JM, 2004). Passive transport can be divided into two sub-types. The first two involves spontaneous movement of membrane permeable substances across the membrane utilizing the laws of simple diffusion. The second type of non-energy dependent transport is facilitated diffusion where the movement of membrane impermeable substances across the membrane is aided via transporters and via co-transport of other charged ions (Dobson PD, 2008; Visentin M, 2011). Both passive and carrier-mediated drug transport processes are known to coexist in tissues and regulate drug concentrations within subvascular sites (Sugano K, 2010; Lau YY, 2007; Varghese Gupta S, 2011).

Conversely, active transport requires energy and may involve transporting the drug against their concentration gradient, involving multiple saturable carriers (Choo EF, 2000; Hinoshita E, 2000; Conrad S, 2002; Krishnamurthy P, 2006). The primary active transporters utilize adenosine triphosphate (ATP) to produce energy for transport. The transport protein itself consists of an ATPase, which hydrolyzes ATP for the required energy. However, a secondary active transport mechanism also exists where the transporter protein does not have a direct ATP coupling and utilizes the potential gradient created when ions are transported across the membrane by primary active transport, but these are mostly found in bacteria or protozoans (Boiangiu CD, 2005; Simon J, 2008). Although, a few of these active ion-pumps have been of potential importance in cancer therapeutics, e.g. proton pump inhibitors (Harguindey S, 2009). In general, drug transporters that are of clinical significance have been divided into two main classes; the solute carrier family (SLC) of passive transporters and the ATP binding cassette (ABC) family of active transporters [Table-2 & Table-3].

3.2.1 The ABC transporters

The drug-efflux function of ABC transporters enables extrusion of a wide range of substrates from the inside to the outside of a cell membrane or organelle (Jones PM, 2009; Locher KP. 2009; Degorter MK, 2011). They are known to transport lipids and sterols, ions and small molecules, drugs and large polypeptides. P-gp (ABCB1) is ubiquitously expressed in a number of important organs such as liver, intestine, lymphocytes, placenta and the brain endothelial cells. P-gp can transport mainly cationic or electrically neutral substrates as well as a broad spectrum of amphiphilic substrates. The ABCC family members confer MDR to organic anion compounds, and MRP1 is more ubiquitous than MRP-2. Interestingly, their expression can either be at the apical (AP) or on the basolateral (BL) membranes of epithelial or endothelial barriers. The ABCG2 transporter, also known as BCRP (breast cancer resistance protein) are also expressed on apical surfaces and confer resistance to Topoisomerase inhibitors and doxorubicin [Table-2].

The best characterized ABC-transporter is P-glycoprotein (also known as P-gp, MDR-1 or ABCB1) (Brinkmann U, 2001; Fromm MF. 2003; Kroetz DL, 2003). MDR-1 displays a broad substrate spectrum comprising of both neutral and cationic organic compounds. Another ABC-transporter, recently cloned from a drug resistant breast cancer line, is BCRP (a.k.a. ABCG2) and substrate specificities and tissue localization of BCRP have been found to be similar to that of MDR-1 (Jonker JW, 2000; Krishnamurthy P, 2006). BCRP is also referred to as a half transporter since it has one transmembrane domain and functions as a dimer to transport a variety of drugs. The immunosuppressant cyclosporine-A and verapamil, a calcium channel antagonist, are competitive inhibitors of MDR-1 mediated efflux (also referred to as MDR-modulators) and have often been used in the laboratory to determine MDR-1 specific drug-efflux (Eilers M, 2008; Roy U, 2009). A newly discovered group of ABC transporters is the MDR associated proteins (MRPs) also referred to as the ABCC family of transporters (Gradhand U, 2008). MRPs are found to cotransport drugs along with glutathione (GSH) or transport GSH-drug conjugates and glucuronide-drug conjugates. Amongst the nine members of the MRP transporters family, the first five (MRP-1, MRP-2, MRP-3, MRP-4 and MRP-5) are frequently associated with the efflux of therapeutic agents. MRP-1, MRP-2 and MRP-3 transport hydrophilic anionic compounds, large molecules and peptidomimetics; however, both MRP-4 and MRP-5 transport small polar compounds such as nucleosides, cyclic nucleotides and nucleoside analogs (Schuetz JD, 1999). The overexpression of ABC transporters had been shown to result in chemotherapeutics being pumped out of cells faster than they can enter, and is an well accepted mechanism leading to the development of multidrug resistance (MDR) in cancer cells (Gottesman MM, 2002; Luqmani YA. 2005; Tiwari AK, 2011). Recent studies by us, and others, have also shown that several anti-HIV-1 drugs, especially HIV protease inhibitors (HPIs) and nucleoside analog reverse transcriptase inhibitors (NRTIs) are substrates of ABC-transporters (Choo EF, 2000; Roy U, 2009) and their expression on both lymphocytes and BBB endothelial cells (ECs) can suppress drug entry into the cellular and anatomical reservoirs of HIV-1 (Eilers M, 2008; Tarbell JM. 2010; Shen S, 2010). The polarized expression of MRPs regulates the directional transport of drugs in and out of various tissue compartments. Both P-gp and MRP1 are predominantly expressed in the human lung; thus, these transporters may be pivotal in the protection against toxic compounds.

Gene	Protein	Tissue distribution	Polarity	Representative drug substrates
ABC transporters				
ABCB1	MDR1 (P-gp)	Liver, intestine, kidney, blood–brain barrier, lymphocytes, placenta	AP	Anthracyclines, taxanes, vinca alkaloids, imatinib, etoposide, levofloxacin, erythromycin, cyclosporine, tacrolimus, digoxin, quinidine, verapamil, diltiazem, ritonavir, saquinavir, talinolol, phenytoin, cimetidine, simvastatin, morphine, hydrocortisone
ABCC1	MRP1 (GS-X)	Ubiquitous	BL	Anthracyclines, vinca alkaloids, irinotecan, SN-38, methotrexate, camptothecins, saquinavir, ritonavir, difloxacin, drug-glucuronate/-glutathione/-sulfate conjugates
ABCC2	MRP2 (cMOAT)	Liver, kidney, intestine	AP	Anthracyclines, vinca alkaloids, methotrexate, camptothecins, rifampin, pravastatin, and drug-glucuronate/-glutathione/-sulfate conjugates
ABCG2	BCRP	Liver, intestine, placenta, breast	AP	Anthracyclines, irinotecan, SN38, SN38G, imatinib, tamoxifen

Table 2. *ABC family of drug transporters.* The gene name and common protein names for the most common transporters are shown. Their tissue distribution, expression polarity (apical or basal) and representative drugs that are transported by each of the drug-efflux pumps, are shown. *(Adapted from Bluth MH, 2011)*.URL: http://dx.doi.org/10.2147/PGPM.S18861

3.2.2 The SLC transporters

The solute carrier family functions by facilitative diffusion and secondary active transport (Shitara Y, 2002; Hagenbuch B, 2003; Niemi M, 2004; Lau YY, 2007; Visentin M, 2011). SLC transporters, also known as the organic anion transporter polypeptide (OATP) belong to a large superfamily that comprises of approximately 300 SLC genes classified into 43 families. The SLC transporters transport both endogenous molecules like amino acids, sugars etc. and many exogenous drugs [Table-3]. They are located on the cell membrane as well as on the intracellular membrane of organelles. Except for SLC22A11 (OAT4) all others are expressed on basolateral membranes. They can transport a variety of small molecules and inhibitors of the SLC transporters have proved useful in the treatment of a variety of disorders, including depression, epilepsy and Parkinson's disease (Kuroda M, 2005; Gether U, 2006; Thwaites DT, 2011). Variance in the expression and function of these transporter proteins can significantly impact the PK profile of a number of drugs.

Uptake transporters belong to the SLC family while efflux transporters belong to the ABC family. Many of these drug transporter proteins contain polymorphisms which can significantly alter their function. Within the last decade more information has become available reinforcing the fact that polymorphisms which effect expression or activity of the drug transporters contribute to the variability seen in the drug disposition between individuals. A number of studies have demonstrated the importance of P-gp for drug disposition in humans (Fromm MF, et al, 2003). Chemotherapeutic drugs (e.g. paclitaxel), uricosuric agents (e.g. probenecid), and the leukotrienes (LT) receptor antagonist (e.g. MK-571), are known inhibitors of MRPs (Eilers M, 2008). A number of preclinical and clinical trials are also being carried out to discover new and more effective efflux pump inhibitors (EPIs). Initial studies showed that PSC 833, a P-gp specific EPI was able to increase the efficacy of vincristine and digoxin in rat models (Song, S. 1999). In recent years, both verapamil and cyclosporine-A analogs are showing significant promise as safe and effective EPIs (Bauer F, 2010; Kolitz JE, 2010; O'Brien MM, 2010; Patel NR, 2011).

Gene	Protein	Tissue distribution	Polarity	Representative drug substrates
SLC transporters				
OATP family				
SLC21A3	OATP1A2 (OATP-A)	Ubiquitous, with highest expression in brain and testis	BL	Rosuvastatin, methotrexate, ouabain, D-penicillamine
SLC21A6	OATP1B1 (OATP-C)	Liver	BL	Statin, pravastatin, fexofenadine, and repaglinide, rosuvastatin, ouabain, D-penicillamine, rifampin
SLC21A8	OATP1B3 (OATP8)	Liver	BL	Digoxin, rifampin, ouabain, methotrexate, D-penicillamine, rosuvastatin, cyclosporin
SLC21A9	OATP2B1 (OATP-B)	Ubiquitous	BL	Benzylpenicillin, rosuvastatin
OCT family				
SLC22A1	OCT1	Liver	BL	Metformin, cisplatin, oxaliplatin, imatinib, procainamide, citalopram, cimetidine, quinidine, verapamil, acyclovir
SLC22A2	OCT2	Kidney	BL	Metformin, cisplatin, oxaliplatin, imatinib, procainamide, citalopram, cimetidine, quinidine, amantadine
SLC22A3	OCT3	Brain, liver, kidney, heart, muscle, placenta, and blood vessels	BL	Cimetidine, agmatine, adefovir, catecholamines
OAT family				
SLC22A6	OAT1	Kidney, brain	BL	Methotrexate, salicylate, antiviral agents (eg, acyclovir)
SLC22A7	OAT2	Liver, kidney	BL	Methotrexate, salicylate, tetracyclines
SLC22A8	OAT3	Kidney, brain, muscle	BL	Methotrexate, antiviral agents (eg, acyclovir), cimetidine, pravastatin, salicylate
SLC22A11	OAT4	Kidney, placenta	AP	Methotrexate, cimetidine, salicylate, tetracyclines

Table 3. *SLC family of drug transporters.* The gene name and common protein names, tissue distribution, polarity (apical or basal) and representative drugs transported by each, are shown. *(Addapted from Bluth MH, 2011).*
URL: http://dx.doi.org/10.2147/PGPM.S18861

4. Pharmacogenomics

Even using the same medications, different patients respond in different ways. Defining the changes seen in drug efficacy and toxicity are of crucial significance since PK measurements alone cannot explain such variability (Kuehl P, 2001; Evans WE, 1999; Kroetz DL, 2003; Lai Y, 2011). The intrapatient variability and large population differences suggest that genetic inheritance may be a critical determinant of the therapeutic responses to drugs which are substrates for ABC-transporters and CYP450 enzymes (Ameyaw MM, 2001; Dorne JL, 2002; Evans WE, 2001). Although we know many nongenetic (or epigenetic) factors influence the effects of medications, including age, organ function, concomitant therapy, drug interactions and the nature of the disease, there are now numerous examples of cases in which inter-individual differences in drug response are attributed to sequence variants in genes encoding drug-metabolizing enzymes and drug transporters. Moreover, recent findings demonstrate that genetic differences in both drug metabolizing enzymes and drug transporters ultimately regulate the individualistic differences in drug PK (Evans WE, 2003; Staatz CE, 2010). Because most drug effects are determined by the interplay of several gene products that influence the PK and PD of medications, including inherited differences in drug targets (receptors) and drug disposition (metabolizing enzymes and transporters), the genetic characteristics in different patient populations, as well as within individuals, have become increasingly important in regulating PK. This new field of Medicine is now known as pharmacogenomics (PG).

A gene is considered to be polymorphic when the frequency of a variant allele in a specific population is at least 1% (Sachidanandam R, 2001). More than 1.4 million single-nucleotide polymorphisms (SNPs) were identified in the initial sequencing of the human genome, with over 60,000 of them in the coding region of genes (www.ncbi.nlm.nih.gov/SNP/GeneGt.cgi?geneID=5243). Some of these SNPs have already been associated with substantial changes in the metabolism or effects of medications and some are now being used to predict clinical response. The burgeoning field of PG uses these genome-wide approaches to elucidate the inherited differences between persons and their drug responses (Lamba JK, 2002; MacPhee IA, 2005; Tamura A, 2007a ; Song IS, 2008; Staatz CE, 2010a). It has been suggested that 20 to 95 % of the variability in drug disposition and effect can be attributed to genetics; therefore, considerable efforts to investigate the genetic factors influencing drug response via PG studies hold the promise of personalized medical care in the future. Such an approach focuses on drugs and drug combinations that are optimized to each individual's unique genetic makeup (Tamura A, 2007b; Staatz CE, 2010b). Mutations play a clear role in the functioning of the majority of the body's organs (lung, liver, brain, etc.) in which CYP and ABC transporter expression may regulate drug distribution and clearance. For example, mutations in the ABC transporter, cystic fibrosis transmembrane conductance regulator (CFTR) is responsible for the development of the lung disorder cystic fibrosis, while the cause of Tangier disease, a high cholesterol-related condition, is attributed to mutations in ABCA1 (van der Deen et al., 2005). Other studies provide evidence that genetic polymorphisms exert an effect on interethnic variation and frequency of CYP and multi-drug resistance gene (MDR1) alleles among Orientals, Caucasians and Africans (Iida A, 2002; Lai et al., 2011). Furthermore, interpatient variability in drug response and toxicity to standard doses of the most commonly prescribed chemotherapeutic agents is often explained, in part, by genetic polymorphisms in genes encoding CYP enzymes and ABC transporters. Single nucleotide polymorphisms (SNPs) account for 80% of all sequence variations residing in genes and these sequence variations can result in a multitude of adverse drug reactions (Lee et al, 2010). We may be able to facilitate personalized clinical treatment of pain and opioid addiction by understanding the PK and PD of methadone. Methadone, a P-gp substrate primarily metabolized by CYP3A4 and CYP2B6, has a narrow therapeutic index and large interpatient variability. Genetic polymorphisms in genes coding for the methadone-metabolizing enzymes and P-gp contribute to the interindividual variability of methadone kinetics and methadone blood concentrations (Li et al., 2008). Ensuing discussion illustrates the relevance of cancer pharmacogenomic studies in optimizing chemotherapeutic response by enhancing the efficacy and safety of some select chemotherapy drugs.

4.1 Polymorphisms in the CYP-450 genes

Polymorphisms within the CYP genes include gene deletions, missense mutations, deleterious mutations creating splicing defects or premature stop codon and gene duplications, which can result in abolished, reduced, normal or enhanced enzyme activity (Ball SE, 1999; Lamba JK, 2002; Daly AK. 2006; Bluth MH, 2011) [Table 4]. A number of studies have shown interindividual variability and tissue specificity in the expression of cytochrome P450 gene expression (Koch I, et al, 2002). As a result, patients can be classified into four phenotypes based on the level of a CYP enzyme activity: poor metabolizer (abolished activity), intermediate metabolizer (reduced activity), extensive metabolizer (normal activity), and ultrarapid metabolizer (enhanced activity). Substantial evidence suggests that genetic polymorphisms within the CYP genes have significant impact on drug disposition and/or response. The lack of functional CYP3A5 may not be readily evident, because many medications metabolized by CYP3A5 are also metabolized by the universally expressed CYP3A4. For medications that are equally metabolized by both enzymes, the net rate of metabolism is the sum of that due to CYP3A4 and that due to CYP3A5; the existence of this dual pathway partially obscures the clinical effects of genetic polymorphism of CYP3A5 but contributes to the large range of total CYP3A activity in humans. Notably, the most pharmacologically and clinically relevant CYP polymorphisms are found in *CYP2D6*, *CYP2C9*, and *CYP2C19* genes (Ingelman-Sundburg M. 2004; Bluth MH, 2011). Of the Food and Drug Administration (FDA)-approved drug labels referring to human genomic biomarkers, 62% pertain to polymorphisms in the CYP enzymes, with CYP2D6 (35%), CYP2C19 (17%), and CYP2C9 (7%) being the most common [Table-2]. The genetic basis of CYP3A5 deficiency is predominantly a SNP in intron 3 that creates a cryptic splice site causing 131 nucleotides of the intronic sequence to be inserted into the RNA, introducing a termination codon that prematurely truncates the CYP3A5 protein. Although it is now possible to determine which patients express both functional enzymes (i.e., CYP3A4 and CYP3A5), the clinical importance of these variants for the many drugs metabolized by CYP3A remains unclear. Differences in the *CYP450* genotypes may contribute to the inter-ethnic variations in the disposition and response of substrate drugs (Burk O, 2002; Rettie AE, 2005; Lim HS, 2007). However, pharmacogenetic testing for drug metabolizing enzymes is not yet frequently implemented in the clinic practice (Gardiner SJ, 2005).

The most common functional polymorphisms occurring in few of the major human CYP genes, along with allele frequencies and functional effects, are provided in Table-4. CYP1 genes are mainly expressed in extrahepatic tissues and have been linked to bioactivation of a variety of carcinogens. Multiple SNPs in CYP1 increase their functional activity by inducing gene expression or protein stability and have been linked to ethnic differences in PK (Mcilwain CC, 2006). The CYP1A1 polymrphism, CYP1A1*2C is associated with increased lung cancer risk in African Americans. Their role in estrogen activation has also linked several CYP1A1 genotypes to increased risk of prostate, breast and ovarian cancers.

Common allelic variants	Polymorphism/substitution	Allele frequency (%)[a]			Functional effect[b]
		Caucasian	Asian	African	
CYP1A1					
*CYP1A1*2A*	3698T>C(MspI)	6.6–19.0	33–54	22–28	↑ Inducibility
*CYP1A1*2B*	I462V; 3698T>C(MspI)	–	–	–	↑ Inducibility
*CYP1A1*2C*	I462V	2.2–8.9	28–31	0.0–2.7	↑ Activity
*CYP1A1*3*	3204T>C	0	0	7.6–14.0	Normal
*CYP1A1*4*	T461N	2.0–5.7	–	–	Normal
CYP1A2					
*CYP1A2*1C*	−3860G>A				↓ Inducibility
*CYP1A2*1F*	−163C>A	33	68		↑ Inducibility
*CYP1A2*1K*	Haplotype (−63C>A, −739T>G, −729C>T)	0.5			↓ Inducibility ↓ Activity
CYP2A6					
*CYP2A6*1 × 2*	Gene duplication	1.7		0.4	↑ Activity
*CYP2A6*2*	L160H	1–3		<1	↓ Activity
*CYP2A6*4*	Gene deletion	0.5–1.0	7–22	15–20	Abolished activity
CYP2B6					
*CYP2B6*4*	K262R	5			↑ Activity
*CYP2B6*5*	R487C	11–14	1		↓ Expression
*CYP2B6*6*	Q172H; K262R	16–26	16		↑ Activity
*CYP2B6*7*	Q172H; K262R; R487C	13	0		↑ Activity
CYP2C8					
*CYP2C8*2*	I269F	0.4		18	↓ Activity
*CYP2C8*3*	R139K; K399R	13	0	2	↓ Activity
*CYP2C8*4*	I264M	7.5			↓ Activity
CYP2C9					
*CYP2C9*2*	R144C	13–22	0	3	↓ Activity
*CYP2C9*3*	I359L	3–16	3	1.3	↓ Activity
*CYP2C9*5*	D360E	0	2	0	↓ Activity

Table 4. (Continued)

CYP2C19					
CYP2C19*2	Splicing defect; I331V	15	30	17	Abolished activity
CYP2C19*3	W212X; I331V	0.04	5	0.4	Abolished activity
CYP2C19*17	I331V	18	4		↑ Transcription
CYP2D6					
CYP2D6*3	Frameshift	1–2	<1		Abolished activity (PM)
CYP2D6*4	Splicing defect	20–25	1	6–7	Abolished activity (PM)
CYP2D6*5	Gene deletion	4–6	4–6	4–6	Abolished activity (PM)
CYP2D6*10	P34S; S486T	<2	50	3–9	↓ Activity (IM)
CYP2D6*17	T107I; R296C; S486T	<1		20–34	↓ Activity (IM)
CYP2D6*41	R296C; splicing defect; S486T	1.3	2	5.8	↓ Activity (IM)
CYP2D6*1 × N, N ≥ 2	Gene duplication				↑ Activity (UM)
CYP2D6*2 × N, N ≥ 2	Gene duplication				↑ Activity (UM)
CYP3A4					
CYP3A4*1B	5′ flanking region	2–9	0	35–67	Altered expression
CYP3A4*2	S222P	2.7–4.5	0	0	Substrate-dependent altered activity
CYP3A4*3	M445T	1.1			↓ Activity
CYP3A4*17	F189S	2.1			↓ Activity
CYP3A4*18	L293P	0		1	↑ Activity
CYP3A5					
CYP3A5*3	Splicing defect	90	75	50	Abolished activity
CYP3A5*6	Splicing defect	0	0	7.5	Severely ↓ activity
CYP3A5*7	346Frameshift	0	0	8	Severely ↓ activity
CYP3A7					
CYP3A7*1C	Promoter	3		6	↑ Expression
CYP3A7*2	T409R	8	28	62	↑ Activity

Table 4. Most common functional polymorphisms in major human CYP genes (adapted from Bluth MH, 2011).
DOI: http://dx.doi.org/10.2147/PGPM.S18861

Since both CYP1A2 and CYP2A6 can convert nicotine to cotinine, polymorphisms in these enzymes are associated with nicotine addiction and tobacco-related cancers. The CYP2B6 polymorphisms may affect the PK and therapeutic outcome of anti-HIV agents such as efavirenz and nevirapine. Indeed, the CYP2B6 variant, Q172H is linked to increased breakdown of these anti-HIV drugs in different minority population (Musana AK, 2005). The CYP2C9 accounts for ~20% of total hepatic CYP contents, and the CYP2C9*2 (R144C) and CYP2C9*3 (I359L) variants may affect PK of numerous important pharmaceutical agents such as warfarin, celecoxib, ibuprofen, phenytoin, etc. (Rettie AE, 2005). Interestingly, the CYP2C8*3 (R139K; K39R) is associated with lower activity and decreased clearance of both R- and S-ibuprofen, and polymorphisms in CYP2C19 effect the response of several classes of drugs, including proton pump inhibitors and barbiturates. Although CYP2D6 is involved in the metabolism of ~25% of all drugs, SNPs in this gene is mostly due to changes in activity rather than induction in gene expression. The CYP2D6 genotypes exhibit large interethnic differences and are of significant importance for the dosing of many drugs, including tricyclic antidepressants, antiarrhythmics, neuroleptics, analgesics, antiemetics, and anticancer drugs. CYP3A4 has the highest abundance in the human liver (~40%) and metabolizes over 50% of all currently used drugs. Genetic polymorphisms in CYP3A4 appear to be more prevalent in Caucasians, but a direct clinical association has not been established. The clinical relevance of CYP3A5 polymorphisms are demonstrated by changes in PK of immunosuppressive drugs such as tacrolimus.

4.2 Polymorphisms in drug-transporters

Within the SLC superfamily, genetic variance in organic anion-transporting polypeptides (OATPs) have been most well characterized (Kameyama Y, 2005; Xu G, 2005; Song IS, 2008; Franke RM, 2009). The OATPs are expressed in many tissues like liver, gut and BBB. OATP1B1 is one of the major uptake transporters expressed in hepatocytes and transports drugs like rifampin and statins etc. This protein is encoded by *SLCO1B1*, several allelic variants of which have been characterized and resulted in decreased transporter activity. Another example is OATP-C, which is a liver-specific transporter involved in the hepatocellular uptake of a variety of clinically important drugs. A number of functionally relevant SNPs have been reported in OATP (Xu G, 2005). In *in vitro* experiments several variants showed reduced uptake of the OATP-C substrates estradiol, estrone sulfate and E2-17-βG (Kameyama Y, 2005). Also, OATP-C variants were found to have reduced cell membrane expression compared with the wild-type transporter, especially under inflammatory conditions (Le Vee M, 2008). These studies have implicated SLC and OATP transporters in drug disposition as well as in normal physiological functions such as hormonal signaling.

Polymorphisms within the ABC transporter super family have been well classified and SNPs within *ABCB1* or *MDR-1* gene (coding for P-gp) serves as an excellent example (Hoffmeyer S, 2000; Tanabe M, 2001; Brinkmann U, 2001; Ieiri I, 2004). P-gp genes have a wide range of substrates including anti cancer agents, antiarrhythmics and immunosuppressive drugs (Drescher S, 2002; Hulot JS, 2005; Elens L, 2007; Thervet E, 2008). P-gp expression is widely distributed, liver, the intestines both small and large, and the blood brain barrier (BBB) endothelial cells. In addition, polymophisms in both MRP (ABCCs) and BCRP (ABCG) are expected to affect the pharmocokintics of several drugs, however, a clear pattern of increase or decrease has not yet been decipherable (Tamura A, 2006a & 2006b). Large inter-individual variability in P-gp expression, almost two to eight folds, has been observed in healthy volunteers, leading to significant differences in the bioavailability of P-gp substrate drugs within a population. Individual variations in the expression of ABC transporters may give rise to a change in the bioavailbility of a particular drug and may thus lead to a need for change in dosing. Increasing evidences demonstrate that both genotypic and phenotypic polymorphisms may affect membrane transporters and that this may well be the cause for variability of a drugs PK profile and toxicity in different ethnic groups [Table-5].

Allele variants	Polymorphism/ substitution	Allele frequency (%)*		
		Caucasian	Asian	African
ABCB1				
1236C>T	Silent	34–42	60–72	15–21
2677G>T	A893S	38–47	32–62	15/ND
/A	/T	/1–10	/3–22	
3435C>T	Silent	48–59	37–66	10–27
ABCB1*13	1236C>T/2677G> T/3435C>T haplotype	23–42	28–56	4.5–8.7
ABCC1				
128G>C	C43S		1	
1299G>T	R433S	1.4		
2012G>T	G671V	2.8		
ABCC2				
1271A>G	R412G			
1249G>A	V417I	22–26	13–19	14
3563T>A	V1188E	4–7	1	
4544G>A	C1515Y	4–9		
ABCG2				
34G>A	V12M	2–10	15–18	4–6
376C>T	Q126stop	0	0.9–1.7	0
421C>A	Q141K	9–14	27–35	1–5

Allele variant	Polymorphism/ substitution	Allele frequency (%)*		
		Caucasian	Asian	African
OATP				
SLCO1A2 (OATP1A2)				
38T>C	I13T	11.1	0	2.1
516A>C	E172D	5.3	0	2.1
833A	N278del	0	0	0.6
SLCO1B1 (OATP1B1)				
217T>C	F73L	2	0	0
388A>G	N130D	30	54	74
463C>A	P155T	16	0	2
521T>C	V174A	14	0.7	2
1463G>C	G488A	0		9
2000A>G	E667G	2		34
SLCO1B3 (OATP1B3)				
334T>G	S112A	74		
699G>A	M233I	71		
1564G>T	G522C	1.9		
SLCO2B1 (OATP2B1)				
1457C>T	S486F	1.2	30.9	
OCT				
SLC22A1 (OCT1)				
41C>T	S14F	0	0	3.1
480C>G	G160L	0.65	8.6–13.0	0.5
1022C>T	P341L	0	16	8.2
1201G>A	G401S	1.1	0	0.7
1222A>G	M408V	60	74–81	74
1256delATG	M420del	18	0	2.9

Table 5. Most common functional polymorphisms in major ABC and SLC transporters (adapted from Bluth MH, 2011).
DOI: http://dx.doi.org/10.2147/PGPM.S18861

Although our knowledge of polymorphisms in ABC and SLC transporters and their clinical association to different drug PK is just developing, the most common functional polymorphisms occurring in some of the major transporter genes, along with allele frequencies and functional effects, are provided in Table-5. Sequence diversity and haplotype structure in the human ABCB1 (MDR1, multidrug resistance transporter) gene were previously documented (Kroetz DL, 2003; Pauli-Magnus C, 2004; Wang J, 2006; Kimchi-Sarfaty C, 2007; Elens L, 2007). Numerous functional implications of these genetic polymorphisms in P-gp have also been clearly seen. Several SNPs in the ABCB1 gene, e.g. 1236C>T and 3435C>T are silent polymorphisms occurring outside of the coding region, and do not change the expression of P-gp (Hitzl M, 2001 & 2004). However, these SNPs change protein translation and substrate specificities. It has also been shown to affect its mRNA, may reduce heteronuclear RNA (hnRNA) processing and translation of the protein. Interestingly, these two SNPs have been shown to correlate with ethnic differences in drug disposition (Wang D, 2005). The ABCB1*13 genotype has also been shown to affect inhibition by some of the efflux-pump modulators. Several genetic polymorphisms in the *ABCC1* gene are associated with doxorubicin-induced cardiotoxicity (Wojnowski L, 2005). These SNPs were found to be associated with reduced intestinal expression of P-gp, along with increased oral bioavailability of digoxin. Several of the ABCC genes, which code for the MRP transporters, are known to affect both drug-efflux and apical to basal drug transport (Fellay J, 2002). Several ABCC1 SNPs have been associated with anthracycline-induced cardiotoxicity. The ABCC2 associated SNPs can alter their expression and localization within the cells. Also, several of them, e.g. 3563T>A (V1188E) and 4544G>A (C1515Y), have also been associated with anthracycline-induced cardiotoxicity. Several ABCG2 genetic variants, which code for the BCRP transporter, are also found to change transporter activities and have been associated with MDR tumors. Interestingly, unlike ABCB1 (P-gp), a clear clinical correlation with race has not been established with any of these other ABC-transporters.

Less emphasis has been placed on changes in passive diffusion due to polymorphisms in the SLC genes. Although numerous polymorphisms have been identified and code for altered protein such as SLCO1A2, SLCO1B1, CLCO1B3, etc, most of them have been shown to suppress facilitated diffusion of their substrates and some of these may also affect substrate specificities. However, due to the lack of correlative studies with these SNPs occurring in different OATP transporters, we know very little about their ultimate effects on drug disposition. Also, less is known about the role of polymorphisms in the phase-II enzymes, such as the UGT family members (Guillemette C. 2003; Han JY, 2006; Lo HW, 2007). Genetic variations in UGT genes alter the function or expression of the protein, and potentially modify the glucuronidation capacity of the enzyme. Furthermore, SNPs have been identified in most of the human SULT genes (Glatt H, 2004) which are associated with altered enzymatic activity and have the potential to influence therapeutic response. Two human NAT genes, *NAT1* and *NAT2*, carry functional polymorphisms that influence the enzyme activity (Hein DW. 2002; Walker K, 2009) and bioactivation (via O-acetylation) of aromatic and hetercyclic amine carcinogens. Patients who inherit defective *TPMT* alleles are at significantly increased risk for thiopurine-induced toxicity (e.g. myelosuppression) (Peregud-Pogorzelski J, 2010; Ben Salem C, 2010). Indeed, clinical diagnostic tests are now available for the detection of the SNPs in human *TPMT* gene that lead to decreased or abolished enzyme activity (Nguyen CM, 2011).

The above findings reiterate the fact that both genotypic and phenotypic polymorphisms may affect variability in drug disposition. Further studies of the polymorphisms in human drug-metabolizing enzymes and drug-transporters would shed more light on the subject of pharmacogenomics, and could be used in selecting drugs and dosages according to genetic and specific individual markers in order to individualize drug therapy. Just as for CYP450's, the possibility of defining patient populations and even individual patients on the basis of drug transporter polymorphisms may improve drug safety and efficacy in the future. Positron emission tomography (PET) may serve as a very useful tool in determining the *in vivo* effects of transporters and their polymorphisms (Martínez-Villaseñor D, 2006; Cantore M, 2011). Also in the future it would be valuable to establish a correlation between genotype and phenotype and then assess the effects of polymorphisms on drug transporter expression and function and in turn, effects on drug disposition.

5. Pharmacogenomics: A potent tool for maximizing chemotherapeutic response

5.1 Genetic variations in TMPT may be used to predict toxicity to 6-Mercaptopurine

Thiopurine methyltransferase (TPMT) catalyzes the S-methylation of 6-MP to form inactive metabolites. Genetic variations in the *TPMT* gene have profound effects on the bioavailability and toxicity of 6-MP. It has been demonstrated that about 1 in 300 individuals inherit TPMT deficiency as an autosomal recessive trait. Patients who carry *TPMT* polymorphisms are at risk for severe hematologic toxicities when treated with 6-MP because these polymorphisms lead to a decrease in the rate of 6-MP metabolism (Evans WE, 1991; Lennard L, 1993). Currently, TPMT testing is being used for dose optimization in children with ALL before 6-MP therapy is initiated.

5.2 Genetic variations in UGT1A1: The basis of inter-patient variability with Irinotecan therapy

Irinotecan (Camptosar®; Pfizer Pharmaceuticals; New York, NY, http://www.pfizer.com) has potent antitumor activity against a wide range of tumors, and it is one of the most commonly prescribed chemotherapy agents. However, dose-limiting toxicities of irinotecan interfere with optimal utilization of this important drug. Once consumed the drug requires metabolic activation by carboxylesterase to form the active metabolite 7-ethyl-10-hydroxycamptothecin (SN-38), which in turn inhibits topoisomerase-I. SN-38 is further detoxified via formation of SN-38 glucuronide (SN38G) (Gupta E, 1994). Toxicity of irinotecan has been associated with increased levels of SN-38. Clinical pharmacogenetics of irinotecan is mainly focused on polymorphisms in UDP-glucuronosyltransferase 1A1 (UGT1A1), the enzyme responsible for glucuronidation of SN-38 to the less toxic, inactive metabolite SN38G (Iyer L, 1998 & 1999). Variations in UGT1A1 activity most commonly arise from polymorphisms in the *UGT1A1* promoter region that contains several repeating TA elements. The presence of seven TA repeats (referred to as *UGT1A1*28*), instead of the wild-type number of six, results in reduced UGT1A1 expression and activity (Beutler E, 1998). Clinical trials are ongoing to address the impact of dose on irinotecan safety in patients with different *UGT1A1*28* genotypes (McLeod HL, 2004).

5.3 CYP2D6 allele activity affects clinical outcome of patients treated with tamoxifen

One in eight women above seventy develops breast cancer each year in the United States. Approximately 70 percent of them have estrogen receptor–positive cancer. Many of these women are prescribed tamoxifen following surgical treatment. Tamoxifen is an anti–estrogen drug that prevents relapse of cancer in 50% of patients and reduces the mortality rate by one–third in women with early breast cancer. However, there is a large group of women who do not respond to tamoxifen. CYP2D6 encodes for an enzyme involved in the metabolism of up to 25 percent of all drugs. The enzyme is present in different forms in different people and some lack it entirely. Tamoxifen is a "pro–drug," meaning that it is relatively inactive until the liver recruits the CYP2D6 enzyme and converts it into active molecules. The key role of CYP2D6 in catalyzing the conversion of tamoxifen to its abundant active metabolite endoxifen has been shown to directly affect the clinical outcome of patients treated with tamoxifen. This is because the functional alleles of ÇYP2D6 in some individuals result in abolished, decreased, normal, or ultrarapid CYP2D6 enzyme activity. Women with nonfunctional and reduced-function *CYP2D6* alleles appear to have significantly lower circulating endoxifen concentrations than those with wild-type *CYP2D6*. It has also been shown that use of CYP2D6 inhibitors such as SSRIs and SNRIs has a negative impact on the efficacy of tamoxifen. Together, these studies support the notion that low CYP2D6 activity, caused by genetic polymorphisms or drug interactions, leads to low levels of the active tamoxifen metabolite (Jin Y, 2005; Lim HS, 2007; Hoskins JM, 2009). The effect of CYP2D6 activity on tamoxifen pharmacokinetics also translates into an effect on clinical outcome. Despite conflicting data in some instance, the majority of retrospective studies suggest that the presence of nonfunctional or reduced-function alleles of CYP2D6 is associated with worse outcome of patients receiving tamoxifen. A recent large retrospective analysis of 1325 patients with early-stage breast cancer treated with adjuvant tamoxifen suggests that compared with extensive metabolizer, those with decreased CYP2D6 activity (heterozygous extensive/intermedidate and poor metabolizers) have significantly increased risk of recurrence as well as worse event-free survival and disease-free survival (Schroth W, 2009). In addition, *CYP2D6* genotype has also been shown to influence the efficacy of tamoxifen as a chemopreventive agent, whereby tamoxifen-treated women with poor metabolizer phenotype was associated with a significantly higher incidence of breast cancer compared with controls (Higgins MJ, 2010). Findings from these studies support a role for the *CYP2D6* genotype in the activation of tamoxifen and likelihood of therapeutic benefit from testing for *CYP2D6* genoptype.

6. Consequences of epigenetic factors on PG and PK

Genetic polymorphisms exhibited by many of the Phase-I and Phase-II drug-metabolizing enzymes as well as both passive and active drug-transporters, can alter drug distribution, drug metabolism and drug-drug interactions and are of great clinical relevance. However, a number of other factors may also contribute to the variation in polymorphism activity, including; (1) environmental factors, (2) age, sex and ethnicity of the patient, (3) physiological status, and (4) disease state. Therefore, in addition to genetic variations, changes in CYP450 enzyme functions and ABC and SLC transporter activities are responsible for the occurrence of adverse effects or lack of therapeutic efficacy of drugs in many cases.

6.1 Drug-drug interactions regulate drug disposition

Many coadministered drugs can increase or decrease the activity of various CYP isozymes, by either inducing the biosynthesis of an isozyme (enzyme induction) or by directly inhibiting the activity of the CYP (enzyme inhibition). If one drug inhibits the CYP-mediated metabolism of another drug, the second drug may accumulate within the body to toxic levels. Hence, these drug interactions may necessitate either dosage adjustments or choosing drugs that do not interact with the CYP system (Anglicheau D, 2003). Such drug interactions are especially important to take into account when using drugs of vital importance to the patient. Drugs with important side-effects and drugs with small therapeutic windows may be subject to an altered plasma concentration due to altered drug metabolism. A classical example includes anti-epileptic drugs (Li XQ, 2004; Li Y, 2008). CYP450 enzyme induction can occur following repeated administration of antibiotics such as Rifampin (Zhang HX, 2009). Numerous immunosuppressive drugs such as cyclosporine-A and FK-506, used in organ transplantation, show potent drug interactions and are important in pharmacogenetics (Thervet E, et al, 2008). Certain drugs can cause CYP enzyme inhibition by either binding to the cytochrome component or act to competitively inhibit drug metabolism. The histamine (H2) receptor antagonist, Cimetidine (Tagamet) and the antifungal agent, Ketoconazole (Nizoral) are known to be potent inhibitors of multiple CYPs. Several antibiotics can cause catalytic inactivation of CYPs as well. The Macrolide antibiotics (e.g. erythromycin), which are themselves metabolized by CYPs are known to complex with the cytochrome heme-iron, producing a complex that is catalytically inactive. In addition, Chloramphenicols which are also substrates of CYPs have been shown to inactivate these enzymes by their direct inactivation. It is expected that poor metabolizers would have higher concentrations of a drug that is inactivated by that enzyme pathway and therefore require a lower dose to avoid adverse reactions, whereas ultrarapid metabolizers would require a higher dose to achieve therapeutically effective drug concentrations. The opposite pattern of reactions is expected for a drug that undergoes metabolic activation. Both tobacco use and drugs of abuse, as well as dietary factors can impact CYP450 enzymes and ABC transporters, expression and function. One of the most documented relationships between disease and transporter expression is the association between the overexpression of ABC transporters and the concomitant increased efflux of chemotherapeutic drugs such as vinca-alkaloids, epipodophyllotoxins, and anthracyclines.

6.2 Social and dietary factors regulate drug disposition

Increasing evidence supports the assertion that one mechanism behind clinically significant herb-drug and food-drug interactions is interference at the level of ABC transporters and CYP enzymes (Zhang W, 2005; Marchetti et al., 2011). Naturally occurring compounds may also induce or inhibit CYP activity. For instance, grapefruit, orange, and pimelo juices inhibit CYP3A4 and P-gp function, which impacts metabolism and increases drug bioavailability, and, thus, the strong possibility of overdosing. Approximately 10% of all admissions in general hospitals are the result of inappropriate administration of drugs or combinations of drugs that can cause severe to lethal drug-drug or herb-drug interactions. Grapefruit Juice, regularly used as a digestive and dieuretic agent, is also known to be a potent inhibitor of CYPs (Bailey DG, 1998). The drugs most susceptible to pharmacokinetic interactions with citrus juices are those with a narrow therapeutic index and a reported affect by P-gp or CYP enzymes; thus, physicians and patients should be cognizant of these clinically significant food-drug interactions when prescribing or following drug treatment (Marchetti et al., 2011). The principle compounds in these Citrus fruits, furanocoumarins and flavonoids, cause interactions with over 50% of the most commonly prescribed drugs in major drug classes such as antiallergics, antibiotics, anxiolytics, calcium channel blockers and HIV protease inhibitors (Cuciureanu M, 2010; Kakar SM, 2004; Pillai et al., 2009). In contrast, although regular consumption of these citrus juices may decrease the therapeutically efficacious dose required, co-administration with drugs such as astemizole, terfenadine, or verapamil may severely increase drug plasma levels and result in toxicity or fatality (Bailey et al., 1998; Pillai et al., 2009).

Several other dietary components and supplements influence drug bioavailability. For example, Watercress is also a known inhibitor of CYP2E1, which may result in altered drug metabolism for individuals on certain medications (e.g., chlorzoxazone) (van Erp NP, 2005). St. John's Wort (SJW), a common herbal remedy and antidepressant, can induce CYP3A4, and also inhibit multiple CYP enzymes such as CYP1A1, CYP1B1 and CYP2D6 (Schwarz UI, 2007; Lei HP, 2010; Lau WC, 2011). Clinical studies demonstrated that coadministration of SJW significantly reduced plasma concentrations of drugs including oral contraceptives, warfarin, verapamil and fexofenadine which was associated with both failures of therapies and under treatment (Marchetti et al., 2011). Coadministration of SJW and the HIV protease inhibitor, indinavir, or the cardiac glycoside, digoxin increased intestinal P-gp expression and produced significantly lower plasma area under the concentration-time curves. Chronic administration of SJW and cyclosporine-A significantly reduced plasma levels of cyclosporine-A, and increased acute organ rejection in transplanted patients. Curcumin, curcuminoids and catechins from green tea reduce P-gp expression *in vitro* and reports indicate that piperine, ginsenosides, capsaicin, resveratrol and silymarin inhibit *in vitro* P-gp activity.

Socially used factors such as tobacco and alcohol activate receptors that modulate P-gp and CYP expression. A genetic polymorphism in the regulatory sequences of human CYP2E1 has been associated with increased liver toxicity following ethanol consumption, especially in obese individuals (McCarver DG, 1998). Tobacco smoking also induces CYP1A2 and changes the bioavailability of numerous CYP1A2 substrates such as clozapine and olanzapine (Bartsch H, 2000). Significantly greater non-small cell lung cancer tumors were P-gp positive in smokers compared to non-smokers (Volm et al., 1991). Although it remains unclear if P-gp expression levels definitively play a defensive role towards tobacco-derived agents, there is a correlation between current smoking and resistance to the anthracycline drug doxorubicin. Therefore, significant amount of current literature verifies that drug bioavailability can be modulated by components in foods and herbs that regulate drug-metabolizing enzymes and drug-transporters. Hence, dietary components and herbal supplements has important clinical implications, especially in those individuals containing specific augmenting or suppressing polymorphisms in their CYP450 enzymes and/or ABC-transporters.

6.3 Drug disposition: Effects age, sex and ethnicity

Aging is characterized, in part, by alterations in all stages of pharmacokinetic processes (absorption, distribution, metabolism, and excretion), several of which can affect the safety/efficacy profile of a variety of drugs (McLeod HL, 1992; Aronoff GR, 1999; Bjorkman S. 2006; Corsonello A, 2010). The elderly population is more sensitive to bleeding complications arising from warfarin administration which may be attributed to variations in CYP2C9 function. In addition, elderly patients are especially susceptible to adverse drug reactions due to comorbidity, use of multiple pharmaceutics, and age-related changes in PK (Burk O, 2002; Anglicheau D, 2003). Specific CYPs are inhibited by numerous drugs commonly prescribed to elderly patients, a fact that may help explain significant pharmacological interactions. For instance, the distribution of drugs acting on the CNS can be significantly affected by the changes of BBB permeability which occurs with aging. Several drugs are effluxed via the activity of cerebrovascular P-gp at the BBB; therefore, age-related regression in P-gp function could increase drug levels in the CNS (Corsonello et al., 2010). The CYP450-mediated hepatic drug clearance in neonates, infants and children were found to differ significantly from adults and was a predictor of drug response (Bjorkman S. 2006). The hepatic clearance of drugs in older patients can be reduced more than 40%, some of which may be attributed to alteration in CYP enzyme activity. Although some studies suggest that CYP-mediated activity and enzyme affinity for their substrates are not altered during the aging process, clinically relevant changes in drug-metabolizing enzyme expression have been observed. For instance, a clear age-related decline (20%) in the metabolism of CYP2D6 substrates has been demonstrated (Corsonello et al. 2010; Dorne et al., 2002; O'Connell et al., 2006). Selective serotonin reuptake inhibitors (SSRIs) can inhibit

CYP2D6 activity and therefore reduce the efficiency of drugs that need to be activated by CYP2D6 when coadministered, such as tamoxifen and codeine. The antiplatelet drug clopidogrel is prescribed to prevent stroke and heart attack and it requires CYP2C19 for activation. Omeprazole, a drug used to treat gastroesophageal reflux disease, is both a substrate and an inhibitor of CYP2C19. As a result, individuals with reduced CYP2C19-mediated activity will suffer from impaired clopidogrel bioactivation and enhanced accumulation of omeprazole (Furuta et al., 1998; Li et al., 2004; Roden et al., 2009).

The predominant enzymes involved in phase I hepatic drug metabolism are CYPs, several of which show clear sex-related differences and impact drug clearance (Soldin OP, 2009). Individuals exhibit great variation in biotransformation and although most 'sex-dependent' differences are eliminated with correction for height, as well as weight, composition, and surface area of the body, sex-dependent differences in biotransformation of a few drugs such as nicotine, aspirin, heparin, flurazepam, and chlordiazepoxide have been demonstrated. For instance, the activity of enzymes CYP1A and CYP2E1 is higher in men, while a higher activity of CYP2D6 and CYP3A4 enzymes have been observed in women (O'Connell MB, 2006). A series of physiological changes that are known to affect drug plasma concentrations occur during gestation and pregnancy, one of which causes significant changes in CYP enzyme activity. To date, the PK data amassed pertaining to menopause-related intestinal and hepatic CYP3A4 activity found no significant differences in biotransformation and drug clearance in pre- and postmenopausal women. Sex-related and pregnancy-related changes in drug metabolism and elimination may guide changes in dosage regimen or therapeutic monitoring to reduce possible toxicity and increase drug efficacy (Soldin and Mattison, 2009).

Race related changes in the CYP enzyme and ABC transporter activation and regulation may alter drug accumulation and contribute to the increasing occurrence of adverse drug reactions in elderly patients. Pharmacodynamic differences between races can be associated with changes in drug transporters, and both differences in baseline performance and sensitivity to treatment is attributed to drug efflux from tissues. For instance, some drugs may penetrate the CNS more readily with advancing age thereby increasing their bioavailability. The variation in frequency of SNPs for MDR1 in different racial/ethnic populations has been previously documented. Allelic frequency can differ among these groups (Kim RB, 2001; McLeod H. 2002; Hesselink DA, 2004). The incidence of C/T and C/C genotypes at position 3435 has been found to be much higher in African than in Caucasian or Asian populations (Wang D, 2005; Wang J, 2006). One crucial factor regulating drug levels is African Americans is P-gp function since decreases in P-gp expression has been linked to increased drug serum concentrations and extended drug residence time within the brain (Tirona RG, 2001). While only 26% of Caucasians and 34% of Japanese were homozygous for the C allele, 83% of Ghanaians and 61% of African Americans were homozygous for the C allele (Xie XG, 2001. Certain common allelic variants of CYP3A4 were found to be highly prevalent in different minority populations (Lamba JK, 2002a & 2002b Koch I, 2002). Population distribution and effects on drug metabolism of a genetic variant in the promoter region of CYP3A4 were also previously documented (Ball SE, 1999; Schaeffeler E, 2001). In fact, the functional decline in P-gp may play a role in the increased sensitivity to selected benzodiazepines such as flurazepam reported in patients with specific P-gp SNPs. Therefore, individualized prescriptions for patients should incorporate knowledge from basic pharmacology, race or ethnicity, clinical practice and pharmacosurveillance (Sim SC, 2005; Corsonello et al., 2010). Therefore, age, sex and race related changes in the CYP enzyme and ABC transporter activation and regulation may alter drug accumulation and contribute to the increasing occurrence of adverse drug reactions.

6.4 Patient health status dictate drug disposition

The most noteworthy condition which alter drug bioavailability in patients is chronic renal failure (CRF) which has been shown to significantly reduce renal clearance of drugs which are predominantly metabolized by the liver and intestine (Bjorkman S, 2006). Patients with CRF exhibit decreased volume of distribution for a variety of drugs due to reduced renal and skeletal muscle mass and decreased tissue binding. In both preclinical and clinical studies, drug transporters such as P-gp and CYPs are affected. In fact, CRF causes a 40 to 85 % downregulation of hepatic and intestinal CYPs with high levels of hormones, cytokines, and uremic toxins also reducing CYP activity. The alteration in these enzymes and proteins affects drug bioavailability and increases the risk for adverse drug reactions (Dreisbach and Lertora 2008; Dreisbach 2009). In transplant patients on cyclosporine-A or tacrolimus, studies have shown changes in both CYP3A4 and P-glycoprotein activity in healthy controls and patients (Lemahieu WP, 2004). In addition to the condition or disease alone regulating enzyme activity and transporter expression, consideration should be applied during treatment for patients on multiple medications (van der Deen M, 2005). P-gp can regulate drug uptake in the CNS and is expressed constitutively in endothelial cells that form the BBB. The expression, however, can be activated or inhibited by other compounds or modified under pathological conditions. For instance, antipsychotics, antiepileptics, or antidepressants that are P-gp substrates can interact at the P-gp level and may be responsible for some documented cases of drug resistance. An induction of P-gp expression decreases psychotropic drug uptake in the central nervous system, which ultimately reduces drug efficacy (Wikinski, 2005). While the health of a patients during treatment may be primarily shaped by their disease and drug disposition, social factors will also influence treatment outcome and should be taken into account during therapeutic decisions.

7. Drug efflux-drug metabolism alliance

There is considerable overlap in the substrate selectivity and tissue localization of specific groups of CYP450 enzymes and ABC transporters (Benet LZ, 2001 & 2004). Common substrates, inhibitors and inducers for CYP3A and P-gp clearly implicate that both common regulatory mechanisms and cross-talk between this CYP iso-enzyme and drug-efflux pump can ultimately regulate drug disposition. Interestingly, in CYP3A4-transfected Caco-2 cells the expression of several efflux transporters, e.g. P-gp, MRP1, and MRP2 were upregulated, especially after stimulation of cells with either the protein kinase-A (PKA) inducer sodium butyrate or the protein kinase-C (PKC) inducer phorbol ester 12-O-tetradecanoylphorbol-13-acetate (PMA) (Cummins, CL, 2001 & 2002). In an *in vivo* intestinal perfusion model, these investigators had also shown modulation of intestinal CYP3A metabolism by P-gp (Cummins, CL, 2003). This has led to the hypothesis that both drug-transporter and drug-metabolizing enzymes act as a coordinated barrier against xenobiotic agents. Several animal studies using mdr1a (−/−) knockout mice have demonstrated P-gp's importance in limiting drug absorption and decreasing bioavailability. Human clinical studies investigating the importance of intestinal CYP3A and P-gp through inhibition or induction of these proteins have provided further evidence of this interaction. Recent *in vitro* studies using CYP3A4-expressing Caco-2 cells reveal that the role of P-gp in the intestine not only limits parent drug absorption, but also increases the access of drug to metabolism by CYP3A through repeated cycles of absorption and efflux. These early findings suggested a biochemical link or coregulation of the drug-efflux and drug-metabolism functions in cells (Benet LZ, 2001; Cummins CL, 2002). A number of recent studies further corroborate this dynamic interplay between different ABC-transporters and different Cyp450 enzymes (Lam JL, 2006; Lee NH, 2010). These studies, carried out in cellular systems, isolated organ, whole animal and human studies, have elucidated the importance of these interacting processes. The importance of this phenomenon with respect to the intestine and the liver, characterizing inhibition and induction of apical and basolateral transporters and how drug metabolism can change independent of any change in the metabolic enzymes, has been effectively shown.

8. Conclusions

As alluded to in the previous section, drug-drug interactions, environmental and physiological factors significantly contribute to inter-individual variability in drug PK. However, these differences are not sufficient to explain the significant heterogeneity associated with patient responses to therapeutic agents and their narrow therapeutic indices. Continued investigation and adaptation of PG with respect to understanding PK should provide improved benefit to therapeutic efficacy versus side effect profiles of many drugs currently available. Studies are being translated to clinical practice via molecular diagnostics (genotyping) and identifying relevant inherited variations that may better predict patient response to chemotherapy. Among these, nucleotide repeats, insertions, deletions, and SNPs, which can alter the amino acid sequence of the encoded proteins, RNA splicing and gene transcription particularly in drug-metabolizing enzymes and drug transporters have been actively explored with regard to functional changes in phenotype (altered expression levels and/or activity of the encoded proteins) and their contribution to variable drug response. Recent studies also indicate that information on combination of polymorphisms that are inherited together (haplotype analysis) can often result in better correlation with phenotypes than with individual polymorphisms. The potential is enormous for PG to yield a powerful set of molecular diagnostic methods that will become routine tools with which clinicians will select medications and drug doses for individual patients. Gene-expression profiling and proteomic studies are evolving strategies for identifying genes that may influence drug response. Thus, patient oriented PG will provide a very unique approach towards increasing the therapeutic efficacies of numerous anti-cancer, anti-viral as well as anti-diabetic drugs. Furthermore, an effective re-evaluation of new drug design toward the generation of specific therapies focused on drugs that are not critically affected by the Cyp450 enzymes and the drug-transporter biology may eventually lead to personalized and individualized medicine. However, there are a number of issues which must be considered before developing strategies that target these inherited determinants of drug effects. One formidable challenge would be the fact that these inherited components are often polygenic and a complex interplay between genetic and epigenetic factors may ultimately dictate drug disposition. Therefore, the limitations of the current PG approaches will be the lack of complete knowledge and understanding of the complex mechanisms of drug distribution and drug-drug interactions. Another very important hurdle in correctly delineating the pharmacogenetic traits that regulate individualistic differences is the need for well characterized *in vivo* models. Studies in transgenic and knockout animals are proving highly efficacious in this respect, but only accounts for monogenic traits. Patient populations, with race, gender and ethnicity specified, who have been uniformly treated and systematically evaluated for drug action and toxicities, will be highly instrumental in making it possible to quantify the role of different CYP450 enzymes and ABC-transporters, objectively. The marked population heterogeneity has deterred a clear understanding of the effects of specific genotypes and their importance in determining efficacy. The effects of a medication for one population or disease may not as effective for another population; therefore, PG relations must be validated for each therapeutic indication and in different racial and ethnic groups, which will indeed be a daunting task. However, since genotyping methods are improving rapidly, it will be possible to test for thousands of polymorphisms which determine patient responses. In a clinical setting, it should be easy to collect patient samples and carry out a panel of genotypes and test for those which are important determinants of drug disposition. With the advent of new computer programming and new softwares to delineate pathways and interactions, it will be possible to simplify the complexities of the alliances between drug metabolizers and drug transporters. We believe that in the near future, genotyping results will be of great clinical value only if they are interpreted according to the patient's diagnosis. An effective and safe treatment option can then be recommended by the physician.

9. Acknowledgements

We would like to thank Mrs. Nancy Busija (MA, CCC-SLP) for critical reading and editing of the chapter. Time allotted to this chapter was supported by funds from Tulane University Medical Center (TUMC) and Tulane Cancer Center (TCC) given to Dr. Mondal.

10. References

Abdel-Tawab M, Werz O, Schubert-Zsilavecz M. Boswellia serrata: an overall assessment of in vitro, preclinical, pharmacokinetic and clinical data. Clin Pharmacokinet. 2011 Jun 1;50(6):349-69. Review.

Allabi AC, Gala JL, Horsmans Y, et al. Functional impact of CYP2C9*5, CYP2C9*6, CYP2C9*8, and CYP2C9*11 in vivo among black Africans. Clin Pharmacol Ther. 2004;76:113-118.

Ameyaw MM, Regateiro F, Li T, et al. MDR1 pharmacogenetics: frequency of the C3435T mutation in exon 26 is significantly influenced by ethnicity. Pharmacogenetics 2001;11:217-21.

Anglicheau D, Flamant M, Schlageter MH, et al. Pharmacokinetic interaction between corticosteroids and tacrolimus after renal transplantation. Nephrol Dial Transplant 2003; 18 (11): 2409-14

Aragon-Ching JB, Zujewski JA. CNS metastasis: an old problem in a new guise. Clin Cancer Res. 2007 Mar 15;13(6):1644-7. Review.

Aronoff GR, Berns JS, Brier ME, et al. Drug Prescribing in Renal Failure: Dosing Guidelines for Adults. 4th ed. Philadelphia, PA: ACP-ASIM; 1999.

Avila MD, Morgan JP, Yan X. Genetically modified mouse models used for studying the role of the AT2 receptor in cardiac hypertrophy and heart failure. J Biomed Biotechnol. 2011;2011:141039. Epub 2011 Apr 27. Review.

Awad WA, Aschenbach JR, Setyabudi FM, Razzazi-Fazeli E, Böhm J, Zentek J. In vitro effects of deoxynivalenol on small intestinal D-glucose uptake and absorption of deoxynivalenol across the isolated jejunal epithelium of laying hens. Poult Sci. 2007 Jan;86(1):15-20.

Bailey DG, Malcolm J, Arnold O., & Spence JD. Grapefruit-juice drug interactions. British Journal of Clinical Pharmacology.1998. 46, 2, pp. 101 – 110.

Baiocchi M, Biffoni M, Ricci-Vitiani L, Pilozzi E, De Maria R. New models for cancer research: human cancer stem cell xenografts. Curr Opin Pharmacol. 2010 Aug;10(4):380-4. Epub 2010 Jun 17. Review.

Ball SE, Scatina J, Kao J, et al. Population distribution and effects on drug metabolism of a genetic variant in the 50 promoter region of CYP3A4. Clin Pharmacol Ther 1999; 66 (3): 288-94

Bartsch H, Nair U, Risch A, Rojas M, Wikman H, Alexandrov K. Genetic polymorphisms of CYP genes, alone or in combination, as a risk modifier of tobacco-related cancers. Cancer Epidemiol Biomarkers Prev. 2000;9:3-28.

Basnet P, Skalko-Basnet N. Curcumin: an anti-inflammatory molecule from a curry spice on the path to cancer treatment. Molecules. 2011 Jun 3;16(6):4567-98. Review.

Bauer F, Kuntner C, Bankstahl JP, Wanek T, Bankstahl M, Stanek J, Mairinger S, Dörner B, Löscher W, Müller M, Erker T, Langer O. Synthesis and in vivo evaluation of [11C]tariquidar, a positron emission tomography radiotracer based on a third-generation P-glycoprotein inhibitor. Bioorg Med Chem. 2010 Aug 1;18(15):5489-97.

Ben Salem C, Ben Salah L, Belajouza C, Bouraoui K. Azathioprine-induced severe cholestatic hepatitis in patient carrying TPMT*3C polymorphism. Pharm World Sci. 2010 Dec;32(6):701-3

Benet LZ, Cummins CL, Wu C-Y. Unmasking the dynamic interplay between efflux transporters and metabolic enzymes Int. J. Pharm. 2004, 277, 3– 9

Benet LZ, Cummins CL. The drug efflux-metabolism alliance: biochemical aspects. Adv Drug Deliv Rev 2001; 50 Suppl. 1: S3-11

Benet LZ. The drug transporter-metabolism alliance: uncovering and defining the interplay. Mol Pharm. 2009 Nov-Dec;6(6):1631-43. Review.

Beutler E, Gelbart T, Demina A. Racial variability in the UDP-glucuronosyltransferase 1 (*UGT1A1*) promoter: a balanced polymorphism for regulation of bilirubin metabolism? Proc Natl Acad Sci USA 1998;95:8170–8174.

Bjorkman S. Prediction of cytochrome p450-mediated hepatic drug clearance in neonates, infants and children: how accurate are available scaling methods? Clin Pharmacokinet 2006; 45 (1): 1-11

Bluth MH, Li J. Pharmacogenomics of drug metabolizing enzymes and transporters: implications for cancer therapy Pharmacogenomics and Personalized Medicine. 2011;4: 11 – 33

Board PG. The use of glutathione transferase-knockout mice as pharmacological and toxicological models. Expert Opin Drug Metab Toxicol. 2007 Jun;3(3):421-33.Review.

Bogard KN, Peterson NT, Plumb TJ, Erwin MW, Fuller PD, Olsen KM. Antibiotic dosing during sustained low-efficiency dialysis: special considerations in adult critically ill patients. Crit Care Med. 2011 Mar;39(3):560-70. Review.

Boiangiu CD, Jayamani E, Brügel D, Herrmann G, Kim J, Forzi L, Hedderich R, Vgenopoulou I, Pierik AJ, Steuber J, Buckel W. Sodium ion pumps and hydrogen production in glutamate fermenting anaerobic bacteria. J Mol Microbiol Biotechnol. 2005;10(2-4):105-19. Review.

Booth RA, Ansari MT, Loit E, Tricco AC, Weeks L, Doucette S, Skidmore B, Sears M, Sy R, Karsh J. Assessment of thiopurine S-methyltransferase activity in patients prescribed thiopurines: a systematic review. Ann Intern Med. 2011 Jun 21;154(12):814-23, W-295-8. Review.

Borst P, Evers R, Kool M, Wijnholds J. A family of drug transporters: the multidrug resistance-associated proteins. J Natl Cancer Inst 2000;92:1295-302.

Brinkmann U, Roots I, Eichelbaum M. Pharmacogenetics of the human drugtransporter gene MDR1: impact of polymorphisms on pharmacotherapy. Drug Discov Today 2001;6:835-9.

Brockmeier D. Estimating reduced availability due to first pass elimination from relative total clearance and renal clearance. Eur J Clin Pharmacol. 1988;35(4):397-400.

Brown AS, James OF. Omeprazole, ranitidine, and cimetidine have no effect on peak blood ethanol concentrations, first pass metabolism or area under the time-ethanol curve under 'real-life' drinking conditions. Aliment Pharmacol Ther. 1998 Feb;12(2):141-5.

Burk O, Tegude H, Koch I, et al. Molecular mechanisms of polymorphic CYP3A7 expression in adult human liver and intestine. J Biol Chem 2002;277 (27): 24280-8

Cantore M, Capparelli E, Berardi F, Perrone R, Colabufo NA. Clinical Pharmacokinetic and Metabolism of PET Radiotracers for Imaging P-glycoprotein in Chemoresistant Tumor of Colorectal Cancer. Curr Drug Metab. 2011 Jul 25. [Epub ahead of print].

Cascorbi I, Haenisch S. Pharmacogenetics of ATP-binding cassette transporters and clinical implications. Methods Mol Biol. 2010;596:95-121.

Choo EF, Leake B, Wandel C, et al. Pharmacological inhibition of P-glycoprotein transport enhances the distribution of HIV-1 protease inhibitors into brain and testes. Drug Metab Dispos 2000;28:655-60.

Conrad S, Kauffmann HM, Ito K, et al. A naturally occurring mutation in MRP1 results in a selective decrease in organic anion transport and in increased doxorubicin resistance. Pharmacogenetics. 2002;12: 321–330.

Corsonello A, Pedone C, & Antonelli Incalzi R. Age-related pharmacokinetic and pharmacodynamic changes and related risk of adverse drug reactions. Current Medicinal Chemistry.2010.17, 6, pp. 571 - 584.

Cuciureanu M, Vlase L, Muntean D, Varlan I, & Cuciureanu R. Grapefruit juice—drug interactions: importance for pharmacotherapy. Revista medico-chirurgicala a Societatii de Medici si Naturalisti din Iasi.2010. 114, 3, pp. 885 - 891.

Cummins CL, Jacobsen W, Benet LZ. Unmasking the dynamic interplay between intestinal P-glycoprotein and CYP3A4. J Pharmacol Exp Ther 2002; 300 (3): 1036-45

Cummins CL, Mangravite LM, Benet LZ. Characterizing the expression of CYP3A4 and efflux transporters (P-gp, MRP1, and MRP2) in CYP3A4-transfected Caco-2 cells after induction with sodium butyrate and the phorbol ester 12-O-tetradecanoylphorbol-13-acetate Pharm. Res. 2001, 18, 1102– 1109

Cummins CL, Salphati L, Reid MJ, Benet LZ. In vivo modulation of intestinal CYP3A metabolism by P-glycoprotein: studies using the rat single-pass intestinal perfusion model J. Pharmacol. Exp. Ther. 2003, 305, 306– 314

Daly AK. Significance of the minor cytochrome P450 3A isoforms. Clin Pharmacokinet 2006; 45 (1): 13-31

Davidson AL, Dassa EO, & Chen J. Structure, function, and evolution of bacterial ATP-binding cassette systems. Microbiology and Molecular Biology Reviews, 2008. 72, 2, pp. 317 - 364.

Degorter MK, Xia CQ, Yang JJ, Kim RB. Drug Transporters in Drug Efficacy and Toxicity. Annu Rev Pharmacol Toxicol. 2011 Jan 17. [Epub ahead of print]

Desta Z, Ward BA, Soukhova NV, et al. Comprehensive evaluation of tamoxifen sequential biotransformation by the human cytochrome P450 system in vitro: prominent roles for CYP3A and CYP2D6. J Pharmacol Exp Ther. 2004;310:1062–1075.

DiazGranados N, Zarate CA Jr. A review of the preclinical and clinical evidence for protein kinase C as a target for drug development for bipolar disorder. Curr Psychiatry Rep. 2008 Dec;10(6):510-9. Review.

Dobson PD, Kell DB. Carrier-mediated cellular uptake of pharmaceutical drugs: an exception or the rule? Nat Rev Drug Discov. 2008 Mar;7(3):205-20. Review.

Dorne JL, Walton K, Slob W, & Renwich AG. Human variability in polymorphic CYP2D6 metabolism: is the kinetic default uncertainty factor adequate? Food and Chemical Toxicology.2002. 40, pp. 1633 – 1656.

Dossing M, Pilsgaard H, Rasmussen B, Poulsen HE. Time course of phenobarbital and cimetidine mediated changes in hepatic drug metabolism. Eur J Clin Pharmacol 1983;25:215-22.

Dreisbach AW, & Lertora JJ. The effect of chronic renal failure on drug metabolism and transport. Expert Opinion on Drug Metabolism and Toxicology.2008. 4, 8, pp. 1065 – 1074.

Dreisbach AW. The influence of chronic renal failure on drug metabolism and transport. Clinical Pharmacology and Therapeutics.2009. 86, 5, pp. 553 – 556.

Drescher S, Schaeffeler E, Hitzl M, et al. MDR1 gene polymorphisms and disposition of the P-glycoprotein substrate fexofenadine. Br J Clin Pharmacol 2002; 53 (5): 526-34

Durán JM, Cano M, Peral MJ, Ilundáin AA. D-mannose transport and metabolism in isolated enterocytes. Glycobiology. 2004 Jun;14(6):495-500. Epub 2004 Mar 19.

Eilers M, Roy U, Mondal D. MRP (ABCC) transporters-mediated efflux of anti-HIV drugs, saquinavir and zidovudine, from human endothelial cells. Exp Biol Med (Maywood). 2008 Sep;233(9):1149-60.

Elens L, Capron A, Kerckhove VV, et al. 1199G>A and 2677G>T/A polymorphisms of ABCB1 independently affect tacrolimus concentration in hepatic tissue after liver transplantation. Pharmacogenet Genomics 2007; 17 (10): 873-83

Evans W, Schentag J, Jusko J (editors): Applied Pharmacokinetics (3rd edition). San Francisco, CA. Applied Therapeutics, 1992.

Evans WE, Horner M, Chu YQ et al. Altered mercaptopurine metabolism, toxic effects, and dosage requirement in a thiopurine methyltransferase-deficient child with acute lymphocytic leukemia. J Pediatr 1991;119:985–989.

Evans WE, Johnson JA. Pharmacogenomics: the inherited basis for interindividual differences in drug response. Annu Rev Genomics Hum Genet 2001;2:9-39.

Evans WE, McLeod HL. Pharmacogenomics: drug disposition, drug targets, and side effects. N Engl J Med 2003; 348 (6): 538-49

Evans WE, Relling MV. Clinical pharmacokinetics-pharmacodynamics of anticancer drugs. Clin Pharmacokinet. 1989 Jun;16(6):327-36. Review.

Evans WE, Relling MV. Pharmacogenomics: translating functional genomics into rational therapeutics. Science 1999;286:487-91.

Fasolo A, Sessa C. Translational research in phase I trials. Clin Transl Oncol. 2009 Sep;11(9):580-8. Review.

Fellay J, Marzolini C, Meaden ER, et al. Response to antiretroviral treatment in HIV-1-infected individuals with allelic variants of the multidrug resistance transporter 1: a pharmacogenetics study. Lancet 2002;359: 30-6.

Fesler P, Mimran A. Estimation of glomerular filtration rate: what are the pitfalls? Curr Hypertens Rep. 2011 Apr;13(2):116-21. Review.

Franke RM, Scherkenbach LA, Sparreboom A. Pharmacogenetics of the organic anion transporting polypeptide 1A2. Pharmacogenomics. 2009;10:339–344.

Fromm MF. Importance of P-glycoprotein for drug disposition in humans. Eur J Clin Invest 2003; 33 Suppl. 2: 6-9

Furuse M. Molecular basis of the core structure of tight junctions. Cold Spring Harb Perspect Biol. 2010 Jan;2(1):a002907. Review.

Furuta T, Ohashi K, Kamata T, Takashima M, Kosuge K, Kawakaki T, Hanai H, Kubota T, Ishizaki T, & Kaneko E. Effect of genetic differences in omeprazole metabolism on cure rates for Helicobacter pylori infection and peptic ulcer. Annals of Internal Medicine.1998. 129, pp. 1027 – 1030.

Gardiner SJ, Begg EJ. Pharmacogenetic testing for drug metabolizing enzymes: is it happening in practice? Pharmacogenet Genomics. 2005;15:365-369.

Gether U, Andersen PH, Larsson OM, Schousboe A. Neurotransmitter transporters: molecular function of important drug targets. Trends Pharmacol Sci. 2006 Jul;27(7):375-83.

Glatt H, Meinl W. Pharmacogenetics of soluble sulfotransferases (SULTs). Naunyn Schmiedebergs Arch Pharmacol. 2004;369: 55–68.

Goteti K, Brassil PJ, Good SS, Garner CE. Estimation of human drug clearance using multiexponential techniques. J Clin Pharmacol. 2008 Oct;48(10):1226-36. Epub 2008 Jun 16.

Gottesman MM, Fojo T, Bates SE. Multidrug resistance in cancer: role of ATP-dependent transporters. Nat Rev Cancer. 2002;2:48–58.

Gradhand U, Kim RB. Pharmacogenomics of MRP transporters (ABCC1-5) and BCRP (ABCG2). Drug Metab Rev. 2008;40:317–354.

Guengerich FP. Cytochrome p450 and chemical toxicology. Chemical Research in Toxicology.2008. 21, 1, pp. 70 – 83.

Guillemette C. Pharmacogenomics of human UDP-glucuronosyltransferase enzymes. Pharmacogenomics J. 2003;3(3):136–158.

Gulinello M, Putterman C. The MRL/lpr mouse strain as a model for neuropsychiatric systemic lupus erythematosus. J Biomed Biotechnol.2011;2011:207504. Epub 2011 Feb 10. Review.

Gupta E, Lestingi TM, Mick R et al. Metabolic fate of irinotecan in humans: correlation of glucuronidation with diarrhea. Cancer Res 1994;54:3723–3725.

Haber PS, Gentry RT, Mak KM, Mirmiran-Yazdy SA, Greenstein RJ, Lieber CS. Metabolism of alcohol by human gastric cells: relation to first-pass metabolism. Gastroenterology. 1996 Oct;111(4):863-70.

Hagenbuch B, Meier PJ. The superfamily of organic anion transporting polypeptides. Biochim. Biophys. Acta 2003, 1609, 1– 18

Han JY, Lim HS, Shin ES, et al. Comprehensive analysis of UGT1A polymorphisms predictive for pharmacokinetics and treatment outcome in patients with non-small-cell lung cancer treated with irinotecan and cisplatin. J Clin Oncol. 2006;24:2237–2244.

Hans H. (Editor). "The laboratory mouse". The handbook of experimental animals. Elsevier Academic Press. 2004

Harguindey S, Arranz JL, Wahl ML, Orive G, Reshkin SJ. Proton transport inhibitors as potentially selective anticancer drugs. Anticancer Res. 2009 Jun;29(6):2127-36. Review.

Hartmann B, Czock D, Keller F. Drug therapy in patients with chronic renal failure. Dtsch Arztebl Int. 2010 Sep;107(37):647-55; quiz 655-6. Epub 2010 Sep 17. Review.

Hein DW. Molecular genetics and function of NAT1 and NAT2: role in aromatic amine metabolism and carcinogenesis. Mutat Res. 2002; 506–507:65–77.

Hesselink DA, van Gelder T, van Schaik RH, et al. Population pharmacokinetics of cyclosporine in kidney and heart transplant recipients and the influence of ethnicity and genetic polymorphisms in the MDR-1, CYP3A4, and CYP3A5 genes. Clin Pharmacol Ther 2004; 76 (6): 545-56

Higgins MJ, Stearns V. CYP2D6 polymorphisms and tamoxifen metabolism: clinical relevance. *Curr Oncol Rep*. 2010;12:7–15.

Hinoshita E, Uchiumi T, Taguchi K, et al. Increased expression of an ATP-binding cassette superfamily transporter, multidrug resistance protein 2, in human colorectal carcinomas. Clin Cancer Res. 2000;6:2401–2407.

Hitzl M, Drescher S, van der Kuip H, et al. The C3435T mutation in the human MDR1 gene is associated with altered efflux of the P-glycoprotein substrate rhodamine 123 from CD56+ natural killer cells. Pharmacogenetics 2001; 11 (4): 293-8

Hitzl M, Schaeffeler E, Hocher B, et al. Variable expression of P-glycoprotein in the human placenta and its association with mutations of the multidrug resistance 1 gene (MDR1, ABCB1). Pharmacogenetics 2004; 14 (5): 309-18

Hoffmeyer S, Burk O, von Richter O, et al. Functional polymorphisms of the human multidrug-resistance gene: multiple sequence variations and correlation of one allele with P-glycoprotein expression and activity in vivo. Proc Natl Acad Sci U S A 2000;97:3473-8.

Hoskins JM, Carey LA, McLeod HL. CYP2D6 and tamoxifen: DNA matters in breast cancer. *Nat Rev Cancer*. 2009;9:576–586.

Hulot JS, Villard E, Maguy A, et al. A mutation in the drug transporter gene ABCC2 associated with impaired methotrexate elimination. Pharmacogenet Genomics. 2005;15:277–285.

Ieiri I, Takane H, Otsubo K. The MDR1 (ABCB1) gene polymorphism and its clinical implications. Clin Pharmacokinet. 2004;43:553–576.

Iida A, Saito S, Sekine A, et al. Catalog of 605 single-nucleotide polymorphisms (SNPs) among 13 genes encoding human ATP-binding cassette transporters: ABCA4, ABCA7, ABCA8, ABCD1, ABCD3, ABCD4, ABCE1, ABCF1, ABCG1, ABCG2, ABCG4, ABCG5, and ABCG8. J Hum Genet. 2002;47:285–310.

Ingelman-Sundberg M. Human Cytochrome P450 (CYP) Allele Nomenclature Committee [online]. URL: http://www.cypalleles.ki.se/[2009]

Ingelman-Sundburg M. Pharmacogenetics of cytochrome P450 and its applications in drug therapy: the past, the present and future. Trends Pharmacol Sci. 2004;25:193-200.

Iyer L, Hall D, Das S et al. Phenotype-genotype correlation of in vitro SN-38 (active metabolite of irinotecan) and bilirubin glucuronidation in human liver tissue with *UGT1A1* promoter polymorphism. Clin Pharmacol Ther 1999;65:576–582

Iyer L, King CD, Whitington PF et al. Genetic predisposition to the metabolism of irinotecan (CPT-11). Role of uridine diphosphate glucuronosyltransferase isoform 1A1 in the glucuronidation of its active metabolite (SN-38) in human liver microsomes. J Clin Invest 1998;101:847–854.

Jin Y, Desta Z, Stearns V, et al. CYP2D6 genotype, antidepressant use, and tamoxifen metabolism during adjuvant breast cancer treatment. *J Natl Cancer Inst*. 2005;97:30–39.

Johanson CE, Stopa EG, McMillan PN. The blood-cerebrospinal fluid barrier: structure and functional significance. Methods Mol Biol. 2011;686:101-31. Review.

Jones PM, O'Mara ML, George AM. ABC transporters: a riddle wrapped in a mystery inside an enigma. Trends Biochem Sci. 2009 Oct;34(10):520-31..

Jonker JW, Smit JW, Brinkhuis RF, et al. Role of breast cancer resistance protein in the bioavailability and fetal penetration of topotecan. J Natl Cancer Inst. 2000;92:1651–1656.

Kakar SM, Paine MF, Stewart PW, & Watkins PB. "6′,7′-Dihydroxybergamottin contributes to the grapefruit juice effect. Clinical Pharmacology and Therapeutics.2004. 75, 6, pp. 569 – 579.

Kameyama Y, Yamashita K, Kobayashi K, et al. Functional characterization of SLCO1B1 (OATP-C) variants, SLCO1B1*5, SLCO1B1*15 and SLCO1B1*15+C1007G, by using transient expression systems of HeLa and HEK293 cells. Pharmacogenet Genomics. 2005;15:513–522.

Kennedy AJ, Ellacott KL, King VL, Hasty AH. Mouse models of the metabolic syndrome. Dis Model Mech. 2010 Mar-Apr;3(3-4):156-66. Review.

Khan N, Adhami VM, Mukhtar H. Review: green tea polyphenols in chemoprevention of prostate cancer: preclinical and clinical studies. Nutr Cancer. 2009;61(6):836-41. Review.

Kim RB, Leake BF, Choo EF, et al. Identification of functionally variant MDR1 alleles among European Americans and African Americans. Clin Pharmacol Ther 2001; 70 (2): 189-99

Kimchi-Sarfaty C, Oh JM, Kim IW, et al. A "silent" polymorphism in the MDR1 gene changes substrate specificity. Science 2007; 315 (5811): 525-8

Kolitz JE, George SL, Marcucci G, Vij R, Powell BL, Allen SL, DeAngelo DJ, Shea TC, Stock W, Baer MR, Hars V, Maharry K, Hoke E, Vardiman JW, Bloomfield CD, Larson RA; Cancer and Leukemia Group B. P-glycoprotein inhibition using valspodar (PSC-833) does not improve outcomes for patients younger than age 60 years with newly diagnosed acute myeloid leukemia: Cancer and Leukemia Group B study 19808. Blood. 2010 Sep 2;116(9):1413-21..

Kooman JP. Estimation of renal function in patients with chronic kidney disease. J Magn Reson Imaging. 2009 Dec;30(6):1341-6. Review.

Krishnamurthy P, Schuetz JD. Role of ABCG2/BCRP in biology and medicine. Annu Rev Pharmacol Toxicol. 2006;46:381–410.

Kroetz DL, Pauli-Magnus C, Hodges LM, et al. Sequence diversity and haplotype structure in the human ABCB1 (MDR1, multidrug resistance transporter) gene. Pharmacogenetics 2003; 13 (8): 481-94

Kuehl P, Zhang J, Lin Y, et al. Sequence diversity in CYP3A promoters and characterization of the genetic basis of polymorphic CYP3A5 expression. Nat Genet. 2001;27:383-391.

Kukanich B. Pharmacokinetics of acetaminophen, codeine, and the codeine metabolites morphine and codeine-6-glucuronide in healthy Greyhound dogs. J Vet Pharmacol Ther. 2010 Feb;33(1):15-21.

Kuroda M, Kusuhara H, Endou H, Sugiyama Y. Rapid elimination of cefaclor from the cerebrospinal fluid is mediated by a benzylpenicillin-sensitive mechanism distinct from organic anion transporter 3. J Pharmacol Exp Ther. 2005 Aug;314(2):855-61.

Lai Y, Zhang J, Wang YX, Wang XD, Li JL, Zeng YJ & Huang M. CYP3A5*3 and MCR-1 C3435T single nucleotide polymorphisms in six Chinese ethnic groups. Pharmazie, 2011. 66, 2, pp. 136 - 140.

Lam JL, Okochi H, Huang Y, Benet LZ. In vitro and in vivo correlation of hepatic transporter effects on erythromycin metabolism: characterizing the importance of transporter-enzyme interplay Drug Metab. Dispos. 2006, 34, 1336– 1344

Lamba JK, Lin YS, Schuetz EG, et al. Genetic contribution to variable human CYP3A-mediated metabolism. Adv Drug Deliv Rev 2002; 54 (10): 1271-94 (b).

Lamba JK, Lin YS, Thummel K, et al. Common allelic variants of cytochrome P4503A4 and their prevalence in different populations. Pharmacogenetics 2002; 12 (2): 121-32 (a).

Lau WC, Welch TD, Shields T, Rubenfire M, Tantry US, Gurbel PA. The effect of St John's Wort on the pharmacodynamic response of clopidogrel in hyporesponsive volunteers and patients: increased platelet inhibition by enhancement of CYP3A4 metabolic activity. J Cardiovasc Pharmacol. 2011 Jan;57(1):86-93.

Lau YY, Huang Y, Frassetto L, Benet LZ. Effect of OATP1B transporter inhibition on the pharmacokinetics of atorvastatin in healthy volunteers Clin. Pharmacol. Ther. 2007, 81, 194– 204

Le Vee M, Gripon P, Stieger B, Fardel O. Down-regulation of organic anion transporter expression in human hepatocytes exposed to the proinflammatory cytokine interleukin 1beta. Drug Metab Dispos. 2008 Feb;36(2):217-22.

Lee CR, Pieper JA, Frye RF, Hinderliter AL, Blaisdell JA, Goldstein JA. Tolbutamide, flurbiprofen, and losartan as probes of CYP2C9 activity in humans. J Clin Pharmacol. 2003 Jan;43(1):84-91.

Lee NH. Pharmacogenetics of drug metabolizing enzymes and transporters: effects on pharmacokinetics and Pharmacodynamics of anticancer agents. Anticancer Agents in Medicinal Chemistry.2010. 10, 8, pp. 583 - 592.

Lei HP, Yu XY, Xie HT, Li HH, Fan L, Dai LL, Chen Y, Zhou HH. Effect of St. John's wort supplementation on the pharmacokinetics of bupropion in healthy male Chinese volunteers. Xenobiotica. 2010 Apr;40(4):275-81.

Lemahieu WP, Maes BD, Verbeke K, et al. CYP3A4 and P-glycoprotein activity in healthy controls and transplant patients on cyclosporin vs tacrolimus vs sirolimus. Am J Transplant 2004; 4 (9): 1514-22

Lennard L, Gibson BE, Nicole T et al. Congenital thiopurine methyltransferase deficiency and 6-mercaptopurine toxicity during treatment for acute lymphoblastic leukaemia. Arch Dis Child 1993;69:577–579.

Li XQ, Andersson TB, Ahlstrom M, & Weidolf L. Comparison of inhibitory effects of the proton pump-inhibiting drugs omeprazole, esomeprazole, lansoprazole, pantoprazole, and rabeprazole on human cytochrome P450 activities. Drug Metabolism and Disposition. 2004. 32, pp. 821 - 827.

Li Y, Kantelip JP, Gerritsen-van Schieveen P, & Davani P. Interindividual variability of methadone response: Impact of genetic polymorphism. Molecular Diagnosis and Therapy. 2008. 12, 2, pp. 109 - 124.

Lijnen HR. Murine models of obesity and hormonal therapy. Thromb Res. 2011 Feb;127 Suppl 3:S17-20. Review.

Lim HS, Ju Lee H, Seok Lee K, et al. Clinical implications of,CYP2D6 genotypes predictive of tamoxifen pharmacokinetics in,metastatic breast cancer. J Clin Oncol. 2007;25:3837–3845.

Lo HW, Ali-Osman F. Genetic polymorphism and function of glutathione S-transferases in tumor drug resistance. Curr Opin Pharmacol. 2007;7:367–374.

Locher KP. Review. Structure and mechanism of ATP-binding cassette transporters. Philos Trans R Soc Lond B Biol Sci. 2009 Jan 27;364(1514):239-45. Review.

Luo FR, Paranjpe PV, Guo A, et al. Intestinal transport of irinotecan in Caco-2 cells and MDCK II cells overexpressing efflux transporters Pgp, cMOAT, and MRP1. Drug Metab Dispos. 2002;30:763–770.

Luqmani YA. Mechanisms of drug resistance in cancer chemotherapy. Med Princ Pract. 2005;14 Suppl 1:35-48. Review.

MacPhee IA, Fredericks S, Holt DW. Does pharmacogenetics have the potential to allow the individualisation of immunosuppressive drug dosing in organ transplantation? Expert Opin Pharmacother 2005; 6 (15):2593-605

Mager DE, Woo S, Jusko WJ. Scaling pharmacodynamics from in vitro and preclinical animal studies to humans. Drug Metab Pharmacokinet. 2009;24(1):16-24. Review.

Marchetti, S., Mazzanti, R., Beijnen, JH., & Schellens, JHM. (2007). Concise Review: Clinical relevance of drug-drug and herb-drug interactions mediated by ABC transporter ABCB1 (MDR1, P-glycoprotein). The Oncologist, 12, 927 - 941.

Martínez-Villaseñor D, Gerson-Cwilich R. [PET/CT tomography. Usefulness in oncology]. Cir Cir. 2006 Jul-Aug;74(4):295-304. Review.

Mathijssen RH, van Alphen RJ, Verweij J, et al. Clinical pharmacokinetics and metabolism of irinotecan (CPT-11). Clin Cancer Res. 2001;7:2182–2194.

Matsuhisa K, Kondoh M, Takahashi A, Yagi K. Tight junction modulator and drug delivery. Expert Opin Drug Deliv. 2009 May;6(5):509-15.

McCarver DG, Byun R, Hines RN, Hichme M, Wegenek W. A genetic polymorphism in the regulatory sequences of human CYP2E1: association with increased chlorzoxazone hydroxylation in the presence of obesity and ethanol intake. Toxicol Appl Pharmacol. 1998;152:276-281.

McIlwain CC, Townsend DM, Tew KD. Glutathione S-transferase polymorphisms: cancer incidence and therapy. Oncogene. 2006;25: 1639–1648.

McLeod H. Pharmacokinetic differences between ethnic groups. Lancet 2002;359:78.

McLeod HL, Evans WE. Pediatric pharmacokinetics and therapeutic drug monitoring. Pediatr Rev. 1992 Nov;13(11):413-21. Review.

McLeod HL, Watters JW. Irinotecan pharmacogenetics: is it time to intervene? J Clin Oncol 2004;22:1356–1359

McLeod HL, Yu J. Cancer pharmacogenomics: SNPs, chips, and the individual patient. Cancer Invest. 2003;21(4):630-40. Review.

Mehdipour AR, Hamidi M. Brain drug targeting: a computational approach for overcoming blood-brain barrier. Drug Discov Today. 2009 Nov;14(21-22):1030-6. Epub 2009 Jul 30. Review.

Michel MC, Chapple CR. Basic mechanisms of urgency: preclinical and clinical evidence. Eur Urol. 2009 Aug;56(2):298-307. Epub 2009 May 26. Review.

Miyagawa F, Gutermuth J, Zhang H, Katz SI. The use of mouse models to better understand mechanisms of autoimmunity and tolerance. J Autoimmun. 2010 Nov;35(3):192-8. Epub 2010 Jul 23. Review.

Murray M, Reidy GF. Selectivity in the inhibition of mammalian cytochromes P-450 by chemical agents. Pharmacol Rev 1990;42:85-101.

Musana AK, Wilke RA. Gene based drug prescribing: Clinical implications of the cytochrome P450 genes. Wisconsin Medical J. 2005;104:61-66.

Nagar S, Remmel RP. Uridine diphosphoglucuronosyltransferase pharmacogenetics and cancer. Oncogene. 2006;25:1659–1672.

Nagasubramanian R, Innocenti F, Ratain MJ. Pharmacogenetics in cancer treatment. Annu Rev Med. 2003;54:437-52. Epub 2001 Dec 3. Review.

Nelson, DR. The Cytochrome P450 Homepage. Human Genomics. 2009. 4, 59-65. URL: http://drnelson.uthsc.edu/CytochromeP450.html

Nguyen CM, Mendes MA, Ma JD. Thiopurine methyltransferase (TPMT) genotyping to predict myelosuppression risk. PLoS Curr. 2011 May 15;3:RRN1236.

Niemi M, Schaeffeler E, Lang T, et al. High plasma pravastatin concentrations are associated with single nucleotide polymorphisms and haplotypes of organic anion transporting polypeptide-C (OATP-C, SLCO1B1). Pharmacogenetics 2004; 14 (7): 429-40

Nieminen TH, Hagelberg NM, Saari TI, Neuvonen M, Neuvonen PJ, Laine K, Olkkola KT. Grapefruit juice enhances the exposure to oral oxycodone. Basic Clin Pharmacol Toxicol. 2010 Oct;107(4):782-8.

O'Connell MB, Frye RF, Matzke GR, St Peter JV, Willhite LA, Welch MR, Kowal P, & LaValleur J. Effect of conjugated equine estrogens on oxidative metabolism in middle-aged and elderly postmenopausal women. Journal of Clinical Pharmacology.2006. 46, pp. 1299 – 1307.

O'Brien MM, Lacayo NJ, Lum BL, Kshirsagar S, Buck S, Ravindranath Y, Bernstein M, Weinstein H, Chang MN, Arceci RJ, Sikic BI, Dahl GV. Phase I study of valspodar

(PSC-833) with mitoxantrone and etoposide in refractory and relapsed pediatric acute leukemia: a report from the Children's Oncology Group. Pediatr Blood Cancer. 2010 May;54(5):694-702.

Patel NR, Rathi A, Mongayt D, Torchilin VP. Reversal of multidrug resistance by co-delivery of tariquidar (XR9576) and paclitaxel using long-circulating liposomes. Int J Pharm. 2011 Sep 15;416(1):296-9. Epub 2011 Jun 15.

Peregud-Pogorzelski J, Tetera-Rudnicka E, Kurzawski M, Brodkiewicz A, Adrianowska N, Mlynarski W, Januszkiewicz D, Drozdzik M. Thiopurine S-methyltransferase (TPMT) polymorphisms in children with acute lymphoblastic leukemia, and the need for reduction or cessation of 6-mercaptopurine doses during maintenance therapy: the Polish multicenter analysis. Pediatr Blood Cancer. 2011 Oct;57(4):578-82. doi: 10.1002/pbc.23013.

Pillai U, Muzaffar J, Sen S, & Yancey A. Grapefruit juice and verapamil: a toxic cocktail. Southern Medical Journal.2009. 102, 3, pp. 308 – 309.

Potschka H. Targeting regulation of ABC efflux transporters in brain diseases: a novel therapeutic approach. Pharmacol Ther. 2010 Jan;125(1):118-27. Epub 2009 Nov 5. Review.

Reichel A. Addressing central nervous system (CNS) penetration in drug discovery: basics and implications of the evolving new concept. Chem Biodivers. 2009 Nov;6(11):2030-49. Review.

Rettie AE, Jones JP. Clinical and toxicological relevance of CYP2C9: drug-drug interactions and pharmacogenetics. Annu Rev Pharmacol Toxicol. 2005;45:477-494.

Richardson RM, Larson PS, Bankiewicz KS. Gene and cell delivery to the degenerated striatum: status of preclinical efforts in primate models. Neurosurgery. 2008 Oct;63(4):629-442; dicussion 642-4. Review.

Ritschel WA & Kearns GL: Handbook of Basic Pharmacokinetics, 5th edition. Washington, DC. APhA, 1999.

Roden DM, & Stein CM. Clopidogrel and the concept of high-risk pharmacokinetics. Circulation.2009. 119, pp. 2127 – 2130.

Roy U, Chakravarty G, Honer Zu Bentrup K, Mondal D. Montelukast is a potent and durable inhibitor of multidrug resistance protein 2-mediated efflux of taxol and saquinavir. Biol Pharm Bull. 2009 Dec;32(12):2002-9.

Sachidanandam R, Weissman D, Schmidt SC, et al. A map of human genome sequence variation containing 1.42 million single nucleotide polymorphisms. Nature 2001;409:928-33.

Sai K, Kaniwa N, Itoda M, et al. Haplotype analysis of ABCB1/MDR1 blocks in a Japanese population reveals genotype-dependent renal clearance of irinotecan. Pharmacogenetics. 2003;13:741–757.

Salphati, L.; Benet, L. Z. Effects of ketoconazole on digoxin absorption and disposition in rat Pharmacology 1998, 56, 308– 313

Sausville EA, Burger AM. Contributions of human tumor xenografts to anticancer drug development. Cancer Res. 2006 Apr 1;66(7):3351-4, discussion 3354. Review.

Savage DB. Mouse models of inherited lipodystrophy. Dis Model Mech. 2009 Nov-Dec;2(11-12):554-62. Review.

Schaeffeler E, Eichelbaum M, Brinkmann U, et al. Frequency of C3435T polymorphism of MDR1 gene in African people. Lancet 2001;358:383-4.

Schellens JH, Maliepaard M, Scheper RJ, et al. Transport of topoisomerase I inhibitors by the breast cancer resistance protein. Potential clinical implications. Ann NY Acad Sci. 2000;922:188–194.

Schroeder MA, DiPersio JF. Mouse models of graft-versus-host disease: advances and limitations. Dis Model Mech. 2011 May;4(3):318-33. Review.

Schroth W, Goetz MP, Hamann U, et al. Association between CYP2D6 polymorphisms and outcomes among women with early stage breast cancer treated with tamoxifen. *JAMA*. 2009;302:1429–1436.

Schuetz JD, Connelly MC, Sun D, et al. MRP4: a previously unidentified factor in resistance to nucleoside-based antiviral drugs. Nat Med 1999;5:1048-51.

Schwarz UI, Hanso H, Oertel R, Miehlke S, Kuhlisch E, Glaeser H, Hitzl M, Dresser GK, Kim RB, Kirch W. Induction of intestinal P-glycoprotein by St John's wort reduces the oral bioavailability of talinolol. Clin Pharmacol Ther. 2007 May;81(5):669-78.

Serwer LP, Noble CO, Michaud K, Drummond DC, Kirpotin DB, Ozawa T, Prados MD, Park JW, James CD. Investigation of intravenous delivery of nanoliposomal topotecan for activity against orthotopic glioblastoma xenografts. Neuro Oncol.2011 Sep 27. [Epub ahead of print]

Shen S, Zhang W. ABC transporters and drug efflux at the blood-brain barrier. Rev Neurosci. 2010;21(1):29-53. Review.

Shitara Y, Sugiyama D, Kusuhara H, Kato Y, Abe T, Meier PJ, Itoh T, Sugiyama Y. Comparative inhibitory effects of different compounds on rat oatpl (slc21a1)- and Oatp2 (Slc21a5)-mediated transport Pharm. Res. 2002, 19, 147– 153

Sim SC, Edwards RJ, Boobis AR, et al. CYP3A7 protein expression is high in a fraction of adult human livers and partially associated with the CYP3A7*1C allele. Pharmacogenet Genomics 2005; 15 (9): 625-31

Simon J, van Spanning RJ, Richardson DJ. The organisation of proton motive and non-proton motive redox loops in prokaryotic respiratory systems. Biochim Biophys Acta. 2008 Dec;1777(12):1480-90.

Soldin OP, & Mattison DR. Sex differences in pharmacokinetics and pharmacodynamics. Clinical Pharmacokinetics. 2009. 48, 3, pp. 143 - 157.

Song IS, Shin HJ, Shim EJ, et al. Genetic variants of the organic cation transporter 2 influence the disposition of metformin. Clin Pharmacol Ther. 2008;84:559–562.

Song S, Suzuki H, Kawai R, Sugiyama Y. Effect of PSC 833, a P-glycoprotein modulator, on the disposition of vincristine and digoxin in rats Drug Metab. Dispos. 1999, 27, 689– 694

Srinivas SP. Cell signaling in regulation of the barrier integrity of the corneal endothelium. Exp Eye Res. 2011 Sep 24. [Epub ahead of print].

Staatz CE, Goodman LK, & Tett SE. Effect of CYP31 and ABCB1 single nucleotide polymorphisms on the pharmacokinetics and pharmacodynamics of calcineurin inhibitors: Part I. Clinical Pharmacokinetics, 2010. 49, 3, pp. 141 –171.(a)

Staatz CE, Goodman LK, Tett SE. Effect of CYP3A and ABCB1 single nucleotide polymorphisms on the pharmacokinetics and pharmacodynamics of calcineurin inhibitors: Part II. Clin Pharmacokinet 2010;49 (4): 207-21. (b)

Sugano K, Kansy M, Artursson P, Avdeef A, Bendels S, Di L, Ecker GF, Faller B, Fischer H, Gerebtzoff G, Lennernaes H, Senner F. Coexistence of passive and carrier-mediated processes in drug transport. Nat Rev Drug Discov. 2010 Aug;9(8):597-614. Review.

Tamura A, Wakabayashi K, Onishi Y, et al. Re-evaluation and functional classification of non-synonymous single nucleotide polymorphisms of the human ATP-binding cassette transporter ABCG2. Cancer Sci. 2007;98:231–239.(a)

Tamura A, Watanabe M, Saito H, et al. Functional validation of the genetic polymorphisms of human ATP-binding cassette (ABC) transporter ABCG2: identification of alleles that are defective in porphyrin transport. Mol Pharmacol. 2006;70:287–296.(b)

Tanabe M, Ieiri I, Nagata N, et al. Expression of P-glycoprotein in human placenta: relation to genetic polymorphism of the multidrug resistance (MDR)-1 gene. J Pharmacol Exp Ther 2001; 297 (3): 1137-43

Tarbell JM. Shear stress and the endothelial transport barrier. Cardiovasc Res. 2010 Jul 15;87(2):320-30. Epub 2010 Jun 12. Review.

Tassaneeyakul W, Veronese ME, Birkett DJ, Doecke CJ, McManus ME, Sansom LN, Miners JO. Co-regulation of phenytoin and tolbutamide metabolism in humans. Br J Clin Pharmacol. 1992 Dec;34(6):494-8.

Thervet E, Anglicheau D, Legendre C, et al. Role of pharmacogenetics of immunosuppressive drugs in organ transplantation. Ther Drug Monit 2008;30 (2): 143-50

Thwaites DT, Anderson CM. The SLC36 family of proton-coupled amino acid transporters and their potential role in drug transport. Br J Pharmacol. 2011 Apr 18. doi: 10.1111/j.1476-5381.2011.01438.x. [Epub ahead of print]

Tirona RG, Leake BF, Merino G, et al. Polymorphisms in OATP-C: identification of multiple allelic variants associated with altered transport activity among European- and African-Americans. J Biol Chem.2001;276:35669–35675.

Tiwari AK, Sodani K, Dai CL, Ashby CR Jr, Chen ZS. Revisiting the ABCs of multidrug resistance in cancer chemotherapy. Curr Pharm Biotechnol. 2011 Apr;12(4):570-94. Review.

Tóth A, Veszelka S, Nakagawa S, Niwa M, Deli MA. Patented in vitro blood-brain barrier models in CNS drug discovery. Recent Pat CNS Drug Discov. 2011 May 1;6(2):107-18. Review.

Townsend DM, Findlay VL, Tew KD. Glutathione S-transferases as regulators of kinase pathways and anticancer drug targets. Methods Enzymol. 2005;401:287-307.Review.

Umar A, Della'Zanna G, Lubet R. Further thoughts on preclinical animal models for cancer prevention: when is it best to start treatment? What are potential histopathologic endpoints? Semin Oncol. 2010 Aug;37(4):339-44. Review.

US National Center for Biotechnology Information. Single nucleotide polymorphism [online]. Available from: www.ncbi.nlm.nih.gov/SNP/GeneGt.cgi?geneID=5243 [Accessed 2009 Feb 23]

van der Deen, M., de Vries, EGE., Timens, W., Scheper, RJ., Timmer-Bosscha, H., & Postma, DS. (2005). ATP-binding cassette (ABC) transporters in normal and pathological lung. Respiratory Research, 6, 1, pp. 59 – 75.

van Erp NP, Baker SD, Zhao M, et al. Effect of milk thistle (Silybum marianum) on the pharmacokinetics of irinotecan. Clin Cancer Res. 2005;11:7800–7806.

van Waterschoot RA, Schinkel AH. A critical analysis of the interplay between cytochrome P450 3A and P-glycoprotein: recent insights from knockout and transgenic mice. Pharmacol Rev. 2011 Jun;63(2):390-410. Epub 2011 Apr 13. Review.

Varghese Gupta S, Gupta D, Sun J, Dahan A, Tsume Y, Hilfinger J, Lee KD, Amidon GL. Enhancing the Intestinal Membrane Permeability of Zanamivir: A Carrier Mediated Prodrug Approach. Mol Pharm. 2011 Sep 22. [Epub ahead of print]

Verbeeck RK, Musuamba FT. Pharmacokinetics and dosage adjustment in patients with renal dysfunction. Eur J Clin Pharmacol. 2009 Aug;65(8):757-73. Epub 2009 Jun 20. Review.

Visentin M, Chang MH, Romero MF, Zhao R, Goldman ID. Substrate- and pH-specific antifolate transport mediated by OATP2B1-SLCO2B1. Mol Pharmacol. 2011 Oct 21. [Epub ahead of print]

Volm M, Mattern J, & Samsel B. Overexpression of P-glycoprotein and glutathione S-transferase-pi in resistant non-small cell lung carcinomas of smokers. British Journal of Cancer.1991. 64, 700 – 704.

Wacher VJ, Wu CY, Benet LZ. Overlapping substrate specificities and tissue distribution of cytochrome P450 3A and P-glycoprotein: implications for drug delivery and activity in cancer chemotherapy. Mol Carcinog. 1995;13:129–134.

Walker K, Ginsberg G, Hattis D, Johns DO, Guyton KZ, Sonawane B. Genetic polymorphism in N-Acetyltransferase (NAT): Population distribution of NAT1 and NAT2 activity. J Toxicol Environ Health B Crit Rev. 2009;12(5-6):440-72. Review.

Wang D, Johnson AD, Papp AC, et al. Multidrug resistance polypeptide 1 (MDR1, ABCB1) variant 3435C>T affects mRNA stability. Pharmacogenet Genomics 2005; 15 (10): 693-704

Wang J, Sonnerborg A, Rane A, et al. Identification of a novel specific CYP2B6 allele in Africans causing impaired metabolism of the HIV drug efavirenz. Pharmacogenet Genomics. 2006;16:191-198.

Watanabe, T.; Maeda, K.; Kondo, T.; Nakayama, H.; Horita, S.; Kusuhara, H.; Sugiyama, Y. Prediction of the hepatic and renal clearance of transporter substrates in rats using in vitro uptake experiments Drug Metab. Dispos. 2009, 37, 1471– 1479

Wee B, Charles N, Holland EC. Animal models to study cancer-initiating cells from glioblastoma. Front Biosci. 2011 Jun 1;17:2243-58. Review.

Wikinski, S. Pharmacokinetic mechanisms underlying resistance in psychopharmacological treatment. The role of P-glycoprotein. Vertex. 2005. 16, 64, pp. 438 – 441.

Wilhelm I, Fazakas C, Krizbai IA. In vitro models of the blood-brain barrier. Acta Neurobiol Exp (Wars). 2011;71(1):113-28. Review.

Wojnowski L, Kulle B, Schirmer M, et al. NAD(P)H oxidase and multidrug resistance protein genetic polymorphisms are associated with doxorubicin-induced cardiotoxicity. Circulation. 2005;112:3754–3762.

Wong J, Brugger A, Khare A, Chaubal M, Papadopoulos P, Rabinow B, Kipp J, Ning J. Suspensions for intravenous (IV) injection: a review of development, preclinical and clinical aspects. Adv Drug Deliv Rev. 2008 May 22;60(8):939-54.Epub 2008 Feb 7. Review.

Xiangdong L, Yuanwu L, Hua Z, Liming R, Qiuyan L, Ning L. Animal models for the atherosclerosis research: a review. Protein Cell. 2011 Mar;2(3):189-201. Epub 2011 Apr 6. Review.

Xie HG, Kim RB, Wood AJ, et al. Molecular basis of ethnic differences in drug disposition and response. Annu Rev Pharmacol Toxicol.2001;41:815–850.

Xu G, Bhatnagar V, Wen G, et al. Analyses of coding region polymorphisms in apical and basolateral human organic anion transporter (OAT) genes [OAT1 (NKT), OAT2, OAT3, OAT4, URAT (RST)]. Kidney Int. 2005;68:1491–1499.

Yates CR, Krynetski EY, Loennechen T, et al. Molecular diagnosis of thiopurine S-methyltransferase deficiency: genetic basis for azathioprine and mercaptopurine intolerance. Ann Intern Med 1997;126:608-14.

Zaragoza C, Gomez-Guerrero C, Martin-Ventura JL, Blanco-Colio L, Lavin B, Mallavia B, Tarin C, Mas S, Ortiz A, Egido J. Animal models of cardiovascular diseases. J Biomed Biotechnol. 2011;2011:497841. Epub 2011 Feb 16. Review.

Zhang HX, Huang Y, Frassetto LA, Benet LZ. Elucidating rifampin's inducing and inhibiting effects on glyburide pharmacokinetics and blood glucose in healthy volunteers: unmasking the differential effects of enzyme induction and transporter inhibition for a drug and its primary metabolite Clin. Pharmacol. Ther. 2009, 85, 78– 85.

Zhang W, Han Y, Lim SL, & Lim LY. Dietary regulation of P-gp function and expression. Expert Opinion in Drug Metabolism and Toxicology.2009. 5, 7, pp. 789 – 801.

6

Application of Pharmacokinetics/Pharmacodynamics (PK/PD) in Designing Effective Antibiotic Treatment Regimens

Ghada F. Ahmed[1] and Ayman M. Noreddin[2,*]
[1]University of Minnesota
[2]Hampton University
USA

1. Introduction

Designing antibiotic dosing regimens is often not optimal and the dose-response relationship for most antibiotics is not well-known[1]. Both Pharmacokinetics (PK) and Pharmacodynamics (PD) are characteristics of antimicrobial agents that should be considered in the development of effective antibiotic therapy. By linking the concentration time profile at the site of action to the drug effect (PK/PD), the effect of varying dosage regimens against pathogens could be simulated enabling the identification of effective dosage strategies. It is known that inadequate antibiotic dosing could not only lead to a therapeutic failure, but also to the development of bacterial resistance. Importantly, the evolution of resistance in pathogenic bacteria combined with the decreasing interest from the pharmaceutical industry in developing new antibiotics has created a major public health problem[3]. Therefore, the activities to maintain the effects of existing antibiotics and prolong their useful life span have a high priority.

PK/PD analysis proved to be a useful tool for investigating effective therapies that minimize the emergence of antibiotic tolerance. Although the European Medicine Agency and FDA clearly recommends PK/PD assessment for new compounds, there are no standardized procedures for such analyses for antibiotics[3]. For characterizing the PD of an antibiotic, bacterial growth and death under antibiotic exposure have to be investigated. Since these are difficult to measure in human tissues, animal and *in vitro* models have been developed.

Although animal models provide similar growth conditions for bacteria and imitate the characteristics of human infection, they exhibit different PK and drug disposition profiles compared to humans[4]. In contrast, *in vitro* models have the advantage of simulating human PK and bacterial resistance analysis. Therefore, they are considered adequate for the investigation of antimicrobial activity[4].

Frequently, the pharmacodynmic relationship is reduced to a single parameter, the Minimum inhibitory concentration (MIC), even though antibiotics with the same MIC can

* Corresponding Author

have different PD functions[1]. Differences in the kill profiles exhibited by antibiotics is hypothesized to be influenced by disparities of their PD characteristics that- if not taken into account during the design of treatment regimens- may lead to therapeutic failure and development of resistance.

In this study, five antibiotics of five different classes were considered for PK/PD analysis. The antibiotics were Ciprofloxacin (a fluorquinolone that acts by inhibiting bacterial DNA gyrase enzyme), Ampicillin (a beta-lactam antibiotic acts by inhibiting bacterial cell wall synthesis), and finally Rifampin, Streptomycin, and Tetracycline (protein synthesis inhibitors). The antibiotics were further classified according to their pharmacodyamic properties into concentration dependent antibiotics (Ciprofloxacin, Rifampin and Streptomycin), and time dependent antibiotics (Ampicillin and Tetracycline).

PK/PD simulations using STELLA® (Version 9.1, isee system inc, NH, USA) were used to investigate the effect of various PD parameters on the achievement of the therapeutic outcome and in designing effective dosing regimen that help overcome the development of resistance to the antibiotic.

2. Pharmacokinetic analysis

The PK of the antibiotics was assumed to follow one compartment disposition characteristics with a first order elimination rate constant. The drug was given in a dose that gave an initial plasma concentration equivalent to 5 times the MIC and the plasma concentration was allowed to decrease mono-exponentially to a minimum of 0.5 times the MIC over 8 hours according to the following equation

$$C_t=C_0 \exp\{-kt\} \quad (1)$$

Where C_t is the plasma concentration at time t, C_0 is the initial plasma concentration and k is the first-order elimination rate constant.

Doses were administered as multiple IV boluses with a time interval of 8 hours. The system was assumed to be at a steady state. The volume of distribution was assumed to be fixed (equals 1); since the data were obtained from an *in vitro* experiment. Clearance (k*v) was then assumed to be equivalent to the value of the elimination rate constant k. For this analysis, Ciprofloxacin, Ampicillin, Rifampin, Streptomycin and Tetracycline were the considered antibiotics.

3. Pharmacodynamic analysis

3.1 Effect of exposure to antibiotics on the bacterial net growth rate

The net growth rate under certain antibiotic pressure could be described by the following equation:-

$$\Psi(a) = \Psi\max - \mu(a) \quad (2)$$

Where is the net growth rate at antibiotic concentration a, is the growth rate of the bacteria in absence of antibiotic, and is the death rate of the bacterial population exposed to an antibiotic concentration a. Therefore, the net growth rate of the bacterial population under antibiotic treatment could be described by the following model:-

$$\Psi(a)=\Psi\max-\frac{(\Psi\max-\Psi\min)\times(\frac{a}{zMIC})^{k}}{(\frac{a}{zMIC})^{k}-\frac{\Psi\min}{\Psi\max}} \qquad (3)$$

Whereis the minimum net growth rate of the bacteria at high antibiotic concentration, a is the antibiotic concentration, zMIC is the pharmacodynamic MIC (concentration of the antibiotic at which the net bacterial growth rate was calculated to be zero), and K is the Hill coefficient which is a measure of the steepness of the sigmoidal relationship between antibiotic concentration and the net growth rate.

The model was constructed to evaluate the effect of the antibiotics against a single micro-organism (E. coli); and therefore, the maximum growth rate is assumed to be constant.

The minimum growth rate, zMIC as well as the Hill coefficient will, however, change due to different antibiotic treatments. Bacterial net growth rate against the antibiotic concentration was analyzed for the aforementioned antibiotics.

4. PK/PD analyses

The bacterial population was modeled during the mono-exponential growth phase. The change in bacterial density was modeled according to the following equation:-

$$dx/dt = \text{growth rate} - \text{kill rate due to antibiotic}$$

Where x is the bacterial density measures in colony forming units per mL (CFU/mL)

Time plots of the logarithm to the base 10 of the bacterial density were generated and the effect of the PD parameters (MIC, K, minimum growth rate, and maximum growth rate) on the achievement of the target treatment outcome was investigated through a sensitivity analysis in STELLA®. The target treatment outcome was defined as three $\log_{10}$ decrease in the bacterial density over a 24 hour course of the treatment.

4.1 Design of antibiotics treatment strategies

Antibiotics are generally classified to concentration dependent and time dependent agents. In the current analysis, treatment strategies were constructed and tested under different scenarios. Results from the simulation were used to conclude on the most appropriate treatment option for different classes of antibiotics.

Increasing the MIC by two fold and four folds supported the simulation of bacterial resistance against the antibiotic treatments. The outcome target of the treatment is to achieve three $\log_{10}$ decrease in the bacterial density over a 24 hours course of treatment through the given dosage regimen. Towards that target, two treatment strategies were used. The first was to increase the area under the antibiotic concentration time curve above the minimum inhibitory concentration (AUC>MIC) through increasing the administered dose, while the second was to increase the percentage of time during which the drug concentration is above the MIC relative to the dosing interval (% t>MIC) through decreasing the dosing interval with smaller maintenance doses. Both scenarios were applied to each of the investigated antibiotics and the outcomes of the treatment regimens were compared.

5. Results

5.1 The pharmacokinetic model

The disposition of the antibiotics was shown to follow a one compartment model with a first order elimination rate. The achievement of the steady state was assumed form the beginning of therapy. (Figure 1a and 1b)

The antibiotics were given as multiple intravenous boluses every 8 hours over a course of 24 hours.

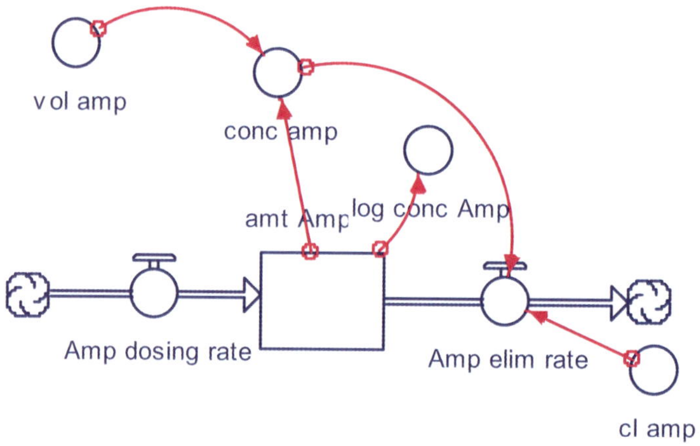

Fig. 1a. STELLA® model simulating the one compartment PK model with first order elimination rate constant for Ampicillin

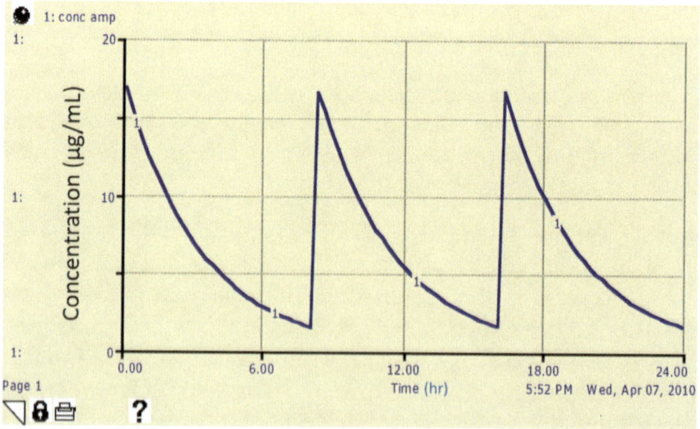

Fig. 1b. Simulation of the Ampicillin steady state concentration time profile form the PK model.

5.2 Pharmacodynamic analysis

5.2.1 Effect of antibiotic concentration on the bacterial net growth rate

Changing antibiotic concentration is assumed to be affecting the net growth rate of the bacteria cultured in the *in vitro* system. The infection was therefore assumed to occur in the central compartment. The pharmacodynamic parameter estimates for the five considered antibiotics are displayed in Table 1. STELLA® model (Figure 2) was created to determine the effect of changing drug concentration on the net bacterial growth rate according the pharmacodynamic function expressed in equation 3.

PD parameter/ drug	Max. growth rate (h^{-1})	Min. growth rate (h^{-1})	K	zMIC (μg/mL)
Ciprofloxacin	0.75	-6.5	1.1	0.017
Ampicillin	0.75	-4.0	0.75	3.4
Rifampin	0.75	-4.3	2.5	12.0
Streptomycin	0.75	-8.8	1.9	18.5
Tetracycline	0.75	-8.1	0.61	0.67

Table 1. Pharmacodynamic parameter estimates[1]

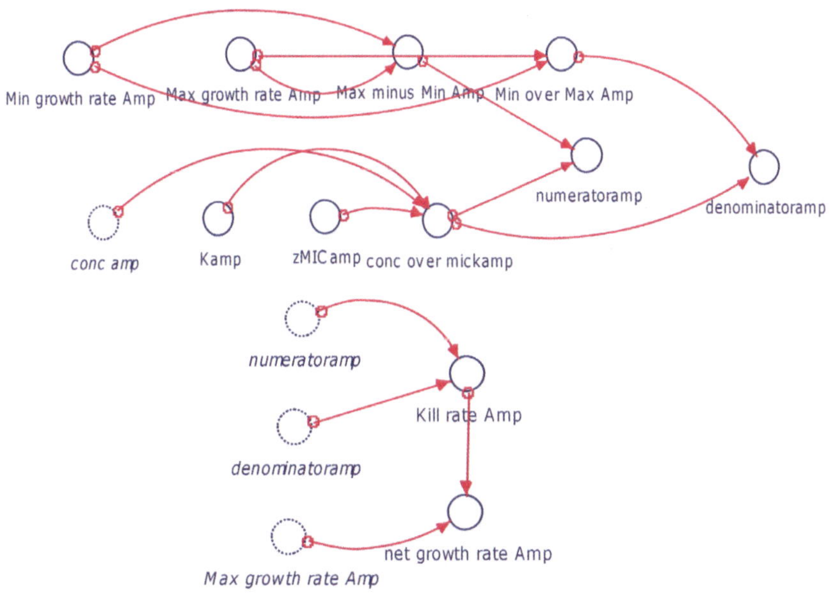

Fig. 2. Sketch of the STELLA® model used to assess the pharmacodynamic effect of the antibiotic Ampicillin.

Bacterial net growth rate against the antibiotic concentration displayed a nonlinear inhibitory PD function with increasing antibiotic concentration. It is assumed that the four PD parameters (MIC, K, minimum growth rate, and maximum growth rate) contribute to the shape of the PD curve.

It is noticed that concentration dependent antibiotics (Ciprofloxacin, Rifampin, and Streptomycin) showed a sharper decrease in the net growth rate in relation to antibiotic concentration (greater K value), while time dependent antibiotics (Ampicillin and Tetracycline) showed slower decline with respect to increase in concentration (lower K values) (Figure 3). Additionally, Figure 4 shows that three antibiotics with the same MIC values and minimum growth rate against a specific microorganism can have different microbiological activity depending on the value of the Hill coefficient K.

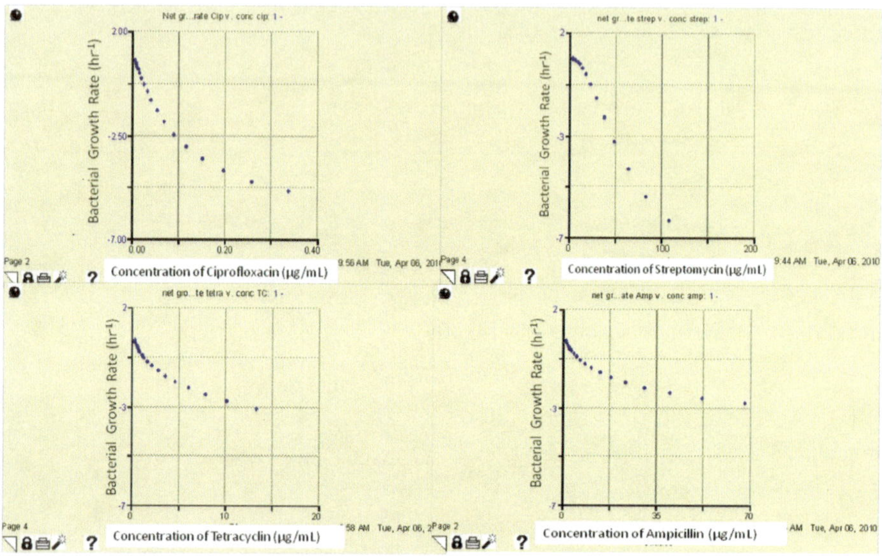

Fig. 3. Effect of antibiotic concentration on bacterial net growth rate

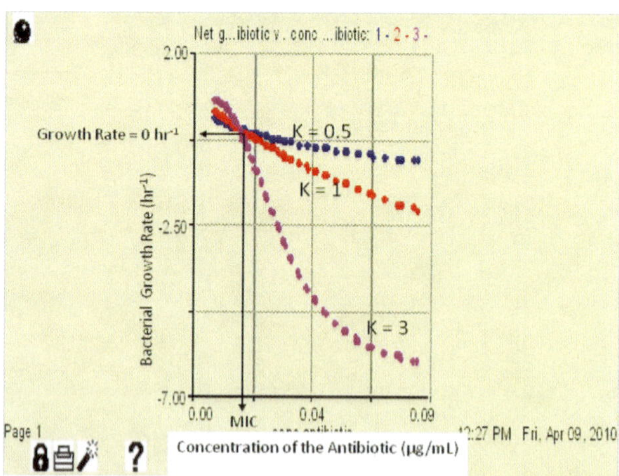

Fig. 4. Pharmacodynamic sensitivity analysis shows the effect of three antibiotics with the same MIC and minimum growth rate on the bacterial net growth rate due to different values of Hill coefficient (K).

5.3 PK/PD analysis

Change in the bacterial density over time was modeled using STELLA® as in figures 5a and b. the model assumes that bacterial growth over time follows an exponential pattern.

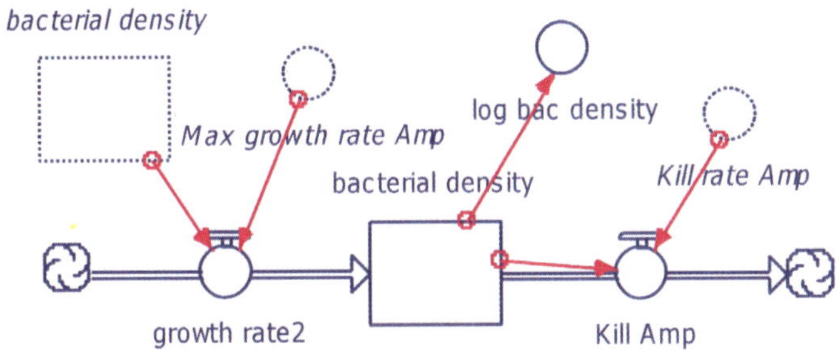

Fig. 5a. STELLA® model constructed to investigate the change in bacterial density over time.

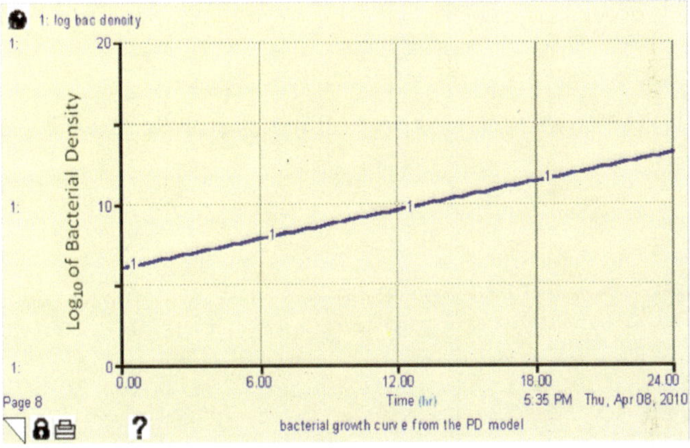

Fig. 5b. Bacterial growth curve from the PD model.

The drug effect was added to the previous model through the inclusion of a first order kill rate. This resulted in a decline in the $\log_{10}$ bacterial density over time. The decline was found to be governed by the magnitude of the PD model parameters. The effect of the Hill coefficient, the minimum growth rate, and the maximum growth rate was investigated for both concentration dependent and time dependent agents. The values of the PD parameters that were used in the sensitivity analysis are reported in Table 2. The results from the sensitivity analysis are shown in Figures 6, 7 and 8. It is noticed that as K increases, there is a sharper decline in the bacterial density due to a faster rate of killing. In addition, on the single dose level, ciprofloxacin showed greater rate of killing compared to ampicillin (Figure 6).

Similarly, minimum growth rate achieved under high antibiotic concentration was related to the treatment outcome. Increased minimum growth rate under certain high antibiotic pressure, led to a decreased antibiotic efficacy. This could be attributed to development of resistance. It is also noticed that the effect was greater for concentration dependent antibiotics than the for time dependent agents (Figure 7).

PD parameter	Hill coefficient (K)	Minimum growth rate (h^{-1})	Maximum growth rate (h^{-1})
Scenario 1	0.5	-3	0.75
Scenario 2	1	-6	1.2
Scenario 3	3	-9	2

Table 2. Pharmacodynamic parameters incorporated in the sensitivity analysis

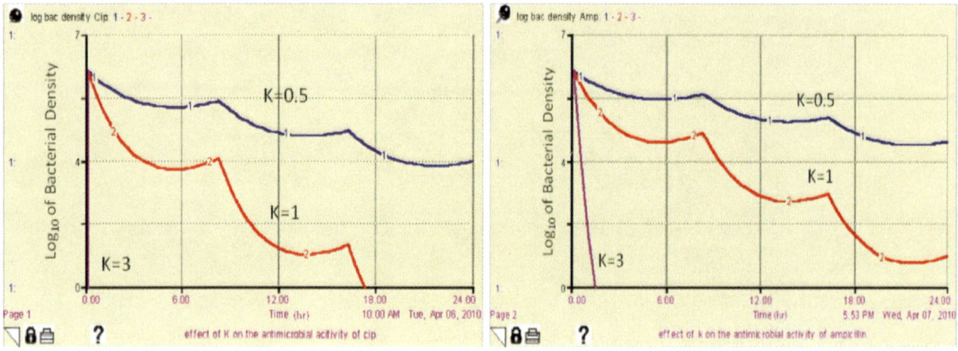

Fig. 6. Effect of the Hill coefficient (K) on the treatment outcomes for both Ciprofloxacin and Ampicillin.

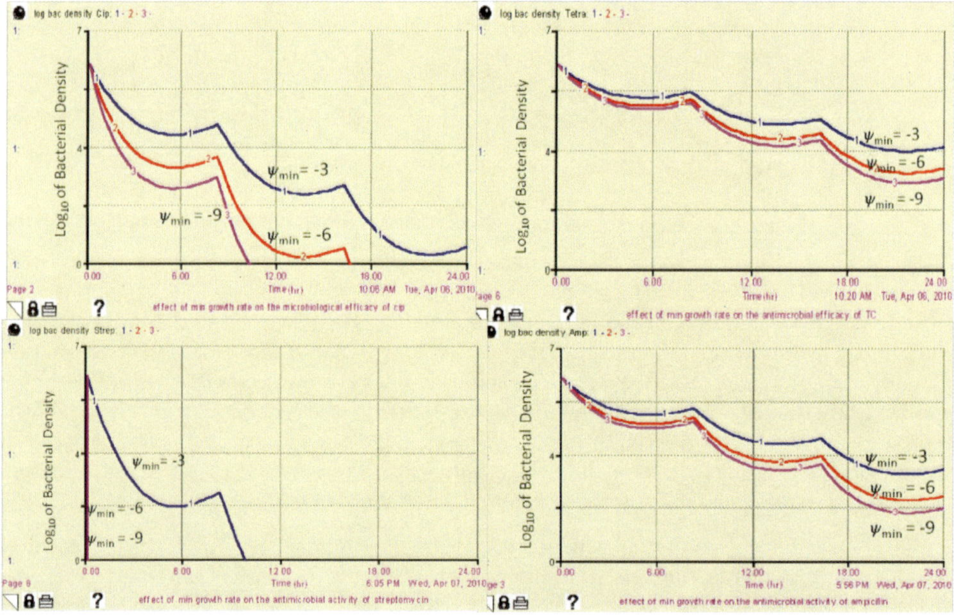

Fig. 7. Effect of variation of minimum growth rate achieved under high antibiotic concentration on the treatment outcomes for the investigated antibiotics.

In addition to the previously mentioned PD parameters, maximum growth rate of the bacteria achieved in the absence of antibiotic was an influential parameter. Change in that parameter could be considered when the effect of the antibiotic on different bacterial strains is a point of interest. Moreover, it could be important for a single microbial strain. For instance, it is known that the growth rate of the bacterial biofilm is reduced compared to the planktonic cultures due to the development of a matrix of extracellular polymeric substance that is referred to as a slime[2]. This will result in reduced penetration of the antibiotics as well as nutrients. Figure 8 augments that by showing that the increase in the maximum growth rate led to a more susceptible micro-organism and a faster kill by the antibiotic.

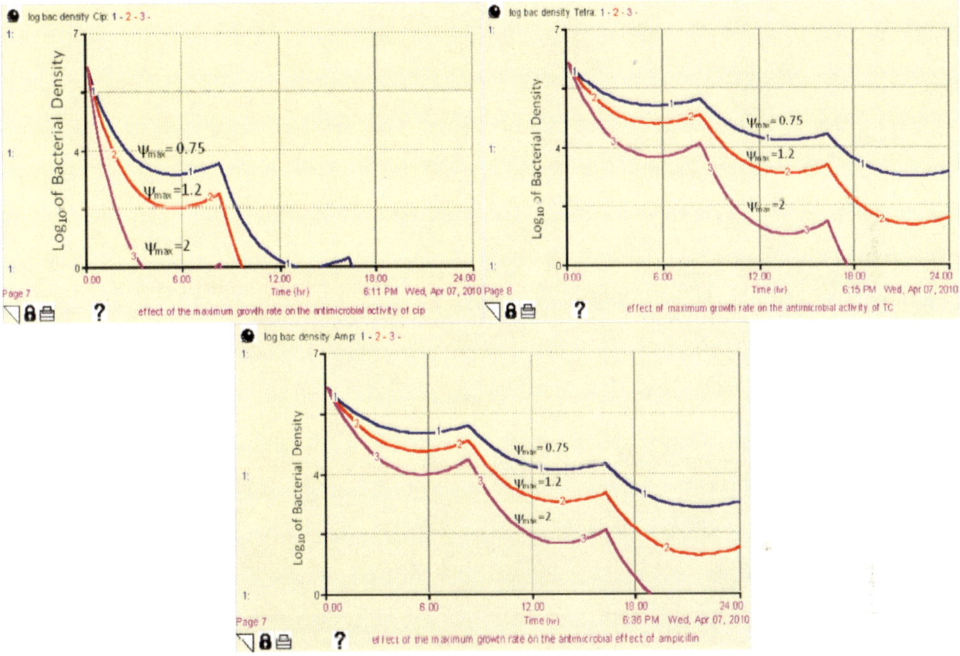

Fig. 8. Effect of variation of maximum growth rate of the microorganism on the treatment outcome with Ciprofloxacin, Tetracycline and Ampicillin.

6. Development of microbial resistance

Development of microbial resistance is a major challenge that faces antibiotic treatments and causes reduction in the treatment efficacy. In order to simulate cases of bacterial resistance, MIC values were allowed to vary two and four fold from the original MIC through conducting a zMIC sensitivity analysis (Table 3). The pharmacokinetic profiles of the five antibiotics were simulated using the previously mentioned one compartment disposition model. It is noticed that as the MIC increases, the level of resistance of the microorganism increases, thus an expected reduction in the rate of kill will occur. Under such circumstances, the antibiotic may no longer be effective in eradicating the microorganism as shown in Figure 9

MIC (µg/mL) /antibiotic	Scenario 1	Scenario 2	Scenario 3
Ciprofloxacin	0.017	0.034	0.068
Ampicillin	3.4	6.8	13.6
Rifampin	12	24	48
Streptomycin	18.5	37	74
Tetracycline	0.67	1.34	2.68

Table 3. MIC values incorporated in the sensitivity analysis for simulating the development of resistance.

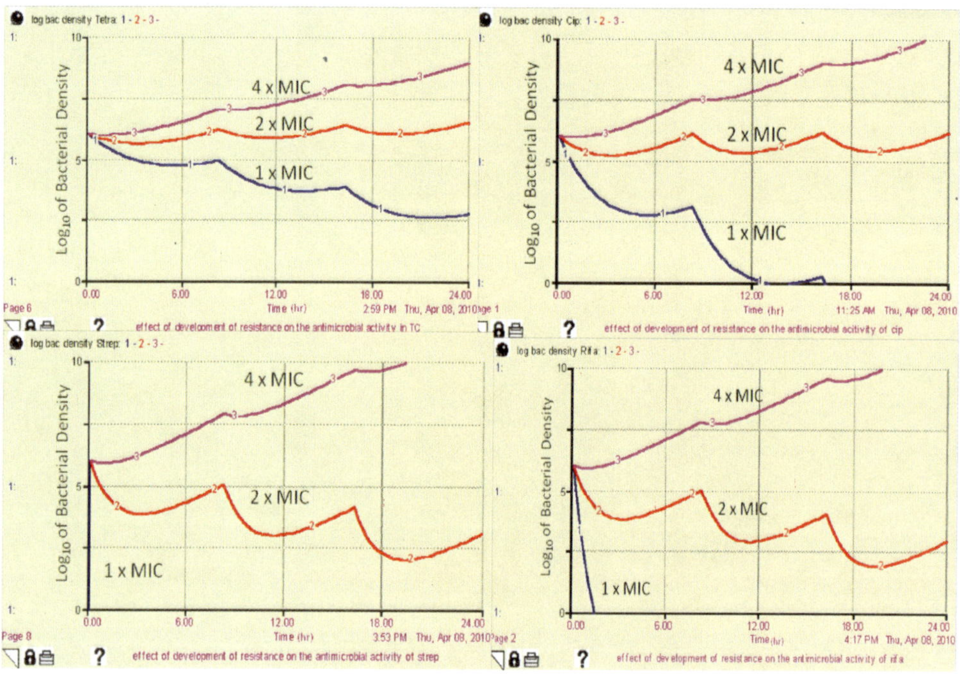

Fig. 9. Effect of the development of resistance (simulated through increasing zMIC) on the antimicrobial outcome for the different antibiotics.

7. Design of treatment strategies

Each of the five antibiotics was allowed to follow two treatment scenarios to overcome the emergence of the resistant microbe (Figure 10) and the treatment outcome was then evaluated. Treatment modalities included two protocols: the first implemented a method to increase the AUC/MIC by increasing the doses of the antibiotic. The second allowed the percentage of time that the drug concentration stays above the MIC to increase by decreasing the dosing interval while giving small maintenance doses of the antibiotic. Shown in Figure 10 is a representation of the concentration profiles expected from the treatment scenarios and in Figures 11a, b, and c are the simulated treatment outcomes expected from each protocol for three of the antibiotics.

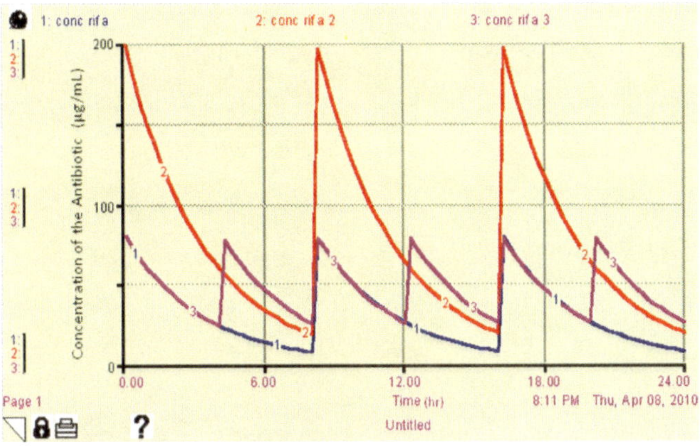

Fig. 10. Simulation of the concentration time profile for the treatment scenarios proposed to overcome resistance. 1. Represents original treatment protocol. 2. Represents increasing AUC>MIC scenario and 3. Represents the case of increased % t>MIC

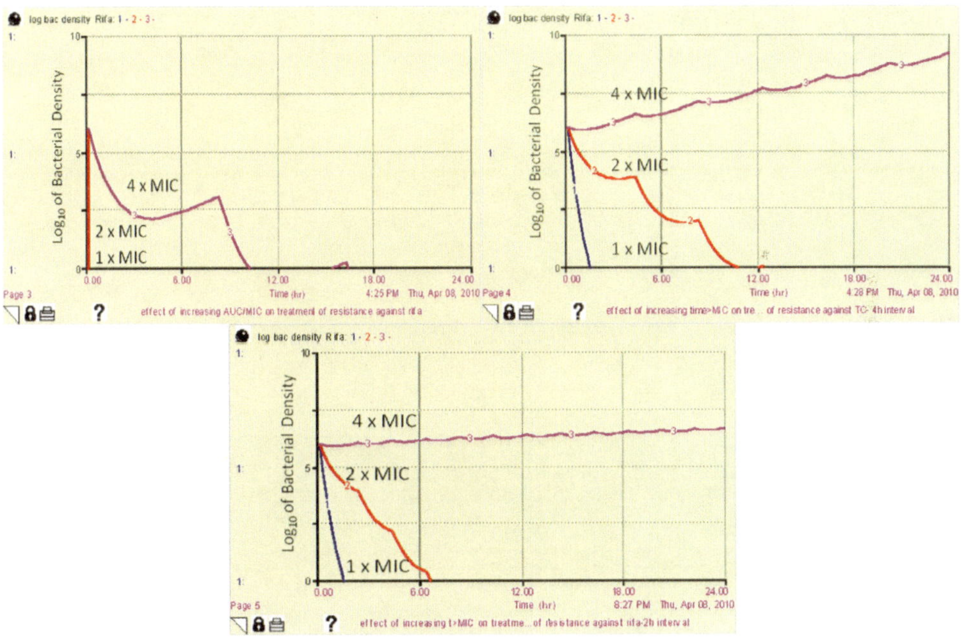

Fig. 11a. Simulation of the target outcome for the two treatment scenarios used against the Rifampin resistance. Upper left: increasing the dose of Rifampin 1.5 folds over 8 hours interval. Upper right: decreasing the dosing interval to 4 hours while maintaining the original dose. Down: decreasing the dosing interval to 2 hours while maintaining the original dose.

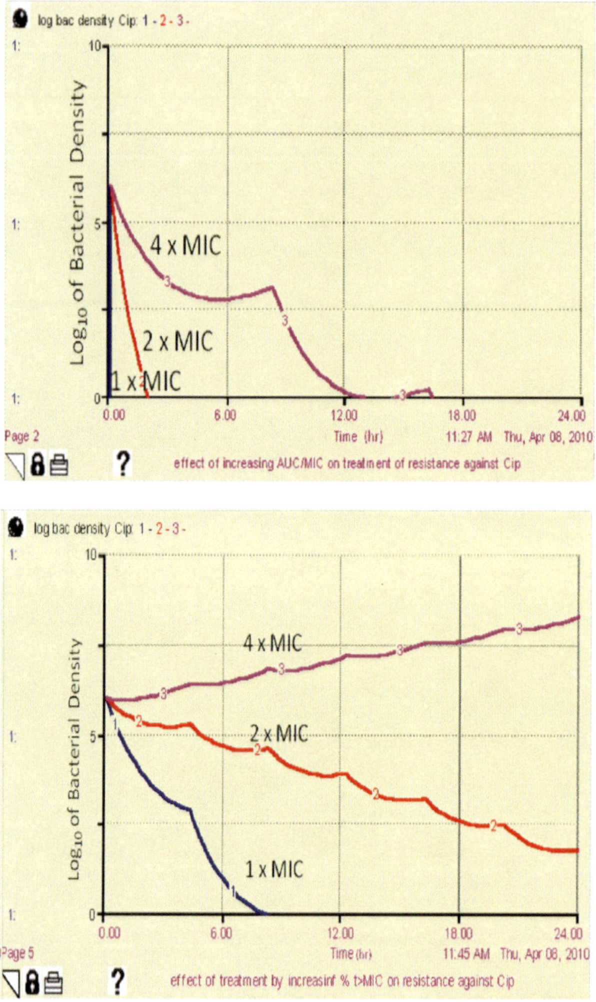

Fig. 11b. Simulation of the treatment outcomes obtained after implementation of the two treatment scenarios with Ciprofloxacin. Left side curve represents increasing the dose by four times over 8 hours dosing interval. Right side curve represents decreasing the dosing interval by 4 hours while maintaining the original dose.

Rifampin is known to be a concentration-dependent antibiotic. Increasing the exposure to the drug above the MIC (by 1.5 fold increase in the dose) improved the treatment outcome, yet increasing the percentage of time relative to the dosing interval (tau) that the drug concentration was above the MIC- by decreasing tau from 8 hours to 4 and 2 hours simultaneously- did not achieve the target outcome even when the dosing interval decreased to 2 hours. Ciprofloxacin- a fluoroquinolone known to be a concentration dependent antibiotic- displayed similar results to Rifampin upon increasing exposure above MIC (four fold increase in the dose) compared to t>MIC (reducing the dosing interval to 2 hours).

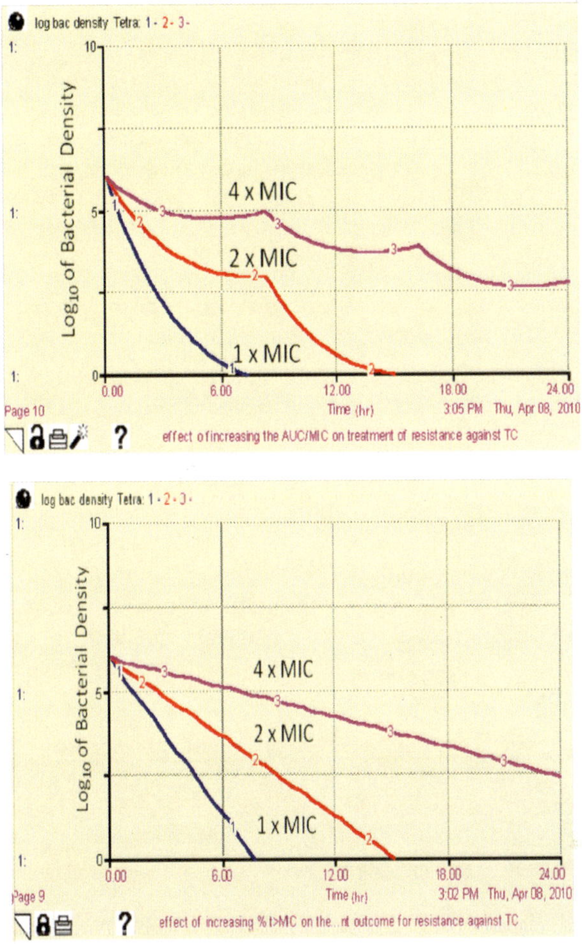

Fig. 11c. Simulation of the treatment outcomes achieved after increasing Tetracycline dose (four folds over 8 hours dosing interval, left side curve), or decreasing the dosing interval (2 hours, while maintaining original dose, right side curve).

On the other hand, the efficacy of Tetracycline is known to be time dependent. Therefore, increasing the percent of time the drug stays above MIC relative to the dosing interval seems to be more relevant than increasing the exposure above the MIC. Surprisingly, the two scenarios have achieved nearly the same treatment outcome for microbial resistance against Tetracycline. Both treatment scenarios succeeded to achieve the target outcome of three $\log_{10}$ reduction in bacterial density by the end of the antibiotic treatment.

8. Discussion

This study addressed the complex relationship between the exposure to antibiotics and the growth and death rates of bacteria. PK/PD simulations using STELLA® showed that although MIC is an important PD parameter, it is not the only parameter that governs the interaction of the antibiotic and the bacteria. Other PD parameters should additionally be taken into consideration when designing antibiotic dosage regimens. For instance, Figure 4 showed that three antibiotics with the same MIC (the concentration corresponding to a net growth of zero) could show different microbiological activity depending on the magnitude of the Hill coefficient (K). Other PD parameters to be considered are the minimum growth rate and the maximum growth rate, which can capture effects that cannot be accounted for by solely considering the MIC and can importantly affect the therapeutic outcomes.

Pharmacodynamic simulations of the antibiotics concentration against net bacterial growth showed that the shape of the sigmoidal functions differs among antibiotics from different classes with some of them showing greater sensitivity to changing concentrations (Ciprofloxacin and Streptomycin) than others (Tetracycline and Ampicillin). The shape of the pharmacodynamic function is determined by the values of PD parameters displayed in Table 2.

Additionally, using a STELLA® model for the change in bacterial density over time, it was found that the parameters that govern the PD function have a profound effect on the microbiological activity. The Hill coefficient influences the sensitivity of the bacteria to the change in the antibiotic concentration as was shown in Figure 4. Assuming a PK model in which the drug reaches steady state form the beginning of the treatment, a concentration that is above the MIC most of the time, and all other parameters are equal, the simulation predicts that antibiotics with a high Hill coefficient are more effective than those with a low value of the coefficient.

Considering the minimum bacterial net growth rate at high antibiotic concentrations, the simulation predicts that antibiotics that induced lower values of minimum bacterial net growth rate are more effective than those with higher values. Increase in the minimum bacterial net growth rate could be atrributed to the development of resistance or to the utilization of ineffective therapy against a specific bacterial strain.

Maximum growth rate in the absence of antibiotic is another important parameter to consider in the design of antibiotic treatment. That PD parameter is subject to change when treating different micro-organisms or if the nature of infection by the same microbe has been changed. Regarding the later condition, biofilm infection could be considered as a change in the nature of the infection by the same micro-organism[5]. It is well-known that biofilm is a type of persistent infections that is developed in chronic disease statuses and is characterized by a slower rate of growth compared to acute infections[2]. This phenomenon is also observed in the *in vitro* systems- where the planktonic cultured bacteria exhibit a faster rate of growth compared to the biofilm cultured ones[6]. Therefore, increasing the maximum growth rate in the sensitivity analysis has led to a faster kill by different antibiotics due to the greater exposure of the bacteria to the antibiotic compared to the slowly growing biofilm infection.

Interestingly enough, estimates of the parameter K was higher for antibiotics that are concentration dependent (Ciprofloxacin, Rifampin, and Streptomycin) compared to those that are time dependent (Ampicillin and Tetracycline) which means that the formers are characterized by a steeper pharmacodynamic function. The steeper the function, the more dramatically the bacterial killing is sensitive to the change in antibiotic concentration above the MIC. Therefore, it could be a reasonable assumption that for antibiotics that have grater K, increasing the concentration above MIC (AUC/MIC) is the most effective strategy to improve the treatment outcomes. This hypothesis was fully augmented by the PK/PD simulation shown in both Figures 11a and b. Increasing the % t>MIC for Rifampin by reducing the dosing interval to 4 hours and even 2 hours did not achieve the target outcome for the resistant strain as did the increase in the AUC/MIC. Furthermore, Ciprofloxacin achieved the target therapeutic outcome only when the dose increased allowing AUC>MIC to increase. It is worth mentioning that the magnitude of the dose increase for concentration dependent antibiotics appears to be related to the PD parameter K (the Hill coefficient); since Rifampin- has a K value of 2.5 compared to 1.1 for Ciprofloxacin- has achieved the target therapeutic outcome upon 1.5 fold increase in the dose compared to a four folds increase for Ciprofloxacin. In another way, one can conclude that as K increases, as the antibiotic efficacy is more sensitive to small changes in concentration.

On the other hand, it was assumed that lower values of K could be associated with time dependence of the antibiotics. This assumption is not fully supported by the current simulation, since for Tetracycline (k=0.61) both scenarios of increasing the AUC/MIC and % t>MIC worked well and achieved comparable therapeutic outcomes. It is worth mentioning, however, that the maintenance dose used in the former scenario (12.08 μg every 8 hours) was four times higher than that used in the later scenario (2.95 μg every 2 hours). Although it is known that longer dosing intervals are more convenient and can improve patient adherence to therapy, drug toxicity is an important consideration as well. In case where toxicity is expected from higher doses of a time-dependent antibiotic, the strategy of dividing the doses into smaller fractions for shorter dosing intervals may be considered.

Finally, it should be noted that this model may suffer some limitations due to many causes. The model assumes that the kill rate increases with increasing antibiotic concentration, however in reality, the development of an adaptive resistance- a mechanism by which the bacteria becomes increasingly refractory to the antibiotic treatment- may lead to the decrease in kill rate with time and therefore limit such assumptions. Moreover, the constitutive and inducible immune defense of the human body contributes to the efficacy of the antibiotic treatment protocols in a way that could not be fully represented by the current PK/PD analysis under *in vitro* conditions.

9. References

[1] Roland R. Regoes, Camilla Wiuff, Renata M. Zappala, Kim N. Garner, Fernando Baquero, and Bruce R. Levin. Pharmacodynamic Functions: a Multiparameter Approach to the Design of Antibiotic Treatment Regimens. *Antimicrobial agents and chemotherapy*. October 2004, 48: 3670–3676

[2] Hall-Stoodley L, Costerton JW, Stoodley P. Bacterial biofilms: from the natural environment to infectious diseases. *Nature Reviews. Microbiology*. February 2004, 2 (2): 95–108.

[3] Marc H. Scheetz, Kristin M. Hurt, Gary A. Noskin and Catherine M. Oliphant. Applying antimicrobial pharmacodynamics to resistant gram-negative pathogens. *Am J Health-Syst Pharm.* July 2006, 63: 1346-1360

[4] Julia Gloede, Christian Scheerans, Hartmut Derendorf and Charlotte Kloft. In vitro pharmacodynamic models to determine the effect of antibacterial drugs. *J Antimicrob Chemother.* 2010, 65: 186–201

[5] Daniel J Hassett, Thomas R Korfhagen, Randall T Irvin, Michael J Schurr, Karin Sauer, Gee W Lau, Mark D Sutton, Hongwei Yu and Niels Hoiby. *Pseudomonas aeruginosa* biofilm infections in cystic fibrosis: insights into pathogenic processes and treatment strategies. *Expert Opin Ther Targets.* 2010, 14:117-30

[6] Thien-Fah C. Mah and George A. O'Toole. Mechanisms of biofilm resistance to antimicrobial agents. Trends in Microbiology. 2001, 9:34-39

Pharmacokinetics and Drug Interactions of Herbal Medicines: A Missing Critical Step in the Phytomedicine/Drug Development Process

Obiageri O. Obodozie
Department of Medicinal Chemistry and Quality Control, National Institute for Pharmaceutical Research and Development, Abuja, Nigeria

1. Introduction

Discovering and developing safe and effective new medicines is a long, difficult and expensive process involving multi-billion dollar investments in Research and Development by research-based pharmaceutical industries yearly. On average, it will cost a pharmaceutical company up to $800m and upwards of 15 years to get one new medicine from the laboratory to the pharmacist's shelf. Only five in 5,000 compounds that enter preclinical testing will actually progress into human clinical trials, and of these five, only one is likely to be approved by the regulatory authorities using new drug approvals systems that are extremely rigorous, costly and time-consuming (1).

One of the regulatory requirements for an investigational new drug (IND) approval is pre-clinical pharmacokinetics of the new drug entity. However, for the majority of herbal remedies used in ethnomedical or conventional medical practice, data on their disposition and biological fate in humans are lacking or in paucity. It is vital in the drug development chain, to understand the disposition of these herbal products and how they interact with conventional drugs before their launch in the market, in order to ensure the rational use of herbal medicines. For natural products, the additional challenge currently is in their pharmacokinetics, arising from the multiplicity of components, inability to identify biological markers and lack of knowledge of the fate of the agents and/or their metabolites in vivo. Are these processes currently largely ignored in drug development, due to the rigor, cost and time consumption of the conventional drug development process? The clinical consequences of diminished drug efficacy can be as devastating as those of enhanced drug toxicity. Also sometimes, the clinical effect may not be obvious in a short term study and therefore may go unrecognized, possibly leading to the inappropriate discontinuation of an effective medication or the unnecessary addition of other drugs. Does the extent and volume of botanical - drug interactions observed in today's medical care and understanding the processes involved therein, make it a critical area for in-depth attention in pharmaceutical research & development?

Herbal medicines are classified as dietary supplements and the Food and Drug Administration (FDA) regulatory requirements for their approval are not as stringent as those for new chemical entities yet these are products with pharmacological properties with the potential to cause harm.

The term 'Herbal products' has become a colloquial term which commonly refers to all types of preparations obtained from herbs, spices, roots, stems, leaves and other non-botanical materials of natural origin. They can be used therapeutically as prescription or over-the-counter medicines or even as cosmetics orally or topically. Plants are important sources of medicines and plant derived drugs came into use in modern medicine through the uses of plant materials as indigenous cure in folklore or traditional systems of medicine. The use of plant extracts and herbs as medicines preparations has been since the beginning of recorded time, probably originating from ancient China and Egypt. Over 80,000 species of plants are in use throughout the world. In the last century, roughly 121 pharmaceutical products were formulated based on the knowledge of plant use in traditional medicine from various sources and presently about 25% of pharmaceutical prescriptions in the United States contain at least one plant-derived ingredient.

Herbal medicine, phytotherapy, phytomedicine, nutraceuticals, natural product medicine, complimentary & alternative medicine, ethnomedicine, botanicals, herbal medicinal product, dietary supplements and phytopharmaceuticals are all terms used interchangeably to denote the use of botanicals in healthcare and are therefore used as such in this text. Increasing number of patients and consumers are using plant-based therapeutic products as complementary therapy in the treatment and management of chronic ailments such as tuberculosis, diabetes, hypertension, HIV/AIDS, cancer and diseases of endemicity and high recrudescence especially malaria, as well as other social conditions like obesity, cigarette smoking and drug abuse. This upsurge in the use of phytomedicines is a global phenomenon, with more than 80% of people in Africa and Asia using herbal medicines and an increasing number in the Western world. It is estimated that 60% to 70% of the American population is taking botanical products (2).

The World Health Organisation promotes the use of herbal medicine, thus herbal medicine has become big business. Many Americans use complementary and alternative medicine (CAM) to prevent or alleviate common illnesses, with the effect that in the United States, botanical products are now a $1.5 billion per year industry. In 2005, trade in herbal medicine was worth 14 billion USD in China, 5 billion USD in Western Europe in 2003-2004 and 160 million USD in Brazil in 2007. In Africa where all types of plant derived medicines and dietary supplements (both domestic and foreign) are seen, the volume of trade in botanicals is unquantified.

In recent times many factors have contributed to the current surge in phytomedicine use. The therapeutic superiority of many plant extracts over single isolated constituents, as well as the bioequivalence of many phytopharmaceuticals with synthetic chemotherapeutics is well documented (3). The gradual transition from the long-standing use of monodrug therapy in classical medicine to the new concept of a multidrug and multitarget therapy is greatly promoting phytotherapeutics. There is a gradual shift from the orthodox use of mono-substance therapy and an increasing transition to multidrug therapy of patients with drug combinations, such as is done presently for the treatment of diabetes, cancer, acquired immune deficiency syndrome (AIDS), malaria, tuberculosis or hypertension (4, 5).

The rationalization for this strategy is based on therapeutic experiences that the use of drug combinations can target the multiple aetiologies, disease dynamics and/or complications that are seen in many ailments better than each of the components separately, while promoting patient compliance. Also there is the consideration that a complex pathophysiological process can be influenced more effectively and with fewer or no severe side-effects by a combination of several low-dosage compounds or the corresponding extracts than by a single large dosage isolated compound. Phytotherapy has long followed and developed these strategies by using mono-extracts or extract combinations containing mixtures of bioactive compounds that complement one another to elicit an efficacy of superior power. It is also believed that these components do primarily activate self-healing and protective processes of the human body (especially the immune system, which can then properly fight foreign invaders), promote the balancing of regulatory process in the body and help to destroy offending pathogens without toxic side effects, rather than attacking and directly destroying the damaging agents.

Most consumers often consider herbal therapies as accessible and affordable therapeutic alternatives to orthodox therapy without any safety concerns and sometimes even as the only effective therapeutic way left to treat certain disorders that have defied conventional drugs or promote and maintain health. The above factors have led to a situation where the concomitant administration of phytomedicines and orthodox drugs has become inevitable. One of the consequences of concurrent use of herbal medicines and orthodox drugs is the possibility of interactions. The interaction of drugs with herbal medicines is a significant safety concern, especially for drugs with narrow therapeutic indices (e.g. warfarin and digoxin), drugs with long-term regimens and drugs used in the management of life-threatening conditions due to the fact that an alteration in the pharmacokinetics and/or pharmacodynamics of the drug by herbal remedies could bring about potentially severe and perhaps even life-threatening adverse reactions. Because of the clinical significance of drug interactions with herbs, it is important to identify drugs and compounds in development that may interact with herbal medicines. This can be achieved by incorporating timely herb-drug interaction studies using appropriate in vitro and in vivo approaches in order to identify such drugs has important implications for drug development.

With the availability of over 30000 over-the-counter products, more than 1000 different chemical substances that are constituents of prescription drugs and hundreds of herbs, vitamins, and minerals, the possibilities of drug interaction are endless. A drug interaction is defined as any modification caused by another exogenous chemical (drug, herb, or food) in the diagnostic, therapeutic, or other action of a drug in or on the body. The risk for drug interactions increases with the number of products consumed: for 2 products, the risk is 6%; for 5 products, 50%; and for 8 or more products, 100% (6). The use of complimentary alternative medicine alongside conventional therapy continues to grow rapidly especially in the developed countries. It is estimated that less than a third of Americans taking botanical products inform their physicians of such use (7). In oncology therapy alone, about 72% of cancer patients taking herbal medicines with their conventional treatments do not inform their physicians (8) and 27% of them were at risk for developing herb – drug interaction (9).

Because the issue of botanical-drug interaction has not been well appreciated and is definitely under-studied, today, our understanding of the interactions between drugs and herbs and between drugs and food has not advanced much, therefore much research is still required in herbal therapy to examine individual plant constituents and to determine how plants interact with drugs and foods. Therefore in our effort to understand the potential therapeutic role of botanicals and promote their safe use, one must not only focus on evaluating toxicity, efficacy, mechanism of action but also on their safe and appropriate use particularly with respect to the research and knowledge on botanical-drug interactions.

A general lack of knowledge of the interaction potentials of concurrent use of botanicals with prescription and/or over-the-counter medicines, poses a great challenge for health care professionals and a safety concern for consumers. Although most people especially in developing countries believe that herbs are harmless plants, about a third of our drugs (including digitalis, morphine, atropine, and several chemotherapeutic agents) were developed from plants. So, indeed, herbs can be potent products. Herbs can affect body functions; therefore, when they are taken concurrently with orthodox drugs, interactions are possible, impacting on the clinical effects of the latter. That natural products are largely unregulated contributes to the misconception that they are safe, with the effect that patients don't feel the need to tell their physicians that they are using them, and physicians don't routinely ask patients if they are taking them.

2. Selected clinically relevant botanical–drug interactions

Although our knowledge of interactions of phytomedicines with conventional drugs in patients is still relatively young and not well understood, many case reports, controlled clinical and in vitro studies constitute strong evidence that support the assumption that significantly more of the large inter-individual variations in the response to treatment seen in medical practice can be attributed to botanical–drug interactions. This assumption is supported by several studies which show that some herbal medicinal products have the capacity to influence plasma levels of drugs (10, 11), giving rise to clinical problems of unexpected toxicities and under-treatment seen in different groups of patients. Factors relating to co-administered drugs (dose, dosing regimen, administration route, pharmacokinetic and therapeutic range), herbs (species, dose, dosing regimen, and administration route) and patients (genetic polymorphism, age, gender and pathological conditions) largely determine the extent and thus the clinical relevance of drug interactions with herbs (12). In general terms, the appearance of enhanced drug effects and/or adverse effects is usually associated with a doubling or more in drug plasma concentration (13). However, less marked changes may still be clinically important for drugs with a steep concentration–response relationship or a narrow therapeutic index. In most cases, the extent of drug interactions with herbs varies markedly among individuals, depending on inter-individual differences in drug metabolizing enzymes and transporters, co-medication with other drugs, age and many of other factors (14).

Several clinically important botanical-drug interactions have been reported leading to altered efficacy and/or toxicity, adverse reactions that are sometimes life threatening or lethal (15). Often times, the evidence of interactions with dietary supplements is often based on presumed pharmacologic activity, data derived from in vitro or animal studies, or anecdotal single case reports and to a lesser extent, well-designed clinical studies. Tamarind, an Asian fruit used not only in ayuverdic medicine but also as a food flavouring agent, has been shown to significantly increase the extent of absorption of a single 600mg dose of aspirin in six healthy volunteers, posing potential danger if a large amount of aspirin is ingested concomitantly with tamarind. Ginseng induced mania when used concomitantly with phenelzine (16). An enhanced hypoglycemic effect has also been reported when a meal containing garlic and *Mormodica charantia L.* (balsampear) *family: curcubitaceae,* a herb traditionally used in the treatment of type 2 diabetes was consumed with chlorpropamide (17).

The over-the-counter antidepressant herb St John's Wort (SJW) is probably the most studied of all herbal preparations when considering interactions with orthodox drugs. Several clinically relevant drug–drug interactions have been reported between SJW and a wide range of drugs. Chronic administration of SJW together with cyclosporin A has been associated with a significant reduction in cyclosporin plasma levels and a higher risk for acute organ rejection in transplanted patients (18, 19). In healthy volunteers, administration of SJW together with the protease inhibitor indinavir produced an approximately 57% lower plasma AUC of indinavir (20). Co-administration of SJW with digoxin produced an18% lower plasma AUC of digoxin and a 40% higher expression level of intestinal P-gp (21). Other drugs with reported clinically relevant interactions with St. John's Wort include tacrolimus, warfarin, verapamil, fexofenadine, imatinib, (ethinylestradiol/desogestrel), loperamide, or selective serotonin-reuptake inhibitors (e.g. sertraline, paroxetine, and nefazodone) with attendant clinical implications such as under-treatment and failure of therapies (22, 23)

Ginkgo is a popular herbal product used to improve cognitive function in alzeihmer and dementia as well as to improve blood flow and improve impaired memory in vascular disease. Several reports of bleeding associated with its concurrent use with drugs like aspirin, warfarin, acetaminophen, or an ergotamine caffeine preparation have been documented (24, 25). Matthew MK, reported the association of a recent use of Gingko biloba with the occurrence of cerebral haemorrage in a patient who had been stabilized for five years on warfarin (26). Also, a combined use of ginkgo with a thiazide diuretic may precipitate high blood pressure and coma when combined with trazodone (27, 28). Grapefruit juice is another botanical product that has widely been reported to affect the plasma concentrations and bioavailabilities of conventional drug products ingested with it, such that the FDA includes documented information on drug-grape fruit juice interactions in the product insert of certain medications including statins, drugs for blood pressure reduction, some antiretroviral agents (29) and the Health Canada in 2002 advised the public not to consume grape fruit juice with medications for anxiety, depression among others (30).

As part of the drug development process,' before 'studies studies from our laboratories have investigated possible interactions of the concomitant administration of various natural products being developed as phytomedicines and various drugs routinely used in the treatment of co-morbidities in the respective disorders. The alteration in bioavailability and pharmacokinetic parameters of paracetamol by an investigational antimalarial phytomedicine (AM-1), when concomitantly administered in humans was reported by us (31). AM-1 an extract from the plant *Nauclea latifolia* Smith (family:Rubiaceae) used in the treatment of uncomplicated malaria was orally administered to healthy volunteers with and without 500mg of acetaminophen. Almost a 50% reduction in the area under the curve of paracetamol was observed in the presence of 500mg capsules of AM-1

Niprisan® an anti-sickling phytomedicine has been shown to also significantly affect the systemic concentrations of paracetamol when both products were concomitantly administered (32), as well as the pharmacokinetic disposition of chloroquine and metronidazole in animal studies (33).

Pharmacokinetic Parameters	Metronidazole alone	Metronidazole + Niprisan	% Diff.	Metronidazole +Nifadin	% Diff	Metronidazole + AM1	% Diff.
$t_{1/2a}$ (h)	1.788 ± 0.08	2.145 ± 0.21	20↑	1.908 ± 0.12	7 ↑	3.062± 0.41	71 ↑
Ka (h^{-1})	0.392 ± 0.02	0.340± 0.04	13 ↓	0.351 ± 0.02	10 ↑	0.255± 0.04	35 ↓
Cmax (μg/ml)	3.109 ± 0.11	4.989 ± 0.16	60 ↑	7.243 ± 0.25	133 ↑	5.490± 0. 66	77 ↑
tmax (h)	0.833 ± 0.11	2.417 ± 0.43	190↑	1 ± 0.00	20↑	0.583 ± 0.08	30 ↓
$AUC_{0\to24}$ (μg.h/ml)	13.135 ± 0.41	19.781 ± 1.10	50↑	29.520 ± 0.91	124 ↑	21.553± 0.77	64 ↑
$AUC_{0\to\infty}$ (μg.h/ml)	18.794 ± 0.76	28.364 ± 2.02	51↑	42.111 ± 2.03	124 ↑	28.424± 3.50	51 ↑
Vd (L)	2.449 ± 0.12	1.875 ± 0.11	25↓	1.208 ± 0.03	50↓	1.791 ± 0.13	27 ↓
Cl_T (L/h)	0.427 ± 0.02	0.231 ± 0.04	45↓	0.180± 0.01	57↓	0.188± 0.05	56 ↓

Table 1. Effect of Niprisan, AM-1, and Nifadin on the pharmacokinetic parameters of Metronidazole in rats.

Pharmacokinetic parameters	Chloroqine alone value	Chloroquine + Niprisan	% Diff	Chloroqine + Nifadin	% Diff	Chloroquine + AM1	% Diff.
$t_{1/2a}$ (h)	4.5612± 0.69	5.2760 ± 0.71	3↑	35.567± 2.5147	680 ↑	2.7301 ± 0.21	40↓
Ka (h^{-1})	0.1691± 0.02	0.1454 ± 0.05	14↓	0.020± 0.0011	88↓	0.2610 ±0.0178	54 ↑
Cmax (μg/ml)	5.2287± 0.69	1.8709 ± 0.19	64 ↓	2 ± 0.00	62 ↓	2.9785 ± 0.10	43 ↑
tmax (h)	0.9167± 0.06	2.3333 ± 0.33	155	1.4139 ± 0.11	54↑	0.9167 ± 0.08	0
$AUC_{0\to24}$ (μg.h/ml)	30.1470± 0.18	17.3477 ± 0.38	42 ↓	19.5059 ± 0.59	35↓	18.8178 ± 1.21	38 ↓
Vd (L)	1.4978± 0.19	3.5924 ± 0.22	139 ↑	5.7563 ± 0.11	284 ↑	2.2360 ± 0.24	49 ↑
Cl_T (L/h)	0.1531± 0.04	0.247 ± 0.01	61↑	0.0908 ± 0.04	40↓	0.2472 ± 0.01	61 ↑
$t_{1/2\beta}$ (h)	9.5048± 1.73	10.9652 ± 0.64	15↑	88.9772 ± 13.49	836↑	6.2434 ± 0.52	34 ↓
k_β (h^{-1})	0.07351± 0.01	0.0632 ± 0.001	14↓	0.0086 ± 0.001	88↓	0.1144 ± 0.01	56 ↑

Table 2. Effect of Niprisan, AM-1, and Nifadin on the pharmacokinetics parameters of chloroquine (CQ) in rats

Not all botanical-drug interactions result in undesirable effect, while some studies have shown a lack of interaction in the concurrent use of some botanical-drug combinations, other interactions may have beneficial effect on drug therapy. In the presence of the extract of Chinese medicinal plant *Tripterygium wilfordi*, the dose of cyclosporine needed for 100% kidney allograft survival in animals was reduced by 50% - 75% (34). The adverse effect of 'statins' therapy arises from a decreased biosynthesis of endogenous coenzyme Q10 leading to depleted tissue levels, the co-administration of coenzyme Q10 with statin in this therapy reduces the adverse effect (35). In women receiving long-term phenothiazine or buyrophenone therapy, researchers found that intake of 800 mg daily of mistletoe extract silymarin was associated with a significant improvement in liver function tests due to a decrease in malondialdehyde (a polyunsaturated fatty acid oxidation product). Thus the coadministration of this herbal product in the psychoactive therapy has the potential to prevent drug-induced hepatotoxicity (36).

Recently, we have also shown that the concomitant administration of three first line antiretroviral drugs (lamivudine, stavudine and nevirapine) and a plant - based immune booster from *Andrographis paniculata* Nees (Acanthaceae) known in north-eastern India as 'king of bitters', used in the management of HIV/AIDS as an immune stimulant, precipitated interactions observed as beneficial changes in food and water intake as well as the haematological and biochemical indices including CD4, in the presence of the herb (37). There was observed steady increase in red blood cells, white blood cells, food and water intake without an associated increase in cholesterol and high density lipoprotein levels and a decrease in platelet counts. Concomittant administration of this herb with the first line antiretrovirals can ameliorate the anemia and lipodystrophy associated with the use of these drugs. A good review of reported cases and clinical studies of drugs that interact with herbal medicinal products can be found in (38, 13).

3. Challenges to botanical-drug interactions research

In spite of growing concern and examples of herb-drug interactions, little systematic research has been published or funded in this area. An important limiting factor that has majorly led to this situation is the reliability of the existing evidence. A survey of 44 of the leading dietary supplement manufacturers in 2003 revealed that only 10 of 15 respondents considered interactions to be an important issue, and only 2 allocated funds to study herbal-drug interactions (39). Poor reliability of the It was reported in a study that of one hundred and eight cases of suspected interactions studied, 68.5% were classified as 'unable to be evaluated', 13% as 'well-documented' and 18.5% as 'possible' interactions (40). One of the major reasons for this unreliability of reports of the clinical evidence on interactions between herbal and conventional drugs is the inherent scientific and clinical challenges in the use of herbal medicines.

3.1 Predictability of herb-drug interactions

Predicting the potential for a botanical medicine to interact with other drugs can be possible, applying the same principles and study designs as for new chemical entities (NCEs) to evaluate the potential inductive/inhibitory effects of herbal extracts on metabolic enzymes and transporters. However, while it may be easier to define the overall pharmacokinetic and/ or pharmacodynamic mechanisms of interactions for NCEs, especially with those drugs mainly metabolized by CYPs, the prediction of drug interactions with herbs appears to be more difficult and complex (41). Predictability is complexed by factors mainly associated with the drug, and herb (active ingredients complex and not well characterised as well as poorly understood mechanisms of action). Every herbal product is a complex mixture of multiple secondary metabolites / constituents contained in a preparation regarded as one single active substance, even when the preparation is made from a single herb. Masimirembwa et al, using LC MS/MS analysis of six herbal extracts, observed peaks predictive of over 300 chemical species for each herb (42). Each constituent may have a different modulatory potential for the same enzyme and/or modulate a different enzyme. Potentially therefore, a herb may increase, reduce or not affect the effect of a co-administered drug through a combination of simultaneous activities on the same drug target. The inhibition/induction of metabolic enzymes by herbal medicines may vary depending on the herb's method of preparation (different extraction methods may yield different types and quantities of constituents from the same herb). In the work of Gwaza et al, 2mg/ml methanolic extract of the African potato *Hypoxis obtuse* had greater inhibitory effects than same concentration of the water extract. Similar effect was also obtained with the extracts of *Dicoma anomala* (43). Dosing, route of administration, oral bioavailability of the product and other factors are equally confounding factors.

Most often, herbal medicinal products are ingested in a chronic manner by its users, thus a predicted interaction outcome from a single exposure with a target conventional drug may be different in clinical situation. Other drug and patient related factors such as presence of extra-hepatic metabolism; and active transport in liver, age, disease, renal and hepatic functions and genetic polymorphisms are as for conventional drugs and all contribute to the final outcome of drug interaction with herbal medicines. A pharmacological basis of qualitative prediction may be on the 'rule of thumb' simply by comparing the biological effects of the drugs that is, if both products are expected to give similar response, then a potentiation of effect may be expected and vice versa. Also if a drug is a substrate for CYP3A4 and P-gp, its potential for interaction with herbal medicines would be high.

3.2 Lack of consistency in the quality of herbal medicinal products

In a study of 81 published studies on randomized controlled trials of herbal drug interactions, only 15% reported performing tests to quantify actual contents of the herbal supplements used in the studies (43). There are reports of disparity in content of constituents among different brands of echinacea, ginseng, St John's Wort and of particular concern is the fact that inconsistency is also observed even within the same product and same batch (45). Conflicting results of studies of the effect of St John's wort on CYP3A4 are evident. While three enzyme marker studies indicated a potent inducing effect of St John's wort (300 mg three times daily × 14 days) on CYP3A4 activity (46, 47) two others found no effect (both 300 mg three times daily, one for 3 days (48), the other for 8 days (49) on CYP2D6 or 3A4 activities. Lack of batch-to-batch uniformity in the composition and quality of the herbal medicinal products used might explain the discrepancy. Most of these inconsistencies can be attributed to the fact that when compared with conventional drugs, herbal medicines present additional challenges related to quality;

- No established methods to establish the quality of herbal medicines
- Lack of stringent methods for Batch - to - Batch controls
- Susceptibility to environmental contamination

- Herbal medicines are prone to counterfeit practises
- Quality of product prone to seasonal variation & regional source

Thus, there is often great disparity in reported patient response to the use of same herbal medicinal product. The results from many of the published interaction studies therefore may be of little value, since the identity, purity, quality, strength, and composition of the supplements is not always confirmed.

3.3 Lapses in the phytomedicine drug development process

The current phytodrug development process has introduced gaps and lapses that are unfavourable to botanical - drug interaction studies as an integrated step. The argument often is concerning the usefulness of such studies especially where these products have been used therapeutically for centuries without such information. The World Health Organization promotes drug development from traditional medicines partly due to the saving in time and cost that makes the products affordable and accessible, leading to cheaper and cost-effective primary healthcare it offers its teeming population of users. The fast tracking is based on the assumption that the substantial experience from the long history of human use increases the chances that a remedy will be effective and safe, and that precautions will be known. Conventional drug development is slow and expensive and often the finished products are unavailable and unaffordable to resource-limited countries, unless when made available by donors from high-income countries, under heavily subsidized schemes (50). For most phytomedicines, drug development from complimentary and alternative medicines usually follows a "reverse pharmacology" approach (51, 52).

The first step is to select a remedy for development, through a retrospective treatment-outcome study or an ethnobotanical survey to identify medicinal plants used in the treatment of target disease conditions. This step usually will yield insufficient clinical information but is often a good guide to identification of plants and remedies for a given ailment (53, 54). This is because the traditional medicine practitioners often do not have enough records as regards observed patient status as well as progress and treatment outcome and their perception of the efficacy and limitations of their remedies is subjective. Generally also their ability to accurately diagnose a disease condition may be inadequate because a lot of similar symptoms which may present in entirely different disease conditions may be treated with the same remedy. Thus often times, same remedies are employed in the treatment of 'fevers', 'stomach pains', et cetera. Therefore a lot of the information collected at this stage is largely vague, needing evidence-driven scientific evaluation.

The second step usually spins off the first. Following the analyses of the collated remedies, treatment claims and subsequent plants identification, two essential elements are added to the ethnobotanical survey by performing an organized treatment of a fairly large sample size, aimed at generating clinical information and evidence of efficacy in the presentation and progress of an episode of the target disease and statistically correlating treatment with reported clinical recovery as the marker of effectiveness.

Step three involves further research on a selected candidate remedy, to determine the possible pharmacological basis for the therapeutic claim through bioassays. Also at this pre-clinical stage, standardization and characterization of raw materials, intermediates and extracts are commenced, to generate quality control specifications data and chemical finger printing and identification of markers that can be used for monitoring of batch - to – batch uniformity.

The last step is clinical studies, usually involving a dose optimization observational study that will help select the safest and most efficacious dose through a dose-response phenomenon and finally a randomized controlled trial to compare the phytomedicine to the gold standard treatment for the target disease is conducted.

This 'short – cut' approach facilitates the production of standardized phytomedicines faster and more cheaply than conventional drugs. In recent times, advances in this drug development strategy employs great efforts in standardization of mono- and multi-component phyto-preparations using all available high-tech methods, screening of extracts and their constituents by integration of modern molecular biological bioassays and controlled clinical studies, aimed at evidence based phytotherapy. However, it is still deficient in pertinent steps that involve systematic studies in the systemic effect of the phytomedicines inclusive of pharmacokinetic, bioavailability and drug interaction investigations.

For any medicine, efficacy and safety are the major issues thus before proceeding to clinical studies, it is important to establish that the remedy is safe. Safety of medicines in comprehensive sense would consist of not just the absence of toxicity but also the ability to use it effectively in a manner that avoids adverse reactions, therapeutic failure, minimizing risk-benefit ratio associated with its use while promoting rational drug use. WHO guidelines state that: "If the product has been traditionally used without demonstrated harm, no specific restrictive regulatory action should be undertaken unless new evidence demands a revised risk-benefit assessment." The guideline relies heavily on evidence of traditional use or recent clinical experience as sufficient proof for safety (55, 56) and also arguing that often times, the same plants are traditionally used both as a food and as a medicine and no toxicological tests are required for foods, which are usually consumed in greater quantities than medicines (57). This may not be sufficient reason to de-emphasis detailed safety studies for herbal medicinal products because, one may argue that most often herbs are used as spices and condiments in foods at smaller quantities than when used as medicines, meaning that they will be consumed in smaller quantities as foods than as medicines. The differences in dosing can introduce variation in an observed response. For example, *Zingiber officinale* has been used and tested as an antinauseant and antispasmodic agent with very good results (58). Ginger has been shown to be a potent inhibitor of thromboxane synthetase and thus prolongs bleeding time and persons taking warfarin or other drugs that affect platelet activity have been advised to refrain from taking ginger in tablet form (59). Using ginger as a spice does not give same effect. Therefore, even when preliminary field studies show that a herbal medicinal preparation is of common and ancient use, with no known important side effects, to avoid or minimize toxic drug–herb interactions, it is important to identify the interaction potential of such herb(s) using proper in vitro and in vivo models in the early stages of drug development. The essence is to obtain enough information that may be useful for providing warning and proper advice to patients in clinical practice and improve the safe utilization of the herb.

In the past, the focus to address the above issues has been on scientific standardization and appropriate regulatory controls in the manufacture of phytomedicines in the following areas:

- application of all available modern, high-tech methods to standardize phytopreparations before conducting systematic pharmacological investigations and clinical studies

- using new molecular biological assays for screening of extracts and plant constituents to evaluate their exact pharmacological profiles, to elucidate the pharmacological basis of the claimed actions of the constituents of an extract and bioassay guided fractions thereby gain a better understanding of the various mechanisms underlying these pharmacological effects
- controlled clinical studies paralleled by pharmacokinetic and bioavailability studies (60).

However in addition, we propose one more research focus in the area of;

- incorporation of conventional principles in studies addressing additional safety concerns such as herb-drug interaction for the clinical use of herbal medicines, early in the drug development process

3.4 Poor knowledge of pharmacokinetics of botanicals

There is limited information on the pharmacokinetics of herbal medicines even though their use either alone or in addition to conventional drugs is increasing. One of the major reasons is that for most of these multicomponent mixtures, their active ingredient(s) are not known. In addition, there is the difficulty of measuring the quantities of the actives in systemic circulation due to very low concentrations, arising from the very small amount per dose in the final product. These challenges have lead to the situation that most herb - drug interaction studies and case reports in literature only evaluate the outcome of adding a herbal medicinal product to an existing conventional drug therapy and monitoring changes in pharmacokinetics and/or clinical response of the orthodox drug. The reverse is rarely the case. Therefore, a better understanding of the pharmacokinetics of herbal medicines is needed to support the predictability of botanical - drug interactions. Giant strides in the availability of specific high-tech analytical methods and equipment has resulted to the fact that complex extracts and phytopreparations can be analyzed today, to quantify the major active compounds, which are supposed to be responsible for the efficacy of an extract. The effectiveness of these modern tools and processes has been illustrated in several reports (61). Also, they meet the quality standards of drug authorities with high reproducibility of pharmacological studies subjected to good clinical practice (GCP) and conform to clinical trials requirements (62).

4. Mechanisms of herbal-drug interactions

Basically, the same principles and mechanisms responsible for drug-drug interactions are still involved in interactions between phytomedicines and drugs, resulting in pharmacokinetic and pharmacodynamic interactions. Herbal medicinal products or botanicals share the same metabolic and transport proteins, including cytochrome P450 enzymes (CYP), glucuronosyltransferases (UGTs), and P-glycoprotein (Pgp), with over-the-counter and prescription medicines increasing the likelihood of drug—botanical interactions. In other words, herbal products can interact with drugs by affecting the biological processes that regulate their metabolism and elimination.

The family of enzymes known as the cytochrome P450s (CYPs) are involved in 75% of drug metabolism. These monooxygenase enzymes are located mainly in intestinal and liver cells and catalyzes several phase I metabolic processes of many prescription drugs. Of its many subtypes, CYP3A4 is one of the most important, being responsible for about 50% of CYP450

– mediated metabolism. Thus natural products interfering with actions and/or quantities of CYP3A4 have the potential to affect a high percentage of drugs to variable extents. One way that a natural product can alter the action of an enzyme is to modulate by up or down regulating it. Also precipitators may affect bioavailability by modulating absorption or first pass metabolism, altered protein binding, or pharmacological effect. Interactions between herbals and medications can be caused by either pharmacodynamic or pharmacokinetic mechanisms.

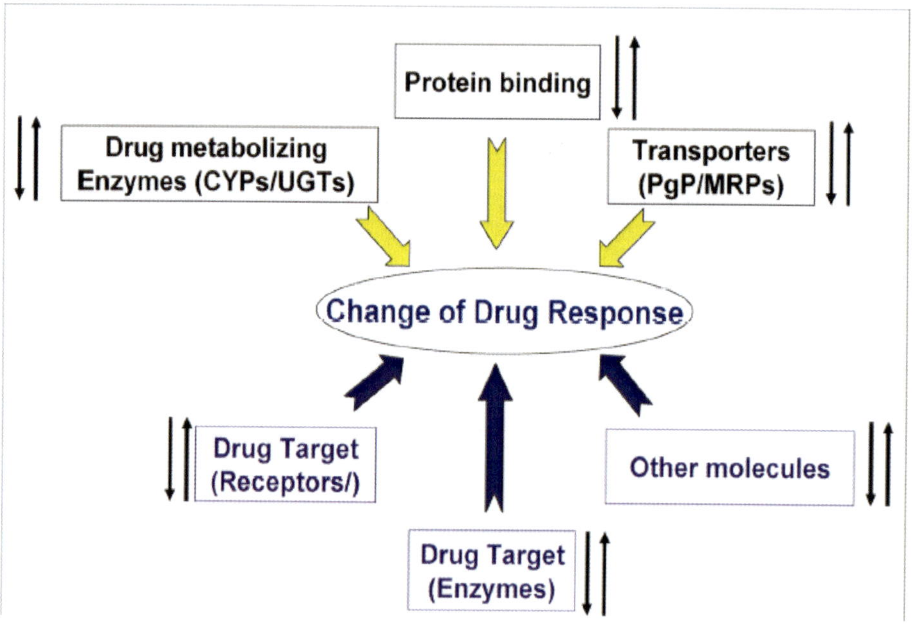

Fig. 1. Possible mechanisms for drug interactions with combined herbal medicines. (ref 63)

Pharmacodynamic interactions can occur when a herbal product produces additive, synergistic, or antagonist activity in relation to the conventional drug with no change in the plasma concentration of either herbal product or drug. Such interactions are related to the pharmacological activity of the interacting agents and can affect organ systems, receptor sites, or enzymes. A pharmacodynamic interaction may occur when herbals that possess antiplatelet activity are administered with antiplatelet/ anticoagulant drugs, thus increasing the risk for bleeding. When Kava, a herbal that depresses the central nervous system (CNS) was administered concomitantly with CNS depressant drug alprazolam, a semicomatose state was induced (64). When a sedative botanical like valerian is co-administered with diazepam or other such sleep inducing agents, a potentiation of sleeping effect could occur. In addition, herbals with the potential to cause organ toxicity may cause further risk of toxicity when drugs with similar toxicity are administered concurrently, such as when the hepatotoxic herbal comfrey is given with large and prolonged doses of acetaminophen (65). An example of an antagonistic interaction is when an herbal with high caffeine content, such as guarana, is administered with a sedative-hypnotic.

In pharmacokinetic interactions on the other hand, the herbal changes the absorption, distribution, metabolism, protein binding, or excretion of a drug which results in altered levels of the drug or its metabolites. The resultant alterations caused by the combination of drugs may or may not alter the dose-response relationship despite the change in the plasma levels and /or drug disposition profile of the drugs because an observable pharmacodynamic change will depend on the degree of change in systemic concentration.

Absorption. Absorption of drugs can be impaired when herbs that contain hydrocolloidal fibers, gums, and mucilage are taken together. Examples of such herbs include psyllium, rhubarb, flaxseed, marshmallow and aloe gel. These herbals can bind to drugs preventing their absorption and, subsequently, reduce systemic availability of the compounds. Psyllium a herb with high content of mucilage, used in the treatment of constipation, inhibits the absorption of lithium (66). Herbal laxatives such as aloe latex, buckthorn, cascara sagrada, rhubarb, and senna can cause loss of fluids and potassium and can potentially increase the risk of toxicity with digoxin (67) as well as reduction in the action of drugs that have a narrow therapeutic index (eg, digoxin, warfarin) due to the diarrhea (68).

Distribution. Salicylates can displace highly protein-bound drugs such as warfarin and carbamazepine from plasma proteins thereby increasing the adverse/toxic effects of the drugs. Meadowsweet and black willow herbs contain salicylates and can potentially interact with such drugs (69). Potential pharmacokinetic interactions can occur with displacement of a drug from protein binding sites. Drug displacement of highly protein-bound drugs by another compound may result in increased activity of the displaced drug. Although displacement of protein-bound drugs has been described as a mechanism for potential drug interactions, there are no documented reports of herbal-drug interactions attributable to displacement of drugs from protein-binding sites.

Metabolism. Licorice when used as an herb, not a sweetener decreases the metabolism of corticosteroids and the anticoagulant action of warfarin is enhanced by ginkgo and possibly by many other herbs (70). Change in renal clearance of a drug is another potential mechanism for producing herbal-drug interactions. Herbals that can inhibit tubular uptake or in other ways that can interfere with the renal clearance of a drug should be considered as having potential to produce pharmacokinetic herbal drug interactions (71).

Two important processes involved in drug disposition in man have been implicated in most of the current evidence of herbal-drug interactions. Several of the documented herb-drug interactions are pharmacokinetic in nature, involving metabolizing enzymes related to oxidative metabolism by the cytochrome P-450 system (CYP) and / or the efflux drug transporter Pglycoprotein, with fewer evidence of the involvement of other enzymes such as glutathione S-transferases and uridine diphosphoglucuronyl transfereases (UGTs) and more than half of all medications undergo metabolism by CYP3A4 substrates (72). Besides CYP3A4 which has been shown to be involved in most herbal - drug interactions, other CYP isoenzymes, which have been found to be involved in significant pharmacokinetic reactions in humans, include CYP1A2, CYP2C9, CYP2C19, CYP2D6, CYP2E. Because some herbals and various drugs may be substrates of the same CYP isoenzyme, either of them may inhibit or induce the activity of the enzyme when ingested concomitantly, the choice of which is dependent on the enzyme –substrate affinity and concentration among other factors.

The other important system that significantly contributes to drug disposition in human is the P-glycoprotein drug transporter. It is a glycoprotein encoded by the MDR1 gene and functions as a transmembrane efflux transporter that pumps drugs out of cells as they try to get into the intestinal wall from the gut lumen where they again become available for oxidative elimination from the body. They are found mainly in organs responsible for drug absorption or elimination, such as the intestine, liver, and kidneys and also present in many tissues. This drug efflux therefore limits the rate and extent of drug absorption from the intestinal tract. Altered expression or activity of several drug transporters and drug-metabolizing enzymes can lead to lower therapeutic efficacy or greater toxicity. The P-glycoprotein has high transport capacity and broad substrate specificity thus it can transport a wide number of clinically relevant drugs with structurally different features and belonging to different classes such as several anticancer drugs, some HIV protease inhibitors, H_2 receptor antagonists, antiarrhythmics—(cardiac glycosides and calcium channel blockers), immunosuppressive immunosuppressive agents, corticosteroids, antiemetic and antidiarrheal agents, analgesics, antibiotics, anthelmintics, antiepileptics, sedatives, antidepressants.

Drugs that are substrates of CYP3A4 often affect P-glycoproteins as well (73), thus the interplay of both intestinal P-gp and CYP3A4 has a strong effect on the bioavailability of most orally administered drugs including proton pump inhibitors (PPIs), cyclosporine, midazolam, talinolol, statins, HIV protease inhibitors and verapamil (74, 75, 76). Therefore concomitant intake of herbal medicinal products that are P-gp and/or CYP3A4 substrates with othodox drugs has a higher potential for interaction. Studies have shown that in cancer therapy several anticancer drugs (such as vincristine, vinblastine, vinorelbine, irinotecan, etoposide, docetaxel, and paclitaxel), as well as certain supportive care agents concomitantly and commonly used by cancer patients, such as ondansetron, fentanyl, morphine, loperamide, and domperidone can modulate P-glycoprotein and/or CYP isoenzymes (77). Thus, the modulation of intestinal and hepatic Pgp and CYP enzymes by herbal medicines represents a potentially important mechanism by which the bioavailability of co-administered drugs can be modulated.

Inhibition or induction of metabolizing enzymes or drug transporters involved in the systemic disposition of drugs is the mechanism of most pharmacokinetic interactions elicited by herbs or their active constituents. Inhibition occurs when herb is able to decrease the normal activity level of a metabolic enzyme or drug transporter via a competitive or noncompetitive mechanism. Induction on the other hand is a much slower process involving gene regulation and expression. The herbal product activates increase in the mRNA leading to increased expression of the corresponding gene or drug transporter. Discontinuation of the precipitator usually brings enzyme levels back to normal, making the process reversible. Induction of the enzymes involved in the metabolism and transport of chemotherapeutic drugs irinotecan or imatinib is responsible for the lower plasma levels observed when each is concurrently administered with St John's Wort (78, 79). On the other hand, inhibition of CYP3A4 by grapefruit juice was responsible for the increase in plasma levels of felodipine when a 5mg tablet was taken with the juice (80). Some botanicals that actively inhibit CYP enzymes include evening primrose oil, kava, garlic, *Ginkgo biloba, Echinacea purpurea,* milk thistle, while Pgp activity was shown to be inhibited by curcumin, , piperine, green tea, quercetin, and silymarin (81 - 83). Ginseng and ginsenosides inhibit both CYP enzyme and Pgp.

In a broad sense, the mechanisms behind induction of metabolizing enzymes will include processes that involve enhanced translational efficiency, increased gene transcription rates, improved enzyme stability and ligand binding / other enzyme-related actions. However, the most commonly encountered is that involving the activation of certain nuclear receptors in man. This mechanism has been further elucidated, giving rise to new possibilities for the identification of herbal preparations capable of causing induction because the mechanistic knowledge about induction processes can be an aid in the prediction of clinically relevant interactions.

Pregnane X receptor (PXR), the constitutive androstane receptor (CAR), and the vitamin D-binding receptor (VDR) are nuclear receptors that have been identified to be involved in the induction of metabolizing enzymes and some drug transporters. After activation by endogenous or exogenous ligands, these receptors form heterodimers with the 9-*cis* retinoic acid receptor (RXR) and bind to xenobiotic response elements in the target genes (84). Because of this, the transcription of the target genes is increased, leading to detoxification and elimination of xenobiotics.

PXR, is one of the main transcriptional regulators of CYP3A4 and Pgp, while possessing some transcriptional control over CYP2B6, CYP2C9, sulfotransferase (SULT), UGT1A1, glutathione S-transferases (GST), and MRP-2. Studies have shown that the activation of PXR is one of the main mechanisms behind induction of metabolizing enzymes and drug transporters by herbal medicines (85). The inductive capacity of SJW is mediated via this mechanism. Hyperforin, a bioactive constituent in St John's wort, forms a complex with the ligand-binding domain of human PXR thereby activating the PXR and consequently inducing CYP3A4 and CYP2C9 expression (86, 87). Studies using gene reporter assays or measuring mRNA levels of CYP3A4 in human hepatocytes have also shown that gugulipid, or its chemical constituents guggulsterones, derived from the Mukul myrrh tree, hops, two traditional Chinese medicines (TCMs), Wu Wei Zi (*Schisandra chinensis* Baill) and Gan Cao (*Glycyrrhiza uralensis* Fisch), and their selective constituents, carotenoids, especially β-carotene, and retinol have the potential to induce CYP3A4 by activation of PXR (88-90).

Both P-gp and CYP3A4 are abundantly expressed in the villus tip of enterocytes and hepatocytes, correspondingly, both intestine and liver express significant concentrations of PXR. This is important because the transcriptional regulation of drug metabolizing enzymes is cell-mediated and tissue-selective, thus significant inductions will not be found in tissues that have low concentrations of the receptors and enzymes when in contact with the relevant ligands. Known ligands of human PXR include rifampicin, dexamethasone, clortrimazole, and paclitaxel and all are established inducers of CYP3A4 (91).

Metabolizing enzymes are also induced to a lesser extent by other nuclear receptors such as CAR and VDR. *CYP2B* gene is the main target of CAR but the expression of other hepatic genes, such as *UGT1A1* and *CYP2C9* and MDR-1 is also modulated by this receptor (92, 93). VDR is the receptor responsible for modulating cytogenesis and cell death in response to 1α, 25-dihydroxy vitamin D_3 as the ligand. In addition, it also regulates CYP3A4, CYP2B6 and CYP2C9 (94). Though PXR has been shown to mainly regulate CYP3A4 expression while CAR regulates CYP2B expression, it is clear that one type of nuclear receptor has the ability to modulate the expression of several enzymes, meaning that the specificity is not absolute but rather there is some overlap in both the nuclear transcription function as well as the ligand-binding capacity and the extent of induction will vary depending on the ligand, tissue involved. Consequently, more than one enzyme modulated by different receptors may be responsible for an observed effect in a herb induced interaction. For example, PXR, CAR and the aryl hydrocarbon receptor (AhR) are all known to modulate the overall UGT1A1 response to flavonoids, though the AhR is mainly responsible for the UGT1A1 expression (95).

In vitro screening for potential inhibition or induction of CYP enzymes by various herbals is gaining momentum (96), but data about the inductive capacity of herbal medicinal products and their interaction with nuclear receptors is scarce and mainly focused on PXR. However, with the discovery of the mechanistic processes involving nuclear receptors in the induction of metabolizing enzymes and drug transporters drug transporters, recent efforts to address these challenges are more optimistic.

5. Investigating herb–drug interaction

FDA requires that the extent of metabolism for all new drugs be defined, the CYP enzymes involved in the formation of its major metabolite be identified and their potency for enzyme inhibition evaluated. This is with a view to complying with the regulatory requirement that a warning towards such interactions be added in the product insert and label (97). Thus, in the discovery of conventional drugs, new chemical entities (NCEs) are tested for inhibitory effects on CYP3A4, potent inhibition is associated with a potential for drug-drug interactions. Similarly, there is a need to identify the potentials for herbal medicinal products to interact with drugs in the early stages of drug development using proper in vitro and in vivo models, so as to improve their safe use in clinical practice.

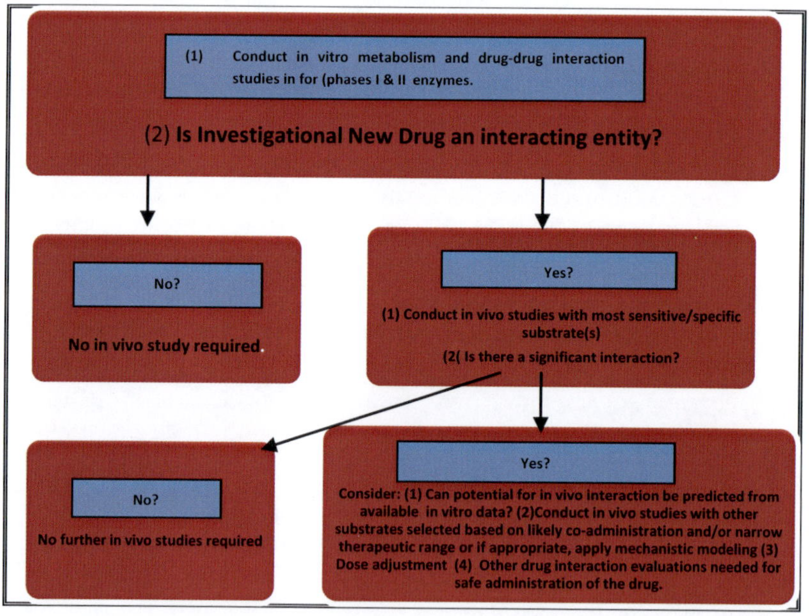

Fig. 2. Simplified schematic representation of the FDA recommended approach to evaluating Investigational New Drugs for possible drug-drug interactions (DDIs).

Although there are challenges of content of numerous constituents of unknown pharmacokinetics and pharmacology inherent in herbal agents that limit the application of methods used in screening conventional drugs, several of these methods can be adapted for determining whether a phytomedicine will affect metabolic enzymes and drug transporter systems thereby deduce its interaction potential. For example, an inhibition study can be adapted from the FDA guidance document on drug / drug interaction as shown in figure 3.

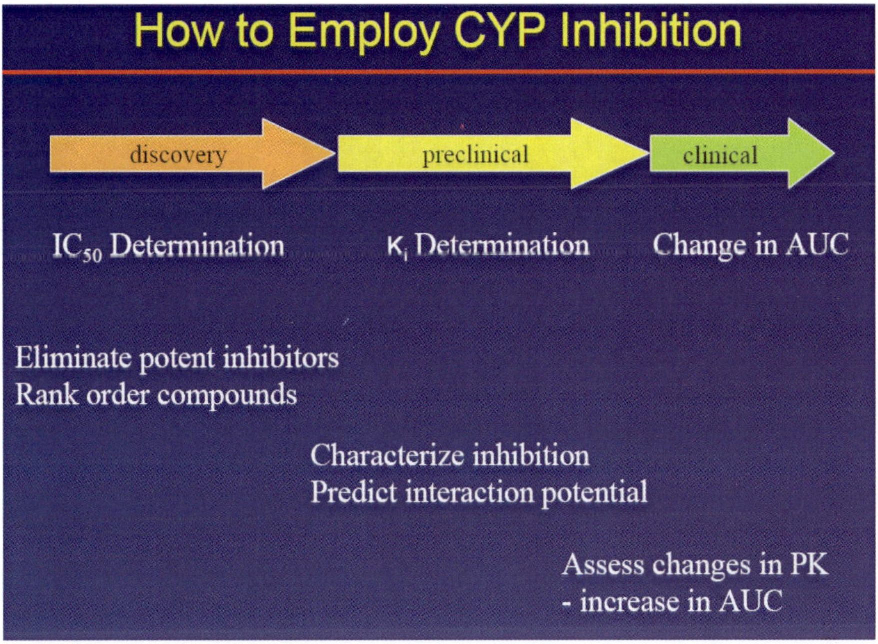

Fig. 3. Schematic representation on how to employ CYP inhibition at different stages of drug development process

Likelihood	Ki (μM)	I/Ki
Probable	<1	>1
Possible	1<Ki<50	0.1<1/Ki<1
Unlikely	>50	<0.1

Table 3. Inhibition studies Interpretation: Potential for in vivo inhibition.

Compounds with Ki< 1μM are generally predicted to cause drug / drug interaction hence in vivo studies recommended. Hyperforin one of the constituents of St John's wort, purpoted to be the active constituent and the most potent agonist of PXR, has a Ki of 27nM (98).

In vitro models generally use subcellular fractions of human liver tissues, whole-cell models of isolated human hepatocytes, liver slices, or human cell lines (99). Changes in the activity or concentration of enzymes or transporters can be demonstrated through use of selective chemical inhibitors of specific CYP enzymes or transporter systems. For metabolic studies, the major models usually are subcellular fractions (liver microsomes, cytosols and homogenates), precision-cut liver slices, isolated and cultured hepatocytes or liver cell lines, and cDNA-expressed enzymes while human gastrointestinal absorption and cancer cell lines, as well as membrane vesicles and cDNA expressed drug transporters are widely used for transport studies (100, 101).

High throughput screening has been successfully adapted to the study of drug-herb, herb-CYP and herb/P-gp interactions (102). This has an advantage that a large number of herbs, their bioactive fractions and constituents can be screened at the same time in a multiple well plate (see figure 4), thereby providing in vitro inhibition data as a criterion for further investigation. This method has been used in our laboratories to study in vitro, inhibition studies involving the inhibition of CYP-specific marker reactions by test herbal medicinal products. These phytomedicines are being developed for use in the treatment and management of malaria, HIV infection, diabetes and sickle cell disease respectively.

The products were investigated at two concentrations for CYP-specific marker reactions using recombinant CYP3A4 and fluorescent based marker reactions. Inhibition of the CYP activity by more than 20% was considered significant and in such cases, the IC_{50} (the concentration of product bringing about 50% inhibition of enzyme activity) value was determined. All the products had inhibition greater than 50%, some comparable to the troleandomycin, a known inhibitor of CYP3A4. Their IC_{50} ranged from 0.004 - 0.060mg/ml and was compared with that of ketoconazole, a potent inhibitor of CYP3A4 with an IC_{50} of 0.016mg/ml (Obodozie et al, unpublished data).

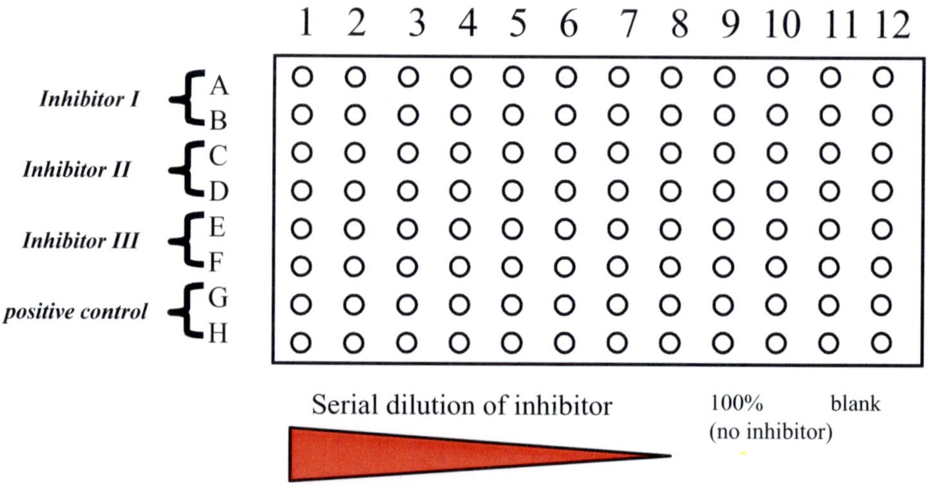

Fig. 4. Design of HTS for CYP Inhibition (*ref. 102*)

The IC_{50} curves for four of the five products and control inhibitor is shown in figures 5a - 5e

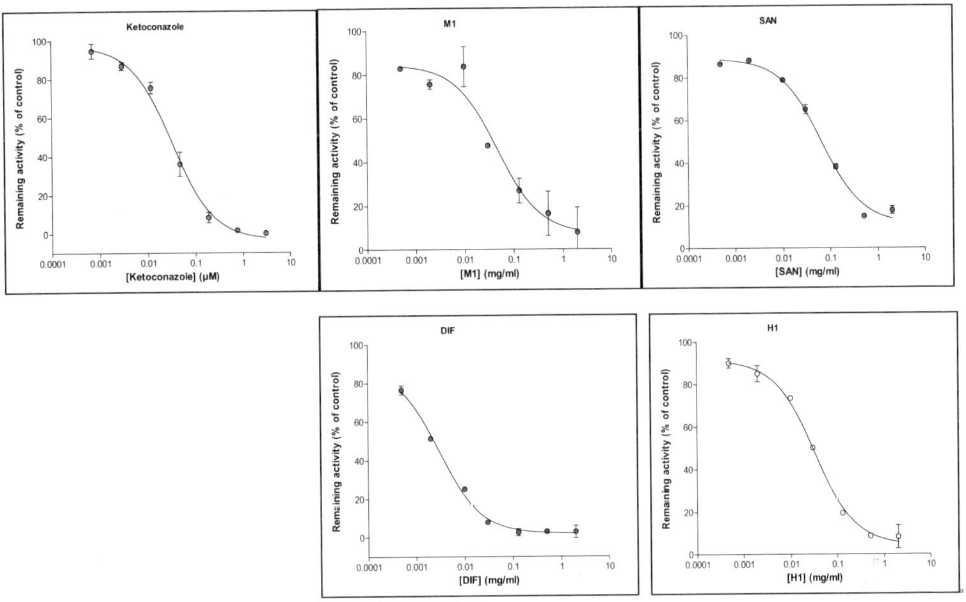

Fig. 5. (a – e): IC_{50} Curves for some natural products and control inhibitor. [a] M1=AM-1 extract from *Nauclea latifolia,* [b] SAN=NIPRISAN [c] D1F= Fraction component of the extract of *Vernonia amygdalina* and [d] HI=extract *Andrographis paniculata*

If absorbed, these products are predicted to result in significant clinical drug-herb interactions. Therefore further in vivo studies are necessary as recommended by FDA approach (see figure 2).

Other in vitro methods involve the use of in silico methods to determine the interactions potential of CYPs, Phase II enzymes, P-gp with botanicals, often by the use of rule-based modelling, and structure–activity relationships (103, 104).

Often times, to obtain enough information that is useful for a test herbal product in evaluating how the herb may affect CYPs and P-gp, various methods may be used in combination. For example, in an in vitro study performed to investigate the inductive properties of several flavonoids, including quercetin, resveratrol, and curcumin to activate nuclear receptors and to induce metabolizing enzymes using primary cultures of human hepatocytes of 17 individuals, it was found that only quercetin led to an increase in the quantity of CYP3A4 mRNA. To further elucidate the involvement of PXR, a reporter gene assay with hPXR was used. Quercetin did not show a significant increase in luciferase activity, suggesting that CYP3A4 was induced by mechanisms not involving PXR (105). Kava-kava also increases CYP3A4 mRNA levels in hepatocytes with enhanced luciferase activity, others like grapeseed extract, ginseng and garlic stimulates only CYP3A4 mRNA without increasing luciferase activity indicating that that the induction CYP3A4 by some herbs may not always be mediated via PXR.

Each of these models has very different cost, reliability, advantages and limitations. For example, some models will maintain the structure and integrity of isolates and cellular cultures with a loss in quality and quantity of the target enzymes. Thus they may be useful for the study of Phase I and II reactions (106, 107) but not suitable for inhibition and transport studies (108) due to the rapid down regulation of certain enzymes and transporters which occurs after isolation of hepatocytes. Primary liver cell cultures have been used for a long time to study inductive potentials of products but its major set back is the availability, quality and inter-individual variation of human liver tissue and the fact that it can only give information about the inductive capacity and not about the nuclear receptor involved. The development of reporter gene assays has reduced some of the challenges associated with the use of human liver tissue.

Making decisions on whether an herbal-drug interaction occurs based on data from in vitro or animal test models is inadequate. When drug interactions with a herbal medicinal product is suspected to be likely based on in vitro results or significant in animal studies, they should be confirmed with further well conducted in vivo studies and in human to validate the clinical significance. Such studies are needed because most often in vitro assays do not necessarily correlate with in vivo and human metabolism. This is most important for herbal medicines which usually contain multiple constituents because the entity that is precipitating enzyme modulation in vitro may not be systemically available due to instability in the GIT, unabsorbed or is inactive prodrug.

As reported earlier, the in vitro studies using rCYP3A4 and paracetamol as the substrate showed AM-1as a potent inhibitor of the enzyme indicating that an increase in paracetamol (acetaminophen) blood levels will be likely if both drugs are co-administered. However, further in vivo studies in human volunteers showed reduction in AUC of paracetamol when both products were concurrently administered (31). Grapefruit juice, a potent inhibitor of intestinal CYP3A4 precipitated lower AUC of etoposide when both were taken concomittantly orally in humans, contrary to the expected increase in oral bioavailability of the CYP3A4 substrate. The involvement of another mechanism, possibly an inductive effect of grapefruit juice on Pgp-mediated transport of etoposide may have been responsible for this lower AUC (109). Another example is the use of in vitro preparations of liver microsomes to predict drug interaction potentials. These results may not agree with in vivo studies because human liver microsomes are not able to predict enzyme induction due to inability of microsomal preparations to synthesize new proteins thus may not give an indication of potential induction in vivo. An example of this is the case of St John's Wort which has been shown to induce both CYP3A4 through an action on PXR in vivo, as well as Pgp and CYP2C19 but in vitro, it inhibits CYP2D6, CYP 2C9 and CYP3A4 (110, 111).

Animal models are widely used for the evaluation of drug–herb interactions. Such models include the use of wistar rats, rabbits, mice, transgenic mice et cetera. Caution should be exercised in the interpretation and extrapolation of in vivo results obtained from animal models to humans because the species differences in nuclear receptors and inductive processes make extrapolation difficult. Also there are observed species differences in the ligand-binding domains (LBDs), especially in the LBD of PXR of wild-type laboratory animals that may produce discrepancies between in vivo animal and human study data. The report by Bakare-Odunola et al (112), showed that metronidazole pharmacokinetic parameters were significantly altered by concomitant administration of the antimalaria phytomedicine AM-1, such that AUC and maximum serum concentration were increased by over 100% and Vd and Cl were similarly reduced in rats, another study showed no significant alteration in the oral bioavailability of the same drugs when concurrently administered to healthy human volunteers (113).

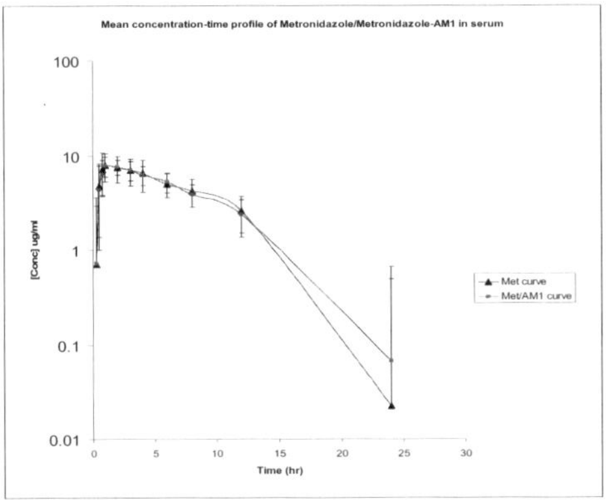

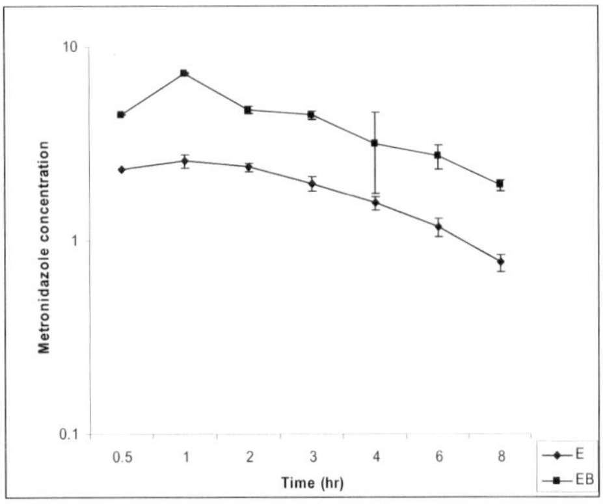

(a) (b)

Fig. 6. (a – b): (a) Serum concentration-time curve of metronidazole in human volunteers following oral administration of two tablets of 200mg metronidazole (flagyl®) alone and after concurrent administration with 400mg AM1 (b) Serum concentration-time curve of metronidazole in rats following oral administration of 7.5mg/kg metronidazole alone and after co-administration with 16mg/kg NIPRD AM-1

Not with standing, results from animal studies can also be source of useful information especially when human transgenic animals are used (114).

Clinical studies on drug-herb interaction usually employ the use of human participants and most are designed to monitor pharmacokinetic interactions. The studies follow principally three basic designs, while the first and third give an idea of the involvement of specific enzyme in an interaction, the second provides general information on the effect of the herb on a target drug. Several well conducted clinical studies some popularly used botanicals demonstrate these methods.

(I) The use of probe drugs that are known to be metabolized by specific enzymes and monitoring the change in AUC of the probe drug with and without the test herbal product.

The effect of different herbal drugs on various metabolizing enzymes and transporters in humans have bee shown. Artemisinin was shown to be a potent inhibitor of CYP1A2 activity by decreasing the paraxanthine levels when co-administered with caffeine in humans (115). *Citrusaurantium*, *Panax*ginseng, *Echinaceapurpurea,* milk thistle, and saw palmetto extracts taken by healthy volunteers all had no effect on the activity of CYP3A4, CYP1A2, CYP2E1, and CYP3A4 measured using model substrates (116). Meanwhile the disposition profile of some substrates for other enzymes CYP3A4, CYP1A2, CYP2E1, and CYP2D6 were not affected by gingko when administered to healthy volunteers or elderly patients (117, 118). FDA recommended substrates for specific enzymes include Theophylline/caffeine for CYP 1A2, S-warfarin/Lorstan for CYP 2C9, Desipramine for CYP2D6, mizodolam, buspirone, felodipine, simvastatin, lovarstatin for CYP3A4 while fexofenadine and digoxin are P-gp substrates.

(II) Administering the test herbal product with and without a target conventional drug and monitoring the change in pharmacokinetic profile of the latter.

Mills et al have given a good review the effects of St John's Wort on the pharmacokinetics of some conventional drugs (119). One of the renowned cases of herb - drug interaction is the effect of garlic preparations on the plasma concentrations of antiretroviral drugs saquinavir and ritonavir. The effect of garlic supplements on the pharmacokinetics of saquinavir was reported by Piscitelli et al. Garlic preparations decreased the mean AUC and the mean C_{max} of saquinavir by 51% and 54% respectively (120), while not having effect on neither ritonavir concentrations nor the metabolism of acetaminophen in healthy volunteers (121, 122). Ritonavir is now known to be a CYP3A4 inhibitor, an effect that has prompted its use in antiretroviral therapy with positive therapeutic benefit in boosting (by inhibition of CYP3A4) other protease inhibitors and enhancing their bioavailability (saquinavir, lopinavir) as well as reducing hepatic clearance (indinavir, amprenavir, and atazanavir).

Administering the test herbal without a target conventional drug or enzyme probe and monitoring the change in an enzyme activity marker before and after treatment.

Omeprazole hydroxylation, a CYP2C19 mediated action was shown to be induced in healthy male subjects by *Ginkgo biloba*, one of the most widely used herbal products, indicating that the effect of omeprazole could be reduced with the concurrent adminstration of Gingko (123). The effect of P. Ginseng on the 6-B-hydroxycortisol to cortisol ratio, a marker of CYP3A4 activity was evaluated in twenty healthy human participants before and after a 14 day intake of 100mg of P. Ginseng standardized to contain 4% ginsennosides. The results suggested that there was no induction of CYP3A4 activity (124)

6. Risk factors for herbal-drug interactions

The risk of having an herbal-drug interaction is based on a variety of factors related to patient, dosing regimen, co-administered drug and herb, and not solely based on the pharmacologic and pharmacokinetic characteristics of the herbal. One important factor that increases the likelihood of having a herbal-drug interaction is concomitant use of a herbal product with drugs that have a narrow therapeutic index because while a doubling or more in drug plasma concentration has the potential for enhanced drug effects and/or appearance of adverse effects (125), less marked changes may still be clinically important for such drugs with steep concentration–response relationship. Drugs in this category include digoxin, antiepileptic drugs, antineoplastic agents, immunosuppressants and warfarin.

Patient populations who are at increased risk for having herbal-drug interactions include the elderly, critical care patients, patients undergoing surgical procedures, patients with liver or renal disease, and patients receiving multiple medications. In most cases, the extent of drug interactions with herbs varies markedly among individuals, with gender and genetic polymorphism as additional factors for the inter-individual differences.

In persons using herbal products chronically, hepatic and intestinal metabolism or drug transport may be affected by the same herb differently for the same substrate. In vitro data obtained in human hepatocyte cultures, showed that St John's Wort a known CYP3A4 inhibitor, can induce greater docetaxel metabolism in patients using the herb chronically (126). The oral bioavailability of midazolam after echinacea intake was significantly greater, while in contrast, multiple dosing of the same herb in volunteers for 8 days resulted in a significantly lower AUC and 34% increase in systemic clearance of the drug (127). CYP3A4 was inhibited by single dose administration of ritonavir, chronic administration resulted in an induction of same enzyme (128). Herb related factors that are risk factors in drug interactions with herbal medicinal product include species, dose, dosing regimen, and administration route (13)

7. Conclusion

The metabolism of a drug can be altered by another drug or foreign chemical, and such interactions can often be clinically significant. Cytochrome P450 (CYP) enzymes, a superfamily of enzymes found mainly in the liver, are involved in the metabolism of a plethora of xenobiotics and have been shown to be involved in numerous interactions between drugs and food, herbs and other drugs. The observed induction and inhibition of CYP enzymes by natural products in the presence of a prescribed drug has (among other reasons) led to the general acceptance that natural therapies can have adverse effects, contrary to the popular beliefs in countries where there is an active practice of ethnomedicine. Majority of the classes of conventional drugs have been shown to be affected by different types of botanical preparations leading to various consequencies, including treatment failure, adverse / toxic effects and even death. In order to improve the safety of ethnomedicines use alongside conventional therapies in public healthcare, it is necessary to understand how the former will interact with the latter, early in drug development. It is also necessary to predict early so as to eliminate regulatory obstacles and avoid market pressure for recalls that may have been induced by adverse effects linked to interactions.

It is possible and highly recommended that the conventional industrial preclinical platform be used to evaluate herbal extracts for metabolism based drug-herb interactions, thereby incorporating such studies into drug development for phytomedicines. Although the presence of numerous active ingredients in herbal medicines, foods and dietary supplements complicate experimentation, the observable interactions with CYP enzymes warrant systematic studies, so that metabolism-based interactions can be predicted and avoided more readily. Over the years, there has been great advances in the availability of "high tech" tools, in vitro and in vivo study designs and analytical equipment that can be adapted for use in such studies. Pharmaceutical research must go beyond focusing on pharmacological efficacy of botanicals but also in studies that improve their effectiveness in order for humanity to fully benefit from their inherent therapeutic potentials.

8. References

[1] DiMasi JA, Hansen RW, Grabowski HG: The price of innovation: new estimates of drug development costs. Journal of Health Economics 2003, 22:151-185.

[2] Eisenberg DM, Davis RB, Ettner SL, et al. Trends in alternative medicine use in the United States, 1990-1997: results of a follow-up national survey. *JAMA*. 1998;280: 1569-1575.

[3] Abdel-Aziz, H.; Wadie, W.; Kelber, O.; Weiser, D.; Khayyal, M.T. Evidence for the effectiveness of stw5 (iberogast) in an experimental model of ulcerative colitis. Personalisierte Therapeutika – Traum oder Wirklichkeit? 4. - 7. Oktober 2010 Tagungsband 2010; Book of Abstracts

[4] World health Organisation. Antiretroviral therapy for HIV infection in adults and adolescents Recommendations for a public health approach: 2010 revision.
[5] Ho, D. "Time to hit HIV, early and hard". (1995). The New England journal of medicine 333 (7): 450–451.
[6] Kuhn M. Pharmacotherapeutics: A Nursing Process Approach. Philadelphia, Pa: FA Davis; 1998.
[7] Sparreboom A, Cox MC, Acharya MR et al. Herbal remedies in the United States: potential adverse interactions with anticancer agents. J Clin Oncol 2004; 22:2489–2503.
[8] McCune JS, Hatfield AJ, Blackburn AA et al. Potential of chemotherapy-herb interactions in adult cancer patients. Support Care Cancer 2004;12:454–462.
[9] Izzo AA. Herb-drug interactions: an overview of the clinical evidence. Fundam Clin Pharmacol 2005;19:1–16.
[10] Delgoda R, Westlake AC. Herbal interactions involving cytochrome p450 enzymes: a mini review. Toxicol Rev 2004;23: 239–249.
[11] Zhou S, Lim LY, Chowbay B. Herbal modulation of P-glycoprotein. Drug Metab Rev 2004; 36:57–104.
[12] Dresser, G.K. et al. (2000) Pharmacokinetic-pharmacodynamic consequences and clinical relevance of cytochrome P450 3A4 inhibition. Clin. Pharmacokinet. 38, 41–57.
[13] Hu, Z. et al. (2005) Herb–drug interactions: a literature review. Drugs 65, 1239–1282
[14] Zhou, S. et al. (2003) Interactions of herbs with cytochrome P450. Drug Metab Rev. 35, 35-98
[15] Elvin-Lewis, M. (2001) Should we be concerned about herbal remedies. J. Ethnopharmacol. 75, 141–164
[16] Mustapha A. Yakassai IA, Aguye IA. Effect of Tamarindus indica L. on the bioavailability of aspirin in healthy human volunteers. Eur J Drug Metab Pharmacokinet 1996; 21: 223-226.
[17] Aslam, M. and Stockley, I.H. Interaction between curry ingredient (karela) and drug (chlorpropamide). 1979; Lancet 1, 607.
[18] Bauer S, Stormer E, Johne A, et al. Alterations in cyclosporin A pharmacokinetics and metabolism during treatment with St John's wort in renal transplant patients. Br J Clin Pharmacol 2003;55:203-211.
[19] Ruschitzka F, Meier PJ, Turina M, et al. Acute heart transplant rejection due to Saint John's wort. Lancet 2000;355:548-549.
[20] Piscitelli SC, Burstein AH, Chaitt D, et al. Indinavir concentrations and St John's wort. Lancet 2000;355:547-548.
[21] Greiner B, Eichelbaum M, Fritz P, et al. The role of intestinal P-glycoprotein in the interaction of digoxin and rifampin. J Clin Invest 1999;104:147-153.
[22] Zhou S, Chan E, Pan SQ, et al. Pharmacokinetic interactions of drugs with St John's Wort. J Psychopharmacol 2004;18:262-276.
[23] Gordon, J.B. (1998) SSRIs and St. John's Wort: possible toxicity? Am. Fam. Physician. 57, 950.
[24] Rowin J, Lewis SL. Spontaneous bilateral subdural hematomas associated with chronic Ginkgo biloba ingestion. Neurology. 1996;46:1775-1776.
[25] Gianni LM, Dreitlein WB. Some popular OTC herbals can interact with anticoagulant therapy. US Pharmacist. 1998;23:80, 83–84, 86.

[26] Matthews MK Jr. Assosiation of Gingko biloba with intracerebral haemorrhage. Neurology 1998; 50: 1933-1934.
[27] Galluzzi, S. et al. (2000) Coma in a patient with Alzheimer's disease taking low dose trazodone and Ginkgo biloba. J. Neurol. Neurosurg. Psychiatr. 68, 679–680.
[28] Shaw, D. et al. (1997) Traditional remedies and food supplements. A 5-year toxicological study (1991–1995). Drug Saf. 17, 342–356.
[29] <Physicians' Desk Reference at http://pdrel.thomsonhc.com/pdrel/librarian >
[30] Health Canada is advising Canadians not to take certain drugs with grapefruit juice: http://www.hc-sc.gc.ca/english/protectio/warnings/2002/2002_49e.htm
[31] Obodozie O, Mustapha K, Inyang U (2004) Alteration of oral salivary pharmacokinetics of paracetamol by an investigational anti malarial phytomedicine, in healthy human volunteers. Eur J Drug Metabol Pharmacokinet 29(3):193–197.
[32] Adzu B, Haruna A, Maman M, Wambebe C, Gamaniel K. Effect of Niprisan on oral dose pharmacokinetics of paracetamol in rats. Eur j Drug Metab Pharmacokinetic 2001; 26: 201-204
[33] Obodozie OG, Mustapha KB, Taibat-Odunola M, Garba M. The Effect of Phytomedicines on the Single Dose Pharmacokinetics of Metronidazole and Chloroquine The 47th Annual Meeting of the American Society of Pharmacognosy: Natural Products on Target., Washington DC, August 2006, Abstract No P-243
[34] Wang J, Xu R, Chen Z, Fidler JM. Immunosuppressive activity of Chinese medicinal plant Tripterygium wilfordi. I. Prolongation of rat cardiac and renal allograft survival by the PG27 extract and immunosuppressive synergy in combination therapy with cyclosporine. Transplantation 2000; 70: 447-455
[35] Rundek T, Naini A, Sacco R, Coates K, DiMauro S. Atorvastatin decreases the coenzyme Q10 level in the blood of patients at risk for cardiovascular disease and stroke. Arch Neurol. 2004; 61(6):889-892.
[36] Palasciano G, Portincasa P, Palmieri V, et al. The effect of silymarin on plasma levels of malondialdehyde in patients receiving long-term treatment with psychotropic drugs. Curr Ther Res. 1994;55(5):537-545.
[37] Obodozie OO, Adelakun TA, Tarfa FD, Tijani AY, Busu SM, Inyang US. Evaluation of the effect of co-administration of selected first line Antiretroviral agents with an investigational herbal immune booster in healthy rats. FIP Pharmaceutical Sciences 2010 World Congress in Association with the AAPS Annual Meeting and Exposition, New Orleans, USA: Nov. 2010. Abstract # 3804
[38] Zhou S, Koh H-L, Gao Y, Gong Z-Y, Lee EJD. Herbal Bioactivation. Life Sci 2004; 74: 935 – 968.
[39] Thompson Coon J, Pittler M, Ernst E. Herb-drug interactions: survey of leading pharmaceutical/herbal companies. Arch Intern Med. 2003;163(11):1371.
[40] Fugh-Berman, A., Ernst, E., 2001. Herb–drug interactions: review and assessment of report reliability. British Journal of Clinical Pharmacology 52 (5), 587–595.
[41] Houston, J.B. (1994) Utility of in vitro drug metabolism data in predicting in vivo metabolic clearance. Biochem. Pharmacol. 47, 1469–1479
[42] Masimirembwa C, Gamaniel K.S, Mustapha K.B, Adzu B, Obodozie O, Moyo S and Thelingwani R. Herbalomics and drug-herb interactions – towards the safe and efficacious use of traditional medicines in Africa. African Network for Drug/

Diagnostics Discovery and Innovation (ANDI). Conference and high level forum/stakeholders meeting. Nairobi, October 2010. Abstract #150

[43] Luther Gwaza In vitro toxicological evaluation and chemical characterization of herbal medicines used in Zimbabwe MPhil Thesis, University of Zimbabwe Harare, Zimbabwe.2008

[44] Wolsko PM, Solondz DK, Phillips RS, et al. Lack of herbal supplement characterization in published randomized controlled trials. *Am J Med* 2005;118(10):1087-1093.

[45] Lam YWF, Huang S, Hall SD (eds). Herbal Supplements - Drug Interactions: Scientific and Regulatory Perspectives. Drugs and the Pharmaceutical Sciences 2006; 162: 40-4

[46] Roby CA, Anderson GD, Kantor E, et al. St. John's wort: effect on CYP3A4 activity. Clin Pharmacol Ther. 2000;**67**: 451–457.

[47] Kerb R, Bauer S, Brockmöller J, Roots I. Urinary 6-(hydroxycortisol excretio rate is affected by treatment with hypericum extract (Abstract) Eur J Clin Pharmacol. 1997;**52**(Suppl):A186.

[48] Markowitz JS, DeVane CL, Boulton DW, et al. Effect of St. John's wort (Hypericum perforatum) on cytochrome P-450 2D6 and 3A4 activity in healthy volunteers. Life Sci. 2000; 66(9):133–139.

[49] Ereshefsky B, Gewertz N, Lam YWF, et al. Presented at the 39th Annual Meeting of the New Clinical Drug Evaluation Program. Boca Raton, FL: 1999. Determination of SJW differential metabolism at CYP2D6 and CYP3A4, using dextromethorphan probe methodology.

[50] The Global fund. Affordable Medicines Facility – Malaria http://www.theglobalfund.org/en/amfm/

[51] Merlin L Willcox, Bertrand Graz, Jacques Falquet, Chiaka Diakite, Sergio Giani, Drissa Diallo. A "reverse pharmacology" approach for developing an anti-malarial phytomedicine. 2011, Malaria Journal, 10(Suppl 1):S8

[52] Patwardhan B, Mashelkar RA, Patwardhan B, Mashelkar RA: Traditional medicine-inspired approaches to drug discovery: can Ayurveda show the way forward? Drug Discovery Today 2009, 14:804-811.

[53] Graz B, Falquet J, Elisabetsky E: Ethnopharmacology, sustainable development and cooperation: The importance of gathering clinical data during field surveys. Journal of Ethnopharmacology 2010, 130:635-638.

[54] Graz B, Diallo D, Falquet J, Willcox M, Giani S: Screening of traditional herbal medicine: first, do a retrospective study, with correlation between diverse treatments used and reported patient outcome. Journal of Ethnopharmacology 2005, 101:338-339.

[55] WHO: Expert Committee on specifications for pharmaceutical preparations: Thirty-fourth report. Geneva: World Health Organisation; 1996.

[56] WHO: Guidelines for the Appropriate Use of Herbal Medicines. Manila: WHO Regional Office for the Western Pacific; 1998.

[57] Willcox ML, Gamaniel SK, Matsabisa MG, Randriasamimanana JR, Wambebe CON, Rasoanaivo P: Guidelines for the pre-clinical evaluation of the safety of traditional herbal antimalarials. In Traditional Medicinal Plants and Malaria. Boca Raton: CRC Press;Willcox M, Bodeker G, Rasoanaivo P. 2004.

[58] Bone ME, Wilkinson DJ, Young Jr, et al. Ginger root, a new antiemetic: the effect of ginger root on postoperative nausea and vomiting after major gynecological surgery. Anaesthesia. 1990;45:669–671.
[59] Backon J. Ginger: inhibition of thromboxane synthetase and stimulation of prostacyclin: relevance for medicine and psychiatry. Med Hypothesis. 1986; 20:271–278.
[60] A presentation at the 24th International Symposium on the Chemistry of Natural Products and the 4th International Congress on Biodiversity, held jointly in Delhi, India, 26–31 January 2004.)
[61] Amagaya S, A. Iizuka, B. Makino, M. Kubo, Y. Komatsu, F.-Ch. Cheng, T. I. Ruo, T. Itoh, K. Terasawa. *Phytomedicine* **8**, 338–347 (2001).
[62] Williamson EM and F. J. Evans. *Drugs* **60**, 1305–1314 (2000).
[63] Shu-Feng Zhou, Zhi-Wei Zhou, Chun-Guang Li, Xiao Chen, Xiyong Yu, Charlie Changli Xue and Adrian Herington. Identification of drugs that interact with herbs in drug development. Drug Discovery Today 2007; 12: 664-673
[64] Almeida, J.C. and Grimsley, E.W. (1996) Coma from the health food store: interaction between Kava and alprazolam. Ann. Intern. Med. 125, 940–941
[65] Natural Medicine Comprehensive Database. August, 2005. http://www.naturaldatabase.com (accessed August 31, 2005).
[66] Perlman BB. Interaction between lithium salts and ispaghula husk. Lancet. 1990; 17; 335(8686):416.
[67] Kuhn MA. Herbal remedies. Herb-drug interactions. Crit Care Nur. 2002; 22(2):22-32.
[68] Valli G, Giardina EG. Benefits, adverse effects and drug interactions of herbal therapies with cardiovascular effects. J Am Coll Cardiol. 2002; 3: 39(7):1083-1095.
[69] Kuhn M, Winston D. Herbal Therapy and Supplements: A Scientific and Traditional Approach. Philadelphia, Pa: JB Lippincott; 2001.
[70] Brinker F. Herb and Drug Contraindication and Interaction. 2nd ed. Sandy, Ore: Eclectic Institute, Inc; 2001.
[71] Dietary Supplements—A Framework for Evaluating Safety. Institute of Medicine. National Academic Press, 2005. pp. 235-246.
[72] Boullata J. Natural Health Product Interactions with Medication. *Nutr Clin Pract.* 2005; 20(1):33- 51.
[73] Drug Interactions. *Med Lett Drugs Ther* 2003;34(1158):46-48.
[74] Pauli-Magnus C, Rekersbrink S, Kloz U, et al. Interaction of omeprazole, lansoprazole and pantoprazole with P-glycoprotein. Naunyn-Schmiederbergs Arch Pharmacol 2001;364:551-557.
[75] DuBuske LM. The role of P-glycoprotein and organic anion-transporting polypeptides in drug interactions. Drug Saf 2005;28:789-801.
[76] Sankatsing SUC, Beijnen JH, Schinkel AH, et al. P glycoprotein in human immunodeficiency virus type 1 infection and therapy. Antimicrob Agents Chemother 2004;48:1073-1081.
[77] Dagenais C, Graff CL, Pollack GM. Variable modulation of opioid brain uptake by P-glycoprotein in mice. Biochem Pharmacol 2004;67:269-27.
[78] Hu Z, Yang X, Ho PC et al. St. John's Wort modulates the toxicities and pharmacokinetics of CPT-11 (irinotecan) in rats. Pharm Res 2005;22:902–914.
[79] Frye RF, Fitzgerald SM, Lagattuta TF et al. Effect of St John's wort on imatinib mesylate pharmacokinetics. Clin Pharmacol Ther 2004;76: 323–329.

[80] Lundahl J, Regardh CG, Edgar B and Johnsson G (1995). Relationship between time of intake of grapefruit juice and its effect on pharmacokinetics and pharmacodynamics of felodipine in healthy subjects. Eur. J. Clin. Pharmacol., 49: 61-67.

[81] Zou L, Harkey MR, Henderson GL. Effects of herbal components on cDNA-expressed cytochrome P450 enzyme catalytic activity. Life Sci 2002;71:1579–1589.

[82] Zhang S, Morris ME. Effect of the flavonoids biochanin A and silymarin on the P-glycoprotein-mediated transport of digoxin and vinblastine in human intestinal Caco-2 cells. Pharm Res 2003;20: 1184–1191.

[83] Limtrakul P, Khantamat O, Pintha K. Inhibition of P-glycoprotein function and expression by kaempferol and quercetin. J Chemother 2005;17:86–95.

[84] Mangelsdorf DJ, Evans RM. The RXR heterodimers and orphan receptors. Cell 1995;83:841–850.

[85] Lehmann JM, McKee DD, Watson MA et al. The human orphan nuclear receptor PXR is activated by compounds that regulate CYP3A4 gene expression and cause drug interactions. J Clin Invest 1998;102: 1016–1023.

[86] Chen Y, Ferguson SS, Negishi M et al. Induction of human CYP2C9 by rifampicin, hyperforin, and phenobarbital is mediated by the pregnane X receptor. J Pharmacol Exp Ther 2004;308:495–501

[87] Moore LB, Goodwin B, Jones SA et al. St. John's wort induces hepatic drug metabolism through activation of the pregnane X receptor. Proc Natl Acad Sci U S A 2000;97:7500–7502.

[88] Brobst DE, Ding X, Creech KL et al. Guggulsterone activates multiple nuclear receptors and induces CYP3A gene expression through the pregnane X receptor. J Pharmacol Exp Ther 2004;310:528–535.

[89] Mu Y, Zhang J, Zhang S et al. Traditional Chinese medicines Wu Wei Zi (Schisandra chinensis Baill) and Gan Cao (Glycyrrhiza uralensis Fisch) activate pregnan X receptor and increase warfarin clearance in rats. J Pharmacol Exp Ther 2006;316:1369–1377.

[90] Ruhl R, Sczech R, Landes N et al. Carotenoids and their metabolites are naturally occurring activators of gene expression via the pregnane X receptor. Eur J Nutr 2004;43:336–343.

[91] Kliewer SA, Goodwin B, Willson TM. The nuclear pregnane X receptor: a key regulator of xenobiotic metabolism. Endocr Rev 2002;23:687–702.

[92] Wei P, Zhang J, Egan-Hafley M et al. The nuclear receptor CAR mediates specific xenobiotic induction of drug metabolism. Nature 2000;407: 920–923.

[93] Ueda A, Hamadeh HK, Webb HK et al. Diverse roles of the nuclear orphan receptor CAR in regulating hepatic genes in response to phenobarbital. Mol Pharmacol 2002;61:1–6.

[94] Drocourt L, Ourlin JC, Pascussi JM et al. Expression of CYP3A4, CYP2B6, and CYP2C9 is regulated by the vitamin D receptor pathway in primary human hepatocytes. J Biol Chem 2002;277:25125–25132.

[95] Sugatani J, Yamakawa K, Tonda E et al. The induction of human UDP-glucuronosyltransferase 1A1 mediated through a distal enhancer molecule by flavonoids and xenobiotics. Biochem Pharmacol 2004;67: 989–1000.

[96] Yale SH, Glurich I. Analysis of the inhibitory potential of Ginkgo biloba, Echinacea purpurea, and Serenoa repens on the metabolic activity of cytochrome P450 3A4, 2D6, and 2C9. J Altern Complement Med 2005;11:433–439.
[97] Food and Drug Administration (FDA) of the United States. Drug Metabolism/Drug Interaction Studies in the Drug Development Process: Studies in vitro. http://www.fda.gov
[98] Moore, L.B. et al. (2000) St. John's wort induces hepatic drug metabolism through activation of the pregnane X receptor. Proc. Natl. Acad. Sci. U. S. A. 97, 7500–7502
[99] MacGregor JT, Collins JM, Sugiyama Y, et al. In vitro human tissue models in risk assessment: report of a consensus-building workshop. Toxicol Sci. 2001 Jan; 59(1):17-36.
[100] Streetman, D.S. et al. (2000) Phenotyping of drug-metabolizing enzymes in adults: a review of in vivo cytochrome P450 phenotyping probes. Pharmacogenetics 10, 187–216.
[101] Rodrigues, A.D. (1994) Use of in vitro human metabolism studies in drug development. Biochem. Pharmacol. 48, 2147–2156.
[102] Crespi CL and Stresser DM. Fluorometric screening for metabolism-based drug–drug interactions. *J. Pharmacol. Toxicol. Methods* **44**, 325–331 (2000).
[103] Ekins, S. and Wrighton, S.A. (2001) Application of in silico approaches to predicting drug-drug interactions. J. Pharmacol. Toxicol. Method 45, 65–69.
[104] Lewis, D.F.V. (2001) COMPACT: a structural approach to the modelling of cytochromes P450 and their interactions with xenobiotics. J. Chem. Technol. Biotechnol. 76, 237–244.
[105] Raucy JL. Regulation of CYP3A4 expression in human hepatocytes by pharmaceuticals and natural products. Drug Metab Dispos 2003;31:533–539.
[106] Goodwin, B. et al. (2001) Regulation of the human CYP2B6 gene by the nuclear pregnane X receptor. Mol. Pharmacol. 60, 427–431
[107] Moore, L.B. et al. (2000) St. John's Wort induces hepatic drug metabolism through activation of the pregnane X receptor. Proc. Natl. Acad. Sci. U. S. A. 97, 7500–7502
[108] Li, A.P. (2004) In vitro approaches to evaluate ADMET drug properties. Curr. Top. Med. Chem. 4, 701–706
[109] Reif S, Nicolson MC, Bisset D et al. Effect of grapefruit juice intake on etoposide bioavailability. Eur J Clin Pharmacol 2002;58:491–494.
[110] Obach RS, Inhibition of human cytochrome P450 enzymes by constituents of St. John's Wort, an herbal preparation used in the treatment of depression. J Pharmacol Expl Ther 2000; 294: 88-95
[111] Budzinski JW, Foster BC, Vandenhoek S, Amason JT. An invitro evaluation of human cytochrome P450 3A4 inhibition by selected commercial extracts and tinctures.Phytomedicine 2000; 7: 273 -282.
[112] Bakare-Odunola MT, Mustapha KB, Garba M, Obodozie OO, Enemali IS. The influence of Nifadin, Niprisan, Niprd/92/001/1-1 (AM-1) 0n the pharmacokinetics of metronidazole in rats. Eur J Mrug Metab Pharmacokinet 2010; 25: 55-58
[113] Obiageri O. Obodozie, Benjamin U. Ebeshi, Kudirat B. Mustapha, Rukaiyatu A. Kirim, Margaret Ekpenyong and Uford S. Inyang. The effects of an investigational antimalarial agent, NIPRD-AM1 on the single dose pharmacokinetics of metronidazole in healthy human volunteers. Eur J Drug Metab Pharmacokinet 2011; 35: 103-108

[114] Xie W, Barwick JL, Downes M et al. Humanized xenobiotic response in mice expressing nuclear receptor SXR. Nature 2000; 406:435–439.
[115] Tashinga E. Bapiro, Ann-Charlotte Egnell, Julia A. Hassler, Collen Masimirembwa 2001, Drug Metabolism and Disposition; 29(1): 30-35 Application of Higher Thoroughput Screening (HTS) Inhibition Assays to evaluate the Interaction of Antiparasitic drugs with Cytochrome P450s
[116] Gurley BJ, Gardner SF, Hubbard MA et al. In vivo assessment of botanical supplementation on human cytochrome P450 phenotypes: Citrus aurantium, Echinacea purpurea, milk thistle, and saw palmetto. Clin Pharmacol Ther 2004; 76:428–440.
[117] Yin OQ, Tomlinson B, Waye MM et al. Pharmacogenetics and herb-drug interactions: experience with Ginkgo biloba and omeprazole. Pharmacogenetics 2004;14:841–850.
[118] Gurley BJ, Gardner SF, Hubbard MA et al. Clinical assessment of effects of botanical supplementation on cytochrome P450 phenotypes in the elderly: St John's wort, garlic oil, Panax ginseng and Ginkgo biloba. Drugs Aging 2005;22:525–539.
[119] Mills E, Montori VM, Wu P et al. Interaction of St John's Wort with conventional drugs: systematic review of clinical trials. BMJ 2004;329: 27–30.
[120] Piscitelli SC, Burstein AH, WELden N, Gallicano KD, Falloo J. The effect of garlic supplements on the pharmacokinetics of saquinavir.Clin Infect Dis 2002; 34:234 - 238.
[121] Gallicano K, Foster B, Choudhri S. Effect of short-term administration of garlic supplements on single-dose ritonavir pharmacokinetics in healthy volunteers. Br JClin Pharmacol 2002; 55: 199-202.
[122] Gwilt PR, Lear CL, Tempero MA et al. The effect of garlic extract on human metabolism of acetaminophen. Cancer Epidemiol Biomarkers Prev 1994;3:155–160.
[123] Yin OQ, Tomlinson B, Waye MM et al. Pharmacogenetics and herb-drug interactions: experience with Ginkgo biloba and omeprazole. Pharmacogenetics 2004;14:841–850.
[124] Anderson GD, Rosito G, Mohustsy MA, Elmer GW. Drug interaction potential of soy extract and Panax ginseng. J Clin Pharmacol 2003; 43:643-648.
[125] Fugh-Berman, A. (2000) Herb–drug interactions. Lancet 355, 134–138.
[126] Komoroski BJ, Parise RA, Egorin MJ et al. Effect of the St. John's wort constituent hyperforin on docetaxel metabolism by human hepatocyte cultures. Clin Cancer Res 2005;11:6972–6979.
[127] Gorski JC, Huang SM, Pinto A et al. The effect of echinacea (Echinacea purpurea root) on cytochrome P450 activity in vivo. Clin Pharmacol Ther 2004;75:89–100.
[128] Greenblatt DJ, von Moltkke LL, Daily JP, Harmatz JS, Shader RI. Extensive impairment of of triazolam and alprazolam clearance by short-term low dose ritonavir: the clinical dilemma of concurrent inhibition and induction. J Clin Psychopharmacol; 1999,19, 293-296.

8

Pharmacokinetics of Antimicrobials in Food Producing Animals

S. K. Bhavsar and A. M. Thaker
Department of Pharmacology and Toxicology, College of Veterinary Science and Animal Husbandry, Anand Agricultural University, Anand, Gujarat, India

1. Introduction

Pharmacokintics deals with study of absorption, distribution, metabolism and excretion (ADME) of drugs. Pharmacokinetics, the study of time course of drug concentrations in the body, provides means of quantifying ADME parameters. In a clinical situation pharmacokinetics provides the practitioners a useful tool to design optimally beneficial drug dosage regimen for patient. Understanding pharmacokinetic principles allows clinician to make more rational therapeutic decisions. It also provides conceptual understanding to utilize withdrawal time to prevent drug residues that remain in the milk and edible tissues of food producing animals.

Various steps involved in governing fate of drugs must be defined and quantified concentration of free, non-protein bound drug dissolved in serum or plasma is taken as reference point for pharmacokinetic analysis. Serum or plasma drug concentrations generally retract extra cellular fluid drug concentrations. A drug generally be present at its site of action in a tissue at sufficient concentration for a specific period to produce pharmacologic effect. This understanding is important in veterinary medicine where specific difference in any of ADME process significantly affect the extent and/or time course of drug absorption and disposition in the body.

The concentration of antimicrobial achieved at site of infection depends on systemic availability of the drug, which varies with the dosage form and route of administration. The chemical nature and physicochemical properties of the drug influence the extent of absorption, pattern of distribution and rate of elimination. Effective antimicrobial therapy depends on triad of bacterial susceptibility, pharmacokinetic characteristics of the drug and the dosage regimen.

Antimicrobials are administered either as flock medication in poultry and individually or group in swine and cattle. Systemic antimicrobial treatment is given orally through medicated feed or water, or by injections. Antimicrobials used in animals are generally the same to antimicrobials used in humans. Tetracyclines constitute the antimicrobials class quantitatively most used in animals followed by macrolides, lincosamides, penicillins, sulfonamides, aminoglycosides, fluoroquinolones, cephalosporins and phenicols. The most common antimicrobial drug used as growth promoters include macrolides (tylosin and spiramycin), polypeptides (bacitracin), glycolipids (bambermycin), streptogramins (virginiamycin), glycopeptides (avoparcin), quinoxalines (carbadox and olaquindox) and ionophores (monensin and salinomycin).

In human and veterinary practice the primarily concern in antimicrobial drug selection and use is the therapeutic outcome. Larger than therapeutic doses may lead to potential toxicity. Clinicians involved in the treatment of diseases in food animals have additional concern of the persistence of drug residue in the edible tissues after the disease has been treated. Adulteration of food supply with antimicrobial agents and other chemicals is growing concern to general public.

2. Beta-lactam antibiotics: Penicillins, cephalosporins and related drugs

Beta-lactam constitutes one of the most important and frequently used antimicrobial agents. The penicillins, cephalosporins, carbapenems, monobactams and β-lactamase inhibitors are referred to as beta-lactams antibiotics.

2.1 Penicillins

The Penicillins are a large group of naturally occurring and semi-synthetic antibiotics. The penicillins are organic acids available as sodium or potassium salts. The Penicillins (Pk_a 2.7) are predominantly ionized in plasma. Penicillins in general have relatively small apparent volumes of distribution (0.2-0.3 L/kg) and short half-lives (0.5-1.2 hours) in all species of domestic animals.

Penicillins are hydrolyzed & inactivated in the acidic pH of the stomach and therefore not absorbed orally except penicillin-V, aminopenicillins (ampicillin & amoxicillin) and isoxazolylpenicillins (cloxacillin, dicloxacilin & oxacillin). Aminopenicillins are absorbed poorly in horses and ruminants. Following oral administration, absorption of ampicillin in adult horses is only 2-3.5% (Sarasola & Mc Kellar, 1994; Ensink, et al, 1996). Systemic availability of oral amoxicillin is higher (2-10%) than ampicillin in adult horses. (Ensinic, et al, 1996; Wilson, et al, 1998). Serum concentrations of penicillins generally peak within 2 hrs of PO administration. Penicillins in aqueous solution are rapidly absorbed from parenteral administration. Penicillins suspended in vegetable oil vehicles or sparingly soluble penicillins (procaine penicillin G and benzathine penicillin G) administered parenterely absorbs slowly resulting in longer persistence of plasma and tissue drug concentrations.

Penicillins are widely distributed in body fluids & tissues. Protein binding of penicillins is low to moderate ranging from 30-60%. The penicillins have moderate volume of distribution and gets diffuse into extracellular fluid easily. Sufficient concentrations are achieved for susceptible bacteria in kidneys, synovial fluid, liver, lung, skin and soft tissues (Strover et al., 1981; Brown et al., 1982). Penicillins cross biologic membranes poorly. Entry of penicillin across blood-brain, placental, mammary or prostatic barriers is enhanced by inflammation or massive dose.

Penicillins are generally excreted unchanged except penicillin G, penicillin V, nafcillin, ticarcillin and aminopenicillins, which are metabolized to some extent by hydrolysis of β-lactam ring. The metabolites are inactive. Penicillins are eliminated entirely by Kidney (Glomerular filtration and tubular secretion), which results in very high level in the urine except nafcillin, which is excreted mainly in bile. Active tubular secretion of penicillins can be comparatively inhibited by organic acids such as probenicid. Penicillins are also eliminated in milk in trace amounts and may persist for 90 hours. Penicillin residue in milk has been detected after intrauterine infusion also.

2.2 Cephalosporins

The pharmacokinetic characteristics of cephalosporins are typical of penicillins. Very few cephalosporins (cephalexin, cepharidine, cefadroxil & cefachlor) are acid stable and given orally. Pro-drug formations of such drugs enhance oral bioavailability. Cefadroxil is absorbed better in the foal than adult horses (Dufee et al., 1989). Most of the other cephalosporins are either administered IV or IM. Peak plasma concentration usually observes at ~ 30 min after parenteral administration.

Cephalosporins are widely distributed through most body fluids & tissues including kidneys, lung, joints, bone & soft tissues except prostate & CNS. The volume of distribution is <0.3 L/kg. Protein biding for most cephalosporins is low in animals compare to human. For example ceftriaxone & cefazolin has high (85-95%) protein binding in human as compared to dogs (19-25%) (Popick et al., 1987).

Cephalosporins are minimally metabolized in the liver. Several Cephalosporins like cephalothin, cephapirin, cephacetrile & cefotaxime are deacitylated to less active derivatives except ceftiofur, which is transformed to desfuroyl ceftiotur, which is largly responsible for its antibacterial efficacy. Most of the cephalosporins are excreted by renal tubular secretion except cefoperazone, which is largly excreted in the bile. In general cephalosporins have half-lives of 1 to 2 hours except some third generation cephalosporins like ceftiofur having half-life of 3-6 hr in cattle, 4 hours in dogs and 2.5 hr in horses. The pharmacokinetic parameters of some cephalosporins given to food animals like cattle, sheep and goat are given in Table 1.

2.3 Other Beta-lactam antibiotics

2.3.1 Carbepenems

Carbepenems differ from penicillins by the substitution of a CH_2 group for the sulphur in the five- membered ring attached to β-lactam ring. They have very broad spectrum of activity and are resistant to most β - lactamases. It includes imipenem, doripenem, ertapenem, meropenem and biopenem. The carbepenems are not absorbed orally, hence must be given parenterally. Following IV Injection, they are widely distributed to extra cellular fluid throughout body & achieve therapeutic concentrations in most tissues. Carbepenems have low volume of distribution like penicillins & cephalosporins.Following IM administration imipenem has excellent bioavailability (>95%) and distributed widely throughout body except CSF. Imipenem gets largely eliminated through kidneys and gets metabolized in renal tubules by a dihydropeptidase enzyme. Cilastatin, an inhibitor of renal dipeptidase decrease renal metabolism of impenem, leading to increase in elimination half-life and decrease excretion of the drug largely in urine in active form. Half-life of carbepenem in patients having normal renal function is about 1 hour.

Cephalosporin	Animal species	Route	Dose (mg/kg)	C_{max} (μg/ml)	Vd (L/kg)	$T_{1/2}$ (hr)	AUC (0-∞) (μg x h/ml)	Cl (ml/min/kg	F (%)	Reference
Cephapirin	Cows (lactating)							12.7		Prades et al., 1988
Cephalexin	Calves				0.32	2.0		1.9		Garg et al., 1992
Cefazolin	Calves				0.17	0.62		5.8		Soback et al., 1987
Ceftriaxone	Goat	IV	20	-	0.58	1.50	77.51	4.50	-	Tiwari et al., 2009
		IM	20	21.51	0.53	2.03	66.78	3.04	59	
	Sheep	IV	10	-	0.41	1.21	42.65	3.91	-	Swati et al.,2010
		IM	10	15.53	0.43	2.24	47.68	2.22	64	
					0.30			3.7		Guerrini et al., 1985
	Calves (Buffalo)	IV	10	-	0.48	1.27	40.0	4.40	-	Gohil et al, 2009
		IM	10	15.8	1.53	4.38	29.67	4.01	70.2	
	Calves (Cow)	IV	10	-	0.44	1.58	57.35	3.15	-	Maradiya et al., 2010
		IM	10	15.34	1.16	5.02	28.15	2.71	47	
Cefepime	Goat	IV	10	-	0.52	2.71	78.38	2.19	-	Patni et al., 2008
		IM	10	15.75	-	4.89	93.12	1.27	69	
	Sheep	IV	20	-	0.42	2.54	135.5	2.48	-	Patel et al., 2010
		IM	20	26.34	1.11	5.17	140.90	0.15	103	
	Calves (Cow)	IV	5	-	0.57	3.70	47.73	1.81	-	Patel et al., 2006a
		IM	5	8.61	0.99	6.71	47.45	1.72	98	Patel et al., 2006b
Cefoxitin	Calves					1.12				Soback, 1988
Ceftazidime	Sheep				0.36	1.60				Rule at al., 1991
Cefoperazone	Calves					0.89				Carli et al., 1986
	Sheep	IV	47		0.16			2.7		Guerrini et al., 1985
Moxalactam						2.40				Soback, 1989

Table 1. Pharmacokinetic parameters of selected cephalosporins administrated to food producing animals.

2.3.2 Monobactams

Monobactums are simple monocyclic β-lactam compounds active only against bacteria or anaerobes. Aztreonam is a synthetic monobactam. It is not absorbed orally. It is administrators IV or IM having extensive distribution throughout body including CSF. It is having elimination half-life of 1.6 hour in man.

2.3.3 β-lactamase inhibitors

Beta lactamase enzyme production is a major factor in constitutive or acquired resistance of bacteria to β-lactam antibiotics. These drugs are combined with penicillins & cephalospirins to prevent degradation. It includes clavulanic acid, sulbactam and tazobactam.

Clavulanic acid is a synthetic compound. It is combined with amoxillin (4:1) or ticarcillin (15:1). Clavulanic acid is well absorbed following oral administration having bioavailability more than 60%. It has widespread tissue distribution in extra cellular fluid but penetration in milk and CSF is poor. It gets largely eliminated unchanged in urine. Sulbactam (penicillinic acid sulfonate) is synthetic derivative of 6-aminopenicillinic acid. It is combined with either ampicillin or cefoperazone. The combination of sulbactam ampicillin gets absorbed after IM injections, distributes well into tissues and penetrates CSF through inflamed meninges. It is poorly absorbed orally but a pro-drug "sultamicillin" having double esters linkage of sulbactam with ampicillin gets absorbed from small intestine. Tazobactam is combined with piperacillin (piperacillin: tazobactam, 8:1) having pharmacokinetic properties similar to β-lactam drugs.

3. Tetracyclines

Tetracyclines are a group of broad- spectrum antibiotics having a nucleus of four cyclic rings. The tetracyclines are crystalline amphoteric substances that can exist as acid or base salts. The tetracyclines are strong chelating agents. Its chelation with calcium causes tooth discoloration. Tetracyclines include chlortetracycline, oxytetracycline, tetracycline, doxycycline and minocycline.

Tetracyclines have low absorption following oral administration except doxycycline. The tetracyclines are relatively lipophilic drugs that remains ionized in the gastrointestinal tract. Oral absorption of tetracyclines gets drastically reduced in the presence of food (Neilsen and Gurd-Hansen 1996). Its oral absorption decrease with co-administration of food, dairy products, polyvalent cations (Ca^{++}, Mg^{++}, Fe^{++}, Al^{+++}), Kaolin/pectin preparations, ion containing supplements and antacids. Tetracyclines (oxytetracycline) can be administrated IV or IM. All tetracycline produce varying degree of tissue irritation on parenteral administration. The bioavailability of orally administrated oxytetracycline is 5% compared to 37% for chlortetracycline in non fasting calves. The long acting formulation of oxytetracycline used for IM administration to food animals have long acting effect due high dosage and prolonged persistence at the site of IM injection as a result of tissue irritation (Nouws et al.,1990). The bioavailability of most tetracyclines is very poor following oral administration in pigs. Intravenous administration of oxytetracycline is preferred over IM injection in horses as it results in higher and more persistent serum concentration.

Tetracyclines bind to plasma proteins at varying degrees in different species of animals. Tetracyclines are widely distributed in most tissues including kidney, liver, lungs, bile and bones. Tetracyclines have volume of distribution in excess of 1.0 L/kg indicating higher drug concentration intracellular or binding to tissues. Tetracyclines are more lipophilic than other classes of antibiotics hence it can cross lipid membrane easily. Minocycline and doxycycline attain high concentration in brain, ocular tissues, spinal fluid and prostate than other tetracyclines. Doxycycline has high affinity for intracellular accumulation than other tetracyclines (Davis et al., 2006). Tetracyclines cross the placenta and enter foetal circulation and are secreted in milk of lactating animals.

With exception of lipid soluble tetracyclines (doxycycline, minocycline), the tetracycline antibiotics are not metabolized to a significant extent in the body. About 60% of the dose gets eliminated in urine via glomerular filtration and 40% in faeces. Doxycycline gets excreted largely in the large intestine. Doxycycline & minocycline undergo entero-hepatic circulation, which contributes to their longer half-life (6-10 hr) than tetracycline that are eliminated mainly by renal excretion.

4. Aminoglycosides

The aminoglycosides are bactericidal natural and semi-synthetic antibacterials primarily used for treatment of gram negative infections and staphylococci. The group consists of hexose nucleus to which amino sugars are attached by glycosidic linkages. The aminoglycosides are basic polycations with pKa value ranging from 7.2 to 8.8. The chemical structure determines the antimicrobial activity, resistance patterns and inherent propensity to cause toxicosis. The group includes drugs like gentamicin, amikacin, kanamycin, apramycin, tobramycin, neomycin, streptomycin, dihydrostreptomycin, paromomycin and spectinomycin.

The pharmacokinetics of the aminoglycosides is similar across most veterinary species. However, variability within each animal population is large that necessitates close monitoring of serum concentrations to optimize efficacy and minimize toxicosis. Equines receiving multiple doses of parenteral amino-glycosides require therapeutic drug monitoring (Martin & Riviere, 1998)

Aminoglycosides are poorly absorbed (<10%) from gastrointestinal tract because of their highly polar and cationic nature. Aminoglycosides given orally to young animals (neonate) with enteritis, significant absorption occur leading to violative tissue residues. The aminoglycosides are well absorbed following IM or SC injection. The peak serum concentration is achieved within 30 to 45 minutes following extravascular administration. Intravenous and intraperitoneal routes produce rapid effects but should be avoided because of serious side effects. Following intrauterine or intramammary infusion to cows, gentamicin is well absorbed and results in prolonged tissue residues. Absorption is extremely rapid and complete, if aminoglycosides are instilled into body cavities that contain serosal surfaces.

Aminoglycosides are extensively distributed in extracellular fluid, as these are large molecules and highly ionized at physiological pH. They are poorly lipid soluble and have limited capacity to enter cells and penetrate cellular barriers. These drugs attain very low concentration in cerebrospinal, respiratory and ocular fluid. In the renal tubular cells and the endolymph and perilymph of inner ear, aminoglycoside attain high concentration causing nephro and oto-toxicity, respectively. Their apparent volume of distribution is relatively small (<0.35L/Kg). The amino glycosides binds poorly (<20%) to plasma proteins. Gentamicin is distributed into synovial fluid in normal horses; local inflammation may increase drug concentration in the joint.

The aminoglycosides are not metabolized and are excreted largely as such (~90%) in urine by glomerular filtration. Plasma elimination half lives are short (1-2 hr) in domestic animals having normal renal function. It increases to 24-48 hr in patients having renal insufficiency. The disposition of aminoglycosides varies among animals because of differences in glomerular filtration rates. The prolonged terminal elimination phase of aminoglycosides has major implications for veterinary therapeutics in food producing animals. Aminoglycosides accumulate in renal cortex for prolonged periods of time, resulting in tissue residues even after short periods of administration.

5. Fluoroquinolones

Fluoroquinolones are synthetic antibacterial agents introduced in veterinary medicine in the 1980s. Currently available quinolones contain basic structure of 4-quinolone (Short for 4-oxo-1,4- hydroquinoline) with carboxylic acid moiety. Fluoroquinolones are amphoteric molecules having pKa ranging from 6.0-6.5 (Carboxy group) and 7.5-8 (nitrogen of piperazine group). Fluoroquinolones at physiological pH occurs as zwitterions. Fluoroquinolones commonly used in veterinary medicine inciude enrofloxacin, difloxacin, orbifloxacin, marbofloxacin, ibafloxacin and danofloxacin. Other compounds having potential interest in veterinary practice include ciprofloxin, levofloxacin, moxifloxacin, gatifloxacin and pradofloxacin.

The fluoroquinolones have good rate and extent of absorption after oral administration in monogastric animals and pre-ruminant calves. Presence of food has little effect on oral absorption. In dogs, cats and pigs, oral absorption of fluoroquinolones approaches to 100%, but in large animals it is less. Enrofloxacin is more lipid soluble than ciprofloxacin and has a higher oral bioavailability than ciprofloxacin in horses and small animals. The oral bioavailability of enrofloxacin is 63% (Giguere et al., 1996) in adult horses and 42% in foals (Bermingham et al., 2000). Absorption is complete following IM and SC Injection of fluoroquinolones. The pharmacokinetic parameters of some fluoroquinolones given to food animals like cattle, sheep, goat, pig and chicken are given in Table 2.

Following absorption, fluoroquinolones show rapid and extensive tissue distribution due to hydrophilic nature and low (<50%) protein binding. In general, fluoroquinolones concentration in interstitial fluid, skin and bones are 35-100% of those obtained in serum, where as bronchial secretions and prostatic concentrations are two to three times of corresponding serum concentrations. Penetration into CSF is approximately 25% of serum concentration (Davis et al., 2002). Fluoroquinones attain high intracellular concentrations in macrophages and neutrophils. Intracellular concentrations are 4 - 10 times greater than plasma concentrations.

The fluoroquinolones are largely eliminated uncharged in the urine by glomerular filtration and active tabular secretion, except difloxacin, which is excreted largely (80%) in faeces. Parent compound as well as metabolites of some fluoroquinolones is excreted in bile and urine. Enrofloxacin undergoes de-ethylation to active metabolite ciprofloxacin. In cattle the proportion of ciprofloxacin in plasma was 25 - 41% following administration of enrofloxacin (Davis et al., 2002). The ciprofloxacin concentration residues were present in tissue of chicken 12 days after dosing of enrofloxacin (Anadon et al., 1995). Pefloxacin gets completed metabolized to active metabolite norfloxacin. The elimination half-life (3-6 hr) of fluoroquinolones is dependent on the drug and animal species.

Fluoro quinolone	Animal species	Route	Dose (mg/kg)	C_{max} (μg/ml)	Vd (L/kg)	$T_{1/2\beta}$ (hr)	AUC (0-∞) (μg x h/ml	F (%)	Reference
Ciprofloxacin	Sheep	IV	5	-	1.67	1.88	8.40	-	Patel et al., 2004
		IM	5	0.95	3.40	3.67	5.48	68	
	Calves (cow)	IV	5	-	1.67	1.80	7.90	-	Bhavsar et al., 2004
	Calves (Buffalo)	IV	5	-	1.98	1.25	4.56	-	Sarvaiya et al., 2006
	Pigs	IV	3.06	0.17	3.83	2.57	2.88	37	Nouws et al., 1988
	Chicken	PO	5	4.67	2.0	9.0	78.04	70.0	Atta and Sharif, 1997
Levofloxacin	Poultry (Broiler)	IV	10	-	3.25 (Vdss)	3.18	11.33	-	Varia et al., 2009
		PO	10	0.93	-	3.64	6.70	59.5	
Enrofloxacin	Cattle	SC	12.5	0.96	-	6.79	14.95	-	Davis et al., 2006
		IV	8	0.81	-	7.28	7.51	-	Ter Hune et al., 2005
		IV	5		1.63	1.68	7.42		Kaartinen et al., 1997
		IM	5	0.73		5.9		82	
		SC	5	0.98		5.55		137	
			2.5		2.98	2.82	5.28		Bergante et al., 1999
	Goat	IV	5	6.7	1.3	1.1	6.7		Rao et al., 2002
	Sheep	-	5	2.69	1.15	4.8	57.5	98.07	Bermingham and Papich, 2002
		IM	2.5		2.18	3.73	5.47	85.0	Mengozzi et al., 1996
		PO	2.5	0.78	1.3	3.8	10.4	60.6	Pozzin et al., 1997
	Pig	IM	2.5	0.61	3.5	7.73	9.94	95	Richez et al., 1997
			2.5	0.75	3.95	5.5	5.03	101	Pijpers et al., 1997
	Chicken	IV	10.0	1.88 (PO)	5.0 (IV)	5.6	16.17	89.2	Knoll et al., 1999
		PO	10.0	1.5	-	14	35	-	Da Silva et al., 2006
Danofloxacin	Cattle	IV	6	1.7		4.21	9.72	-	Ter Hune et al., 2005
		IM	1.25	0.28	2.04	2.25	132.85	289	Shem-Tov et al., 1998
		IM	5	0.82		2.9	4.7	78	Mann and Frame, 1992
	Goat	SC	1.25	0.33	3.8	4.67	2.29	110	Aliabdi and lees, 2001
	pig	IM	5	0.8	-	8.0	6.0	76	Mann and Frame, 1992
Marbofloxacin	Goat	IM	2	1.9	1.3 (Vdss)	7.2	8.44	100.7	Waxman et al., 2001

Table 2. Pharmacokinetic parameters of selected fluoroquinolones administrated to food producing animals.

6. Sulphonamides and potentiated sulphonamides

The sulphonamides are oldest antimicrobial compounds, derivatives of sulphanilamide which was obtained from the azo dye "prontosil". Sulphonamides are white crystalline powders that are quite insoluble. They are more soluble at an alkaline pH than an acidic pH. Solubility of sulphonamides increases in the presence of another sulphonamide in the solution because it follow law of independent solubility. The sodium salts of sulphonamides are readily soluble in water. These solutions are highly alkaline (used for parenteral preparation) in reaction except sodium sulphonamide which is near neutral and used for ophthalmic instillation. The pKa values of sulphonamies range are from 10.4 (sulfanilamide) to 5.0 (sulfisoxazole). They exist in lipid soluble non-ionised form in biologic fluids of pH lower than their pKa. Sulphonamides commonly used in veterinary medicine include sulphadimethoxine, sulphamethazine (sulphadimidine), sulphaquinoxaline, sulphamerazine, sulphathiazole, sulphasalazine, sulphadiazine, Sulphabromomethazine, sulphaethoxypyridazine, sulphisoxazole and sulphachlorpyridazine. The potentiated sulphonamides are combination of a sulphonamide with diaminopyrimidine compounds (trimethoprim or ormethoprim). Potentiated sulphonamide combinations used in veterinary practice includes Trimethoprim - sulphadiazine, Trimethoprim - sulphamethaxazole, Trimethoprim - sulphachlorpyridazine and ormetoprim - sulphadimethoxine.

Most sulphonamides (except gut acting and topical sulphonamides) get well absorbed following oral administration. The absorption rate is affected by the solubility of sulphonamides and presence of ingesta in the gastrointestinal tract. In general dogs, cats and birds absorb sulphonamides rapidly, pigs takes some time and ruminants require much longer time. In ruminants, age and diet markedly affect oral trimethoprim and sulphadiazine disposition in calves. Orally administered sulphadiazine (30mg/kg) was absorbed slowly in calves fed milk diets, with absorption slightly higher in ruminating calves. Trimethoprim was absorbed in pre-ruminant calves but not absorbed in mature ruminants after oral administration (Shoaf et al., 1987).

Sulphonamides are widely distributed throughout body including soft tissues, CNS (cerebrospinal fluid) and joints (synovial fluid). Plasma protein binding varies from 15 -90 % depending on sulphonamide to sulphonamide and species to species. Extensive (>80%) protein binding increases half-life. Sulfonamides are weak acids and timethoprim is a weak base. Trimethoprim has higher volume of distribution than sulfonamide due to ion trapping of trimethoprim in tissues. Calculation of dosages of sulphonamides to maintain steady state of 100 μg/ml requires consideration of the extent of protein binding, apparent volume of distribution and half-life as it varies between individual within a species.

Sulphonamides and trimethoprim are metabolized faster and more extensively by herbivores than carnivore or omnivores. Acetylation of NH_2 group on N-4 is a major mechanism of metabolism. Hydroxylation of methyl group on the pyrimidine ring and carboxylation also occurs. Ruminants metabolize sulphonamides by acetylation pathways and acetylated metabolites are the major urinary metabolites in cattle, sheep and swine. Acetylated metabolites are less soluble than the parent compound and increase risks of renal tubular injury due to precipitation and crystal formation. The canines' lacks the ability to acetyl ate sulphonamides, relying on alternate metabolic pathway. Glucuronide conjugation and aromatic hydroxylation are two additional pathway for sulphonamide metabolism. Sulphonamide metabolites are therapeutically inactive (N 4- acetyl metabolites) or have reduced therapeutic activity (hydroxy metabolites).

Sulfonamides are excreted in urine. Renal excretion mechanisms include glomerular filtration of free drug in the plasma, active carrier-mediated proximal tubular excretion of ionized unchanged drug and metabolites and passive reabsorption of nonionized drug from distal tubular fluid. Urinary alkalization increases both the fraction of dose that is eliminated by renal excretion and the solubility of sulphonamides in the urine.

7. Peptide antibiotics: Polymyxins, glycopeptides and bacitracin

7.1 Polymyxins

Polymyxins are group of N-mono-acetylated decapeptides. Polymyxin B and polymyxin E (colistin) are chemically related and therapeutically useful. The polymyxins are not absorbed into the body when given orally. Polymyxin B sulfate or colistin methane sulphonate sodium is given parenterally for systemic therapy. Following absorption polymyxins bind moderately (70-90%) to plasma proteins. Polymyxins bind extensively to muscle tissues. It binds to mammalian cell membrane and accumulates following long term dosing. They are slowly excreted unchanged by glomerular filtration in the urine. The polymyxins are highly nephrotoxic damaging the renal tubular epithelial cells.

7.2 Glycopeptides

Vancomycin, teicoplanin and avoparcin are glycopeptide antibiotics. The former two have been considered as the drugs of "last resort" to treat serious infections due to drug resistant gram-positive bacteria in human. Vancomycin and avoparcin are used in veterinary medicine in some countries.

Vancomycin is poorly absorbed following oral administration. Its tissue distribution is poor following parenteral administration. Most of the intravenously administered drug is excreted through the kidneys, with small proportion excreted in bile. Vancomycin hydrochloride is given IV as infusion and it requires monitoring in patients with renal impairment. Teicoplanin is not absorbed after oral administration. Absorption and distribution into tissue and extracellular fluid is excellent following IM Injection. It gets eliminated entirely in urine.

7.3 Bacitracin

It is polypeptide product derived from *Bacillus subtilis*. It is bactericidal to Gram-positive bacteria but has little activity on Gram-negative organisms. It is highly nephrotoxic after parenteral administration. It is only used for topical treatment of superficial infections of the skin and mucosal surfaces. In veterinary medicine it is used at low dose as growth promoter in chicken.

8. Lincosamides, pleuromutilins and streptogramins

8.1 Lincosamides

Lincosamides are a group of monoglycoside antibiotics containing amino-acid like side chain. It includes lincomycin, clindamycin and pirlimycin. Lincosamides are basic compounds with pKa of 7.6. They have high lipid solubility and large apparent volume of distribution.

Lincomysin is rapidly but incompletely absorbed following oral administration (20-50%) in pigs (Hornish *et al,* 1987). Peak levels are achieved within 60 minutes following oral administration and 2-4 hr after IM Injection. It is well distributed in tissues (liver, kidney, muscle & skin) with low levels in CSF (Vd: 1-1.3 L/kg). Following oral administration most of the drug gets excreted through faeces (85%) and remainder in urine. Following IM Injection 38% gets excreted in faeces and 49% in urine.

Clindamycin is 7- chlorolincomycin having better antibacterial effect compared to lincomycin. Clindamycin absorb better from gastrointestinal tract than lincomycin. It is distributed well to tissues and attains high intracellular concentration (Vd: 1.6-3.1 L/kg). It also achieves effective concentration in bone. Following parenteral administration half life ranges from 3.2 hr (IV) to 5-7 hr (IM or SC). It has excellent bioavailability (80-100%) following IM Injection.

8.2 Pleuromutilins

Tiamulin and valnemulin are semisynthetic derivatives of naturally occurring diterpene antibiotic pleuromutilin. Tiamulin hydrogen fumarate is used for oral administration whereas tiamulin base is used for Injection. Valnemulin hydrochloride is used as medicated feed premix. Tiamulin gets rapidly absorbed after oral administration in monogastric species but gets inactivated in rumen if given orally to ruminants. It has half life of 25 minutes following parental administration (Ziv et al., 1983). It gets concentrated into milk as it is more lipophilic having pKa- 7.6. Valnemulin bioavailability exceeds 90% in pigs when given with feed.

8.3 Streptogramins

Streptogramins are a group of natural (virginiamycin, pristinamycin) or semisynthetic (quinupristin/dalfopristin) cyclic peptides. Virginiamycin is used in veterinary medicine as growth promoter (5-20 ppm). It is not absorbed after oral administration. Its use as growth promoter has been banned in several countries because of resistance in enterococcal isolates.

9. Macrolides, azalides and ketolldes

The macrolide antibiotics are a group of structurally similar compounds containing 12-20 atoms of carbon in lactone ring. Various combinations of deoxy sugars are attached to lactone ring by glycosidic linkages. Macrolides used in veterinary medicine include erythromycin, tylosin, spiramycin, tilmicosin and tulathromycin. Other macrolides like oleandomycin and carbomycin have been used as feed additives for growth promotion in food animals.

9.1 Erythromycin

It is base having pKa of 8.8. It is poorly soluble in water and unstable in gastric acid. Erythromycin base is absorbed well following oral administration but it is highly susceptible to degradation from gastric acids. Erythromycin base in entric-coated formulation or erythromycin estolate or stearate or phosphate or ethyl-succinate ester can be given orally. The stearate form is hydrolyzed in the intestine to the base and ethylsuccinate and estolate ester forms are hydrolyzed in the body to the active base. The presence of food in the stomach interferes quite markedly with oral absorption. Aqueous solution of erythromycin glucophate and lactobionate forms can be given IV. Pain and irritation at site of Injection prohibits use of erythromycin by SC or IM routes. The drug is well distributed in the body, being concentrated in the tissue like lungs, liver, spleen, heart, kidney and bile, prostatic, seminal, pleural and peritoneal fluids. Prostatic fluid concentrations are approximately half that of serum concentration. Penetration of erythromycin to CSF is low. The drug is largely metabolized by demethylation and metabolites are excreted largely in bile, which is lost in faeces. Urinary excretion is only 3-5% of administrated dose. The drug has half life of 3-4 hr in cattle.

9.2 Tylosin

Tylosin is more extensively used as a feed additive to promote growth in food-producing animals. Tylosin is a weak base (pKa 7.1) and is highly lipid soluble. The drug has good absorption from gastro-intestinal tract. It is widely distributed in tissues like lung, liver, spleen, heart and kidney. It is metabolized in liver and excreted via the bile and feaces. The elimination half-life in dogs and cattle is about 1 hr with apparent volume of distribution of 1.7 and 1.1 L/kg, respectively. The half-life is longer (4 h) in sheep, goat and pigs.

9.3 Tilmicosin

It is semisynthetic derivative of tylosin. It has slow absorption and low bioavailability (22%) in cows. It has large volume of distribution (>2 L/ kg), with accumulation and persistence in tissues like lung. The drug administrated to cow (10 mg/kg, SC) resulted in milk concentration > 0.8 μg/ml for eight to nine days (Ziv et al.,1995)

9.4 Spiramycin

Spiramycin has quite exceptional ability to concentrate in tissues, resulting in tissue concentrations reaching 25-60 times those of serum. Persistence of drug residues for prolonged periods limits its use in food producing animals.

9.5 Tulathromycin

Tulathromycin is an azalide derivative of erythromycin. It is rapidly and extensively absorbed from SC & IM injection in cattle and pigs having bioavailability of 90%. The drug has half-life of 90 hr. The apparent volume of distribution following IV administration is 12 L/Kg. Lung concentrations are 25-80 times higher than serum concentrations.

9.6 Roxithromycin, dirithromycin, clarithromycin and azithromycin

The newer macrolides are acid stable, produce few gastro-intestinal side effects, have higher oral bioavailability and longer elimination half- lives and produce higher therapeutic tissue concentration as compared to erythromycin. Oral bioavailability of azithromycin is 97% in dogs and about 50% in cats and foals. Elimination half-life of azithromycin is 20 hr and 30 hr in foals and cats, respectively. Clarithromycin half-life (4.8 hr) is shorter than azithromycin but longer than erythromycin (1 hr) in foals. The major route of excretion is bile and intestinal tract for azithromycin. The major route of excretion for clarithromycin is kidney. Tissue concentration of azithromycin is 10-100 times of those achieved in serum. The extensive tissue distribution of azithromycin is due to its concentration within macrophages and neutrophils.

9.7 Ketolides

Ketolides are members of a new semisynthetic 14 membered ring macrolide, with a 3-keto group instead of a α-L cladinose on the erythronolide A ring. It includes telithromycin and cethromycin, which are given orally. Their pharmacokinetics display a long half-life as well as extensive tissue distribution and uptake into respiratory tissues and fluids, allowing once daily dosing

10. Chloramphenicol and derivatives

10.1 Chloramphenicol

Chloramphenicol is a derivative of dichloroacetic acid and contains a nitrobenzene moiety. It is slightly soluble in water and freely soluble in propylene glycol and organic solvents. Chloramphenicol base or its palmitate salt is used for oral administration. Chloramphenicol palmitate is hydrolyzed in the small intestine by estrases, which release the free base form of chloramphenicol to systemic circulation. Chloramphenicol succinate is freely soluble in water and is used for IV or IM administration. It gets hydrolyzed in plasma to produce active drug. Pharmacokinetic parameters of chloramphenicol in food producing animal species are summarized in table 3.

Animal species	Route	Dose (mg/kg)	Formulation	Vd (L/kg)	$T_{1/2\beta}$ (hr)	Reference
Cattle	IV	40	Base	0.35	2.81	Sanders et al., 1988
	IM	90	Base	-	1.35	
	SC	90	Base	-	1.15	
Calves	IV	25	Base in Propylene Glycol	1.03 (1 day old) 0.81 (7 day old) 0.90 (14 day old) 0.69 (28 day old) 1.38 (9 months old)	7.56 (1 day old) 5.96 (7 day old) 4.0 (14 day old) 3.69 (28 day old) 2.47 (9 months old)	Burrows et al., 1983
Sheep	IV	30	Base	0.69	1.70	Dagorn et al., 1990
	IM	30	Base	-	2.71	
	SC	30	Base	-	17.93	
Goats	IV	25	Succinate	1.68	1.22	Kume and Garg, 1986
	IV	25	Succinate	1.96	1.29	
	IM	25	Succinate	3.02	1.46	
	IM	25	Succinate	2.77	1.45	
	IV	10	Succinate	0.31	1.47	Abdullah and Baggot, 1986
Pigs (Adult)	IV	22	base	1.05	1.3	Davis et al., 1972
Piglets	IV	25	Base	0.94	12.7	Martin and Weise, 1988
Chicken	IV	20	Succinate	0.24	8.32	Atef et al., 1991
	IM	20	Succinate	0.44	7.84	
	PO	20	Succinate	0.41	8.26	

Table 3. Pharmacokinetic parameter of chloramphenicol in food producing animal

Chloramphenicol is well absorbed from gastro-intestinal tract in monogastric and pre-ruminant calves. The oral bioavailability in foals is 83%. Chloramphenicol palmitate is poorly absorbed in cats. Chloramphenicol administrated orally to ruminants gets inactivated in rumen. High lipid solubility and low plasma protein-binding (30-46%) enable it to attain effective concentration most tissues and body fluids including cerebrospinal fluid and central nervous system. It also get readily diffuse into milk and pleural and ascetic fluids. It also readily crosses the placenta and achieves high concentration in fetus. The drug has large volume of distribution (1-2.5 L/kg) due to its lipophilic nature.

Chloramphenicol is metabolized in the liver. Phase-II glucuronidation is the principal pathway producing metabolite chloramphenicol glucuronide. Rapid metabolic clearance produces short half-lives in many species and requires frequent administration. The elimination half-life of chloramphenicol varies widely among species. It is short (1hr) in horses (Sisodia et al, 1975) and long (5-6 hr) in cats (Watson, 1991). Most of the absorbed chloramphenicol (80%) gets excreted into the urine as inactive metabolite via tubular secretion.

10.2 Thiamphenicol

Thiamphenicol is a semisynthetic structural analogue of chloramphenicol, in which the p-nitro group has been replaced by a sulfomethoxyl group. Absorption and distribution are similar to those of chloramphenicol. Bioavailability in pre-ruminant lambs and calves is 60 % following oral administration. It is well distributed in the body. Thiamphenicol is not eliminated by hepatic glcronide conjugation but excreted unchanged in the urine. The pharmacokinetics of thiamphenicol follow allometric scaling, in that values of elimination half-life and volume of distribution increase with body size (Castells , 2001).

10.3 Florfenicol

Florfenicol is a fluorinated derivative of thiamphenicol, in which the hydroxyl group has been replaced with fluorine. The oral bioavaibility of florfenicol is 89% in calves. Bioavailability following IM injection and intramammary infusion in lactating dairy cattle is 38% and 54%, respectively. Florfenicol is well distributed into many tissues and fluids including lungs, muscle, bile, kidney and urine. Concentrations in brain and CSF are ¼ to ½ , respectively of the corresponding concentrations in plasma. The drug has volume of distribution of 0.7-0.9 L/kg with low plasma protein binding (13-19%) in cattle. Most of the administrated dose gets excreted as the parent drug (64%) in urine of cattle. Florfenicol amine metabolites persist longer in tissues of cattle and are used as marker residue for withdrawal determination. The elimination half-life is 2-4 hr in cattle. The commercially available formulation of florfenicol is long-acting, so that "flip-flop" kinetics occur, where elimination is prolonged due to slow absorption from the injection site.

11. Miscellaneous antimicrobials

11.1 Ionophore antibiotics

Carboxylic ionophore polyether antibiotics are *streptomyces* products used as growth promoters. Ionophore antibiotics used in veterinary medicine include monensin, lasalocid, maduramicin, narasin and salinomycin.

Following oral administration, monensin gets rapidly and completely absorbed in monogastric animals. In ruminants, oral bioavailability of monensin is 50%. Ionophore antibiotics do not attain higher concentration in tissues even at larger doses. Ionophores are rapidly and extensively metabolized in the liver and the metabolites are excreted in the bile and eliminated in the faeces. Horses are most sensitive to monensin toxicity because of very slow elimination as compared to cattle.

11.2 Nitrofurans

Nitrofurans are broad spectrum antimicrobials. They are used topically because of toxicity following systemic use. Nitrofurans are carcinogenic, hence their use in food animal has been banned in several countries (United States, Canada and European Union) of the world. In veterinary medicine, nitrofurazone is still used in non-food animals for skin infections.

11.3 Nitroimidazoles

The nitroimidazoles like metronidazole, dimetridazole, ronidazole, tinidazole and ipronidazole were once widely used in veterinary medicine but because of potential carcinogenicity, their use is banned in several countries (United States, Canada and European Union). Metronidazole is still used in companion animals against anaerobes & protozoa.

Metronidazole is absorbed rapidly in monogastric animals following oral administration. The drug has oral bioavaibility of 75-85% in horses and 59-100% in dogs (Neff-Devis et al., 1981; Steinman et al., 2000). It is lipophilic and widely distributed in tissues. It penetrates bone, abscesses and the central nervous system. It crosses the placenta and also distributed to milk attaining concentration similar to those in plasma. The drug has volume of distribution of 0.7 to 1.7 L/kg in mares, 0.95 L/kg in dogs and 0.8 L/kg in cow calves. Metronidazole is primarily metabolized in the liver by oxidation and conjugation. Parent drug & metabolites are excreted in urine & faeces. The drug has half-life of 3-4 hr in horses, 8 hr in dogs and 1.9 hr in cow calves. Following oral administration in cow calves and sheep, half-lives were 4.38 & 1.72, respectively. Oral bioavailability in calves was 33.7 percent (Patel et al., 1993; Bhavsar & Malik, 1994).

11.4 Rifamycins

Rifampicin is the most important synthetically modified derivative of natural antibiotics rifamycins. Rifampicin is soluble in organic solvents and water at an acidic pH. The drug gets rapidly absorbed after oral administration in calves, dogs and horses. In horses, bioavailability is low and administration with food prolongs the time to maximum serum concentration. Rifampin is very lipophilic and penetrates most tissues including milk, bone, abscesses and central nervous system. It is well distributed in milk. It crosses placenta and is teratogenic in rodents. The volume of distribution of rifampin in horses is 0.6 - 0.9 L/kg. It is highly bound to plasma proteins. The biotransformation and elimination of rifampin in animals is not well known. The elimination half-life of rifampin in horses is 6-8 hrs after IV injection and 12-13 hrs after oral administration. In dogs, elimination half-life is 8 hrs. Rifampin causes induction of hepatic enzymes in many species.

12. Animal origin foods and antimicrobial drug residues

Food safety is one of the most significant issues for animal produce. During last several years great concern has been shown about the presence of chemical adulterants or residues especially antimicrobials and pesticides in the meat, poultry egg and milk. A chemical residue is either the parent compound or metabolite of that parent compound that may accumulate, deposit or otherwise be stored within the cells, tissues, organs or edible products of an animal following its use to prevent, control or treat animal disease or to enhance production. Residues can also result from unintentional administration of drugs or food additives. Contamination of the food supply with chemical residue is rarely an intentional act and usually results either from failure to observe the correct meat withdrawal or milk discard time for a drug after it has been used to treat a disease process in food animals or from accidental contamination of feed by chemicals or drugs.

12.1 Regulation of drug residue

Livestock and poultry production depends on drugs and other chemicals to protect animal health. Consumers are protected from adverse effects by regulation of chemicals and drugs and the detection of chemical and drug residues in foods of animals' origin through national agencies (FDA in USA, Veterinary Drug Directorate in Canada, Medicines and healthcare products regulatory agency in UK and others). The codex alimentarius committee on residue of veterinary drugs in foods is subsidiary body of the world health organization (WHO) and the food and agriculture organization (FAO). One of the primary functions of the codex alimentarius is the establishment of the internationally acceptable concentrations of the veterinary drugs in food animal products. Extensive toxicological evaluations of the drugs and its metabolite are required before the drug is approved for use in food-producing animals. Based on the results of toxicity tests, regulatory agencies establish an acceptable daily intake (ADI). The ADI represents a level of daily intake of a chemical which, during an entire life time, appears to be without appreciable risk to the health of the consumer. The ADI is used to determine the maximum concentration of a marker residue in edible tissues, honey, milk or eggs that is legally permitted or recognized as acceptable. These acceptable concentrations are also termed as "tolerances" (USA) or "maximum residue limits" (MRL) (Canada and European union).

12.2 Pharmacokinetics and drug residues

Pharmacokinetics is the science of quantitating the change in drug concentration in the body over time as a function of the administered dose. How a drug or combination of drugs behaves in the body after administration not only is important from therapeutic point of view but is of paramount importance in order to prevent residues in the edible tissues after the disease process has been resolved and the animal is slaughtered. For determining withdrawal times of drug, half-life ($t_{1/2}$) of drug is more relevant. The $t_{1/2}$ of a drug by definition is the time taken for 50% of the drug in the animal to be eliminated from the body. It is calculated by the equation.

$$t_{1/2} = \ln 2 / \text{ slope or } t_{1/2} = 0.693 / \text{ slope} \tag{1}$$

Half-life is influenced by biological factors like volume of distribution and elimination rate. The volume of distribution (Vd) is the quantitative estimate of the extent of the distribution of the drug in the body and it influence $t_{1/2}$ of the drug. It is proportionality constant relating the concentration of drug in the serum to the total amount of drug in the body.

$$Vd = \text{amount of drug in the body} / \text{serum drug concentration} \quad (2)$$

In addition to Vd, the clearance (Cl) of the drug also play important role in determining the withdrawal time of the drug. Clearance quantitates the efficiency of the elimination process and is defined as the rate of drug elimination from the body relative to the concentration of drug in the serum.

$$Cl = \text{rate of elimination} / \text{Serum drug concentration} \quad (3)$$

The $t_{1/2}$ dependent on two functions: Volume of distribution and clearance. By combining term, an equation can be derived that reflects the influence of Vd and Cl on the $t_{1/2}$ of a drug.

$$t_{1/2} = \ln 2\ Vd/Cl \text{ or } t_{1/2} = 0.693Vd/Cl \quad (4)$$

For an orally or extrvascularaly administrated drug withdrawal can be derived as

$$\text{Withdrawal time} = 1.44 \ln CC^{o} \text{ (tolerance) } (t_{1/2}) \quad (5)$$

Where C^{o} is the initial concentration of drug in the body derived by ratio bioavailability to Vd.

The above equation is useful to gain a perspective on what the withdrawal time is relative to the terminal half-life. If the drug has a short half-life (eg. penicillin), the withdrawal time is short. However, If a drug (eg. An aminoglycoside) has a prolonged tissue half-life the withdrawal time could be very long. Similarly, a drug with a very low tissue tolerance has a longer withdrawal time.

For lactating dairy cows and goats milk discard times are determined using pharmacokinetic principles. The milk discard or withdrawing time is the time after drug administration when the milk cannot be used for human consumption. This is determined by administering the drug and collecting and analyzing milk until drug concentrations are below the milk tolerance established for that drug. It is based on the half-life of the drug in the milk. Basic drugs like erythromycin have longer discard times than acidic drugs such as penicillin because the former tend to distribute more readily into milk due to pH partitioning phenomenon. Similarly, lipophilic drugs will tend to have longer milk discard times.

13. Conclusion

Food safety is one of the most significant issue faced by livestock owners and consumers of animal derived food. Residues of drugs and chemicals in food of animal origin raise special concern for human safety. Consumer concern about drug residue in animal food has led to reduction in demand in many countries. It has also disturbed international trade of food. Globally, food safety programs are advancing but formal training in drug residue prevention is limited. It is global need that Veterinarians should be acquainted with legal and regulatory issues concerning control of drug and other chemicals residues in food animals. The primary pharmacokinetic parameters used by veterinarians to prevent violative tissue residues are withdrawal time for meat and discard time for milk.

14. Acknowledgement

Authors are grateful to Anand Agricultural University, Anand, Gujarat state, India for providing financial support facilities to conduct pharmacokinetic studies on some cephalosporins and fluoroquinolones in domestic animals. Authors are also thankful to colleagues and post-graduate students for technical support. Authors thank Sejal and Pooja for secretarial assistance in preparing manuscript.

15. References

Abdullah A.S. & Baggot J.D. (1986). Effect of short term starvation on disposition kinetics of chloramphenicol in goats. *Research in Veterinary Science*, Vol.40, No.2, (February 1986), pp.382-385, ISSN: 0034-5288

Anadon A.; Martinez-Larranaga M.R.; Diaz J.; Bringas P.; Martinez M.A.; Fernandez-Cruz M.L. & Fernandez R. (1995). Pharmacokinetics and residues of enrofloxacin in chicken. *American Journal of Veterinary Research*, Vol.56, No.4, (April 1995), pp.501-506, ISSN: 0002-9645

Atef, M.; Atta A.H. & Amer A.M.(1991). Pharmacokinetics of chloramphenicol in normal and *Escherichi coli* infected chickens. *British Poultry Science*, Vol.32, No.3, (March 1991), pp.589-596, ISSN (printed): 0007-1668.

Atta A.H. & Sharif L. (1997). Pharmacokinetics of ciprofloxacin following intravenous and oral administration in broiler chickens. *Journal of Veterinary Pharmacology and Therapeutics*, Vol.20, No.4, (August 1997), pp.326-329, ISSN 0140-7783

Bergante M.A.; Saez P.; Aramayona J.J.; Fraile, L.; Gracia M.A. & Solan C. (1999). Comparitive pharmacokinetics of enrofloxacin in mice, rats, rabbits, sheep and cow. *American Journal of Veterinary Research*, Vol.60, No.8, (August 1999), pp.1111-1116, ISSN: 0002-9645

Bermingham E.C. & Papich M.G. (2002). Pharmacokinetics after intravenous and oral administration of enrofloxacin in sheep. *American Journal of Veterinary Research*, Vol.63, No.7, (July 2002), pp.1012-1017, ISSN: 0002-9645

Bermingham E.C.; Papich M.G. & Vivrette S. (2000). Pharmacokinetics of enrofloxacin after oral and IV administration to foals. *American Journal of Veterinary Research*, Vol.61, No.6, (June 2000), pp.706-709, ISSN: 0002-9645

Bhavsar S.K. & Malik J.K. (1994). Pharmacokinetics of metronidazole in calves. *British Veterinary Journal*, Vol.150, No.4, (July August 1994), pp.389-393, ISSN 1090-0233

Bhavsar S.K.; Verma M.P. & Thaker A.M. (2004). Pharmacokinetics, tissue concentration, and safety of multiple dose Intravenous administration of ciprofloxacin in cow calves. *Journal of Veterinary Pharmacology and Toxicology*, Vol. 3, No 1& 2, (December 2004), pp.27-34, ISSN 0140-7783

Brown M.P.; Stover S.M.; Lelly R.H. & Farver T.B. (1982). Body fluid concentration of ampicillin trihydrate in 6 hours after a single intramuscular dose. *Equine Veterinary Journal*, Vol.14, No.1, (January 1992), pp.83-85, , ISSN: 0425-1644.

Burrows G.E; barto P.B.; Martin B. & Tripp M.L.(1983). Comparitive pharmacokinetics of antibiotics in newborn calves: Chloramphenicol, lincomycin and tylosin. *American Journal of Veterinary Research*, Vol.44, No.6, (June 1983), pp.1053-1057, ISSN: 0002-9645

Carli S.; Montesissa C.; Sonzogni O & Madonna M. (1986). Pharmacokinetics of sodium cefoperazone in calves. *Pharmacological Research Communications*, Vol.18, No.5, (May 1986), pp.481-490, ISSN 0031-6989

Castells G. (2001). Allometric analysis of thiamphenicol disposition among seven mammalian species. *Journal of Veterinary Pharmacology and Therapeutics*, Vol.24, No.3, (June 2001), pp.193-197, ISSN 0140-7783

da Silva R.G.; Reyes F.G.; Sartori J.R. & Rath S. (2006). Enrofloxacin assay validation and pharmacokinetics following a single dose in chickens. *Journal of Veterinary Pharmacology and Therapeutics*, Vol.29, No.5, (October 2006), pp.365-372, ISSN 0140-7783

Dagorn M.; Guillot P. & Sanders P. (1990). Pharmacokinetics of chloramphenicol in sheep after intravenous, intramuscular and subcutaneous administration. *Veterinary Quarterly*, Vol.12, No.3, (August 1990), pp.166-174, ISSN 0165-2176

Davis J.L.; Foster D.M. & Papich M.G. (2006). Pharmacokinetics and tissue distribution of enrofloxacin and its active metabolite ciprofloxacin in calves. *Journal of Veterinary Pharmacology and Therapeutics*, Vol.30, No.6, (October 2006), pp.564-571, ISSN 0140-7783

Davis J.L.; Salmon J.H. & Papich M.G. (2006). Pharmacokinetics and tissue distribution of doxycycline after oral administration of single and multiple doses in horses. *American Journal of Veterinary Research*, Vol.67, No.2, (Febrauary2006), pp.310-316, ISSN: 0002-9645

Davis L.E.; Baggot J.D. & Powers T.E. (1972). Pharmacokinetics of chloramphenicol in domesticated animals. *American Journal of Veterinary Research*, Vol.33, No.11, (November 1972), pp.2259-2266, ISSN 0002-9645

Dufee N.E.; Christensen, J.M. & Craig A.M. (1989). The pharmacokinetics of cefadroxil in the foal. *Journal of Veterinary Pharmacology and Therapeutics*, Vol.12, No.4, (December 1989), pp.323-326, ISSN 0140-7783

Ensink J.M.; Vulto A.G. and vanMiert ASJPAM (1996). Oral bioavailability and in vitro stability of pivampicillin, bacampicillin, talampicillin and ampicillin in horses. *American Journal of Veterinary Research*, Vol.57, No.5, (May 1996), pp.1021-1024, ISSN: 0002-9645

Garg S.K.; Chudhary R.K. and Srivastava A.K.(1992). Disposition kinetics and dosage of cephalexin in cow calves following intramuscular administration. *Annales de Recherches Veterinaires*, Vol.23, No.2, (February 1992), pp.399-402, ISSN 0003-4193

Giguere S.; Sweeny R.W. & Belanger M. (1996). Pharmacokinetics of enrofloxacin in adult horses and concentration of drug in serum, body fluids and endometrial tissue after repeated intragastrically administered doses. *American Journal of Veterinary Research*, Vol.57, No.7, (July 1996), pp.1025-1030, ISSN: 0002-9645

Gohil P.V.; Patel U.D.; Bhavsar S.K. & Thaker A.M.(2009). Pharmacokinetics of ceftriaxone in buffalo calves (*Bubalus bubalis*) following intravenous and intramuscular administration. *Iranian Journal of Veterinary Research*, Vol.10, No.1, (January 2009), pp.33-37, ISSN 1728-1997

Guerrini V.H.; Filippich L.J.; cao G.R. English P.B. & Bourne D.W. (1985). Pharmacokinetics of cefaronide, ceftriaxone and cefoperazone in sheep. *Journal of Veterinary Pharmacology and Therapeutics*, Vol.08, No.2, (June 2002), pp.120-127, ISSN 0140-7783

Hornish R.E.; Gosline R.E. & Nappier J.M. (1987). Comparitive metabolism of lincomycin in in the swine, chicken and rat. *Drug Metabolism Review*, Vol.18, No.2-3, (January 1987), pp.177-214, ISSN 0360-2532

Knoll U.; Glunder G. & Kietzmann M. (1999). Comparitive study of the plasma pharmacokinetics and tissue concentrations of danofloxacin and enrofloxacin in broiler chicken. . *Journal of Veterinary Pharmacology and Therapeutics*, Vol.22, No.4, (August 1999), pp.239-246, ISSN 0140-7783

Kume B.B. & Garg R.C. (1986). Pharmacokinetics and bioavailability of chloramphenicol in normal and febrile goats. *Journal of Veterinary Pharmacology and Therapeutics*, Vol.9, No.3, (September 1986), pp.254-263, ISSN 0140-7783

Maradiya J. J.; Goriya H.V.; Bhavsar S.K., Patel U.D. & Thaker A.M. (2010). Pharmacokinetics of ceftriaxone in cow calves, *VETERINARSKI ARHIV* , Vol. 80, No 1, (January 2010), pp.1-9, ISSN 0372-5480

Martin K. & Weise B. (1988). The disposition of chloramphenicol in colostrums-fed and colostrums-deprived newborn pigs. *Pharmacology and Toxicology*, Vol.63, No.1, (January 1988), pp.16-19, ISSN ISSN 0972-8872

Martin T. & Riviere, J.E. (1998). Population pharmacokinetics in veterinary medicine: potential use for therapeutic drug monitoring and prediction of tissue residues. *Journal of Veterinary Pharmacology and Therapeutics*, Vol.21, No.3, (June 1998), pp.167-189, ISSN 0140-7783

Mengozzi G.; Intorre L.; Bertini S. & Soldani G. (1996). Pharmacokinetics of enrofloxacin and its metabolite ciprofloxacin after intravenous and intramuscular administration to sheep. *American Journal of Veterinary Research*, Vol.57, No.7, (July 1996), pp.1040-1043, ISSN: 0002-9645

Neilsen P. & Gyrd-Hansen N. (1996). Bioavailability of oxytetracycline, tetracycline and chlortetracycline after oral administration to fed and fasted pigs. *Journal of Veterinary Pharmacology and Therapeutics*, Vol.19, No.4, (August 1996), pp.305-311, ISSN 0140-7783

Nouws J.F.; Mevius D.J.; Vree T.B.; Baars A.M. & Laurensen J. (1988). Pharmacokinetics, renal clearance and metabolism of ciprofloxacin following intravenous and oral administration to calves and pigs, *Veterinary Quarterly*, Vol.10, No.3, (September 1988), pp.156-163, ISSN 0165-2176

Nouws J.F.M.; Smulders A. & Rappalini M. (1990). A comparative study on irritation and residue aspect of five oxytetracycline formulations administered to calves, pigs and sheep. *Veterinary Quarterly*, Vol.12, No.3, (September 1988), pp.129-138, ISSN 0165-2176

Patel U.D.; Patni K.Z.; Bhavsar S.K. & Thaker A.M. (2006b). Disposition of cefepime following single dose intramuscular administration in calves. *International Journal of Cow science*, Vol.2, No.1, (January 2006), pp.49-51, ISSN 0973-2241

Patel H.B.; Bhavsar S.K.; Thaker A.M.; Suresh Babu N. and Wadhwani K.N. (2004). Pharmacokinetics of ciprofloxacin following intravenous and intramuscular administration in Sheep. *Journal of Veterinary Pharmacology and Toxicology*, Vol. 3, No 1& 2, (December 2004), pp.35-38, ISSN 0972-8872

Patel H.M.; Bhavsar S.K.; Thaker A.M.; Wadhwani K.N. & Malik J.K. (1993). Disposition kinetics of metronidazole in sheep following oral administration. *Indian Journal of Animal Science*, Vol.63, No.12, (December 1993), pp.1282-1283, ISSN 0367-8318

Patel P.N.;Patel U.D.; Bhavsar S. K. & Thaker A. M. (2010). Pharmacokinetics of cefepime following intravenous and intramuscular administration in sheep, *Iranian Journal of Pharmacology and Therapeutics*, Vol. 9, No 1, (January 2010), pp.7-10, ISSN 1735-2657

Patel U.D.; Bhavsar S. K. & Thaker A. M. (2006a). Pharmacokinetics and dosage regimen of cefepime following single dose intravenous administration in calves , *Iranian Journal of Pharmacology and Therapeutics*, Vol. 5, No 2, (July 2006), pp.127-130, ISSN 1735-2657

Patni K.; Patel U.D.; Bhavsar S. K.; Thaker A. M. & Sarvaiya J.G. (2008). Single dose pharmacokinetics of cefepime after intravenous and intramuscular administration in goats, *Turkish Journal of Veterinary & Animal Science*, Vol. 32, No 3, (March 2008), pp.159-162, ISSN 1300-0128

Popick A.C.; Crouthamel W.G. & Bekersky I. (1987). Plasma protein binding of ceftriaxone. *Xenobiotica*, Vol.17, No.10, (October 1987), pp.1139-1145, ISSN 0049-8254

Prades M.; Brown M.P.; Gronwall R.& Miles N.S. (1988). Pharmacokinetics of sodium cephapirin in lactating dairy cows. *American Journal of Veterinary Research*, Vol.49, No.11, (November 1988), pp.1888-1890, ISSN: 0002-9645

Rao G.S.; Ramesh S.; Ahmad A.H.; Tripathi H.C.; Sharma L.D. & Malik J.K. (2002). Pharmacokinetics of enrofloxacin and its metabolite ciprofloxacin in goats given enrofloxacin alone and in combination with probenecid. *The veterinary Journal*, Vol.163, No.1, (January 2002), pp.85-93, ISSN 1090-0233

Richez P.; Pedersen Morner A.; DeJong A. & Monlouis J.D. (1997). Plasma pharmacokinetics of parenterally administered danofloxacin and enrofloxacin in pigs. *Journal of Veterinary Pharmacology and Therapeutics*, Vol.20, No. 1, (January 1997), pp.41-42, ISSN 0140-7783

Rule R.; Rubio M. & Perelli M.C. (1991). Pharmacokinetics of ceftazidime in shep and its penetration into tissue and peritoneal fluid. *Research in veterinary science*, Vol.51, No.3, (November 1991), pp.233-238, ISSN 0034-5258

Sanders P.; Guillot P & Mourot D. (1988). Pharmacokinetics of long acting chloramphenicol formulation administered by intramuscular and subcutaneous routes in cattle. *Journal of Veterinary Pharmacology and Therapeutics*, Vol.11, No.2, (June 1988), pp.183-190, ISSN 0140-7783

Sarasola P. & Mckeller Q.A. (1994). Ampicillin and its congener prodrugs in the horse(review). *British Veterinary Journal*, Vol.150, No.2, (March-April 1994), pp.173-187, ISSN: 0007-1935

Sarvaiya J.G.; Bhavsar S.K.; Mody S.K.; Thaker A.M.& Tripathi R.M. (2006). Multiple dose pharmacokinetics and safety of Ciprofloxacin in Buffalo calves (*Bubalus bubalis*). *Journal of Veterinary Pharmacology and Toxicology*, Vol. 5, No 1& 2, (December 2006), pp.15-18, ISSN 0972-8872

Shoaf S.E; Schwark W.S. & Guard C.L. (1987). The effect of age and diet on sulfadizine/trimethoprim disposition following oral and subcutaneous administration to calves. *Journal of Veterinary Pharmacology and Therapeutics*, Vol.10, No 4, (December 1987), pp.331-345, ISSN 0140-7783

Shem-Tov M.; Rav-Hon O.; Ziv G.; Lavi E.; Glickman A. & Saran, A. (1998). Pharmacokinetica and penetration of danofloxacin from the blood into milk of cows. *Journal of Veterinary Pharmacology and Therapeutics*, Vol.21, No.3, (June 1998), pp.209-213, ISSN 0140-7783

Sisodia C.S. (1975). A pharmacological study of chloramphenicol in horses. *Canadian Journal of Comparative Medicine*, Vol.39, No.2, (April1975), pp.216-223, ISSN 0008- 4050

Soback S. (1988). Pharmacokinetics of single dose cefoxitin given by the intravenous and intramuscular routes to unweaned calves. *Journal of Veterinary Pharmacology and Therapeutics*, Vol.11, No.2, (June 1988), pp.155-162, ISSN 0140-7783

Soback S. (1989). Pharmacokinetics of single dose administration of moxalactam in unweaned calves. *American Journal of Veterinary Research*, Vol.50, No.2, (February 1989), pp.498-501, ISSN: 0003-1488

Soback S.; Bor A. & Ziv G. (1987). Clinical pharmacology of cefazolin in calves. *Journal of veterinary Medicine Series- A*, Vol.34, No.1, (February 1987), pp.25-32, ISSN: 0003-1488

Strover S.M.; Brown M.P.; lelly R.H.; Fraver T.B. & Knight H.D.(1981). Aqueous procaine penicillin G in the horse: serum, synovial, peritoneal and urine concentrations after single-dose intramuscular administration. *American Journal of Veterinary Research*, Vol.42, No.4, (April 1981), pp.629-631, ISSN: 0002-9645

Swati; Tiwari S.; Patel U. D.; Bhavsar S. K. & Thaker A. M. (2010). Pharmacokinetics and Bioavailability of Ceftriaxone in Patanwadi Sheep, *Vet Scan*, Vol.5, No.2, (December 2010), Article 66, ISSN 0973-6980 (online) (http://vetscan.co.in/v5n2/66-ceftriaxone-sheep.htm)

Ter Hune T.N.; Skogerboe T.L.; Shostrom V.K. & Weigel D.J. (2005). Comparision of pharmacokinetics of danofloxacin and enrofloxacin in calves challenged with Mannheimia haemolytica. *American Journal of Veterinary Research*, Vol.66, No.2, (February 2005), pp.342-349, ISSN: 0002-9645

Tiwari S.; Swati, Bhavsar S.K.; Patel U.D. & Thaker A.M. (2009). Disposition of Ceftriaxone in Goats (*Capra hircus*), Vet Scan, Vol.4, No.2, (December 2009), Article 41 ISSN 0973-6980 (online) (http://vetscan.co.in/v5n2/66-ceftriaxone-sheep.htm)

Varia R.D.; Patel J.H.; Patel U.D.; Bhavsar S.K. & Thaker, A.M. (2009). Disposition of levofloxacin following oral administration in broiler chicken. *Israel Journal of Veterinary Medicine*, Vol.64, No 4, (April 2009), pp.118-121, ISSN 0334-9152

Watson A.D. (1991). Chloramphenicol:(2) clinical pharmacology in dogs and cats. *Australian Veterinary Journal* , Vol.68, No.1, (January 1991), pp.2-5 ISSN 0005-0423

Waxman S.; Rodriguez C.; Gonzalez F.; De Vicente M.L.; San Andres M.I. & San Andres M.D. (2001). Pharmacokinetic behavior of marbofloxacin after intravenous and intramuscular administration in adult goats. *Journal of Veterinary Pharmacology and Therapeutics*, Vol.24, No.6, (December 2001), pp.375-378, ISSN 0140-7783

Wilson W.D.; Spensley M.S.; Baggot J.D. & Hietala S.K. (1988). Pharmacokinetics and estimated bioavailability od amoxiciliin in mares after intravenous, intramuscular and oral administration. *American Journal of Veterinary Research*, Vol.49, No.10, (October 1988), pp.1688-1693, ISSN: 0002-9645

Ziv G. (1983). Clinical pharmacology of tiamulin in ruminants. *Journal of Veterinary Pharmacology and Therapeutics*, Vol.6, No.1, (March 1983), pp.23-_, ISSN 0140-7783

Ziv G.; Shem-Tov M. & Glickman A. (1995). Tilmicosin antibacterial activity and pharmacokinetics in cows. *Journal of Veterinary Pharmacology and Therapeutics*, Vol.18, No.5, (October 1995), pp.340-345, ISSN 0140-7783

9

Comparative Veterinary Pharmacokinetics

Akos Jerzsele
Szent Istvan University-Faculty of Veterinary Science, Department of Pharmacology and Toxicology Hungary

1. Introduction

In veterinary clinical practice the sensitivity of a given animal species to a certain drug can be attributed to pharmacodynamic and pharmacokinetic variations. In contrast to human medicine where individual differences are of primary importance, interspecies and also inter-breed distinctions are crucial in comparative veterinary medicine. Pharmacokinetics describes the behaviour of the drug in the body. Similarly to human nomenclature, the ADME process describes the absorption (other than IV adiministration), the distribution, the metabolism and the elimination of certain drugs. To produce a systemic effect, the drug must be absorbed and distributed to attain therapeutic concentration at the site of action. If the target site is the GI tract, then no absorption is needed after oral application. Significant variations can be seen in the extent of absorption and distribution, the rate and the manner of metabolism and elimination between animal species. Because of pronounced interspecies variations extrapolation of parameters from pharmacokinetic data of human or other animal origin is inappropriate and can be hazardous in case of several drugs. Lack of pharmacokinetic data however, necessitates the empiric application of extrapolated human dosages in many cases. This chapter concentrates on the variations in the ADME process between animals of different species, breed and age.

2. Administration routes in veterinary practice

Administration routes in the veterinary medicine are mainly similar to those in the human medicine with minor differences. Major application routes include intravenous (IV), intramuscular (IM), subcutaneous (SC), oral (PO), topical, intramammary and inhalational administration. *Intravenous (IV) administration* is frequent in all animal species. Drug action is the fastest when applied IV because no absorption is necessary. Drugs applied as an intravenous bolus achieve high plasma levels and produce a quick, immediate action and usually a pronounced effect. Drugs can also be applied IV as a continous infusion with which the surgeon can easily govern the effects of the substance as the concentration and the rate of infusion determines plasma steady state levels. It is a common way of applying intravenous anaesthetics like propofol. Although the IV route has many advantages, it is probably the most toxic way of administration. Drugs administered IV have to be applied slowly and observe the patient for potential side effects. *Intramuscular (IM) and subcutaneous (SC) application* is very frequent in the veterinary medicine. It is common in ruminants, swine, horse, dogs, cats and rabbits. Rate of absorption is determined principally by the administration route, the vascularity and area of the region, the concentration and the ionization of the drug. There are also differences in the localization of the injection. For example, suprascapular IM injection is frequently applied in small animals, as it results in much faster absorption when compared to the gluteal muscles because of better vascularity and the proximity of the periosteum. Depending on the injection site, peak plasma concentrations are usually achieved 20-40 minutes after administration. There are several drugs that are formulated as sustained release preparations. Ampicillin and amoxicillin trihydrate, procaine and benzathine penicillin are antibiotics frequently formulated as depot injections resulting in prolonged absorption and effective plasma levels. These preparations are usually applied with 2-3 day intervals that is a great advantage in food producing animals where restraint is an important and avoidable stress factor. Bioavailability is generally higher or equal to oral administration and it is infrequently 100%. Inactivation or precipitation at the injection site and damage of the tissues are common contributing factors to low IM bioavailability values, like in case of diazepam. *Oral administration* is the most frequent mode of application in animals as food producing animals are primarily treated via this route. In poultry and swine drugs are commonly dissolved in the drinking water or mixed into the feedstuff to treat a large number of animals. Boluses, drenches, oral gels and oral pastes are common dosage forms for the oral treatment of ruminants and horses. Tablets, capsules, oral solutions and suspensions are the primary oral dosage forms in companion animals. Differences in oral bioavailability between animal species are conspicouos, detailed comparative aspects are discussed in the "Absorption of drugs" Chapter. *Topical administration* also raises several comparative pharmacokinetic issues that are discussed in the „Absorption of drugs" Chapter. *Intramammary application* is an important veterinary application route in the treatment and prevention of mastitis in cattle.

3. Absorption of drugs

Once the drug has been administered by any route other than IV it has to be absorbed into the bloodstream to exert its systemic effect. The extent of absorption is termed *bioavailability*, and defined as the ratio of AUC (area under the curve) after extravascular and intravenous administration.

$$F\ (bioavailability) = AUC_{extravascular}/AUC_{intravenous}$$

Depending on the administration route we can talk about oral, intramuscular, subcutaneous, topical etc. bioavailability. As the greatest interspecies differences occur after oral administration, this chapter concentrates on this application route. The extent and rate of absorption depends mainly on the lipophilicity, molecular weight and degree of ionization of the substance at the site of administration. Weak acids (like most of the NSAIDs) are mainly in nonionized form in the acidic environment of the stomach thus their absorption starts in the proximal regions of the GI tract resulting in lower T_{max} values. Weak bases are mainly in ionized form in the stomach, thus their T_{max} values are usually higher. Oral bioavailability can also be influenced via biotransformation by intestinal epithelial cells or by the liver. This is called the „first pass effect". Many drugs are inactivated via this mechanism, examples include lidocaine, diazepam, xylazine, detomidine, medetomidine, morphine or cimetidine. In case of prodrugs, like codeine, cefuroxime-axetil or pivampicillin first pass metabolism is essential in activating the substance. To avoid first pass metabolism the drug can be applied parenterally or rectally as the rectum is not connected to the portal vein. Pharmaceutical formulations can also significantly alter the rate of absorption.

Modified release or coated tablets can delay dissolution of the substance in the gastrointestinal (GI) tract thereby protract absorption. Some examples for these preparations are retard tablets and capsules containing potassium, phenytoin, azythromycin, NSAIDs, sedatives and water soluble vitamins. Oily solutions, emulsions and suspensions can be used for the formulation of depot injections which - if injected subcutaneously or intramuscularly - can provide delayed absorption of the active substance. Chemical modifications are also used to prolong absorption. Ceftiofur is a veterinary third generation cephalosporin that has three different formulations for use in swine and ruminants. Ceftiofur sodium and ceftiofur hydrochloride are rapidly absorbed after intramuscular administration, while the free crystalline acid form have a protracted absorption resulting in approximately 150 hours effective plasma levels against certain respiratory pathogens, like *Pasteurella multocida* or *P. haemolytica.* Additional important factors that affect drug absorption include physical or chemical interaction with feed constituents, increased gastrointestinal motility or inflammation of the GI tract and disruption of GI epithelium. An example for the former phenomenon are the tetracyclines that are well known about their ability to form insoluble complexes with calcium and magnesium ions. Thus, feedstuff containing these ions in a high amount (e.g. milk products) should not be administered together with these antibiotics. Diseases with inherent increased GI motility will result in decreased absorption of the administered drugs. Inflammation of the GI mucosa and disruption of the GI epithelium (e.g. canine or feline parvovirosis) will result in increased absorption of the active substances. Aminoglycosides that are practically not absorbed from the intact GI tract can have much higher bioavailability and can exert systemic toxic effects (ototoxicity and nephrotoxicity) in animals with parvovirosis (Gemer et al., 1983, Riviere&Papich, 2009).

3.1 Differences in oral and parenteral absorption in different animal species

Discriminating monogastric and ruminant, herbivorous, omnivorous and carnivorous animal species is essential when defining comparative pharmacokinetics. Although there are notable differences in the whole ADME process, perhaps oral absorption and metabolism phases show the greatest distinctions. The length and volume of the GI tract in ruminants and horses is much more pronounced when compared to the other important domestic species (poultry, swine, dog and cat). This will result in longer passage time and usually delayed absorption after oral application of drugs. An example for this are the benzimidazole class of anthelminthics. A single oral dosage of these substances (e.g. albendazole, fenbendazole) can provide a protracted duration of action in horses, cattle, sheep and goats to eliminate the most important parasitic worms. In other animal species, multiple oral administration is usually necessary to eliminate the GI parasites. Dogs, cats and swine usually resemble in the rate and extent of oral absorption and these parameters are usually similar to humans. There are several exceptions however, that necessitate pharmacokinetic investigations in the certain species and need to arise precautions when extrapolating dosages or dosing intervals to humans or other species. Namely, oral bioavailability values show pronounced differences between animal species. The frequently applied broad spectrum aminopenicillin, amoxicillin shows an oral bioavailability of 5% in horses (Ensink et al., 1992), 28-33% in swine (Agerso&Friis, 1998), 59-68% in poultry (El Sooud et al., 2004, Jerzsele et al., 2009, Jerzsele et al., 2011) and 60-80% in dogs and cats (Küng et al., 1994).

In *horses*, oral bioavailability of a large number of drugs show great individual variations. Absorption of most antimicrobial agents is significantly hindered by feeding, thus 2-4 hours fasting is essential before applying these drugs. Even in these cases systemic availability can show wide variations between individuals, as in case of metronidazole between 60 and 90% (Baggot et al., 1998). Bioavailability of several drugs can be very low compared to other domestic species. Examples include several antibiotics, like ampicillin and amoxicillin that have 0-1% and 5% oral bioavailability, respectively (Ensink et al. 1992, Ensink et al. 1996). This phenomenon can result in severe dysbacteriosis because of the low extent of absorption and accumulation of the substance in the intestinal lumen. Pivampicillin, an ester of ampicillin can be used to overcome this problem, as the oral bioavailability of this drug is 31-36% (Ensink et al. 1992). In foals *per os* absorption is usually more pronounced, oral bioavailability and age being frequently in a negative correlation. Cefadroxil shows approximately 100% oral bioavailability in neonatal foals that decreases to 15% until 5 months of age (Duffee et al. 1997). Metformin, an antidiabetic substance has also very low oral absorption compared to humans (Hustace et al., 2009). Absorption of drugs from the oral mucosa can be quite significant. Detomidine, a frequently applied veterinary α_2-agonist has significant first pass metabolism resulting in low oral bioavailability if ingested. If applied sublingually however, absorption form the oral mucosa eventuates 22% bioavailability (Kaukinen et al., 2010) which is clinically useful. In horses, subcutaneous injection of drugs is infrequent, intramuscular application is more common. Bioavailability values are similar after these administration routes, although IM administration usually produce lower T_{max} values indicating faster absorption. As IM injections can cause sterile abscesses, IV administration is prevalent, in this case no absorption of the drug is necessary.

In *ruminants* the presence of the reticulorumen has some important clinical consequences. Large volume of the ruminal fluid (60-70L in cattle) dilutes the drugs and decreases their rate of absorption delaying the effect of orally applied medicines. Ruminal microbial flora restricts the oral usage of most antibacterial agents in adult individuals. As calves do not possess a mature ruminal microflora, antibiotics can also be applied orally. The bacterial flora plays an important role in the biotransformation of certain substances, like the already banned chloramphenicol. In several cases, however, ruminal microflora can transform a less active substance to a more active/toxic one. For instance, urea is almost nontoxic to monogastric animals, while highly toxic to ruminants as urea is rapidly transformed to ammonia by the bacterial urease enzyme. Netobimine, an inactive prodrug of the anthelminthic molecule albendazole is converted to its active form, albendazole and albendazole sulfoxide in the rumen (Capece et al., 2001). Anthelmintics as one of the most commonly used medications in ruminants can be administered orally to young and adult ruminants alike. In ruminants, sustained release boluses represent an important group of formulations. These preparations often contain anthelminthics which are released slowly and/or intermittently from the product resulting in excellent activity against gastrointestinal endoparasites. These formulations are retained in the reticulorumen and release the substance for months resulting in a very long withdrawal period.

In *swine* oral administration of drugs via feedstuff or drinking water is a common practice. Pharmacokinetic investigations are frequently conducted, especially in case of antibiotics and anthelminthics. In infectious diseases where bacteria are localized mainly in the GI tract antibiotics with no or very low oral bioavailability have an important role. Colistin and the aminoglycosides are frequently applied in these cases as they have excellent activity against

Enterobacteriaceae, mainly *E. coli* and *S. enterica* and retained in the intestinal lumen. Apramycin is an important exception however, it has 25-30% availability, thus it can also be used for the treatment of systemic or urinary tract infections. Oral bioavailability of amoxicillin is approximately half when compared to those in poultry, dogs and cats. The exact explanation is not yet known, but it can be attributed to acid-catalysed hydrolysis, intestinal enzymes or a carrier mediated uptake mechanism, that can be saturated (Reyns et al., 2007). Thus, increasing dosage decreases oral bioavailability, as described in humans (Arancibia et al., 1988). When using an microencapsulated granule formulation, bioavailability is significantly increased to nearly 100%, that might be an explanation as microencapsulation protects amoxicillin from enzymatic degradation (Anfossi et al., 2002).

Dogs and cats are carnivorous animals, they do not possess basal secretion of hydrochloric acid in the stomach, thus the gastric pH varies in fasted and fed animals. In animals with empty stomach gastric pH can reach values of 5-6, while in fed animals it is declined to 1-2. This phenomenon has clinical pharmacological consequences in some cases. As an example, proton pump inhibitors (like omeprazole) as they need a strongly acidic pH to be activated should be administered along with food. Certain NSAIDs, like the newly developed long acting veterinary coxib, mavacoxib should be administered together with food. The oral bioavailability of mavacoxib in fasted animals is approx. 46.1%, while being 87.4% in fed animals (Cox et al. 2010). Other examples that have greater systemic availability when applied with feeding include doxycycline or ketoconazole. Ketoconazole also needs acidic pH in the stomach to be absorbed thus it should to be given with food (Giguere et al, 2006). In contrast, several substances should be applied to fasted animals, as feeding significantly decreases absorption. Examples are ampicillin (Kung et al., 1995, Kluge et al., 1999), oxytetracycline, chlortetracycline (Giguere et al. 2006) or cimetidine (Le Traon, 2009). Drug formulations can also influence oral bioavailability. In case of amoxicillin oral availability was 77%, 68% and 64% after oral suspension, oral drops and tablet administration, respectively (Küng et al., 1994).

In *poultry* the main administration route of drugs is oral application via drinking water or feedstuff. Oral bioavailability values are mainly similar than those in humans. Infectious diseases where bacteria are localized mainly in the GI tract are less frequent compared to swine as *E. coli* and salmonellae frequently penetrate into the bloodstream. Combinations including colistin (that has a very low bioavailability) and an other antibiotic with good absorption helps inhibiting and destroying bacteria systemically and luminally alike. Intramuscular administration of drugs is uncommon, but it comes into question when valuable breeding animals must be treated. IM bioavailability values are similar to oral. In case of marbofloxacin in ducks, oral and IM bioavailability was 87% and 81%, respectively. In case of amoxicillin in broiler chickens, oral and IM bioavailability was 61% and 77%, respectively. Although veterinary products licensed for poultry frequently have two or more target animal species, pharmacokinetic profile and thus dosage can show significant differences. Clavulanic acid has an IM bioavailability of 76% in turkeys and 87% in chickens. The oral bioavailability of the lactamase inhibitor is 61% in turkeys and 66% in chickens.

3.2 Percutaneous absorption after topical administration

Percutaneous absorption consists of three distinct phases. The drug must be dissolved, penetrate the stratum corneum and the epithelial layer and finally enter the bloodstream.

Lipophilicity is a major determining factor. Several substances have excellent transcutaneous absorption, e.g. the ectoparasiticidal amitraz, avermectins and the organophosphates, lipophilic glucocorticoids, omega fatty acids etc. Absorption can be enhanced by formulation, namely surfactant or organic solvents, like dimethyl sulphoxide (DMSO). These auxiliary substances help penetration of the substances through the outer layer of the skin. Percutaneous absorption is also enhanced by inflammation or excoriation of the skin. It is important to note that there are pronounced differences between animals. Cats have relatively thin skin compared to other domestic species thus absorption from the skin can be more significant. This fact together with the metabolic deficiencies in this species contributes to several important toxicological occurences in cats. Therefore spot on preparations containing pirethroids are highly toxic to cats, because of pharmacokinetic and pharmacodynamic peculiarities.

3.3 Intranasal absorption

Intranasal application is uncommon in the veterinary practice, although there is an increasing number of medicines that are to be applied via this route. The notable advantage of this method is to avoid first pass metabolism and thereby increasing bioavailability. Oxytocin can be applied intranasally to induce labor, promote milk letdown and for the adjunctive treatment of mastitis mainly in swine. Absorption is variable however, IM or SC administration is more common. Another example is diazepam, a frequently applied anticonvulsive benzodiazepine. Nasal bioavailability of diazepam is 41-42% in dogs (Musulin et al., 2011), providing an alternative route next to rectal administration in *status epilepticus*.

3.4 Intramammary absorption

Intramammary application of antibiotics, antiinflammatories and other substances is a common practice in dairy cattle. The large inner surface of the mammary gland provides opportunity for the extensive absorption of lipophilic substances. In mastitis inflammation enhances intramammary absorption as described about cefoperazone (Cagnardi, 2010), probably because of disturbances in epithelial cell lining. Florfenicol, a small, lipophilic molecule has 54% intramammary bioavalability compared to 38% when applied IM (Soback et al., 1995). This phenomenon worth considering as drug residues will be present also in the milk and the edible tissues raising a public health issue if the animal must be slaughtered. Less lipophilic substances are absorbed usually in a negligible amount, especially in healthy animals as proved about cloxacillin *in vitro* by Kietzmann et al. (2010)

4. Drug distribution

After the drugs are absorbed or applied intravenously they are distributed in the body. Certain drugs reach and are retained only in extracellular fluids, some are also penetrating cell membranes and distributed intracellularly and extracellularly alike. Finally, the drug reaches the target cell or tissue and/or its receptor sites. Tissue concentration achieved primarily depend on penetration across capillary membranes. Drug distribution is mainly influenced by the lipophilicity, the molecular weight and the degree of ionization of the substance and tissue blood flow rates. Generally, the more lipophilic, the smaller and less ionized the molecule, it is more completely distributed in the body. Distribution shows significant differences between domestic species, breeds and individuals of a certain breed. This can be attributed to distinctions in body composition. For instance highly lipophilic barbiturates are much more dangerous in greyhounds as they do not possess large volume of fat tissue where the drug could be redistributed. Some substances have such high plasma protein binding or large molecular weight that they are retained in the bloodstream after IV administration. Mannitol in a 5-25% concentration is applied intravenously to treat or prevent pulmonary edema, life threatening acute renal failure and reduce intracranial pressure. As it remains in the intravascular space it establishes an osmotic gradient between intravascular and extracellular compartments resulting in rapid decline in extracellular fluid amount.

For quantitating the extent of drug distribution, the *volume of distribution* (V_d) term need to be introduced. V_d is the volume that would be necessary for the drug to be distributed in the body according to its plasma concentration. Thus, V_d can be described as

$$V_d \text{ (volume of distribution)} = A(t)/C_p$$

where A(t) is the amount of drug in the body, C_p is the plasma concentration and t is time. According to this definition, the larger the V_d, the more extensive the drug distribution with higher tissue concentrations. The above mentioned mannitol has a very low V_d as it does not leave the intravascular space. Thus, V_d is practically equivalent with the blood volume, which is 0.08 L/kg. Drugs with V_d values of 0.3-0.8 L/kg (e.g. penicillins) are distributed in the body and achieving concentrations in tissues similar to the plasma. Drugs with moderate to high V_d are for instance marbofloxacin with a V_d of 1.2 L/kg in the horse (Carretero et al., 2002), or pentoxyfilline in chickens (De Boever et al., 2005). These drugs achieve much higher concentrations in the tissues than in the plasma. Chloroquine has extremely high V_d values in all species including humans. The substance has a V_d of 53.3 L/kg in dogs (Aderounmu et al., 1983) representing an almost complete penetration from the plasma to the tissues.

After distribution, *redistribution* occurs when administering certain drugs. Ultrashort acting, highly lipophilic barbiturates (e.g. thiopental) is applied IV, is rapidly distributed, crosses the blood brain barrier and causes general anesthesia. Meanwhile, the drug is quickly redistributed in high blood flow tissues, mainly the voluntary muscles causing a rapid decline in plasma drug levels. As plasma levels decrease, brain concentrations also decline resulting in awakening of the animal. The substance – as being highly lipophilic – is then accumulated in the fat tissue for a certain amount of time. Thus, readministration of thiopental after awakening is prohibited as the tissues featured in redistribution are already saturated. As mentioned above, animals with low amount of fat, like starving animals, or greyhounds are exposed to risk when applying the thiobarbiturates.

Certain drugs are liable to *accumulation* in different regions of the body. Aminoglycosides for instance have very high affinity to the cortical regions of the kidney, probably because of high phospholipid content of this area as the cationic aminoglycosides have high affinity to these anionic molecules. Certain antifungal agents (e.g. griseofulvin, ketoconazole) can be accumulated in the stratum corneum of the skin achieving high concentrations and providing excellent activity against dermatophytosis and onychomycosis. The pK value of the molecule largely influences its ability to accumulate in certain regions of the body. In case of weak acids pH values above the pK_a result in accumulation in regions with higher pH, while in contrast weak bases tend to accumulate at lower pH values than the pK_a. The clinical relevance of this phenomenon is widely accepted. Alkaline drugs are accumulated in the reticulorumen in ruminants (pH 5.6-6.5), the milk (pH 6.5-6.8) or the intracellular environment (pH~7.0) - regions that have lower pH values compared to the plasma - if they are lipophilic enough to penetrate these membranes. This phenomenon is called „ion trapping". Thus, lipophilic, alkaline drugs, like erythromycin, azythromycin, clarythromycin, clindamycin, minocycline or florfenicol have important clinical role (Davis et al., 2002, Yamazaki et al., 2008) in the treatment of infections caused by intracellular pathogens (*Mycoplasma* spp., *Chlamydia* spp., *Rhodococcus equi* etc.) or mastitis.

Plasma protein binding decreases the extent of distribution as it limits capillary membrane transport of the molecule. Drugs are primarily bound to plasma albumin reversibly, maintaining an equilibrium between bound and free molecules. As the concentration of the free drug declines (because of metabolism, redistribution or excretion) the protein bound ratio acts as a reservoir thereby protracts elimination and increases half-life of the drug. A newly developed third generation cephalosporin, cefovecin has 96-98.7% plasma protein binding in dogs and 99.5-99.8% in cats resulting in long half-lives and prolonged action. Desfuroylceftiofur, the metabolite of ceftiofur, another third generation cephalosporin is highly protein bound and has a moderately long, 10 hour half-life in cattle (Brown et al., 1991) and 8 hour in the horse (Meyer at al., 2009), uncommon to other beta lactams. If the drug is extensively bound to plasma proteins, it raises also toxicological issues. If such kind of drugs are applied together (like NSAIDs with anticoagulants) the competition for albumin results in higher free drug concentrations and more pronounced pharmacological effects, and finally, toxicosis. The same phenomenon can be observed in hypoalbuminaemia. It was reported that anesthesia achieved with propofol, a highly protein bound injectable anesthetic increases free fraction of propranolol by approx. 6% compared to untreated control (Perry et al., 1991). Competition for plasma albumin is one of the most frequent cause of pharmacokinetic interactions in the veterinary medicine. Some examples for drugs extensively protein bound can be found in Table 1.

Drug	**Protein binding (%)**
Cefovecin	98-99.8 (dog, cat)
Ceftiofur	~65% (cattle)
Digitoxin	~88% (dog)
Phenytoin	~78% (dog)
Phenylbutazone	~99% (horse)
Furosemide	~95% (dog)
Propranolol	~92% (dog)
Propofol	95-99%
Warfarin	96.5% (cat)

Table 1. Examples of drugs with extensive plasma protein binding

In the course of distribution drugs are able to penetrate certain *physiological special barriers* in a lesser or higher degree. Clinically relevant barriers include the blood brain barrier (BBB), blood milk, blood prostate, blood testicle and blood placenta barriers. Diffusion through these barriers is mainly affected by lipophilicity, molecular weight, ionization of the substance and the presence of inflammation. Inflamed meninges, mammary gland tissue or prostate markedly increases drug concentration in these areas. Acute or chronic nature of inflammation influences penetration of antibiotics across these barriers. Most of the beta lactams (like penicillin or ampicillin) achieve only low concentrations in the cerebrospinal fluid (CSF), the milk or the prostate. In acute meningitis, mastitis or prostatitis, however, penetration is significantly increased and can achieve inhibitory concentrations. In healthy tissues or those with chronic inflammation this diffusion is worse, and need emerges for the administration of more appropriate antibiotics, like third generation cephalosporin ceftriaxone or the phenicols. In modern veterinary practice usually the latter substances are used in the first line treatment of meningitis (Giguere et al., 2006). Another clinically relevant aspect is the sensitivity of some dog breeds to certain drugs including ivermectin. Ivermectin is a highly lipophilic endectocidal agent that readily crosses the BBB, but a P-glycoprotein mediated efflux mechanism helps to pump out the molecule from the CSF (Schinkel, 1999). Some dog breeds (Collie, Sheltie, Australian Shepherd) however, carry a mutated MDR-1 gene encoding a false P-glycoprotein (Roulet et al., 2003) thereby causing disturbances in this efflux mechanism in sensitive individuals. Selamectin, a derivative of ivermectin is tolerated better thus can also be used in MDR-1 mutant dog patients (Geyer et al. 2009). Other substances for P-glycoprotein are loperamide, domperidone or doxorubicine. Penetration of the blood milk barrier is important in the antibacterial therapy of acute mastitis in cattle. Although inflammation increases the level of antibiotics in the milk, only a limited number of substances is able to achieve therapeutic concentrations in this region. Penethamat, a narrow spectrum penicillin is a drug with excellent penetration is appropriate for intramuscular treatment of Gram-positive mastitis. In contrast, intramuscular injection of ceftiofur resulted in tissue and milk concentrations below detectable limits (Owens et al., 1990). In conclusion it can be pronounced that given parenterally, most of the beta lactams licensed for the treatment of mastitis are usually inappropriate in the sole treatment of the disease, but they do potentiate the efficacy of intramammary applied antibiotics (Ehinger et al., 2006, Owens et al., 1990). Certain lipophilic and alkaline substances however, can reach high concentrations in the mammary tissue and the milk because of excellent lipophilicity and the ion trapping mechanism (see above). For comparison, milk:plasma level ratios are 0.1-0.3 in case of penicillins and first generation cephalosporins, while 4.6 and 8.7 in case of spiramycin and erythromycin, respectively (Giguere et al., 2006). In conclusion it should be emphasized that among certain physiological barriers the BBB is the less permeable and is protected also by pump mechanisms, like P-glycoprotein. For comparison, fluoroquinolones can attain 2-3 times higher concentrations in the prostatic fluid than in the serum, while only 25% of serum levels can be achieved in the CSF (Giguere et al., 2006).

5. Drug metabolism

Metabolism or biotransformation involves a series of reactions that will render the xenobiotic (drug) available for excretion. These enzymatic processes decrease lipophilicity and increase polarity and hence water solubility of the parent molecule which can be eliminated via one of the excretion mechanisms present in the organism. Metabolism immediately begins after absorption and runs parallel with further absorption, distribution and exretion. Biotransformation generally takes place in two phases (Figure 1).

Phase I - or non-synthetising phase - involves chemical reactions that „prepare" the xenobiotic for Phase II, namely oxidative processes (oxidation or reduction), dealkylation or hydroxilation that are prerequisites for conjugation in Phase II. Functional groups converted or attached to the molecule in this Phase are future targets of conjugation. During Phase I the molecule can be inactivated or on the contrary, attain activity. Diazinon, a frequently applied organophosphate in dogs is metabolised into diazoxon in the liver that is more active and more toxic than the parent molecule (Kappers et al., 2001., Costa, 2006). Certain antibiotics can be metabolised into an other active form, like the veterinary enrofloxacin to ciprofloxacin in dogs (Kung et al., 1993) or ceftiofur to desfuroylceftiofur. Those drugs that attain activity after biotransformation are called *prodrugs*. Ramipril and enalapril, two frequently applied angiotensin-convertase enzyme inhibitor is metabolised into active ramiprilat and enalaprilat to exert their pharmacological effects. Febantel, a frequently applied benzimidazole anthelminthic achieves activity when it is metabolised to fenbendazole. Fenbendazole is further converted into oxfendazole, a metabolite with higher activity (Montesissa et al., 1989). Netobimine, an other benzimidazole prodrug is transformed to active albendazole which is rapidly metabolised to albendazole sulfoxide (Gokbulut et al., 2006). In most of the cases however, drugs are converted to an inactive form, like phenobarbital to hydroxy-phenobarbital.

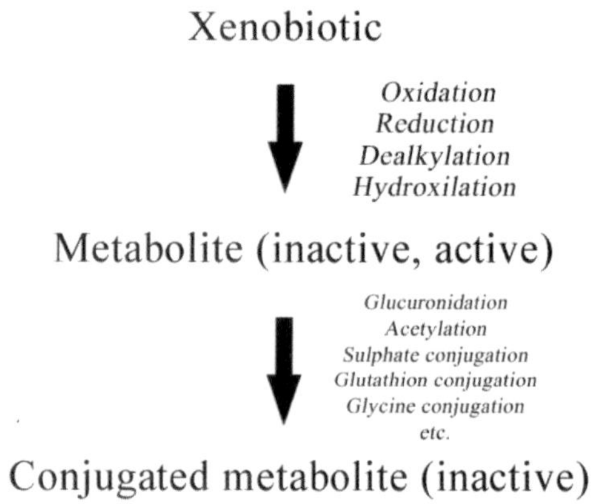

Fig. 1. Summary of Phase I and Phase II metabolic reactions

Phase I metabolic reactions are catalyzed by microsomal enzymes, mainly by the cytochrome P_{450} (CYP_{450}) superfamily. The cytochrome P_{450} enzyme family is located in the smooth endoplasmic reticulum. When the cells are homogenized, these cell organs form vesicles known as microsomes, thus the nomenclature *microsomal enzyme* garniture. Microsomal CYP_{450} enzymes are monooxigenases that account for approx. 70-80% of Phase I metabolic reactions in animals and can be divided into CYP_{450} families and subfamilies. In humans, 18 families are distinguished. There are great differences in activity of the distinct CYP_{450} families in animals and humans. In humans, the largest and widely investigated enzymes belong to the CYP3A1 family. In laboratory animals CYP2E1, CYP1A2 have the highest activity, but CYP4A, CYP2D and CYP3A subfamilies also play important role in metabolic processes (Guengerich, 1997, Fink-Gremmels, 2008). In dogs, CYP1A2 is expressed the most, while CYP2B11 is unique to dogs and account for approx. 20% of CYP_{450} metabolic activity in this species. In chickens, CYP2H1 and CYP3A37 have the highest activity. Not only the presence of certain enzymes but also their activity show great differences between animals. For instance, the highest overall CYP_{450} activity was measured in rabbits (1.77 nmol/mg protein), the lowest in chickens (0.25 nmol/mg protein) (Nebbia et al., 2003, Fink-Gremmels, 2008).

In addition to microsomal CYP_{450} monooxigenases, several enzymes play role in the biotransformation of drugs in animals. Alcohol and aldehyde dehydrogenases, monoamino oxidase (MAO) and enzymes responsible for conjugation in Phase II are also participate in drug metabolism.

Phase II - or synthetising phase - results in conjugation of the molecule with a polar substance, primarily glucuronic acid (glucuronidation), acetic acid (acetylation), less frequently sulphate, glutathion or glycine. This process results in a water soluble, almost exclusively inactive metabolite that can be excreted. In comparative veterinary pharmacokinetic differences in metabolic processes mainly affect Phase II reactions and are discussed in details in the next Chapter.

The primary organ of metabolism is the liver, but several organs have metabolic activity. It is reported in cats (and humans) that propofol is extensively metabolized in the lungs next to the liver making it relatively safe also in patients with hepatic failure (Matot et al., 1993, Dawidowicz et al., 2000). The intestinal tract also has metabolic activity, as several drugs are transformed into active or inactive forms in the intestinal wall. For instance, pivampicillin is hydrolysed to active ampicillin, or cefuroxime-axetil is converted to active cefuroxim. The kidney has also large metabolic capacities. Vitamin D for instance achieves activity in the proximal tubules where it is converted to active dihydroxy-cholecalciferol. Cyclosporin, an immunsuppressive agent is metabolized by renal cytochrome P_{450} enzymes and also causes enzyme induction (Nakamura et al., 1994).

5.1 Comparative veterinary aspects of metabolism

Several domestic animal species show defects in certain metabolic reactions. Phase I reactions show relative similarity among domestic animal species, the clinical relevance of these, usually only quantitative distinctions is not known. Defects in Phase II conjugation reactions, however, result in the clinically most relevant consequences. The most important metabolic pathway is glucuronidation which is present at low levels in cats rendering this species highly sensitive to several substances.

In *cats* glucuronide conjugation is very slow as this species has a low activity of the enzyme glucuronyl transferase. This metabolic defect is known for long to be responsible for the high sensitivity of cats to several drugs (Weisburger et al., 1964). Feline species are one of the most endangered species from a toxicological aspect, drugs potentially toxic to cats include paracetamol (acetaminophen), most of the NSAIDs, especially salicylates, morphine or phenobarbital. Paracetamol toxicosis is a frequently fatal, common household and malicious poisoning in cats. Paracetamol is primarily metabolised by glucuronidation or sulphate conjugation, and in less amount by microsomal enzymes into reactive intermediers, mainly N-acetyl-p-benzoquinine-imine (NAPQI) (Figure 2). In cats however, in the absence of glucuronic acid conjugation, NAPQI is accumulated (Figure 3) and causes methemoglobinaemia, liver necrosis leading to death.

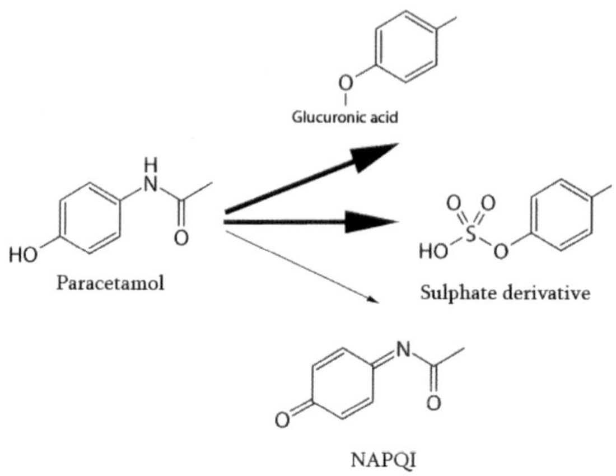

Fig. 2. Paracetamol metabolism in humans and animal species excluding the cat

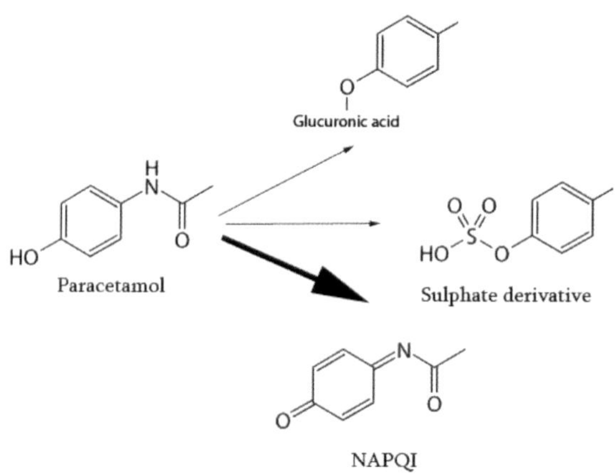

Fig. 3. Paracetamol metabolism in cats

Non-steroidal antiinflammatory drugs like aspirin, ibuprofen, naproxen, diclofenac, phenylbutazone or piroxicam are also conjugated with glucuronic acid in most of the mammalian species. Slow glucuronidation in cats results in long elimination half-lives and consequent gastroduodenal ulcers and renal damage associated with NSAIDs. Diazepam and its several metabolites are also conjugated to glucuronic acid in the liver. Half-lives of diazepam are 2.5-3.2 h and 5.5 h in dogs and cats, and half-lives of nordiazepam (the primary metabolite of diazepam) is 3 h and 21.3 h in dogs and cats, respectively, indicating significant differences between the two species (Plumb, 2005).

In *dogs*, Phase II acetylation reactions are absent, but this has much less importance in veterinary medicine compared to the deficiencies in the cat. These reactions occur when conjugating aromatic amino groups (Williams, 1967), for instance in case of most sulfonamides (Figure 4.). This defect in dogs has an advantage however, as acetylated sulfonamides are less water soluble than the parent compounds and are precipitated in kidney tubules causing renal damage in humans and several animal species. In dogs, however, this side effect is less frequent according to the lack of acetylated metabolites.

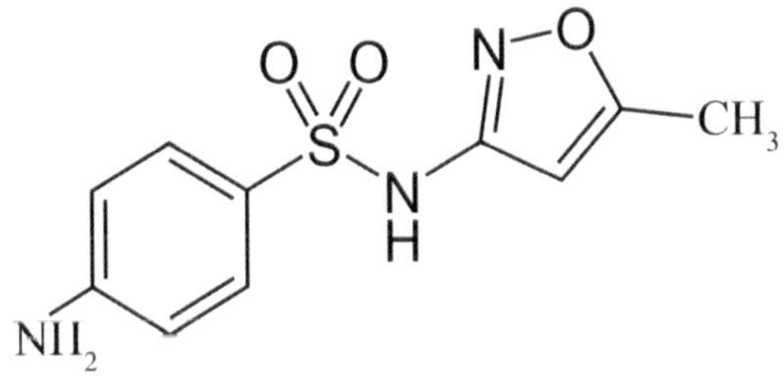

Fig. 4. Sulfametoxazole, an antibacterial agent with an aromatic amino group

In *pigs*, sulphate conjugation is present only in a low extent, but as this pathway is primarily an alternative to glucuronidation, the latter mechanism overcomes this deficiency, resulting in no known clinical importance in the veterinary practice.

5.2 Induction and inhibition of enzymes involved in metabolism

Enzyme induction and enzyme inhibiton are the most important factors affecting drug metabolism. Additional factors include decrease in plasma protein binding or decrease in hepatic blood flow.

Enzyme induction in humans has been experienced for instance in case phenobarbital, phenytoin or rifampin. In animals, inducive capabilities are different. In rats, for instance phenobarbital has much lower while rifampin has negligible effect on CYP3A enzymes (Lu et al, 2001). The most thoroughly studied inducer of CYP_{450} enzymes is phenobarbital, a frequently applied antiepileptic sedative in dogs and cats. In humans it is a potent inducer of CYP3A4, CYP2B6 and CYP2C19. As this medication is given long term (usually lifelong) to veterinary patients, the phenomenon has significant clinical consequences. Phenobarbital accelerates metabolism and thus decreases duration of action of drugs given in conjunction with the barbiturate and metabolised on inducible CYP_{450} enzymes. Examples include amitriptyline, benzodiazepines, phenothiazines, tramadol or fentanyl. As phenobarbital also induces CYP2C19, the enzyme responsible for its own metabolism, the half-life of phenobarbital is subsequently decreased. Therefore, in animals receiving phenobarbital, plasma phenobarbital levels should regularly be checked and dosage adjusted to attain therapeutic levels. Phenytoin is another antiepileptic, that has pronounced enzyme inducer activity. Clinically it is useless in dogs, as it is a strong inducer of microsomal enzymes and therapeutic concentrations can only be achieved in the first days of treatment, after that autoinduction decreases plasma levels rapidly (Frey et al., 1980).

Enzyme inhibition is peculiar to several drugs, like cimetidine, omeprazole, macrolide antibiotics (erythromycin, clarithromycin), ketoconazole, certain fluoroquinolones or chloramphenicol. Omeprazole and lansoprazole are known inhibitors of the human CYP1A subfamily, while pantoprazole has the lowest inhibitory action among the proton pump inhibitors (Masubuchi et al., 1997). These drugs increase half-life of numerous drugs leading to potential side effects. Erythromycin and clarithromycin increases risk of toxicity in case of terfenadine or theophylline. Azithromycin seems to have little potential of CYP_{450} induction. Cimetidine and some fluoroquinolones also increase theophyllin plasma levels by inhibiting CYP1A2 in dogs (Fink-Gremmels, 2008). Ketoconazole increases midazolam plasma levels by interacting with CYP3A4 (Kuroha et al., 2002). One of the most significant metabolic interaction is observed in case of macrolides or pleuromutilins and the ionophore antibiotics. Namely, administration of erythromycin, tiamulin and valnemulin concomittantly with anticoccidial ionophores (monensin, salinomycin, narasin) causes significant increase in mortality, mainly because of decreased elimination of the latter substances. The most frequently investigated interaction is between monensin and tiamulin. According to these data it can be pronounced that tiamulin inhibits biotransformation of monensin on CYP3A subfamily, and very low margin of safety associated with monensin can increase mortality (Nebbia et al.,1999, Szucs et al., 2004).

6. Drug excretion

In the course of metabolism the primary purpose of biotransformation is to increase water solubility of drugs making them capable of elimination. Certain drugs are polar and hydrophilic enough to be excreted unchanged. Examples include the penicillins or the aminoglycosides, that are excreted with the urine in an active form. In point of fact elimination consists of metabolism and excretion, but polar drugs are eliminated mainly by excretion only. Excretion of xenobiotics follows usually first order kinetics, a certain ratio of a drug is eliminated in a certain amount of time. In some cases however, elimination follows zero order kinetics, and only a certain amount of drug is eliminated in a certain amount of time. This happens, when the excretion mechanisms become saturated, for instance in severe renal insufficiency.

Renal excretion is the most important route of elimination. Polar, hydrophilic drugs can be eliminated via the urine and this includes several unchanged (not metabolised) substances. In case of antibiotics it is of great importance, whether the drug is excreted in an active or inactive form when treating urinary tract infections. Antibacterial agents, like penicillins, most of the cephalosporins and aminoglycosides are practically not metabolised, short acting tetracyclines and fluoroquinolones are metabolized in a low extent, but eliminated mainly with the urine. All of the before mentioned substances are effective in the treatment of urinary tract infections, but certainly pharmacodynamic considerations must also be considered. Renal excretion involves passive glomerular filtration and active tubular secretion, mainly in the proximal tubule. The latter requires energy and carrier molecules („organic anion transporters"), and the process can be saturated. As active secretion plays an important role in the excretion of several substances, like most of the beta lactams, inhibiting the process significantly reduces elimination, thus increases half-life of these medicines. Probenecid, a substance inhibiting these carrier mediated transport mechanisms played an important role in prolonging the effect of penicillin (Kampmann et al., 1972).

Probenecid is still used concurrently with several medicines (carbapenems, antiviral agents) to increase their half-life.

Glomerular filtration is a passive process and is significantly hindered by extensive (>80%) plasma protein binding. For instance, cefovecin, a third generation veterinary cephalosporin has over 95% protein binding in dogs and cats, therefore half-lives in these species are very long, 133 h and 166 h, respectively.

Reabsorption in the distal tubule plays an important role in prolonging half-life of drugs. Nonionized, lipophilic substances can diffuse passively from the tubular fluid back to plasma. As several drugs are weak acids or bases, pH of the urine has top priority when predicting tubular reabsorption of these substances. Acidification of the urine increases ionization of weak alkaline substances, while alkalinization increases ionization of weak acids, and these polar molecules are ion trapped in the tubular fluid. This fact helps to govern the elimination of some potentially toxic substances via urine. Excretion of alkaloids, like atropine or caffeine can be enhanced by urine acidifiers. Elimination of acidic substances, like most of the NSAIDs or the barbiturates can be accelerated by alkalizing the urine.

Biliary excretion of xenobiotics is less decisive, than renal excretion and mainly depends on molecular weight. Molecules larger than 500D are usually excreted with the bile in all animal species and humans. Dogs, rats and chickens are „better" biliary eliminators, in these animal species smaller (300-400D) molecules are also excreted via this route. The nature of the xenobiotic largely influences the route of excretion. Certain drugs, like erythromycin, lincomycin, clindamycin, chloramphenicol, ketoconazole, griseofulvin or the methylxanthines are primarily excreted with the bile. Conjugated forms of these substances can be deconjugated in the small intestine by bacterial β-glucuronidase enzymes and can be reabsorbed. This enterohepatic circulation (Figure 5.) can significantly increase half-life of certain drugs, like the xanthine derivatives. Thus, administration of activated charcoal in theophylline or theobromine (chocolate) toxicosis in dogs and cats is highly effective in reducing half-life by binding to intestinal portions of the substance and hindering its reabsorption.

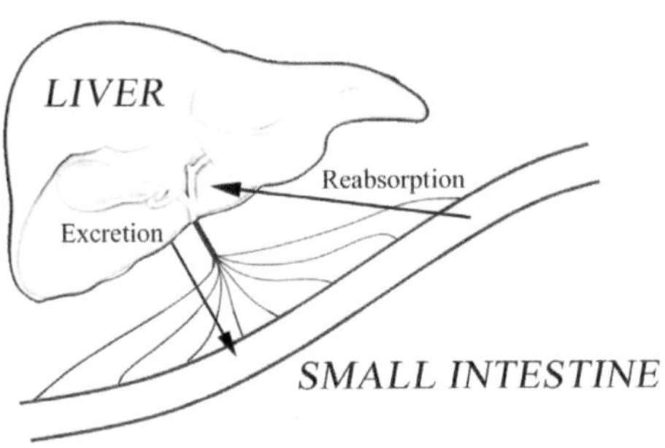

Fig. 5. Enterohepatic circulation of drugs

Elimination via milk and *eggs* is also important in the veterinary medicine. Several lipophilic drugs are excreted partly with the milk. As an example, 3.8% and 6.8% of the dosage of erythromycin and spiramycin, two lipophilic macrolide antibiotics is excreted via the milk, respectively (Giguere et al., 2006). Penethamat can also attain high concentrations in the milk after intramuscular administration. Relatively high drug concentrations in the milk necessitate caution when determining and observing withdrawal time for these substances. Elimination via the eggs is of high practical importance in laying hens. For instance, several anticoccidials, like robenidine must not be applied to egg producing animals, as drug reaches high concentrations and gives an unpleasant taste to the egg.

6.1 Half-life of drugs

Elimination half-life ($t_{1/2}$) is the time when plasma levels of the drug decline to half and is an essential parameter when comparing elimination of drugs between species. The half-life is usually independent from the dosage, as elimination generally follows first order kinetics, and a certain ratio is eliminated from the body in a certain amount of time. As the dosage is increased and excretion capacity becomes saturated, the elimination will show zero order kinetics, and half-lives will be significantly longer. An example for this is acetyl-salycilic acid (aspirin) in cats. Because of this phenomenon, aspirin is usually administered with 48-72 hour intervals to cats if less toxic drugs are not available or not appropriate for the disease condition. As half-life of drugs show pronounced differences, it is crucial in determining dosage and dosing interval and to predict toxic effects in animals. Theobromine for instance that has approx. 7 hours half-life in humans is very slowly eliminated in dogs and cats (dog $t_{1/2}$ is 17.5 h), and frequently causes posioning when chocolate is given to these species. Sulfonamides and trimethoprim are good examples to demonstrate differences in half-lives among species. Trimethoprim for instance has 1.25 h half-life in cattle, 3.2 h in horses, 4.6 h in dogs and 10.6 h in humans. Its partner sulfamethoxasole has 2.3 h half-life in cattle, 4.8 h in horses and 10.1 h in humans. Differences in these parameters necessitate the adaptation in drug dosing in the different species. Similar half-life of sulfonamides and trimethoprim in humans makes it an excellent combination pharmacodynamically and pharmacokinetically. In animals, however, half-life of the sulfonamides and trimethoprim is infrequently similar, thus efficacy of the combination is less pronounced and needs correction in the ratio of the substances in veterinary products. An other important group with pregnant differences are the NSAIDs. Aspirin for instance has 7.5 h elimination half-life in dogs and 37.6 h in cats. This necessitates the prolongation of the dosage interval in cats, as described above. In conclusion it can be stated that half-life of drugs is essential when determining dosage and dosage intervals in each animal species, and prolonged half-lives of certain drugs play a crucial part in evoking toxicoses in animals, especially in those with defects in elimination, like cats.

7. Acknowledgement

I would like to express my gratitude to Dr. József Lehel and Dr. Melinda Donka-Jerzsele for the thorough and critical supervision of this chapter.

8. References

Aderounmu, AF, Fleckenstein, L. (1983). Pharmacokinetics of chloroquine diphosphate in the dog. *Journal of Pharmacology and Experimental Therapeutics*. 226. pp. 633-9.

Agerso, H, Friis, C. (1998). Bioavailability of amoxycillin in pigs. *Journal of Veterinary Pharmacology and Therapeutics.* 21. pp. 41-46.

Anfossi, P. et al. (2002). Relative oral bioavailability of microgranulated amoxicillin in pigs. *Journal of Veterinary Pharmacology and Therapeutics.* 25. pp. 329-334.

Arancibia, A. et al. (1988). Dose-dependent bioavailability of amoxycillin. *Journal Of Clinical Pharmacology Therapy And Toxicology.* 26. pp. 300-303

Baggot, JD. et al. (1988). Clinical pharmacokinetics of metronidazole in horses. *Journal of Veterinary Pharmacology and Therapeutics.* 11. pp. 417-420.

Brown, SA. et al. (1991) Ceftiofur sodium: disposition, protein-binding, metabolism, and residue profile in various species. *Acta Veterinaria Scandinavica.* 87 (suppl). pp. 97–99.

Cagnardi, P. et al. (2010). Cefoperazone sodium preparation behavior after intramammary administration in healthy and infected cows. *Journal of Dairy Science.* 93. pp. 4105-4110.

Capece, BPS. et al. (2001). Effect of ruminal microflora on the biotransformation of netobimin, albendazole, albendazole sulfoxide, and albendazole sulfoxide enantiomers in an artificial rumen. *Journal of Animal Science.* 79. 1288-1294.

Carretero, C. et al. (2002). Pharmacokinetics of marbofloxacin in mature horses after single intravenous and intramuscular administration. *Equine Veterinary Journal.* 34. pp. 360-365.

Cox, SR. et al. (2010). The pharmacokinetics of mavacoxib, a long-acting COX-2 inhibitor, in young adult laboratory dogs. *Journal of Veterinary Pharmacology and Therapeutics.* 33. pp. 461-70.

Costa, LG. (2006). Current issues in organophosphate toxicology. *Clinica Chimica Acta.* 366. pp. 1–13.

Davis, JL. et al. (2002). Pharmacokinetics of azithromycin in foals after i.v. and oral dose and disposition into phagocytes. *Journal of Veterinary Pharmacology and Therapeutics.* 25. pp. 99-104.

Dawidowicz, A. et al. (2000). The Role of Human Lungs in the Biotransformation of Propofol. *Anesthesiology.* 93. pp. 992-997.

De Boever, S. et al. (2005). Pharmacokinetics and oral bioavailability of pentoxyfylline in broiler chickens. *Journal of Veterinary Pharmacology and Therapeutics.* 28. pp. 575-580.

Duffee, NE. et al. (1997). The pharmacokineitics of cefadroxil over a range of oral doses and animal ages in the foal. *Journal of Veterinary Pharmacology and Therapeutics.* 20. pp. 427-433.

Ehinger, AM. et al. Tissue distribution of cefquinome after intramammary and "systemic" administration in the isolated perfused bovine udder. 2006. *The Veterinary Journal.* 172. 1. pp. 147-153.

El-Sooud, KA. et al. (2004). Comparative pharmacokinetics and bioavailability of amoxycillin in chickens after intravenous, intramuscular and oral administrations. *Veterinary Research Communications.* 28. pp. 599-607.

Ensink, JM. et al. (1996). Bioavailability of pivampicillin and ampicillin trihydrate administered as an oral paste in horses. *Veterinary Quarterly.* 18. pp. 117-20.

Ensink, JM. et al. (1992). Bioavailability of oral penicillins in the horse: a comparison of pivampicillin and amoxicillin. *Journal of Veterinary Pharmacology and Therapeutics.* 15. pp. 221-230.

Fink-Gremmels, J. (2008). Implications of hepatic cytochrome P_{450}-related biotransformation processes in veterinary sciences. *European Journal of Pharmacology. 585. pp. 502-509.*

Frey, HH, Löscher, W. (1980). Clinical pharmacokinetics of phenytoin in the dog: a reevaluation. *American Journal of Veterinary Research.* 41. pp. 1635-1638.

Gemer, O. et al. (1983). Absorption of orally administered gentamicin in infants with diarrhea. *Pediatric Pharmacology.* 3. pp. 119-123.

Geyer, J. et al. (2009). Brain penetration of ivermectin and selamectin in mdr1a,b P-glycoprotein- and bcrp- deficient knockout mice. *Journal of Veterinary Pharmacology and Therapeutics.* 32. pp. 87-96.

Giguere, S. et al. (2006). *Antimicrobial therapy in veterinary medicine.* 4th Edition. Blackwell Publishing. Ames, Iowa.

Gokbulut, C. et al. (2006). Plasma disposition and faecal excretion of netobimin metabolites and enantiospecific disposition of albendazole sulphoxide produced in ewes. *Veterinary Research Communications.* 30. 791-805.

Guengerich, FP. (1997). Role of cytochrome P_{450} enzymes in drug–drug interactions, *Advances in Pharmacology.* 43. pp. 7–35.

Hustace, JL. et al. (2009). Pharmacokinetics and bioavailability of metformin in horses. *American Journal of Veterinary Research.* 70. pp. 665-668.

Jerzsele, A. et al. (2011). Oral bioavailability and pharmacokinetic profile of the amoxicillin-clavulanic acid combination after intravenous and oral administration in turkeys. *Journal of Veterinary Pharmacology and Therapeutics.* 34. pp. 202-205.

Jerzsele, A. et al. (2009). Oral bioavailability and pharmacokinetic profile of the amoxicillin-clavulanic acid combination after intravenous and oral administration in broiler chickens. *Journal of Veterinary Pharmacology and Therapeutics.* 32. pp. 506-509.

Jerzsele, A., Semjén, G. (2006). The usage of the amoxicillin-clavulanic acid combination in the veterinary practice. Magyar Állatorvosok Lapja. 7. pp. 419-426.

Kampmann, J. et al. (1972). Effect of some drugs on penicillin half-life in blood. *Clinical Pharmacology and Therapeutics.* 13. pp. 516-519.

Kappers, WA. (2001). Diazinon is activated by CYP2C19 in human liver, *Toxicology and Applied Pharmacology.* 177. pp. 68–76.

Kaukinen, H. et al. (2010). Bioavailability of detomidine administered sublingually to horses as an oromucosal gel. *Journal of Veterinary Pharmacology and Therapeutics.* 34. pp. 76–81.

Kietzmann, M. et al. (2010). Tissue distribution of cloxacillin after intramammary administration in the isolated perfused bovine udder. *BMC Veterinary Research.* 6. 46.

Kluge, K, Ungemach, FR. (1999). Investigation of ampicillin plasma concentration after oral application in dogs. Are recommended dosages sufficient? *Tierarztliche Praxis Ausgabe Kleintiere Heimtiere.* 27. pp. 150-154.

Kung, K. et al. (1993). Pharmacokinetics of enrofloxacin and its metabolite ciprofloxacin after intravenous and oral administration of enrofloxacin in dogs, *Journal of Veterinary Pharmacology and Therapeutics.* 16. pp. 462–468

Kung, K., Wanner, M. (1994). Bioavailability of different forms of amoxycillin administered orally to dogs. *The Veterinary Record.* 135. pp. 552-554.

Kung, K. et al. (1995). Effect of the interval between feeding and drug administration on oral ampicillin absorption in dogs. *Journal Of Small Animal Practice.* 36. pp. 65-68.

Kuroha, M. et al. (2002). Effect of multiple dosing of ketoconazole on pharmacokinetics of midazolam, a cytochrome P-450 3A substrate in beagle dogs. Drug Metabolism and Disposition. 30. pp. 63-68.

Le Traon, G., et al. (2009). Pharmacokinetics of cimetidine in dogs after oral administration of cimetidine tablets. *Journal Of Veterinary Pharmacology And Therapeutics*. 32. pp. 213-218.

Lu, C., A. Li. (2001). Species comparison in P450 induction: effects of dexamethasone,omeprazole, and rifampin on P450 isoforms 1A and 3A in primary cultured hepatocytes from man, Sprague-Dawley rat, minipig, and beagle dog. *Chemico-Biological Interactions*. 134. pp. 271-281.

Masubuchi, N., Okazaki, O. (1997). An evaluation of the CYP1A induction potential of pantoprazole in primary rat hepatocytes: a comparison with other proton pump inhibitors. *Chemico Biological Interactions*. 107. pp. 63-74.

Matot, I. et al. (1993). Pulmonary uptake of propofol in cats. Effect of fentanyl and halothan. *Anesthesiology*. 78. pp. 1157-1165.

Meyer, S, et al. (2009). Pharmacokinetics of intravenous ceftiofur sodium and concentration in body fluids of foals. *Journal Of Veterinary Pharmacology And Therapeutics*. 32. pp. 309-316.

Montesissa, C. et al. (1989). Comparative microsomal oxidation of febantel and its metabolite fenbendazole in various animal species. *Xenobiotica*. 19. 97-100.

Musulin, SE., et al. (2011). Diazepam pharmacokinetics after nasal drop and atomized nasal administration in dogs. *Journal of Veterinary Pharmacology and Therapeutics*. 34. pp. 17–24.

Nakamura, M. et al. (1994). Induction of cytochrome P-450 isozymes in rat renal microsomes by cyclosporin A. *Biochemical Pharmacology*. 48. 1743–1746.

Nebbia, C. et al. (1999). Oxidative metabolism of monensin in rat liver microsomes and interactions with tiamulin and other chemotherapeutic agents: evidence for the involvement of cytochrome P-450 3A subfamily. *Drug Metabolism and Disposition*. 27. pp. 1039-1044.

Nebbia, C. et al. (2003). Comparative expression of liver cytochrome P450-dependent monooxygenases in the horse and in other agricultural and laboratory species, *Veterinary Journal*. 165. pp. 53–64.

Owens, WE. et al. (1990). Determination of milk and mammary tissue concentrations of ceftiofur after intramammary and intramuscular therapy. *Journal of Dairy Science*. 73. pp. 3449-3456.

Perry, SM, et al. (1991). Effect of i.v. anaesthesia with propofol on drug distribution and metabolism in the dog. *British Journal of Anaesthesia*. 66. pp. 66-72.

Plumb, DC. (2005). *Plumb's Veterinary Drug Handbook*. 5th Edition. Blackwell Publishing. Ames, Iowa.

Reyns, T. et al. (2007). Disposition and oral bioavailability of amoxicillin and clavulanic acid in pigs. *Journal of Veterinary Pharmacology and Therapeutics*. 30. pp. 550-555.

Riviere, JE., Papich, MG. et al. (2009). *Veterinary Pharmacology and Therapeutics*. 9th Edition. Wiley-Blackwell Publishing. Ames, Iowa.

Roulet, A. et al. (2003). MDR1-deficient genotype in Collie dogs hypersensitive to the P-glycoprotein substrate ivermectin. *European Journal of Pharmacology*. 460, pp. 85-91.

Schinkel, AH. 1999. P-glycoprotein, a gatekeeper in the blood–brain barrier *Advanced Drug Delivery Reviews*. 36. pp. 179-194.

Soback, S. et al. (1995). Florfenicol pharmacokinetics in lactating cows after intravenous, intramuscular and intramammary administration. *Journal of Veterinary Pharmacology and Therapeutics*. 18. pp. 413-7.

Szucs, G. et al. (2004). Biochemical background of toxic interactions between tiamulin and monensin. *Chemico Biological Interactions*. 147. pp. 151-161.

Weisburger, JH. et al. (1964). The metabolism of N-2-fluorenylacetamide in the cat: Evidence for glucuronic acid conjugates. *Biochemical Pharmacology*. 13. pp. 469-475.

Williams, RT. (1967). Comparative patterns of drug metabolism. *Federation Proceedings*. 26. pp. 1029–1039.

Yamazaki, T. et al. (2008). The intracellular accumulation of phagocytic and epithelial cells and the inhibitory effect on Chlamydophila (Chlamydia) pneumoniae of telithromycin and comparator antimicrobials. *Journal Of Chemotherapy*. 20. pp. 428-430.

Section 2

Methods and Applications

10

Observer-Based Strategies for Anesthesia Drug Concentration Estimation

Jin-Oh Hahn[1], Guy A. Dumont[2] and J. Mark Ansermino[2]
[1]*University of Alberta,*
[2]*University of British Columbia*
Canada

1. Introduction

Knowledge of the anesthesia drug concentration in a patient during a surgical procedure has potential to improve patient monitoring and control of drug administration. High-fidelity estimates of anesthesia drug concentration would allow anesthesiologists to make relevant low-level dose adjustment as well as high-level clinical decisions. The estimated drug concentrations may also be useful for computerized anesthesia delivery, including, but not limited to, targeting/limiting the drug concentration itself (Van Poucke et al., 2004; Gentilini et al., 2002) as well as monitoring and maintaining hemodynamic stability (Rao et al., 2000).

Currently, anesthesia drug concentration is estimated based primarily on a model-based open-loop prediction (Fig. 1(a)), in which the drug concentration is predicted by solving a population-based patient pharmacokinetics (PK) and pharmacodynamics (PD) described in terms of a multi-compartmental model. In the absence of any feedback correction capability, the discrepancy between the real PK of an individual patient and its population-based model counterpart is a major source of errors in drug concentration estimation. The open-loop prediction has been widely used despite this apparent drawback, mainly due to the lack of alternative solutions.

Recently, efforts have been made to improve the fidelity of drug concentration estimation over open-loop prediction. Sartori et al. (2005) proposed a method based on an extended Kalman filter to adapt PD parameters in real-time. Hahn et al. (2011) proposed a robust estimation strategy based on H_∞ control theory. The results strongly suggest that the efficacy of drug concentration estimation can be improved by exploiting the measurements of the clinical effect. Motivated by these pioneering investigations, this chapter aims to study alternative observer design strategies for estimating anesthesia drug concentration. In contrast to open-loop prediction, observer-based approaches can be regarded as closed-loop estimation that exploits the clinical effect measurement for feedback correction (Fig. 1(b)), in order to suppress the adverse influence of patient variability and effectively deal with unknown surgical stimulation (shown as d in Fig. 1) that acts as a disturbance to distort the clinical effect measurement. The specific focus of this chapter is to examine the design and analysis of a robust linear observer (RLO), a robust nonlinear observer (RNO), and an H_∞ observer ($H_\infty O$) in the context of estimating propofol concentrations at the plasma and the effect sites. A depth of hypnosis index called WAV_{CNS} (Zikov et al., 2006) was used to describe the clinical effect of interest for feedback correction. The observers were evaluated against the traditional open-loop prediction using a Monte-Carlo simulation of surgical procedures using a wide range of patient models. $H_\infty O$ boasted the best overall performance with its capacity to deliver statistically significant reduction in plasma and effect site propofol concentration errors over open-loop prediction, regardless of the presence of a surgical stimulation disturbance. RNO was more effective than open-loop prediction in suppressing the effect site propofol concentration error, but its efficacy for plasma propofol concentration was susceptible to surgical stimulation disturbance. RLO was good at reducing the effect site propofol concentration error in the absence of surgical stimulation disturbance, but perfomed poorly in the presence of a surgical stimulation disturbance.

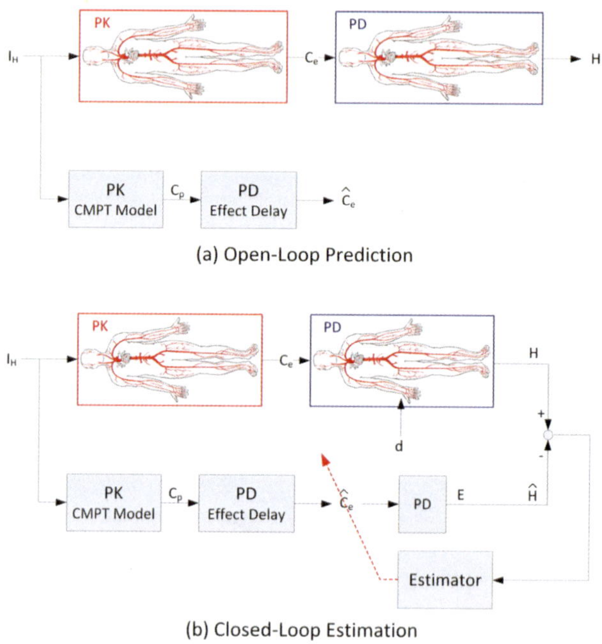

Fig. 1. Open-loop prediction versus closed-loop estimation of anesthesia drug concentration.

This chapter is organized as follows. Section II describes the patient model. Section III details the design of observers for anesthesia drug concentration estimation. Section IV details the Monte-Carlo simulation and statistical analysis to compare the performance of observer-based estimation and open-loop prediction strategies. The results are presented and discussed in Section V, followed by conclusions in Section VI.

2. Patient model

An anesthetized patient can be described by a series connection of a PK model, a PD model, and a monitor model, as shown in Fig. 2. The input to this process is the drug infusion rate (I_H), while the output is the clinical effect measurement (WAV_{CNS}). The surgical stimulation is modeled as an output disturbance, because it counteracts the effect of anesthesia drug in an unpredictable manner and thereby distorts the WAV_{CNS} measurement.

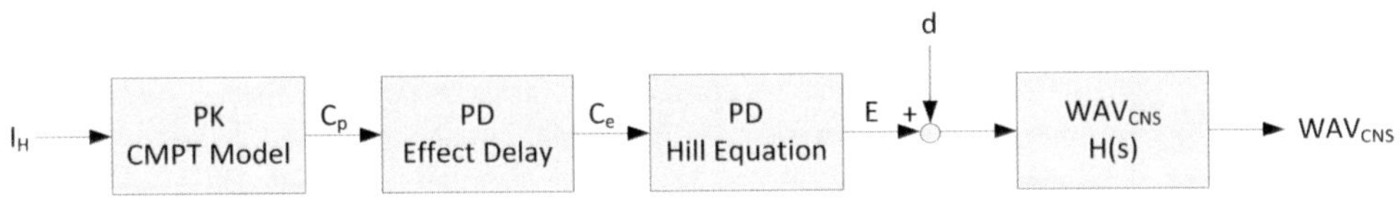

Fig. 2. PK/PD and effect monitor models of anesthesia drug delivery process.

2.1 PK and PD models

A 3-compartment model of propofol developed by Schüttler and Ihmsen (2000) was used to describe the PK (Fig. 3). Denoting x_1, x_2, and x_3 as drug concentrations in the plasma, fast peripheral, and slow peripheral compartments, the state-space representation of the PK is given by (1):

$$\dot{\mathbf{x}}_{PK} = \begin{bmatrix} -(k_{10}+k_{12}+k_{13}) & k_{12} & k_{13} \\ k_{21} & -k_{21} & 0 \\ k_{31} & 0 & -k_{31} \end{bmatrix} \mathbf{x}_{PK} + \begin{bmatrix} V_1^{-1} \\ 0 \\ 0 \end{bmatrix} u = \mathbf{A}_{PK}\mathbf{x}_{PK} + \mathbf{B}_{PK}u, \quad (1)$$
$$C_p = x_1 = \begin{bmatrix} 1 & 0 & 0 \end{bmatrix}\mathbf{x}_{PK} = \mathbf{C}_{PK}\mathbf{x}_{PK}$$

where $\mathbf{x}_{PK}=[x_1\ x_2\ x_3]^T$, $u=I_H$, k_{ij} are the rate constants, and V_1 is the volume of the plasma compartment. To account for the PD lag associated with the distribution of drug into the effect site (i.e. the brain), the following delay-plus-first-order model was used (Zikov et al., 2006):

$$x_4(s) = C_e(s) = e^{-T_d s}\frac{k_d}{s+k_d}C_p(s), \quad (2)$$

where T_d and k_d are respectively the transport delay and the rate of drug distribution from the plasma to the brain. Finally, the saturating Hill equation was used to describe the relation between C_e and the anesthesia effect:

$$E(\bar{C}_e) = \frac{[\bar{C}_e]^{\gamma}}{1+[\bar{C}_e]^{\gamma}}, \quad (3)$$

where $\bar{C}_e = \dfrac{C_e}{EC_{50}}$ is the effect site drug concentration normalized by the 50% effect concentration (EC_{50}), and γ is the cooperativity coefficient.

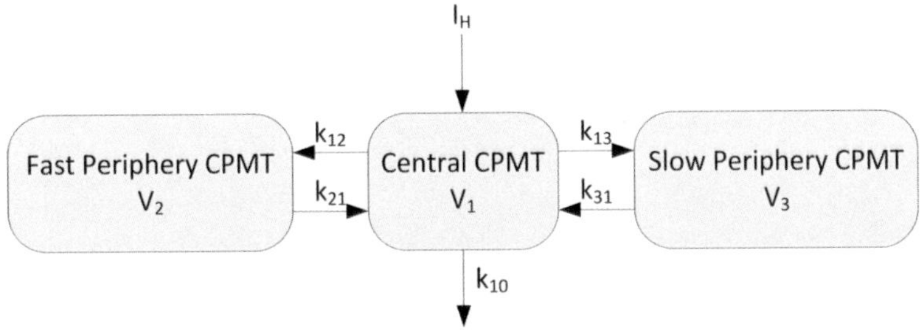

Fig. 3. A 3-compartmental PK model.

2.2 WAV_{CNS} monitor model

The WAV_{CNS} index reflects the combined effect of the anesthesia drug and the unknown surgical stimulation. It takes values ranging from 100 to 0, where WAV_{CNS}=100 corresponds to fully awake state, WAV_{CNS}=50 corresponds to adequate anesthesia, and WAV_{CNS}=0 corresponds to an isoelectric electroencephalogram (EEG). The WAV_{CNS} monitor model derived by Zikov et al. (Zikov et al., 2006) was used:

$$y(s) = WAV_{CNS}(s) = 100 \times \left\{ 1 - \frac{1}{(8s+1)^2}\left[E(s) + d(s) \right] \right\}, \tag{4}$$

where d is the unknown surgical stimulation. Note that maximum (=1) and minimum (=0) clinical effects correspond to WAV_{CNS}=0 and WAV_{CNS}=100, respectively.

2.3 Observer design model

The observer design model is obtained by locally linearizing the PD model in the neighborhood of the operating regime of E=0.5 during the maintenance phase of anesthesia, which yields

$$E(\bar{C}_e) = \frac{\gamma}{4}(\bar{C}_e - 1) + \frac{1}{2} = \frac{\gamma}{4EC_{50}}(C_e - EC_{50}) + \frac{1}{2}. \tag{5}$$

Combining (1), (2), (4), and (5) results in the following observer design model, where the state variables x_5 and x_6 are associated with the WAV_{CNS} monitor model (4):

$$\dot{\mathbf{x}} = \begin{bmatrix} \mathbf{A}_{PK} & 0 & 0 & 0 \\ k_d \;\; 0 \;\; 0 & -k_d & 0 & 0 \\ \mathbf{0}_{1\times3} & 0 & 0 & 1 \\ \mathbf{0}_{1\times3} & -256^{-1}\gamma EC_{50}^{-1} & -4^{-1} & -64^{-1} \end{bmatrix} \mathbf{x} + \begin{bmatrix} \mathbf{B}_{PK} & \mathbf{0}_{5\times1} \\ \mathbf{0}_{3\times1} & 64^{-1} \end{bmatrix} \begin{bmatrix} u(t-T_d) \\ d \end{bmatrix} = \mathbf{Ax} + \mathbf{B}u(t-T_d) + \mathbf{E}d \tag{6}$$
$$\mathbf{y} = \begin{bmatrix} 0 & 0 & 0 & 0 & 1 & 0 \end{bmatrix}\mathbf{x} = \mathbf{Cx}$$

3. Observer design

A patient undergoing anesthesia is subject to a significant amount of uncertainty arising from the inherent inter-patient physiologic variability and unknown surgical stimulation. The population-based PK and PD models have thus limited predictive accuracy (Schüttler & Ihmsen, 2000). Besides, the PK and PD model parameters may fluctuate in response to the individual patient's physiologic condition. Furthermore, the clinical effect measurement is persistently corrupted by unpredictable surgical stimulation. The observer must be designed to be robust against these multiple confounding factors.

3.1 Design strategies

The following alternatives were considered as observers for drug concentration estimation: 1) RLO: a linear observer with a robust feedback gain, 2) RNO: a nonlinear observer with a robust feedback and a nonlinear disturbance rejection gain, and 3) $H_\infty O$: a robust dynamic observer designed based on H_∞ control theory. The RLO was intended to explore the limit of performance of a simple linear observer. The RNO was motivated by the effort to separate the tasks of robustness and disturbance rejection: the linear feedback was designed to achieve robustness against PK/PD model uncertainty, whereas the nonlinear feedback was designed to compensate for the unknown surgical stimulation. The requirements of disturbance rejection and the observer matching condition necessitates the use of WAV_{CNS} and its derivative as measurements in the design of RNO. The purpose of the $H_\infty O$ was to examine if its added complexity is worth exploiting in order to improve the fidelity of drug concentration estimation.

3.2 Robust linear observer (RLO) design

A standard linear observer assumes the following form:

$$\dot{\hat{\mathbf{x}}} = \bar{\mathbf{A}}\hat{\mathbf{x}} + \bar{\mathbf{B}}u + \mathbf{L}(\mathbf{y} - \mathbf{C}\hat{\mathbf{x}}), \tag{7}$$

where the upper bar on a matrix denotes its nominal value. **L** is designed to satisfy the inequality (8) for a positive definite matrix **P** in order to place the closed-loop poles in the left-half plane:

$$(\bar{\mathbf{A}} - \mathbf{LC})^{\mathrm{T}}\mathbf{P} + \mathbf{P}(\bar{\mathbf{A}} - \mathbf{LC}) < \mathbf{0}. \tag{8}$$

Considering the patient model (6) and the observer (7), the propofol concentration estimates provided by the observer are susceptible to the model perturbations included in **E***d* that stem from the PK/PD uncertainty and unknown surgical stimulation. The observer gain matrix **L** must be designed so as to achieve robustness against these confounding factors. It is possible to determine **L** such that the state estimation error is bounded within a prescribed ellipsoid in the presence of model perturbations and/or disturbances by exploiting Theorem 1 below:

Theorem 1 (Set-Theoretic Robustness Condition) (Blanchini & Miani, 2008): Consider the system of the form

$$\dot{\mathbf{x}} = \mathbf{Ax} + \mathbf{Fw}$$

which is subject to a persistent external disturbance **w**. Assume that the disturbance is bounded by $\mathbf{w}^{\mathrm{T}}\mathbf{w} \leq 1$. Then the ellipsoid $\{\mathbf{x}: \mathbf{x}^{\mathrm{T}}\mathbf{P}\mathbf{x} \leq 1\}$ is invariant if $\mathbf{Q} = \mathbf{P}^{-1}$ satisfies the condition

$$\mathbf{QA} + \mathbf{A}^{\mathrm{T}}\mathbf{Q} + \alpha\mathbf{Q} + \frac{1}{\alpha}\mathbf{FF}^{\mathrm{T}} \leq \mathbf{0}$$

for some $\alpha > 0$.

Rewrite (6) as follows where the matrices **A** and **B** are decomposed into their nominal and uncertain parts:

$$\dot{\mathbf{x}} = \mathbf{Ax} + \mathbf{B}u + \mathbf{E}d = (\bar{\mathbf{A}} + \tilde{\mathbf{A}})\mathbf{x} + (\bar{\mathbf{B}} + \tilde{\mathbf{B}})u + \mathbf{E}d. \tag{9}$$

Subtracting (7) from (9) yields the following error dynamics:

$$\dot{\mathbf{e}} = \left(\bar{\mathbf{A}} - \mathbf{LC}\right)\mathbf{e} + \tilde{\mathbf{A}}\mathbf{x} + \tilde{\mathbf{B}}u + \mathbf{E}d = \left(\bar{\mathbf{A}} - \mathbf{LC}\right)\mathbf{e} + \mathbf{Fw}\,. \tag{10}$$

where **F** specifies the uncertainty bound and is chosen such that $\mathbf{w}^T\mathbf{w} \le 1$. Then according to Theorem 1 the state estimation error **e** is bounded within the ellipsoid $\{\mathbf{e}: \mathbf{e}^T\mathbf{P}\mathbf{e} \le 1\}$ if $\mathbf{Q}=\mathbf{P}^{-1}$ satisfies the following inequality for some $\alpha>0$:

$$\mathbf{Q}\left(\bar{\mathbf{A}} - \mathbf{LC}\right)^T + \left(\bar{\mathbf{A}} - \mathbf{LC}\right)\mathbf{Q} + \alpha\mathbf{Q} + \frac{1}{\alpha}\mathbf{F}\mathbf{F}^T \le \mathbf{0}\,. \tag{11}$$

Pre- and post-multiplying (11) by **P** results in (12):

$$\left(\bar{\mathbf{A}} - \mathbf{LC}\right)^T\mathbf{P} + \mathbf{P}\left(\bar{\mathbf{A}} - \mathbf{LC}\right) + \alpha\mathbf{P} + \frac{1}{\alpha}\mathbf{P}\mathbf{F}\mathbf{F}^T\mathbf{P} \le \mathbf{0}\,. \tag{12}$$

Noting that **P** and $\mathbf{PFF}^T\mathbf{P}$ in (12) are positive definite and positive semi-definite, respectively, the inequality (12) is stronger than (8) and the pair of matrices **L** and **P** satisfying (12) automatically satisfies (8). Also, the "size" of **P** is directly related to the size of the error ellipsoid within which the state estimation error is bounded. Therefore, the optimal observer gain **L** for (7) can be determined by finding the pair of matrices **L** and **P** which maximizes the size of **P** while satisfying the set-theoretic robustness condition (12).

The optimal RLO gain design problem can be cast into a linear matrix inequality (LMI) problem by manipulating (12) as follows. The inequality (12) implies that, for any $\mathbf{e}\neq 0$,

$$\mathbf{e}^T\left[\left(\bar{\mathbf{A}} + \frac{1}{2}\alpha\mathbf{I} - \mathbf{LC}\right)^T\mathbf{P} + \mathbf{P}\left(\bar{\mathbf{A}} + \frac{1}{2}\alpha\mathbf{I} - \mathbf{LC}\right)\right]\mathbf{e} + \frac{1}{\alpha}\mathbf{e}^T\mathbf{P}\mathbf{F}\mathbf{F}^T\mathbf{P}\mathbf{e} \le \mathbf{0}\,. \tag{13}$$

Define $\mathbf{Y}=\mathbf{PL}$. Using

$$-\alpha\mathbf{w}^T\mathbf{w} + 2\mathbf{e}^T\mathbf{PFw} = -\alpha\mathbf{w}^T\mathbf{w} + 2\mathbf{e}^T\mathbf{PFw} - \frac{1}{\alpha}\mathbf{e}^T\mathbf{PFF}^T\mathbf{Pe} + \frac{1}{\alpha}\mathbf{e}^T\mathbf{PFF}^T\mathbf{Pe} \le \frac{1}{\alpha}\mathbf{e}^T\mathbf{PFF}^T\mathbf{Pe}\,, \tag{14}$$

the inequality (13) can be converted to the following LMI:

$$\begin{bmatrix} \left(\bar{\mathbf{A}} + \frac{1}{2}\alpha\mathbf{I}\right)^T\mathbf{P} + \mathbf{P}\left(\bar{\mathbf{A}} + \frac{1}{2}\alpha\mathbf{I}\right) - \mathbf{C}^T\mathbf{Y} - \mathbf{YC} & \mathbf{PF} \\ \mathbf{F}^T\mathbf{P} & -\alpha\mathbf{I} \end{bmatrix} \le \mathbf{0}\,. \tag{15}$$

Summarizing, the optimal RLO gain design is equivalent to solving the following LMI:

$$\max tr[\mathbf{P}] \text{ subject to } \begin{bmatrix} \left(\bar{\mathbf{A}} + \frac{1}{2}\alpha\mathbf{I}\right)^T\mathbf{P} + \mathbf{P}\left(\bar{\mathbf{A}} + \frac{1}{2}\alpha\mathbf{I}\right) - \mathbf{C}^T\mathbf{Y} - \mathbf{YC} & \mathbf{PF} \\ \mathbf{F}^T\mathbf{P} & -\alpha\mathbf{I} \end{bmatrix} \le \mathbf{0}\,, \tag{16}$$

where the size of **P** is measured in terms of its trace norm, which is equal to the sum of its eigenvalues.

3.3 Robust nonlinear observer (RNO) design

The RNO to be designed in this chapter assumes the following form:

$$\dot{\hat{\mathbf{x}}} = \bar{\mathbf{A}}\hat{\mathbf{x}} + \bar{\mathbf{B}}u + \mathbf{L}(\mathbf{y} - \mathbf{C}\hat{\mathbf{x}}) + \boldsymbol{\eta}, \quad (17)$$

where **L** is the linear feedback designed to suppress the adverse effect of the PK/PD uncertainty, and $\boldsymbol{\eta}$ is the nonlinear feedback to compensate for the unknown surgical stimulation. The error dynamics is derived by subtracting (17) from (9):

$$\dot{\mathbf{e}} = (\bar{\mathbf{A}} - \mathbf{LC})\mathbf{e} + \tilde{\mathbf{A}}\mathbf{x} + \tilde{\mathbf{B}}u + \mathbf{E}d = (\bar{\mathbf{A}} - \mathbf{LC})\mathbf{e} + \mathbf{Gw} + \mathbf{E}d - \boldsymbol{\eta}, \quad (18)$$

where **G** specifies the uncertainty bound and is chosen such that $\mathbf{w}^T\mathbf{w} \leq 1$. Note that

$$\mathbf{Fw} = \mathbf{Gw} + \mathbf{E}d, \quad (19)$$

which suggests that within the RNO framework the PK/PD uncertainty **Gw** is taken care of by **L**, whereas the surgical stimulation is accounted for by $\boldsymbol{\eta}$, in contrast to the RLO where both of these confounding factors **Fw=Gw+Ed** must be dealt with by **L**.

To exploit $\boldsymbol{\eta}$ to cancel out the effect of d, it is required that the following observer matching condition be satisfied for some function **h**(**x**,u):

$$\mathbf{E}d = \mathbf{P}^{-1}\mathbf{C}^T\mathbf{h}(\mathbf{x},u), \quad (20)$$

where **P** satisfies (8). Note that (20) cannot be satisfied by the output matrix **C** in (6); it violates the positive definite requirement on **P** by imposing $p_{66}=0$. In order to resolve this problem, we assume that WAV_{CNS} and its time derivative are available as sensor measurements:

$$\mathbf{y} = [\mathbf{0}_{4\times4} \quad \mathbf{I}_{2\times2}]\mathbf{x} = \mathbf{Dx}. \quad (21)$$

With this choice of the output, the following constraints are imposed on **P**:

$$p_{16} = p_{26} = p_{36} = p_{46} = 0, \; p_{56}d = 64h_1(\mathbf{x},u), \; p_{66}d = 64h_2(\mathbf{x},u). \quad (22)$$

Then the linear feedback gain **L** of the RNO can be designed by solving the LMI (16) with **F** substituted by **G**, subject to (22). Once a feasible **L** and **P** are obtained from the LMI, the function **h**(**x**,u) is directly obtained from (22).

Assuming that the linear feedback gain **L** and the positive matrix **P** are designed to satisfy (16) with **F** substituted by **G** and the observer matching condition (20), the nonlinear feedback $\boldsymbol{\eta}$ with ρ satisfying $\rho > \|\mathbf{h}(\mathbf{x},u)\|$ guarantees the boundedness of the observer error **e**:

$$\boldsymbol{\eta} = \rho \frac{\mathbf{P}^{-1}\mathbf{D}^T\mathbf{De}}{\|\mathbf{De}\|}, \quad (23)$$

which can be shown by considerng the Lyapunov function $V(\mathbf{e})=\mathbf{e}^T\mathbf{Pe}$. Using the error dynamics (18), the time derivative of V(**e**) becomes:

$$\begin{aligned}\dot{V}(\mathbf{e}) &= \dot{\mathbf{e}}^{\mathrm{T}}\mathbf{P}\mathbf{e} + \mathbf{e}^{\mathrm{T}}\mathbf{P}\dot{\mathbf{e}} \\ &= \mathbf{e}^{\mathrm{T}}\left[\left(\bar{\mathbf{A}}-\mathbf{L}\mathbf{D}\right)^{\mathrm{T}}\mathbf{P} + \mathbf{P}\left(\bar{\mathbf{A}}-\mathbf{L}\mathbf{D}\right)\right]\mathbf{e} + 2\mathbf{e}^{\mathrm{T}}\mathbf{P}\mathbf{G}\mathbf{w} + 2\mathbf{e}^{\mathrm{T}}\mathbf{P}\mathbf{E}d - 2\mathbf{e}^{\mathrm{T}}\mathbf{P}\boldsymbol{\eta} \\ &\le -\alpha\mathbf{e}^{\mathrm{T}}\mathbf{P}\mathbf{e} - \frac{1}{\alpha}\mathbf{e}^{\mathrm{T}}\mathbf{P}\mathbf{G}\mathbf{G}^{\mathrm{T}}\mathbf{P}\mathbf{e} + 2\mathbf{e}^{\mathrm{T}}\mathbf{P}\mathbf{G}\mathbf{w} + 2\mathbf{e}^{\mathrm{T}}\mathbf{P}\mathbf{E}d - 2\mathbf{e}^{\mathrm{T}}\mathbf{P}\boldsymbol{\eta} \\ &\le \underbrace{-\alpha\left(\mathbf{e}^{\mathrm{T}}\mathbf{P}\mathbf{e} - \mathbf{w}^{\mathrm{T}}\mathbf{w}\right)}_{(a)} + \underbrace{2\left\|\mathbf{D}\mathbf{e}\right\|\left(\left\|\mathbf{h}(\mathbf{x},u)\right\| - \rho\right)}_{(b)}\end{aligned} \tag{24}$$

Note that 1) the term (a) is strictly negative whenever **e** is outside of the ellipsoid defined by {**e**: $\mathbf{e}^{\mathrm{T}}\mathbf{P}\mathbf{e}\le 1$}, and 2) the term (b) is always strictly negative. Thus, the time derivative of V(**e**) is strictly negative if $\mathbf{e}^{\mathrm{T}}\mathbf{P}\mathbf{e}\le 1$ is violated. Therefore, the observer error is guaranteed to converge to and be bounded within the ellipsoid {**e**: $\mathbf{e}^{\mathrm{T}}\mathbf{P}\mathbf{e}\le 1$}.

3.4 H$_\infty$ observer (H$_\infty$O) design

The H$_\infty$O was designed as described in Hahn et al. (2011) and the detailed discussion on its design is therefore omitted here. Briefly, the H$_\infty$O assumes the same form as the RLO (6). However, in contrast to the RLO whose observer gain **L** is a constant matrix, the observer gain **L** of the H$_\infty$O is a transfer matrix: **L**=**L**(s), where s is the Laplace variable. Therefore, the state estimation is given by:

$$\dot{\hat{\mathbf{x}}} = \bar{\mathbf{A}}\hat{\mathbf{x}} + \bar{\mathbf{B}}u + \boldsymbol{\upsilon}\,, \tag{25}$$

where the feedback $\boldsymbol{\upsilon}$ is the output of a dynamic system with the clinical effect estimation error as its excitation signal:

$$\dot{\boldsymbol{\xi}} = \mathbf{A}_{\xi}\boldsymbol{\xi} + \mathbf{B}_{\xi}\left(y - \mathbf{C}\hat{\mathbf{x}}\right),\ \ \boldsymbol{\upsilon} = \mathbf{C}_{\xi}\boldsymbol{\xi} + \mathbf{D}_{\xi}\left(y - \mathbf{C}\hat{\mathbf{x}}\right). \tag{26}$$

The transfer matrix between $\boldsymbol{\upsilon}$ and $\tilde{y} = y - \mathbf{C}\hat{\mathbf{x}}$ becomes

$$\mathbf{L}(s) = \mathbf{C}_{\xi}\left[s\mathbf{I} - \mathbf{A}_{\xi}\right]^{-1}\mathbf{B}_{\xi} + \mathbf{D}_{\xi}\,. \tag{27}$$

The objective is to design a feedback gain **L**(s) of the H$_\infty$O that is robust against **Fw**. In the frequency domain, (6) and (25) are expressed as follows:

$$\begin{aligned}\mathbf{x}(s) &= \left[s\mathbf{I} - \bar{\mathbf{A}}\right]^{-1}\bar{\mathbf{B}}u(s) + \left[s\mathbf{I} - \bar{\mathbf{A}}\right]^{-1}\mathbf{F}\mathbf{w}(s) \\ \hat{\mathbf{x}}(s) &= \left[s\mathbf{I} - \bar{\mathbf{A}}\right]^{-1}\bar{\mathbf{B}}u(s) + \left[s\mathbf{I} - \bar{\mathbf{A}}\right]^{-1}\mathbf{L}(s)\tilde{y}(s)\end{aligned} \tag{28}$$

where $\tilde{y}(s) = y(s) - \mathbf{C}\hat{\mathbf{x}}(s)$. Subtracting $\hat{\mathbf{x}}(s)$ from **x**(s) yields the following error dynamics:

$$\mathbf{e}(s) = \mathbf{T}_{\mathbf{ew}}(s)\mathbf{w}(s) = \left\{\mathbf{I} + \left[s\mathbf{I} - \bar{\mathbf{A}}\right]^{-1}\mathbf{L}(s)\mathbf{C}\right\}^{-1}\left[s\mathbf{I} - \bar{\mathbf{A}}\right]^{-1}\mathbf{F}\mathbf{w}(s)\,. \tag{29}$$

Based on (29), the H$_\infty$O can be designed by minimizing the H$_\infty$ norm of the frequency-weighted closed-loop disturbance-to-error transfer function $\mathbf{T}_{\mathbf{ew}}$(s):

$$\min_{\mathbf{L}(j\omega)} \left\| \mathbf{W}_{\mathbf{e}}(j\omega)\mathbf{T}_{\mathbf{ew}}(j\omega) \right\|_{\infty}, \tag{30}$$

where $\mathbf{W}_e(s)$ is a weighting function specifying the desired error bound. The linear fractional transformation (LFT) (Skogestad & Postlethwaite, 1996) can be used to convert (30) to the standard H_∞ optimization set-up (Skogestad & Postlethwaite, 1996) shown in Fig. 4, where $\mathbf{P}(s)$ is given by:

$$\begin{bmatrix} \mathbf{z}(s) \\ \tilde{y}(s) \end{bmatrix} = \mathbf{P}(s) \begin{bmatrix} \mathbf{w}(s) \\ \mathbf{\upsilon}(s) \end{bmatrix} = \begin{bmatrix} \mathbf{W}_{\mathbf{e}}(s)\left[s\mathbf{I} - \bar{\mathbf{A}}\right]^{-1}\mathbf{F} & -\mathbf{W}_{\mathbf{e}}(s)\left[s\mathbf{I} - \bar{\mathbf{A}}\right]^{-1} \\ \mathbf{C}\left[s\mathbf{I} - \bar{\mathbf{A}}\right]^{-1}\mathbf{F} & -\mathbf{C}\left[s\mathbf{I} - \bar{\mathbf{A}}\right]^{-1} \end{bmatrix} \begin{bmatrix} \mathbf{w}(s) \\ \mathbf{\upsilon}(s) \end{bmatrix}, \tag{31}$$

where $\mathbf{z}(s) = \mathbf{W}_e(s)\mathbf{e}(s)$. This chapter employed a simple first-order filter (32) as $\mathbf{W}_e(s)$, which aims at small errors in the low frequency region:

$$\mathbf{W}_{\mathbf{e}4}(s) = k\frac{\tau_2 s + 1}{\tau_1 s + 1} \times \frac{1}{2EC_{50}} \times \left[\mathbf{I}_{4\times4} \quad \mathbf{0}_{4\times2}\right], \tag{32}$$

where k specifies the error bound at steady state, τ_1 specifies the observer bandwidth, and $\tau_2 > \tau_1$. Then the state-space representation (33) of $\mathbf{P}(s)$ is obtained:

$$\begin{aligned} \begin{bmatrix} \dot{\zeta} \\ \dot{\mathbf{e}} \end{bmatrix} &= \begin{bmatrix} -\tau_1\mathbf{I}_{4\times4} & k\frac{1}{\tau_1}\left(1 - \frac{\tau_2}{\tau_1}\right)\mathbf{I}_{4\times4} \quad \mathbf{0}_{4\times2} \\ \mathbf{0}_{6\times4} & \bar{\mathbf{A}} \end{bmatrix} \begin{bmatrix} \zeta \\ \mathbf{e} \end{bmatrix} + \begin{bmatrix} \mathbf{0}_{4\times6} & \mathbf{0}_{4\times6} \\ \mathbf{F} & -\mathbf{I}_{6\times6} \end{bmatrix} \begin{bmatrix} \mathbf{w} \\ \mathbf{\upsilon} \end{bmatrix} \\ \begin{bmatrix} \mathbf{z} \\ \tilde{y} \end{bmatrix} &= \begin{bmatrix} \mathbf{I}_{4\times4} & k\frac{\tau_2}{\tau_1}\mathbf{I}_{4\times4} \quad \mathbf{0}_{4\times2} \\ \mathbf{0}_{1\times4} & \mathbf{C} \end{bmatrix} \begin{bmatrix} \zeta \\ \mathbf{e} \end{bmatrix} + \begin{bmatrix} \mathbf{0}_{4\times6} & \mathbf{0}_{4\times6} \\ \mathbf{0}_{1\times6} & \mathbf{0}_{1\times6} \end{bmatrix} \begin{bmatrix} \mathbf{w} \\ \mathbf{\upsilon} \end{bmatrix} \end{aligned}. \tag{33}$$

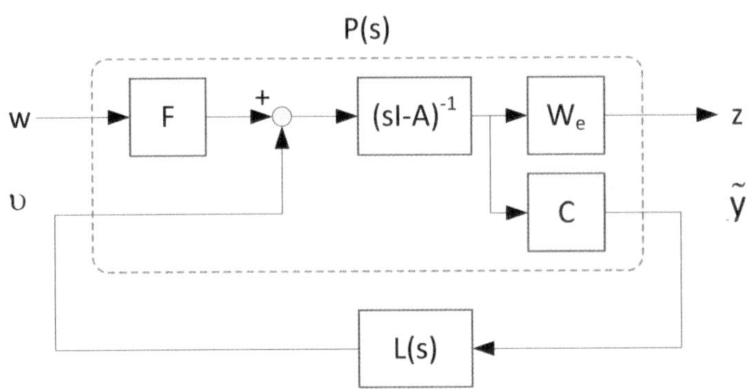

Fig. 4. Standard H_∞ optimization set-up for $H_\infty O$ design.

Based on (33), the optimal $H_\infty O$ can be designed using the D-K iteration (Skogestad & Postlethwaite, 1996). Note that although (33) does not satisfy all the regularity assumptions required for H_∞ optimization (Skogestad & Postlethwaite, 1996), the problem can be resolved by any standard regularization procedure (e.g. Pertew et al., 2006).

4. Methods

4.1 Design of observers

The demographic and PD data of 15 patients aged 18-30 (22+/-3.2) listed in Dumont et al. (2009) were used to obtain a nominal PK and PD model (1)-(4). Then 100 random Monte-Carlo models were created for the nominal model by applying up to +/-15% perturbations to all the PK and PD parameters. The PK/PD variability was specified as follows:

$$\mathbf{Fw} = \tilde{\mathbf{A}}\mathbf{x} + \tilde{\mathbf{B}}u + \mathbf{E}d = diag\{\delta_i\}\mathbf{w}\ , \tag{34}$$

where δ_i, i=1,...,6 were chosen to encompass the resultant effect of up to +/-15% random PK/PD parametric perturbations as well as surgical stimulation of up to +/-20 WAV_{CNS} units.

Before designing the observers, the observability of the system was analyzed by evaluating the observability grammian matrix (35) with the nominal patient model:

$$\mathbf{W}_o = \int_0^\infty \exp\left[\mathbf{A}^T\tau\right]\mathbf{C}^T\mathbf{C}\exp[\mathbf{A}\tau]d\tau\ , \tag{35}$$

using which the relationship between the dominant direction of each eigenvalue and the propofol concentration at each compartment was examined. The condition number of $\mathbf{W}_o$ was also calculated to assess the well-posedness of the observer design problem.

Using the nominal patient model, the observer gain matrix **L** for RLO and RNO were designed by solving the LMI (8) and (16) with α=1 and $\alpha=10^{-5}$, respectively. In the RNO design, the constraint (22) was imposed on **P**. The $H_\infty O$ was designed by applying the D-K iteration procedure to the standard set-up (33). The weighting function (32) was specified as k=5.0, $\tau_1^{-1}=2.0\times10^{-5}$Hz, and $\tau_2^{-1}=1.0\times10^{9}$Hz, which requires the error to be bounded by 20% up to 2.0×10^{-5}Hz, beyond which an increase in size of the error is permitted.

4.2 Monte-Carlo simulation

The 100 randomly created patient models were used for the Monte-Carlo simulation. TCI administration of propofol to target the effect site propofol concentration of 3mcg/ml was chosen as the simulation scenario (Fig. 5). The duration of the simulated procedure was 2000s. The surgical stimulation shown in Dumont et al. (2009) was adopted and applied to the patient models from 1200s to 1700s (Fig. 5). The open-loop-predicted propofol concentrations were calculated by solving the PK and PD models (1) and (2).

4.3 Statistical analysis

From the simulation of each of the 100 random patient models, the following plasma and effect site percentage errors (PE) were calculated for both observer-based estimation (RLO, RNO, and $H_\infty O$) and open-loop prediction:

$$PE_j^s = 100 \times \frac{C_s(j) - \hat{C}_s(j)}{C_s(j)}\ , \tag{36}$$

where PE_j^s denotes the PE for the sample j at the site s (s=p for plasma and s=e for effect site), and $C_s(j)$ and $\hat{C}_s(j)$ are the true versus open-loop predicted or closed-loop estimated drug concentrations for the sample j at the site s. The median absolute PE (MDAPE), mean absolute PE (MNAPE) and maximum absolute PE (MXAPE) were calculated as follows and were used to compare the performance of the observers and its potential over the open-loop prediction: $MDAPE_s = \text{median}\{|PE_j^s|\}$, $MNAPE_s = \text{mean}\{|PE_j^s|\}$, and $MXAPE_s = \max\{|PE_j^s|\}$ (Varvel et al., 1992). The errors were calculated for the induction phase of anesthesia (t<600s) and the entire procedure (t<2000s) in order to examine the effectiveness of the observers against surgical stimulation. The reduction in errors by the observers over the open-loop prediction was assessed in terms of the median value of the 100 observer-estimated MDAPE, MNAPE and MXAPE normalized by their open-loop-predicted counterparts. The statistical significance of the error reduction was determined by applying the two-sample t-test to the 100 pairs of observer-estimated and open-loop predicted MDAPE, MNAPE and MXAPE.

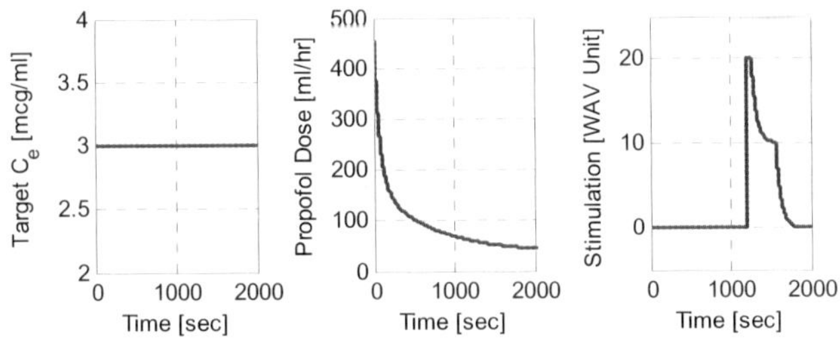

Fig. 5. Propofol effect site TCI scenario for Monte-Carlo simulation.

5. Results and discussion

5.1 Observability analysis and observer design

The effect site propofol concentration x_4 (which is the primary concentration of interest) was associated with the second smallest eigenvalue of $\mathbf{W}_o$, whereas the peripheral compartmental concentrations x_2 and x_3 corresponded to its largest and second largest eigenvalues. This implies that the influence of x_4 on the output (x_5) is relatively weak compared to x_2 and x_3, because x_2 and x_3 can dominate x_4 in terms of output energy through their slowly decaying dynamics (i.e. x_2 and x_3 decay much slower than x_1 and x_4). The condition number of $\mathbf{W}_o$ was very large (approximately 821), indicating that the degree of observability for propofol concentrations in different compartments can be significantly different. Essentially, the observability analysis clearly illustrates that estimating x_4 is inherently a challenging task.

RLO design resulted in $\mathbf{L}$ with optimal tr[$\mathbf{P}$]=6.7×10^8. The real part of the closed-loop eigenvalues ranged from -4.5 to -0.4. RNO design resulted in $\mathbf{L}$ with optimal tr[$\mathbf{P}$]=8.2×10^8. The real parts of the closed-loop eigenvalues range from -2.1×10^2 to -1.2×10^{-4}. H_∞O design resulted in $\mathbf{L}(s)$ that has robust stability margin of ∞ and robust performance margin of 1.1, indicating that the closed-loop system is always stable, and is robust against up to 1.1 times the uncertainty incorporated in the observer design (Balas et al., 2009).

5.2 Performance evaluation and statistical analysis

The distributions of MDAPE, MNAPE, and MXAPE of the propofol concentration errors at the plasma and the effect site are shown in Fig. 6 and Fig. 7 for the induction phase of anesthesia and the entire procedure, respectively. Tables 1-3 summarize mean (SD) of these errors.

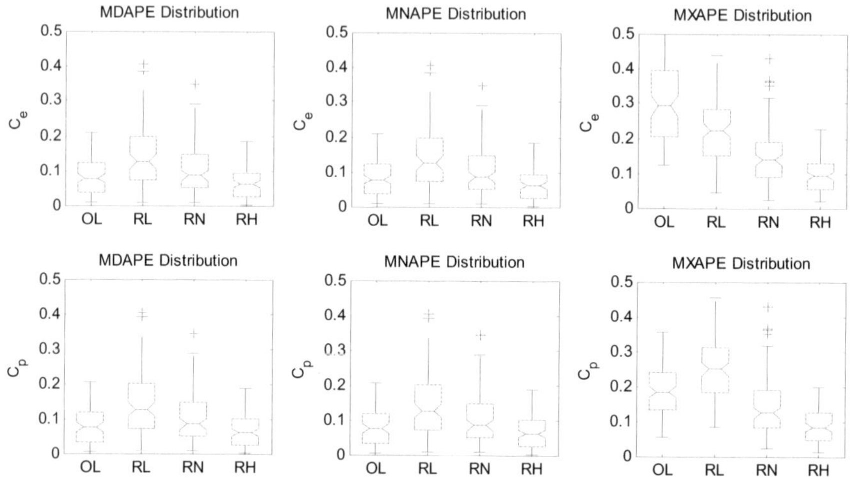

Fig. 6. Distributions of MDAPE, MNAPE, MXAPE during the induction phase of anesthesia. OL: open-loop prediction, RL: RLO, RN: RNO, RH: $H_{\infty}O$.

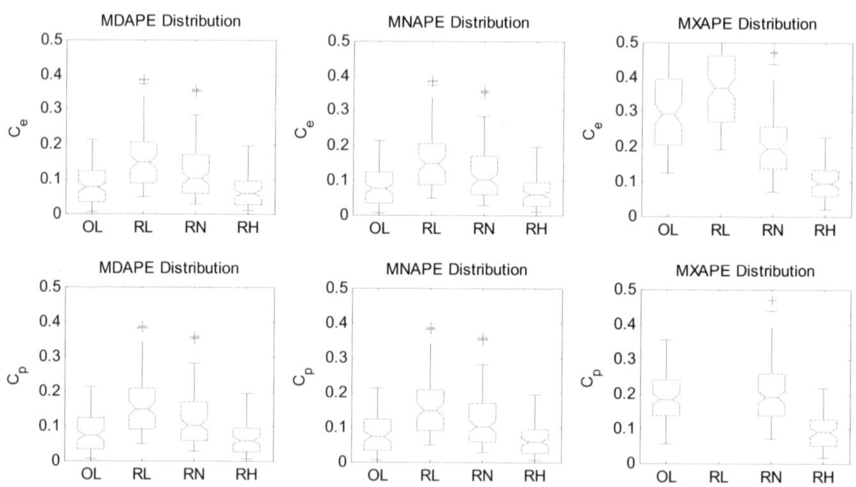

Fig. 7. Distributions of MDAPE, MNAPE, MXAPE during the entire procedure. OL: open-loop prediction, RL: RLO, RN: RNO, RH: $H_{\infty}O$.

The RNO and the $H_\infty O$ outperformed the RLO. Except for its benefit in reducing MXAPE of C_e during the induction phase of anesthesia (by 21%, $p<10^{-5}$; Table 3), the RLO was no better than the open-loop prediction (Table 1 and Table 2). Compared with the open-loop prediction, the RNO was capable of reducing MXAPE of C_e (by 59%, $p<10^{-5}$) and C_p (by 38%, $p<10^{-5}$) during the induction phase of anesthesia (Table 3), and MXAPE of C_e (by 43%, $p<10^{-5}$) during the entire procedure (Table 3). Its MDAPE and MNAPE were as good as those of the open-loop prediction during the induction phase of anesthesia, but they deteriorated more than the open-loop prediction when evaluated for the entire procedure (Table 1 and Table 2). The degraded performance of the observers in the presence of surgical stimulation is expected because it distorts the clinical effect measurement, resulting in an inappropriate feedback correction, whereas the open-loop prediction is not affected by surgical stimulation (see Fig. 1). In contrast to RLO and RNO, the $H_\infty O$ was able to deliver statistically significant reduction in all the PE metrics over the open-loop prediction, regardless of the presence of surgical stimulation (see Table 4). Moreover, the SD of all the metrics for the $H_\infty O$ were significantly smaller than those of the open-loop prediction, indicating that the propofol concentrations provided by the $H_\infty O$ are more reliable. This suggests that, in contrast to the open-loop prediction in which the PK/PD variability directly deteriorates the propofol concentration estimates, the observer's feedback correction based on the clinical effect measurement is viable in suppressing the propagation of the adverse influences of the PK/PD variability into the propofol concentration errors.

	Induction Phase				Entire Procedure			
	OL	RLO	RNO	$H_\infty O$	OL	RLO	RNO	$H_\infty O$
C_e	8.08 (5.61)	14.6 (9.91)	9.70 (6.81)	7.07 (4.96)	8.67 (6.06)	15.1 (10.2)	11.6 (7.78)	6.82 (4.99)
C_p	8.07 (5.65)	14.6 (9.95)	9.70 (6.83)	7.18 (5.06)	8.66 (6.07)	15.1 (10.1)	11.6 (7.77)	6.93 (5.07)

Table 1. Distribution of MDAPE: mean (SD).

	Induction Phase				Entire Procedure			
	OL	RLO	RNO	$H_\infty O$	OL	RLO	RNO	$H_\infty O$
C_e	8.70 (5.06)	14.8 (9.47)	9.51 (6.44)	7.01 (4.80)	8.68 (5.71)	16.3 (8.94)	12.3 (7.60)	6.78 (4.84)
C_p	8.24 (5.18)	14.9 (9.58)	9.48 (6.42)	7.11 (4.90)	8.55 (5.76)	16.6 (9.02)	12.3 (7.58)	6.89 (4.94)

Table 2. Distribution of MNAPE: mean (SD).

	Induction Phase				Entire Procedure			
	OL	RLO	RNO	$H_\infty O$	OL	RLO	RNO	$H_\infty O$
C_e	29.7 (10.8)	22.1 (9.40)	13.9 (7.29)	9.44 (4.81)	29.8 (10.7)	38.1 (12.1)	20.1 (8.61)	10.1 (4.94)
C_p	18.9 (7.11)	25.1 (9.09)	13.2 (7.28)	8.85 (4.83)	19.2 (6.98)	582. (53.7)	19.9 (8.70)	9.61 (4.93)

Table 3. Distribution of MXAPE: mean (SD).

	Induction Phase			Entire Procedure		
	MDAPE	MNAPE	MXAPE	MDAPE	MNAPE	MXAPE
C_e	13% ($p<10^{-10}$)	21% ($p<10^{-10}$)	73% ($p<10^{-10}$)	24% ($p<10^{-10}$)	25% ($p<10^{-10}$)	72% ($p<10^{-10}$)
C_p	11% ($p<10^{-10}$)	15% ($p<10^{-10}$)	59% ($p<10^{-10}$)	22% ($p<10^{-10}$)	21% ($p<10^{-10}$)	56% ($p<10^{-10}$)

Table 4. Reduction of PE metrics over open-loop prediction by $H_\infty O$.

Several important observations can be made from the overall results. First, the observers were effective in reducing MXAPE (except for the RLO in the presence of surgical stimulation, i.e. during the maintenance phase). This is attributed to the philosophy behind the design of robust observers – the observers considered in this chapter were designed to improve the worst-case performance (Skogestad & Postlethwaite, 1996). Due to the design objective of guaranteeing performance and robustness even in extreme situations, the behaviour of these observers on patients whose dynamics are rather close to the nominal design model may not be optimal (this may partly explain why MDAPE and MNAPE metrics of RLO and RNO are not as good as the open-loop prediction).

Second, in spite of its robustified feedback gain, the standard linear observer was not an attractive strategy for anesthesia drug concentration estimation, due to its limited performance in the presence of surgical stimulation. In our attempt to overcome this limitation, we presented an RNO and an $H_\infty O$ as alternatives to the RLO. The RNO could provide a marginal improvement that was not sufficient to justify the cost of additional measurement (i.e. the time derivative of the clinical effect). The $H_\infty O$ exhibited significantly superior performance to RLO and RNO without any extra measurement requirements, by virtue of the additional flexibility in its structure: the feedback gain **L**(s) is a dynamic system rather than a constant matrix as in RLO and RNO. Despite their limited performance in the presence of surgical stimulation, RLO and RNO can still be considered as valid options for applications in the induction phase of anesthesia and the operations involving minor surgical procedures, by virtue of their structural simplicity in implementation in comparison with $H_\infty O$.

From the design perspective, one advantage of the observer-based strategies investigated in this chapter is the explicit specification of the amount of PK/PD uncertainty and surgical stimulation it must tolerate (see the matrix **F** in (16) for RLO and RNO and in (33) for $H_\infty O$) and its systematic use for optimizing the observer performance so that the observer is tuned to appropriately exploit the clinical effect measurement distorted by surgical stimulation, in order to better estimate the drug concentrations over the open-loop prediction in spite of the PK/PD uncertainty.

6. Conclusion

This chapter investigated alternative observer-based strategies for estimation of anesthesia drug concentrations. The design objective was dedicated to robustness of observers against the PK/PD model uncertainty and the unknown surgical stimulation. In this chapter, we considered linear (RLO), nonlinear (RNO), and dynamic ($H_\infty O$) observers. The performance of the observers in comparison with traditional open-loop prediction was evaluated using a

Monte-Carlo simulation of a surgical procedure. Based on the PE-based metrics, it was concluded that the use of $H_\infty O$ is optimal. However, RLO and RNO can be viable alternatives for the induction phase of anesthesia and/or minimally stimulating procedures.

7. Acknowledgment

This research was supported in part by Natural Sciences and Engineering Research Council of Canada and Canadian Institute of Health Research under their Collaborative Health Research Project program.

8. References

Balas, G., Chiang, R., Packard, A., & Safonov, M. (2009). *Robust Control Toolbox User's Guide*, MathWorks, Natick, U.S.A.

Blanchini, F., & Miani, S. (2008). *Set-Theoretic Methods in Control*, Birkhäuser, ISBN 978-0-8176-3255-7, Boston, U.S.A.

Dumont, G.A., Martinez, A., & Ansermino, J.M. (2009). Robust Control of Depth of Anesthesia. *International Journal of Adaptive Control and Signal Processing*, Vol. 23, No. 5, pp. 435-454, ISSN 0890-6327.

Gentilini, A., Schaniel, C., Morari, M., Bieniok, C., Wymann, R., & Schnider, T. (2002). A New Paradigm for the Closed-Loop Intraoperative Administration of Analgesics in Humans. *IEEE Transactions on Biomedical Engineering*, Vol. 49, No. 4, pp. 289-299, ISSN 0018-9294.

Hahn, J.O., Dumont, G.A., & Ansermino, J.M. (2011). Closed-Loop Anesthetic Drug Concentration Estimation Using Clinical Effect Feedback. *IEEE Transactions on Biomedical Engineering*, Vol. 58, No. 1, pp. 3-6, ISSN 0018-9294.

Pertew, A.M., Marquez, H.J., & Zhao, Q. (2006). H_∞ Observer Design for Lipschitz Nonlinear Systems. *IEEE Transactions on Automatic Control*, Vol. 51, No. 7, pp. 1211-1216, ISSN 0018-9286.

Rao, R.R., Bequette, B.W., & Roy, R.J. (2000). Simultaneous Regulation of Hemodynamic and Anesthetic States: A Simulation Study. *Annals of Biomedical Engineering*, Vol. 28, No. 1, pp. 71-84, ISSN 0090-6964.

Sartori, V., Schumacher, P.M., Bouillon, T., Luginbuehl, M., & Morari, M. (2005). On-Line Estimation of Propofol Pharmacodynamic Parameters. *Proceedings of IEEE Engineering in Medicine and Biology Conference*, pp. 74-77, ISBN 0-7803-8740-6, Shanghai, China, September 1-4, 2005.

Schuttler, J., & Ihmsen, H. (2000). Population Pharmacokinetics of Propofol: A Multicenter Study. *Anesthesiology*, Vol. 92, No. 3, pp. 727-738, ISSN 1528-1175.

Skogestad, S., & Postlethwaite, I. (1996). *Multivariable Feedback Control Analysis and Design*, John Wiley & Sons, ISBN 978-0-470-01167-6, Chichester, U.K.

Van Poucke, G.E., Brandon Bravo, L.J., & Shafer, S.L. (2004). Target Controlled Infusions: Targeting the Effect Site While Limiting Peak Plasma Concentration. *IEEE Transactions on Biomedical Engineering*, Vol. 51, No. 11, pp. 1869-1875, ISSN 0018-9294.

Varvel, J.R., Donoho, D.L., & Shafer, S.L. (1992). Measuring the Predictive Performance of Computer-Controlled Infusion Pumps. *Journal of Pharmacokinetics and Biopharmaceutics*, Vol. 20, No. 1, pp. 63-94, ISSN 0090-466X.

Zikov, T., Bibian, S., Dumont, G.A., Huzmezan, M., & Ries, C.R. (2006). Quantifying Cortical Activity During General Anesthesia Using Wavelet Analysis. *IEEE Transactions on Biomedical Engineering*, Vol. 53, No. 4, pp. 617-632, ISSN 0018-9294.

11

Pharmacokinetics and Metabolized Caroteniods in Liver of Single Dose Administration in Fancy Carp (*Cyprinus carpio*)

Bundit Yuangsoi
Department of Fisheries, Faculty of Agriculture
Khon Kaen University, Khon Kaen
Thailand

1. Introduction

The market values of ornamental species are dictated by the qualities of their skin pigmentation, body shape, fin shape and body size (Paripatananont *et al.*, 1999). Among ornamental fish, 'fancy carp' (*Cyprinus carpio*) is being popular worldwide due to the increasing number of hobbyists. One of the frequently found problems includes the color of fancy carp which often turns pale after being raised for a period of time, the fact not preferred by hobbyists. In order to make the fancy carp color remain constantly vivid, certain sort of diet, such as 'carotenoids' is believed to help. However, carotenoids cannot be synthesized by most animals, including fish, and must be obtained from dietary sources (Goodwin, 1984). There has been suggestion to modify alimentary carotenoids and store them in the integument and other tissues.

Once digested, carotenoids are absorbed into the plasma, bound to serum lipoproteins (Ando *et al.*, 1986) and subsequently transported and distributed to various tissues and organs. The liver is the main metabolic and excretory organ for carotenoids (Torrissen and Ingebrigtsen, 1992) and is considered to have the major responsibility for the metabolic of carotenoids. The liver is therefore either catabolizing astaxanthin to other pigments or to metabolites of carotenoids. The exact process of carotenoids metabolism in the liver is unknown. While the available evidence points to the role of the liver in carotenoid metabolism, no studies have attempted to elucidate its role or to quantify its potential in carotenoid clearance.

Once established, pharmacokinetic studies on the given compound, i.e. the fraction of the feeding dose that is absorbed into the circulation, will be an important determinant of its efficiency and safety (Evan, 2004). In this case, this chapter deals with the quantitative aspects of carotenoid uptake, elimination and metabolic of carotenoid in fancy carps. Pharmacokinetics provides a mathematical basis to assess the time course of carotenoids and their effects in the body. It enables the following processes to be quantified:

- **A**bsorption
- **D**istribution
- **M**etabolism
- **E**xcretion

With this background, this chapter presents the reported evidence for the potential role of the liver in carotenoid utilization and investigation outcomes of the pharmacokinetics of the carotenoids in order to determine the absorption and disposition levels of carotenoids that can partially be ascribed to hepatic first-pass of fancy carps.

2. Carotenoids

Carotenoids can be found in plants and animals. These color-generating materials are in plastids that are naturally occurring in chromoplasts of plants and some other photosynthetic organisms like algae, some types of fungus and some bacteria. Though animals cannot produce carotenoids by themselves, they can keep carotenoids as polyunsaturated C40 hydrocarbons which consist of carbon atoms, single bonds along with double bonds. Carotenoids are dissolved in fat called lipophore. Carotenoids are tetraterpenes containing 4 connected isoprenes forming the ring structure. They come in yellow, orange, and red. Light absorption is at 400-600 nm. There are over 600 known carotenoids.

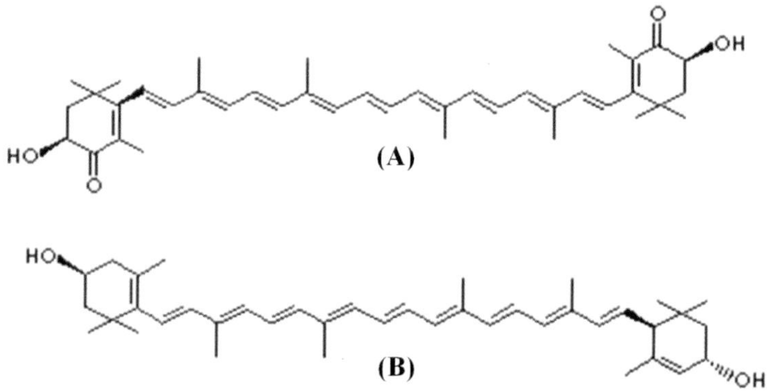

Fig. 1. Chemical structure of carotenoids; A: astaxanthin and B: lutein

Their colors, ranging from pale yellow through bright orange to deep red, is directly linked to their structure. Xanthophylls are often yellow, hence their class name. The double carbon-carbon bonds interact with each other in a process called conjugation, which allows electrons in the molecule to move freely across these areas of the molecule. As the number of double bonds increases, electrons associated with conjugated systems have more room to move, and require less energy to change states. This causes the range of energies of light absorbed by the molecule to decrease. As more frequencies of light are absorbed from the short end of the visible spectrum, the compounds acquire an increasingly red appearance.

3. Digestion and absorption

Carotenoids are lipid soluble and follow the same absorptive path ways as other dietary lipids. This property has been used as a basis for the carotene absorption test, a screening test for lipid malabsorption. Although efficient digestion and absorption of dietary lipid is a prerequisite for optimum absorption of carotenoids, it is suggested that carotenoids are simply absorbed by dietary lipid.

Carotenoid absorption involves several steps from the breakdown of the food matrix and release of carotenoids into the lumen of the gastrointestinal tract through their incorporation into lymphatic lipoproteins. This includes mechanical and chemical disruption of the food matrix, dispersion in lipid emulsion particles, solubilization into mixed bile salt micelles, movement across the unstirred water layer adjacent to the microvilli, uptake by the enterocyte, and incorporation into lymphatic lipoproteins. A perturbation at any point along this chain of events will alter carotenoid bioavailability (Furr and Clark, 1997).

Before absorption, carotenoids must be released from the food matrix, as they are not free in food but are associated with protein in a variety of plant cell structures (Erdman *et al.*, 1993). Once the food is ingested, its mechanical breakdown continues as it is chewed, swallowed, and mixed in the stomach. Gastric hydrolysis of dietary lipids and proteins results in partial release of carotenoids and lipids from the food matrix. The extent of release and the physical-chemical state of the carotenoids in the stomach is not known. Once they are released, however, the lipophilic carotenoids would dissolve in an oily phase of lipid droplets. With mixing, the lipid droplets in the gastric contents become emulsified particles. Thus bile salt and fats are required upon carotenoids absorption process (Simpson and Chichester, 1981).

Shearing forces from normal digestive tract motility bring about the formation of a fine lipid emulsion as the contents of the stomach pass into the duodenum. The emulsion has a triacylglycerol core surrounded by a monomolecular layer of partially digested proteins, polysaccharides and lipids, especially phospholipid and partially ionized fatty acids. The solubility and location of the polar carotenoids (xanthophylls) and the nonpolar carotenoids (carotenes) in emulsions differ. Carotenes are thought to incorporate almost exclusively in the triacylglycerol core of the emulsion, whereas the more polar xanthophylls distribute preferentially at the emulsion surface (Borel *et al.*, 1996). Other lipid soluble nutrients with polar groups such as tocopherol and trans-retinoic acid are also thought to locate at the droplet surface. The significance of location in an emulsion is that the surface components can spontaneously transfer from lipid droplets to mixed micelles, whereas components associated with the emulsion core require digestion of triacylglycerol before transfer (Borel *et al.*, 1996). The enzyme best suited to hydrolyze triacylglycerol in emulsions is pancreatic colipase-dependent lipase which is one reason why pancreatic insufficiency decreases plasma carotenoid concentrations (Leo *et al.*, 1995).

The products of lipid digestion and minor dietary lipids, including the carotenoids, transfer from the emulsion particle to mixed bile salt micelles. Whereas the mechanism of carotenoid solubilization into mixed micelles is unclear, the presence of bile salt micelles is obligatory, as carotenoid absorption is minimal or nonexistent when intraluminal bile salts are below the concentration required for aggregation into micelles (Hollander and Ruble, 1978). A major difference between absorption of other dietary lipid and carotenoids is that the carotenoids seem to have an absolute requirement for bile salt micelles, whereas fatty acids, the major product of lipid digestion, can be absorbed in the absence of micelles.

The solubility of carotenoids in mixed micelles is limited and varies with intraluminal concentration of the carotenoid. Canfield *et a1.*, (1990) studied the incorporation of β-carotene into mixed micelles designed to resemble those seen in the lumen of the small intestine. The incorporation of β-carotene into the micelles varied from approximately 4 to

13% with the percent incorporated decreasing with increasing initial concentration of carotenoid. Whereas the solubility of carotenoids differs in emulsions, the polar and nonpolar carotenoids have similar solubility in bile salt micelles (Borel *et al.*, 1996).

Accumulating of carotenoids in fish could be affected from various factors. Apart from the mentioned external and internal ones; digestibility, absorption, blood flowing by lipoprotein and absorbing of carotenoids in muscle fiber can affect digestibility. Apparent digestibility coefficient (ADC) of astaxanthin in rainbow trout shows that the percentage of ADC is at 70% which is higher than 35-70% of canthaxanthin. Differences of ADC and pigmenting efficiency do not depend only at the type of carotenoid, but also at the geometic isomer of each carotenoids themselves.

Addition of fat in the fodder causes enhanced color change in atlantic salmon (Einen and Skrede, 1998). This goes along with a research study conducted by Choubert *et al.* (1991) which reports that adding more fat results in improvement of carotenoids digestion and retention efficiency in rainbow trout (Nickell and Bromage, 1998). It can be concluded that using fat affects pigmentation regimes. The area where high absorption of carotenoids is found lies in posterior intestine. Absorption ability depends on variation in feed intake and is varied upon different types of fish whose triacyglycerols are packaged in chylomicron in enterocytes and pumped throughout the body by metabolized-like chylomicrons. They associate with lipoprotein which acts as the limiting factor. Superfluous carotenoids were discarded without affecting accumulated ones. However, digestibility depends on types of carotenoids. It is found that astaxanthin is well digested in the form of esterified compared to free form.

Polar carotenoids (xanthophylls) are around emulsion while non-polar carotenoids (carotenes) are found in emulsion. Emulsion, however, consists of triacylglucerol core where monomolecular layer e.g. digested protein, plysaccharides and lipids, particularly phospholipids are found. Specifically in ionized fatty acid, polar carotenoids, carotenoids absorption are highly improved compared to non-polar carotenoids. Such absorption is passive diffusion by concentration gradient. It is also found that adding more fat results in better absorption. Carotenoids found in blood circulation are delivered through lipoprotein. Normally, 75% of plasma carotenoids are delivered via LDL and the rest via VLDL and HDL. Non-polar carotnoids such as α, β-carotene, lycopene are delivered via LDL whilst polar carotenoids such as lutein, astaxanthin are delivered via HDL and LDL (Babin and Vernier, 1989).

4. Distribution of carotenoids among plasma lipoproteins

Carotenoid content and relation concentrations in human blood, the hydrocarbon carotenes (for example, α, β-carotene and lycopenes) are transported primarily on LDL plus VLDL, whereas the xanthohylls (lutein, zeaxanthin, β-cryptoxanthin) are distributed approximately equally between HDL and LDL in human serum (Johnson and Russell, 1992). Parker (1996) suggested that the actual content of β-carotene per unit lipid (triacylglycerol plus cholesterol) may be greater in HDL than in LDL. Parker also noted that although the total surface area of LDL is approximately twice that of HDL in human plasma, the content of xanthophylls (lutein plus zeaxanthin) is greater in HDL than in LDL.

5. Uptake and transport into blood

Being fat-soluble, dietary astaxanthin is assumed to be in micellar form in the intestine, together with bile salts, fatty acids, monoglycerides and other fat-soluble vitamins. It is believed to passively diffuse into the intestinal lumen, together with fatty acids, and the uptake seems to be a slow process taking between 18 and 30 hours (Choubert *et al.*, 1994). The fatty acids are converted into triacylglycerols (TAG), and the astaxanthin, like other xanthophylls (Zaripheh and Erdman, 2002), is incorporated together with TAGs in lipoprotein spheres called chylomicrons. These are then transported into the blood and due to its polarity, astaxanthin is assumed to be attached to the surface of the chylomicron spheres.

In mammals, transport of chylomicrons from the intestinal lumen into the blood is carried out through lymphatic vessels. While being transported along the blood stream, chylomicrons undergo hydrolysis by lipoprotein lipase (LPL), a triacylglycerol lipase found on the surface of endothelial cells of the tissue capillaries, to yield free fatty acids. The fatty acids and monoglycerols that are derived from chylomicrons in this way are subsequently taken up by the tissues or serum albumin. Changes in the lipid composition of a chylomicron modify the affinity of the associated lipoproteins for its surface, causing the chylomicron to change its apolipoprotein signature. When the chylomicrons have lost about 80% of their initial TAG content, they become small enough to pass through the endothelium in the liver, and in addition their apolipoprotein signature can then be recognized by specific receptors in the liver.

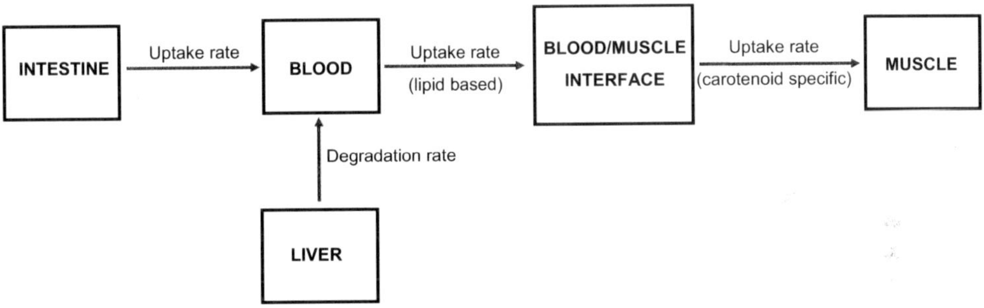

Source: Hannah *et al.*, (2006)

Fig. 2. Variation in pigment level due to variation in intestinal uptake likely accounted for by variation in weight to a substantial degree.

The fate of chylomicron-associated xanthophylls is poorly understood in mammals as well as in fish. It is hypothesized that non-triglyceride components of the chylomicron, including surface molecules such as xanthophylls, may be taken up by extra-hepatic tissues or transferred to other blood lipoproteins. When the chylomicrons reach the liver, however, they still contain a considerable amount of their original carotenoid content. Since fish do not seem to have a lymph system similar to the mammalian one, the chylomicrons are assumed to be transported through the primary blood vessels in the intestine. Aside from this, there is reason to assume that chylomicron-based astaxanthin transport and delivery in salmon are quite similar to that in mammals, as discussed above. Studies in salmon have provided evidence that astaxanthin is strongly associated with a protein likely to be serum albumin. Albumin is the major transporter of free fatty acids released during lipolysis by LPL to tissues (including liver and muscle). This suggests that albumin may acquire astaxanthin from chylomicrons during lipolysis as well as directly from chylomicrons in the bloodstream.

6. Liver metabolism and excretion

The liver is the main metabolic and excretory organ for Carotenoids (Torrissen and Ingebrigtsen, 1992) and is considered to have the major responsibility for the metabolic loss of astaxanthin. The liver secretes bile into the intestine to aid in lipid digestion as well as in the excretion of metabolic breakdown products, and radioactive labelling studies with canthaxanthin found bile radioactivity levels to be 8 times higher than the level in blood. The astaxanthin metabolites in the bile are secreted into the intestine and re-absorbed. Radiolabeling experiments also indicate that either astaxanthin or its metabolites are excreted by the kidneys of salmon and rainbow trout (Hardy *et al.*, 1990). The liver is therefore either catabolizing astaxanthin to other pigments or to metabolites that no longer have a chromophore. The exact process of astaxanthin metabolism in the liver is unknown, as is the case with β-carotene metabolism.

7. Transport and deposition in muscle

Despite numerous studies, the mechanism by which free fatty acids enter cells remains poorly understood. Astaxanthin association with LDLs has been observed in salmon (Aas *et al.*, 2000) and rainbow trout (Chapman *et al.*, 1978), suggesting that astaxanthin-containing LDLs may contribute substantially to the LPL-mediated uptake of astaxanthin by circulating albumin. Astaxanthin is then assumed to be brought to the muscle by circulating albumin. Binding to the muscle cell wall is thought to be non-specific and saturable. After having entered the muscle cell, astaxanthin is deposited in the myotome and binds to actomyosin by weak hydrophobic bonds, forming a complex. The presence of hydroxyl and keto groups at the β-end of the carotenoid increases the binding strength, explaining the higher deposition of astaxanthin compared to other carotenoids in salmon. Metabolites of astaxanthin have also been found in the connective tissues between myotomes.

During VLDL and LDL flow through the blood, some of the TAG found in these lipoproteins is transferred to high density lipoprotein packets (HDL) by the cholesteryl ester transfer protein (CETP) (Tyssandier *et al.*, 2002). Given that astaxanthin is transported along with the TAGs to the HDLs, this mechanism is likely to explain the observed high levels of HDL associated astaxanthin in immature salmon (Aas *et al.*, 2000), where there is no pigment transport out of the muscle. An interesting feature here is that unlike in mammalian systems, Atlantic salmon muscle has been found to express albumin. Carotenoids are highly accumulated around adipose tissue and liver which are considered significant organs to accumulate carotenoids. The level of carotenoids in each organ directly affects the intake.

8. Pharmacokinetics and metabolized caroteniods in liver of single dose administration in fancy carp (*Cyprinus carpio*)

8.1 Fish and feed trial

Mixed sexes of fancy carp with average weight of 26.93 ± 5.14 g/fish were maintained on a non-pigmented diet for a co-variant period of two weeks prior to feeding the experimental diets, tested in four replicates. Each treatment was randomly distributed to each of 20-liter aquarium tanks. The diets were designed to achieve a target level of 200 μg for astaxanthin and lutein per fish.

Astaxanthin was supplied at a finished product concentration of 10% astaxanthin (BASF, Thailand). Lutein from marigolds extract (*Tagetes* spp.) was supplied in a finished product containing 15000 ppm (Kemin Industries, Thailand). After administration of a single dose orally, fish were not fed further meals.

8.2 Sampling procedure

Fish were not fed for 3 days before receiving a single dose feeding. A control liver sample at 0 hr, was taken to measure basal liver astaxanthin and lutein levels prior to experiment. Liver sampling occurred at 15, 30 min 1, 3, 6, 12, 24, 48, 72, 96 and 120 hr after single dose meal, three fish were sampled at each sampling time. Liver was immediately separated from blood and stored at -20° C until samples analysis was performed.

8.3 Carotenoids determination

All experimental diets were extracted with acetone, together with BHT (250 ppm) added as antioxidant, until samples showed no color. After that, petroleum ether was added at 5 ml. and mixed, and water was added in a separating funnel. Mixing was carried out with a careful swirling and the two phases were found separated. In this study, only the hyperphase of diets was collected.

8.4 Liver distribution of carotenoids after its oral administration in fancy carp

Approximately 1 g of each liver was quickly excised after sampling (n 3, each). Each liver sample was rinsed with cold 0.9% NaCl solution, blotted dry with tissue paper and weighed. Then each liver was homogenized with acetone, together with BHT (250 ppm) added as antioxidant, until samples showed no color and saponified by addition of 0.2 ml of 60% KOH, followed by 1 hr incubation at 70°C. The saponified mixture was extracted 3 times with petroleum (containing 250 ppm of BHT. In this study, only the hyperphase was collected then determined maximum absorbance wavelength range over 350-600 nm. Merely the maximum absorbance value (λ max) was recorded and calculated total carotenoids were calculated based on Beer-Lambert's Law (Britton, 1995).

8.5 Instrumentation and chromatographic conditions

The resulting hyperphase of experimental diets and liver from petroleum ether extraction were evaporated under a gentle stream of nitrogen gas. This was followed by redissolving crude carotenoids in petroleum ether and the solution 5 μl were spotted on pre-coated silica gel 60 (10 x 20 cm) with 0.25 mm thickness (Merck, Germany) using a CAMAG Linomat IV (Switzerland) sample applicator. A constant application rate of 4 ul/s was employed and spaces between two spots were 14 mm. The slit dimension was kept at 5 mm x 0.45 mm and 20 mm/s scanning speed was employed. The mobile phase consisted of petroleum ether - diethyl ether - acetone (75:15:10, *v/v/v*). Linear ascending development was carried out in a twin trough glass chamber saturated with mobile phase. The optimized chamber saturation time for the mobile phase was 30 min at room temperature (25 ± 2° C). The length of chromatogram run was 70 mm. Densitometric scanning was performed on CAMAG TLC scanner III in the absorbance mode at 450 nm. The source of radiation utilized was a tungsten lamp (compiled from Mantiri *et al.*, 1996 and Sherma and Bernard, 2003). In order to identify the correct value of astaxanthin, lutein and β-carotene, TLC runs were always conducted including authentic standards for astaxanthin and β-carotene (Sigma); lutein (Chromadex, Canada).

8.6 Pharmacokinetic parameter analysis

The astaxanthin and lutein concentration-time curves from liver best fitted one-compartment pharmacokinetic model. The mean hepatic astaxanthin and lutein concentration-time curves data points of three from each time were then analyzed using pharmacokinetic equation (Evans, 2004).

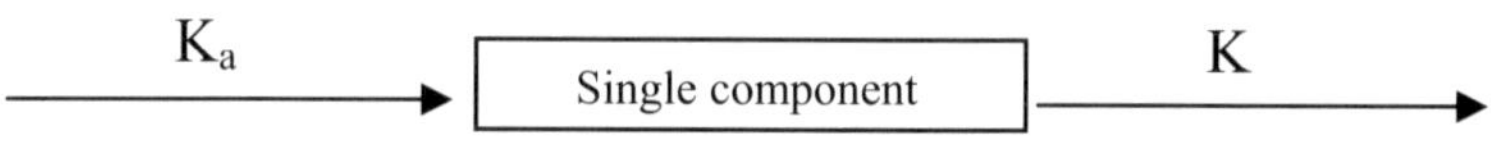

Fig. 3. One-compartment model K_a = absorption rate constant (h^{-1}), k = elimination rate constant (h^{-1})

9. Results

9.1 Pharmacokinetic parameters of fancy carp fed with deprived diets

The astaxanthin and lutein concentration in fancy carp were best described by one compartment model with first order absorption, pharmacokinetic parameters displayed in Table 1. The results showed that hepatic astaxanthin and lutein observed concentration time curve showed a steady rise after post-dosing, a slow increase to the maximum peak at 6 and 24 hr for astaxanthin and lutein, respectively. Astaxanthin and lutein were on a gradual decline after post-dosing.

Parameter	Unit	Parent diets	
		Astaxanthin	Lutein
Vd (area)/kg	ml/kg	1958.80	237.20
CL (area)/kg	ml/hr/kg	8.92	3.50
AUC (area)	µg-hr/ml	5300.00	2082.90
C max (obs)	µg/g	54.20	78.40
T max (obs)	hr	6.0	24.0

Vd (area)/kg: volume of distribution calculations
CL (area)/kg: clearance calculations
AUC (area): area under the serum concentration time curve
C max (obs): maximum observed serum concentrations
T max: observed time at which C max was achieved

Table 1. Pharmacokinetic parameters for astaxanthin and lutein derived from hepatic concentration – time of fancy carp.

Fancy carp fed with an astaxanthin diet developed a maximum concentration of astaxanthin (C max) of 54.20 µg/g occurred at 6 hr (T max) while fancy carp fed with a lutein diet contained lutein hepatic level (C max) of 78.40 µg/g within 24 hr. The volume of distribution (Vd) was 1958.80 and 237.20 ml/kg, respectively. The data illustrated that free astaxanthin was distributed in the liver better than lutein because the high amount of Vd demonstrates the fact that it can disseminate well in liver. However, the area under the curve (AUC) was 5300.00 and 2082.90 µg-hr/ml. AUC, indicating the relationship between hepatic carotenoid concentration and time. It is close to the amount of carotenoids being absorbed in the liver. If the area under the curve (AUC) is elevated, it means that carotenoids can be highly absorbed. Total body clearance (CL) was 8.92 and 3.50 ml/hr/kg, indicating that the clearance of astaxanthin was greater than lutein. This clearance was mainly to eradicate carotenoids. Overall, after fancy carp were fed an astaxanthin diet, they showed better astaxanthin absorption than lutein. When considered together with pharmacokinetic parameter which was Vd and AUC, well dispersion of astaxanthin in liver has been proved.

The results of the present study indicated that hepatic metabolism of astaxanthin and lutein in fancy carp following oral administration single dose feeding shows the faster rate of astaxanthin absorption for the fish fed with an astaxanthin diet compared to lutein diet which was similar to the report of Olsen and Bakker (2006). The absorption of carotenoids depends on disruption of food matrix. These solubility and location of the polar carotenoids (xanthophylls; astaxanthin and lutein) and the non polar carotenoids (carotene) in emulsions are different. Carotenes are thought to incorporate almost exclusively in the triacylglycerol core of the emulsion, whereas the more polar xanthophylls distribute preferentially at the emulsion surface (Furr and Clark, 1997). It has been shown by several authors, including Yonekura and Nagao (2007) that polar carotenoids (xanthophylls) have higher bioavailability characteristics leading to more transfer across the intestine compared to carotenes. This is related to the polar -OH side chains they possess which are absent in carotenes, showing the absorption of β-carotene appeared to be very low compared to astaxanthin and lutein. In this respect, the transfer rate of astaxanthin would be expected to be slightly higher than that of lutein. They also showed an apparent lack of interaction between astaxanthin and lutein on transfer between emulsions and micelles.

9.2 Metabolized serum carotenoids after administration of single dose of carotenoids diets

Analysis of carotenoids distributed to and metabolized in liver and carotenoids derivatives are shown in Table 2.

Parameters	Unit	Lutein metabolited from Astaxanthin diet	Astaxanthin metabolited from Lutein diet
Vd (area)/kg	ml/kg	4349.40	810.40
CL (area)/kg	ml/hr/kg	35.94	1.27
AUC (area)	µg-hr/ml	516.8	14631.10
C max (obs)	µg/g	65.00	40.9
T max (obs)	hr	12.00	24.00

Vd (area)/kg: volume of distribution calculations
L (area)/kg: clearance calculations
AUC (area): area under the serum concentration time curve
C max (obs): maximum observed serum concentrations
T max: observed time at which C max was achieved

Table 2. Pharmacokinetic parameters of metabolized of hepatic astaxanthin and lutein parent diets derived from concentration – time data of fancy carp

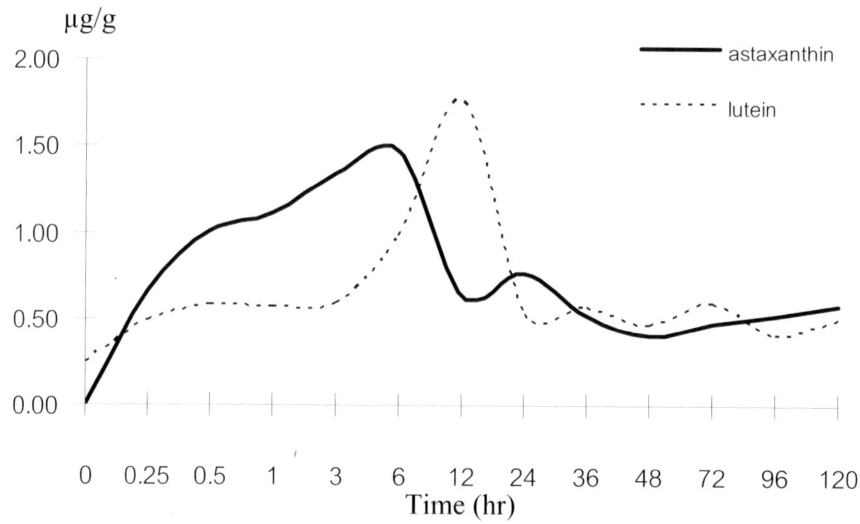

Fig. 4. Hepatic astaxanthin and lutein concentration – time curve for fancy carp administration with a single dose of astaxanthin 200 µg

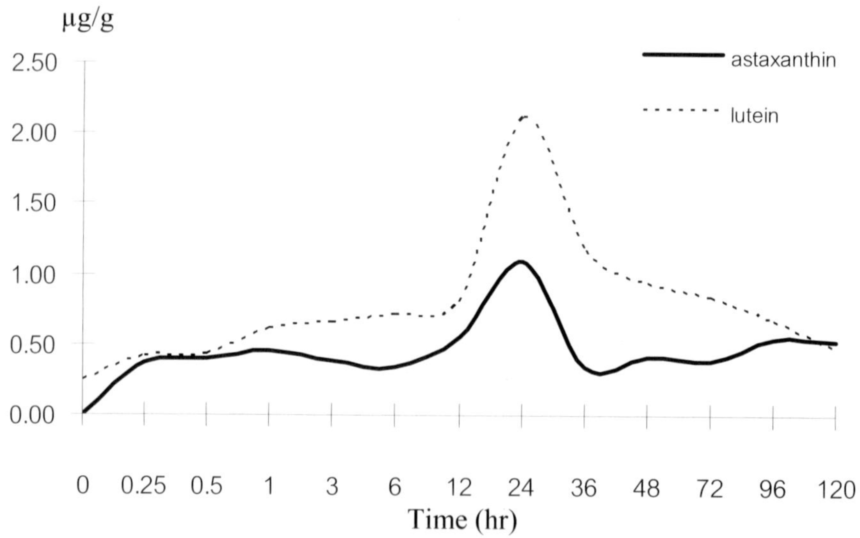

Fig. 5. Hepatic astaxanthin and lutein concentration – time curve for fancy carp administration with a single dose of lutein 200 µg

In this present study, the data showed that the hepatic carotenoids of fancy carp after feeding with an astaxanthin diet were composed of astaxanthin and lutein. Astaxanthin concentration decreased while the time passed, while lutein concentration was increased in liver. In the fancy carp fed with lutein diets, hepatic astaxanthin was found within 24 hr after oral administration feeding. Hepatic astaxanthin concentrations were 40.90 ± 0.03 μg/g. The hepatic astaxanthin concentration continued to increase the serum astaxanthin concentration. It could possibly be assumed that lutein was precursor and converted to astaxanthin, making the level of hepatic astaxanthin concentration higher in liver.

Aquatic animal carotenoids have been reviewed by Goodwin (1984) and Matsuno (2001). Commonly, carotenoids composition in many fishes are β-carotene, β-cryptoxanthin, tunaxanthins, luteins, zeaxanthins, diatoxanthin, alloxanthin, β-echinenone, canthaxanthin, α-doradexanthin, β-doradexanthin and astaxanthins. Carotenoid metabolism in animals takes place as a result of enzymes which catalyse three main types of reaction. These main reaction types are (i) the substitution of carotenoid end groups (often β-end groups) by oxygen functions (-OH and -C=O), (ii) the alteration of end groups, e.g. of β to α and (iii) cleavage of the polyene chain to yield apocarotenoids and even the vitamins A (Davies, 1985).

In this study, after fish were fed with astaxanthin diet, hepatic astaxanthin level was decreased because of metabolic conversions whereas the time hepatic lutein concentration was increased. The results indicated that lutein was carotenoids derived from reductive metabolite of astaxanthin. Based on a minute recovery of radioactivity in lutein after feeding of labeled (3S, 3′S)-astaxanthin, an analogous reductive pathway might also be occurring with gilthead seabeam (Gomes *et al.*, 2002). Lutein and zeaxanthin are metabolized prior to β-carotene, suggesting the precedence of xanthophylls biochemical conversions (Berticat *et al.*, 2000).

By contrast, after fancy carp were fed with lutein diets, hepatic astaxanthin was found within 24 hr after oral administration. This result suggested that lutein was oxidized to astaxanthin. The data shows that carotenoids were derived in liver after being fed with lutein; and that fancy carp can convert lutein to astaxanthin. The results of this present study were similar to other research studies: gold fish fed with lutein and zeaxanthin diets proposed the possible metabolic pathways from lutein and zeaxanthin to astaxanthin (Ohkubo *et al.*, 1999). This indicates that lutein is converted into β-doradexanthin, leading to the formation of astaxanthin by oxidative pathway (Tanaka *et al.*, 1976).

The chapter suggesting that absorbed carotenoids in the liver are rapidly metabolized. Torrissen and Ingebrigsten (1992) recovered a high level of radioactivity in the bile of salmon fed 14C astaxanthin, suggesting a role of the liver in pigment metabolism. This is consistent with earlier findings obtained by Schiedt et al. (1988) who reported that astaxanthin represented only 27% of the total carotenoids recovered. Together, the findings suggest that trout may have an efficient hepatic metabolic capacity for the conversion of these carotenoids. Conversely, it appears that salmon are comparatively slower at metabolic conversion of absorbed carotenoids by the liver as evidenced by the fact that the relative hepatic carotenoid level associated with diet was two-fold higher than in trout. Salmon have either a slower hepatic metabolism, a fundamental shift in the tissue responsible for carotenoid catabolism (e.g. kidney or hind gut), or white muscle pigment uptake potential is lower than in rainbow trout. The liver and kidney appeared to be important sites of carotenoid catabolism based on the relative proportion of the peak chromatogram of the fed carotenoid in rainbow trout and Atlantic salmon. Liver catabolism is suspected to be a critical determinant in carotenoid clearance, with higher catabolism expected in Atlantic salmon than in rainbow trout (Page and Davies, 2006).

In conclusion, this chapter presents the evidence for the potential role of the liver in carotenoid utilization and confirms that the liver plays a significant role in carotenoid metabolism. In addition, the liver appears to be an important organ for the metabolic transformation of carotenoids. Hepatic carotenoids ascribed to first-pass metabolism by pharmacokinetic were designed to investigate dose - response effects on uptake parameters for both astaxanthin and lutein derived from commercial beadlet sources for fancy carp. The first reported evidence for the potential role of the liver in carotenoid utilization showed that liver plays a direct relationship to its potential in metabolism. In addition, the results suggest that the observed discrepancy between absorbed and retained levels of carotenoids can partially be ascribed to first-pass metabolism by the liver, which can be applied in other species research.

10. References

Aas, G.B., B. Bjerkeng, T. Storebakken and B. Ruyter. 2000. Blood appearance, metabolic transformation and plasma transport proteins of (C 14) - astaxanthin in Atlantic salmon (Salmo salar L.) Fish Physiol. Biochem. 21: 325-334.

Ando, S., T. Takeyamaand M. Hatano. 1986. Isolation and characterization of a carotenoid carrying lipoprotein in the serum of Chum salmon (*Oncorhynchus keta*) during spawning migration. Agric. Biol. Chem. 50: 907-914.

Babin, J.N. and G.P. Vernier. 1989. Plasma lipoprotein in fish. J. lipid Res. 30: 467-489.

Berticat, O., G. Negre-Sadargues and R. Castillo. 2000. The metabolism of astaxanthin during the embryonic development of the crayfish Astacus leptodactylus, Eschscholtz. Comp. Biochem. Physiol. 127B: 309-318.

Borel, P., P. Grolier, M. Armand, A. Partier, H. Lafont, D. Lairon and V. Azais-Braesco. 1996. Carotenoids in biological emulsions: solubility, surface-to-core distribution and release from lipid droplets. J. Lipid Res.37: 250-261

Britton, G. 1995. UV/Visible Spectroscopy, pp 13-63. In G. Britton, S. Liaaen-Jensen and H. Pfander.eds. Carotenoids: Spectroscopy,vol 1B. Birkhäuser Verlag. Basel.

Canfield, L.M., T.A. Fritz and T.E. Tarara. 1990. Incorporation of beta-carotene into mixed micelles. Enzymol Methods. 189: 418-422.

Chapman, M.J., S. Goldstein, G.L. Mills and C. Leger. 1978. Distribution and characterization of serum lipoproteins and their apoproteins in rainbow trout (*Salmo gairdneri*). Biochemistry (N. Y.). 17: 4455-4464.

Choubert G., D.L. Noue and J.M. Blanc. 1991. Apparent digestibility of canthaxanthin in rainbow trout, effect of dietary fat level, antibiotics and number of pyloric caeca. Aquaculture 99: 323-329.

Choubert, G., J.C.G. Milicua and R. Gomez. 1994. The transport of astaxanthin in immature rainbow trout *Oncorhynchus mykiss* serum. Comp. Biochem. Physiol. Physiol. 108A: 245-248.

Davies, B.H. 1985. Carotenoid metabolism in animals: a biochemist's view. Pure Appl. Chem. 57: 679-684.

Einen O. and G. Skrede. 1998. Quality characteristics in raw and smoked fillets of Atlantic salmon, *Salmo salar*, fed high-energy diets. Aquac. Nutr. 4: 99-108.

Erdman, J.W., T.L. Bierer and E.T. Gugger. 1993. Absorption and transport of carotenoids. Ann. NY Acad. Sci. 691: 76-85.

Evans, G. 2004. A Handbook of Bioanalysis and Drug Metabolism. CRC Press. Boca Raton, Fla.

Furr, H.C. and R.M. Clark. 1997. Intestinal absorption and tissue distribution of carotenoids. Nutr. Biochem. 8: 364-377.

Gomes, E., J. Dias, P. Silva, L. Valente, J. Empis, L. Gouveia, J. Bowen and A. Young. 2002. Utilization of natural and synthetic source of carotenoids in the skin pigmentation of gilthead seabeam (*Sparus aurata*). Eur. Food Res. Technol. 214: 287-293.

Goodwin, T.W. 1984. The Biochemistry of the Carotenoids. Volume II Animals. Chapman and Hall. New York.

Hannah, R., L. Oyehaug, D.I. Vage and S.W. Omholt. 2006. Carotenoid dynamics in Atlantic salmon. BMC Biology. 4: 1-15.

Hardy, R.W.,O.J. Torrisse and T.M. Scott. 1990. Absorption and distribution of 14C- labeled canthaxanthin in rainbow trout (*Oncorhynchus mykiss*). Aquaculture 87: 331-340.

Hollander, D. and P.E. Ruble. 1978. Beta-Carotene intestinal absorption: bile, fatty acid, pH, and flow rate effects on transport. Am. J. Physiol. 235: 686-691.

Leo, M.A., S. Ahmed, S.I Aleynik, J.H. Siegel, F. Kasmin and C.S. Lieber. 1995. Carotenoids and tocopherols in various hepatobiliary conditions. J. Hepatol. 23: 550-556.

Mantiri, D.M.H., G. Negre-Sadargues, G. Charmantier, J.P. Trilles, J.C.G. Milicua and R. Castillo. 1996. Nature and metabolism of carotenoid pigments during the embryogenesis of the European lobster *Homarus gammarus*. Comp. Biochem. Physiol. 115A: 237-241.

Matsuno, T. 2001. Aquatic animal carotenoids. Fish. Sci. 67: 771-783.

Nickell, D.C. and N.R. Bromage. 1998. The effect of dietary lipid level on variation of flesh pigmentation in rainbow trout (*Oncorhynchus mykiss*). Aquaculture 161: 237-251.

Ohkubo, M., M. Tsushima, T. Maoka and T. Matsuno. 1999. Carotenoids and their metabolism in goldfish (Carassius auratus, Hibuna). Comp. Biochem. Physiol. 124B: 333-340.

Olsen, R.E. and R.T.M Baker. 2006. Lutein does not influence flesh astaxanthin pigmentation in the Atlantic salmon (*Salmo salar* L.). Aquaculture 258: 558-564.

Page, G.I. and S.J. Davies. 2006. Tissue astaxanthin and canthaxanthin distribution in rainbow trout (*Oncorhynchus mykiss*) and Atlantic salmon (*Salmo salar*). Comparative Biochemistry and Physiology, Part A. 143: 125–132.

Paripatananont, T., J. Tangtrongpairoj, A. Sailasuta and N. Chansue. 1999. Effect of astaxanthin on pigmentation of goldfish (*Carassius auratus*). J. World Aquac. Soc. 30: 454-460.

Schiedt, K., M., Vecchi, E., Glinz and T., Storebakken. 1988. Metabolism of carotenoids in salmonids. III. Metabolites of astaxanthin and canthaxanthin in the skin of Atlantic salmon (Salmo salar, L.). Helv. Chim. Acta. 71: 887–896.

Sherma, J. and F. Bernard. 2003. Handbook of Thin Layer Chromatography. Marcel Dekker Inc. New York.

Simpson, K.L., C.O. Chichester. 1981. Metabolism and nutrition significance of carotenoids. Ann. Rev. Nutr. 1: 351-374.

Tanaka, Y., T. Katayama, K.L. Simpson and C.O. Chichester. 1976. Biosynthesis of astaxanthin. XIX. Distribution of α-doradexanthin and metabolism of carotenoids in goldfish. Bull. Jap. Soc. Fish. 42: 885-892.

Torrissen, O.J. and K., Ingebrigsten. 1992. Tissue distribution of 14C-astaxanthin in the Atlantic salmon (Salmo salar). Aquaculture 108: 381–386.

Tyssandier, V., G. Choubert, P. Grolier and P. Borel. 2002. Carotenoids, mostly the xanthophylls, exchange between plasma lipoproteins. Int. J. Vitam. Nutr. Res. 72: 300-308.

Yonekura, L. and A. Nakao. 2007. Intestinal absorption of dietary carotenoids. Mol. Nutr. Food Res. 51: 107-11.

Zaripheh, S. and J.W. Erdman. 2002. Factors that influence the bioavailability of xanthophylls. J. Nutr. 132: 531-534.

Correlation of *in vitro* Dissolution Profiles with *in vivo* Pharmacokinetic Parameters of Some Commercial Brands of Aspirin Tablets Marketed in Nigeria

Emmanuel Adelaja Bamigbola
Department of Pharmaceutics and Pharmaceutical Technology, Faculty of Pharmacy, Niger Delta University, Wilberforce Island, Amassoma, Bayelsa State, Nigeria

1. Introduction

From biopharmaceutical point of view, *in vitro-in vivo* correlation (IV-IVC) is a predictive mathematical treatment describing the relationship between an *in vitro* property of a dosage form (usually the rate or extent of drug release) and a relevant *in vivo* response (e.g. plasma or urine drug concentrations or amount of drug absorbed). IV-IVC is recommended by various regulatory bodies and mostly applicable to drug dosage forms for oral routes and sustained release products. It is a useful tool for drug dosage form development, because a successful correlation can assist in the selection of drug formulation with appropriate and acceptable dissolution criteria, and depending on its predictiveness, it can be used as a forecast or surrogate for further bioequivalence studies. There are different categories of IV-IVC; A, B, C and D.

In biopharmaceutics classification system (BCS), aspirin belong to class 2, and because of its poor water solubility, the dissolution rate is the rate limiting step, which controls the absorption and bioavailability parameters of oral aspirin drug products. This criterion makes aspirin a good candidate for IV-IVC evaluation. *In vitro–in vivo* correlation of four commercial brands of aspirin tablets (one soluble brand and three regular brands) marketed in Nigeria are presented. USPXXI rotating basket apparatus and urinary excretion profiles from eight human volunteers were employed for *in vitro* and *in vivo* assessments respectively. Various dissolution parameters such as percent dissolved in 30 min, dissolution rate constants (k) and time for 50 % dissolution ($DT_{50\%}$) and pharmacokinetic parameters such as cumulative amount excreted up to 8 h (E_8), maximum excretion rate $(dE/dt)_{max}$ and time for maximum excretion rate (T_{max}) were obtained for all the brands.

The soluble aspirin had the highest percent dissolved in 30 minutes and highest dissolution rate constant with shortest time for 50% dissolution compared with other regular aspirin brands. Comparatively, the soluble aspirin had the highest E_8 and highest $(dE/dt)_{max}$ with the shortest T_{max}. Significant rank order correlations were observed between all the *in vitro* dissolution parameters such as percent dissolved at 30 min, dissolution rate constants (k) and time for 50 % dissolution ($DT_{50\%}$) and all the *in vivo* bioavailability parameters such as cumulative amount excreted up to 8 h (E_8), maximum excretion rate $(dE/dt)_{max}$ and time for maximum excretion rate (T_{max}). However, no correlation could be established between the cumulative amount excreted up to 24 h (E_{24}) and any of the *in vitro* dissolution parameters. Moreover statistical analysis showed no significant inter-subject variation among the human subjects that participated in the experiments.

Soluble aspirin tablet exhibited a higher *in vitro* dissolution and *in vivo* bioavailability profiles than regular aspirin tablets. The three regular aspirin brands were not bioequivalent to the soluble brands of aspirin. Good IV-IVC was established for the four brands of aspirin tablets. Therefore, with proper standardization of methods of assessment, *in vitro* dissolution parameters can be used to predict *in vivo* bioavailability of these aspirin tablets marketed in Nigeria.

1.1 Quality assessment of drug products

1.1.1 *In vitro* quality assessment of drug products

The quality of drug product especially oral solid dosage forms such as tablets and capsules are often assessed by carrying out certain in vitro tests as contained in the monographs of various pharmacopoeias. Such test include: assay of active ingredients; weight uniformity; content uniformity; hardness; friability; disintegration and dissolution tests. These are to ensure batch to batch uniformity of quality during manufacturing processes.

The general assumption was that if the physical and chemical integrity of a drug product were assured, satisfactory pharmacologic or therapeutic performance would be obtained [1, 2]

1.1.2 *In vivo* quality assessment of drug products

In addition to the vitro quality assessment of drug products as prescribed in various pharmacopeias, *in vivo* bioavailability requirement is now an essential parameter in quality control of a number of medicinal products, particularly, those which have low or high therapeutic index or those which are poorly water soluble. This became necessary in view of apparent inadequacy of the *in vitro* pharmacopoeia tests which did not take into consideration whether or not the active ingredient would be released from the dosage form, nor at what rate it gets into the biologic system.[3] Many formulations were produced and marketed that satisfied all the required legal standards but which were not therapeutically active.[4]

Events and certain realizations have revealed that percentage chemical strength was not the sole criterion for clinical effectiveness. It became obvious that a dosage form must not only contain the correct amount of labeled drugs, but must also release the drugs on administration for absorption in the patient. So apart from chemical purity and percentage strength, bioavailability, clinical efficacy and safety became additional criteria for effective product development.[5] It is now recognized that various physicochemical properties and formulation factors can influence the biologic availability of medicaments from dosage from in the body system.[1]

1.2 Rate limiting step in drug bioavailability

Systemic absorption of most drug products consists of a succession of rate processes. These processes include: (i) disintegration of the drug product and subsequent release of the drug;

(ii) dissolution of the drug in an aqueous environment: and (iii) absorption across cell membrane into the systemic circulation. In the process of drug disintegration, dissolution and absorption, the rate at which drug reaches the circulatory system is determined by the slowest step in the sequence.

The slowest step in a series of kinetic process is called the rate-limiting step, except for sustained release or prolonged-action products; disintegration of a solid drug product is usually more rapid than dissolution and drug absorption. For drugs that have very poor aqueous solubility for example aspirin, the rate at which the drug dissolves (dissolution) is often the slowest step, and therefore, exerts a rate-limiting effect on drug bioavailability. In contrast, for a drug that has a high aqueous solubility, the dissolution rate is rapid and the rate at which the drug crosses or permeates cell membranes (absorption) is the slowest or rate limiting step [3, 5]

1.3 *In vivo* dissolution and drug bioavailability

In biologic systems, drug dissolution in an aqueous medium is an important condition for systemic absorption and subsequent bioavailability. The rate at which drug with poor aqueous solubility dissolve from an intact or disintegrated solid dosage form in the gastro intestinal tract often controls the rate of systemic absorption of the drug.

Dissolution is the process by which a drug substance is released from the dosage from into a dissolution medium. A drug administered in a tablet or capsule form must be released, dissolved and reach its site of action before it can exert a pharmacological response. Dissolution of drug in the body represents the end of the release process and precedes the absorption of drugs from solid dosage forms. Various theories of tablet dissolution that have been proffered include: (i) the diffusion layer model, (ii) the Noyes-Whitney theory, (iii) the Wagner's, (iv) the Kitazawa, (v) the El-Yazigi, (vi) the Carstensen's theories, (vii) the Danckwert's model [5]

Dissolution kinetics of a drug product can be influenced by various factors such as (i) the physicochemical characteristics of the drug substance e.g. particle size, particle shape, polymorphism, crystal form, salt ester formation; (ii) formulation factors such as the nature and amount of excipients e.g. diluents, disintegrants, binders, lubricants, etc. (iii) manufacturing procedures such as the method of granulation, the size and density of the granules, moisture content, age of the granules, compressional force used in tabletting process, the quality of the personnel, the sophistication of the equipment and level of in-process quality control [4, 5]

Drug in the body particularly, in the gastrointestinal tract, is considered to be dissolving in an aqueous environment. Therefore, temperature of the medium and the agitation rate also affect the rate drug dissolution. The *in vivo* temperature is maintained at a constant temperature of 37°c, and the agitation (primarily peristaltic movement in the gastro-intestinal tract) is reasonably constant [2, 3, 5]

1.4 *In vitro* dissolution tests

Dissolution test is an *in vitro* physicochemical testing of solid oral dosage form. It determines the amount of active ingredient(s) released from a solid oral dosage from, such as from tablets or capsules, using a know volume of dissolution medium, with a predetermined length of time. The general principle of dissolution test is that the solid dosage form is tested under uniform agitation in an attempt to achieve dissolution. Agitation is accomplished by either using stirrer inside the apparatus or rotating the container holding the dosage form. *In vitro* dissolution test can be used to guide formulation development, identify critical manufacturing variables, monitor formulation quality from batch to batch, predict in vitro performance, monitor manufacturing process, assure batch to batch product performance and serve as a surrogate for bioavailability and bioequivalence.

The choice of dissolution apparatus varies from one drug to another, depending on the nature of the drug. Conditions employed for the in vitro dissolution test are made in such a way to give the best and reproducible results for the particular drug under test. Such conditions include the size and shape of the dissolution vessel, the agitation rate, temperature of the dissolution medium which for most dissolution test is temperature of 37°c which is similar to the *in vivo* temperature. The nature and volume of the dissolution media is also important e.g. simulated gastric fluid, simulated intestinal fluid, water, 0.1N Hcl, phosphate and acetate buffer depending on the nature of the drug and the location in the gastro-intestinal tract where the drug is expected to dissolve. The volume of the dissolution medium ranges from 500ml to 1000ml. [6, 7, 5]

There are several official methods of carrying out dissolution test of tablets and capsules e.g. rotating basket method (Apparatus 1); paddle method (Apparatus 2); transdermal product testing (Apparatus 3) transdermal product testing (Apparatus 4); transdermal product testing (Apparatus 5).[2] Other unofficial methods are rotating bottle method; flow-through dissolution method; intrinsic dissolution method, and peristalsis method.[8]

1.5 Bioavailability assessment

Bioavailability of a drug refers to the measurement of the rate and extent of active drug that reaches the systemic circulation. The in vivo behaviours of a dosage form can be explained more precisely by its bioavailability. Bioavailability studies are carried out for both approved drugs and those not yet approved for marketing by drug regulatory agencies. This is to ensure that such drugs are safe and effective for their labeled indications for use and that they meet all applicable standards of identity, strength, quality and purity. *In vivo* bioavailability assessments are also performed for new formulations of active drug ingredients or therapeutic moieties that have full new drug application approvals. Various factors affecting the dissolution of a drug will invariable affect its bioavailability e.g. the physicochemical properties of the drug, formulation factors and manufacturing processes.[9, 5]

1.6 Methods of assessing bioavailability

There are several direct and indirect methods of assessing bioavailability in humans. The selection of a method depends on the purpose of the study, analytical method of drug measurement, and nature of the drug product. The methods are namely:

i. Pharmacokinetic method: this is the measurement of the active drug substance or its metabolite(s) in biological fluids such as blood, plasma, urine, saliva, bile, sweat, milk, breath, feaces and other tissues.

ii. Acute pharmacologic effect. An acute pharmacologic effect such as effect on pupil diameter, heart rate or blood pressure can be useful as an index of drug bioavailability. This may require demonstration of dose related responses.
iii. Clinical observation: such as lack of response (therapeutic failure) good response or toxicity in patience receiving similar drug products may be used to determine drug bioavailability.
iv. iv. In-vitro dissolution test: this is done in selected case where in vitro / in vivo correction has been established for such drug product.

Because the free or therapeutically active drug can be accurately quantified in biological fluids, pharmacokinetic method is often preferred. Among all the body fluids, plasma and urine data gives the most objective information on bioavailability while the rest are less reliable.

The urine method of assessment has some advantages over the blood:

i. Samples are more easily obtained than blood,
ii. Urine collection is more pleasant to the subjects and more convenient,
iii. The concentration of the drugs in the urine is often higher than in the blood, so, simple analytical method (e.g. U.V. spectrophotometer) can be used,
iv. Lack of protein in the urine of a healthy individual obviates the need for denaturation step.

However, the following conditions are necessary for obtaining valid urinary excretion data.

i. Frequent sampling is necessary for a good curve description.
ii. Urine sample should be collected periodically until almost the entire drug has been excreted (a period of approximately seven elimination half lives)
iii. Urinary pH must be kept constant to avoid significant variation in urinary excretion rate.
iv. Subject participating in the study should submit a complete urine specimen i.e. completely emptying the bladder.[10, 1, 11, 2, 5]

1.7 Pharmacokinetic parameters for bioavailability assessment

There are various pharmacokinetic parameters usually employed in evaluating bioavailability when drugs are assessed in biological fluids.

Plasma:

i. AUC- area under the plasma level-time curve and it reflects the total amount of active drug reaching the systemic circulation.
ii. C_{max} - is the maximum plasma drug concentration obtained after administration of drug.
iii. T_{max} – time of maximum plasma concentration, it corresponds to the time required to reach maximum drug concentration. At T_{max}, rate of absorption equals rate of elimination. Absorption continues after T_{max} but at a slower rate.

Urine:

i. $[E]^{\infty}$ - Cumulative amount of drug excreted in the urine over a sufficient period of time (usually above 7 half-lives). It is directly related to the total amount of drug absorbed

ii. $[dE/dt]_{max}$ –Maximum rate of drug excretion, is the maximum rate at which drug is excreted in the urine after the administration of the drug.
iii. T_{max} - Time of maximum urinary excretion rate, it is the time required to reach maximum rate of drug excretion after drug administration.

The AUC and $[E]^{\infty}$ are similar in the sense that they both measure the extend of drug absorption (bioavailability) while T_{max} indicate the rate of drug absorption. C_{max} and $[dE/dt]_{max}$ are analogous in the sense that they reflect both the rate and extent of absorption. If the rate of drug excretion in urine is proportional to the concentration in blood, the curve obtained by plotting [dE/dt] against time will be the same as the plasma concentration-time curve, and T_{max} will be the same. [12, 4, 2, 13, 3, 5]

1.8 *In vitro – in vivo* correlation of aspirin tablets

The formulation and implementation of regulations concerning bioavailability of drugs made considerable attention to be given to correlation of *in vitro* dissolution rate with *in vivo* bioavailability[14]. It has been observed that with proper attention to the operating conditions, dissolution test can become a valuable indicator for potential *in-vivo* performance. *In vitro-in vivo* correlation (IV-IVC) is a predictive mathematical treatment describing the relationship between an in vitro property of a dosage form (usually the rate or extent of drug release) and a relevant *in vivo* response (e.g. plasma drug concentrations or amount of drug absorbed). Establishing an IV-IVC needs an extensive study of drug release from an oral drug delivery system. The study of drug in vitro availability and bioavailability are important part of the IV-IVC procedure for suitable drugs.[15] In order to develop safe and effective drugs and validate their formulation, it is important to identify the exact drug pharmacokinetic parameters and biopharmaceutical properties of the dosage forms.

The main objective of establishing IV-IVC is to use dissolution test as a surrogate for *in vivo* bioavailability studies and reduce the need for expensive human studies.[16, 17] When *in vitro-in vivo* correlations are established on a formulation, dissolution specifications can be used as a means of controlling drug bioavailability and hence a substitute for human bioequivalence studies.[5] There are different categories of IV-IVC; A, B, C and D. Level A correlation represents a point-to-point relationship between *in vitro* dissolution rate and *in vivo* input rate of drug from the dosage form.

Level B correlation utilizes the principle of statistical moment analysis, where the mean *in vitro* dissolution time (MDT_{vitro}) of the product is compared to either mean *in vivo* resident time (MRT) or the mean *in vivo* dissolution time (MDT_{vivo}). Level C correlation, compares one or several dissolution time points ($t_{50\%}$, $t_{90\%}$, etc.) to one or several mean pharmacokinetic parameter such as AUC, t_{max}, or C_{max},

Level D correlation is a rank order and qualitative analysis and is not considered useful for regulatory purposes. It is not a formal correlation but serves as an aid in the development of a formulation or processing procedure.[14]

In the last few years aspirin has become a life saver against cardiovascular complications in addition to its age long usefulness as an analgesic, antipyretic and anti-inflammatory agent.

Aspirin is rapidly absorbed by first order kinetics, following oral administration but is subjected to extensive metabolism to form salicylates which is rapidly and extensively distributed throughout body fluids. The salicylate level in the urine rapidly increases and can be easily detected and analyzed through colorimetric method.[18,19,20,11] In biopharmaceutics classification system (BCS), aspirin belong to class 2 (drug with low solubility but high permeability). Therefore, because, of its poor water solubility, the dissolution rate is the rate limiting step, which controls the absorption and bioavailability parameters of oral aspirin drug products. This criterion makes aspirin a good candidate for IV-IVC study, because any physico-chemical and formulation factors influencing its *in vitro* dissolution profile is expected to affect its in vivo bioavailability. *In vitro–in vivo* correlation of four commercial brands of aspirin tablets (one soluble brand and three regular brands) marketed in Nigeria are presented[21, 22]. Good correlations between various dissolution and bioavailability parameters of some drugs have been documented[12, 23, 24, 25, 26, 27]. However, in some cases, no good correlation could be obtained as reported by some investigators[28, 29, 30]. The following investigations were conducted:

a. *In vitro* dissolution profiles

In vitro dissolution profiles of the four brands of aspirin were evaluated, using USPXXI rotating basket apparatus. The dissolution profiles expressed as percents aspirin dissolved as a function of time for all the brands are shown in Figure 1. Various dissolution parameters such as percent dissolved in 30 min, dissolution rate constants (k) and time for 50% dissolution ($DT_{50\%}$) were obtained for all the brands using standard methods [2]. These are presented in Table 1.

Brand	Percent dissolved at 30 min	Dissolution rate constant, k (hr^{-1})	Time for 50% dissolution, $dt_{50\%}$ (min)
A1	75.71	0.059	11.79
A2	65.75	0.040	17.41
A3	63.47	0.037	18.53
A4	68.90	0.043	16.23

Table 1. Dissolution parameters obtained from the dissolution tests of the various brands of aspirin tablets

Figure 1 shows that A1 exhibited the highest dissolution rate while the other three brands (A2 - A4) has similar dissolution rates ($p < 0.05$). Table 1 shows that overall relative ranking of all the brands in terms of the percent dissolved in 30 min and dissolution rate constant (k) followed the order of A1>A4>A2>A3 while the ranking of time for 50% dissolution ($DT_{50\%}$) follows the reverse order (i.e. A1<A4<A2<A3). A1 is a soluble brand of aspirin containing calcium carbonate which can provide a reactive medium by changing the pH of the environment adjacent to the drug to alkaline, thus making the acidic drug like aspirin form a water soluble salt, thereby enhancing its rapid dissolution. This possibly accounted

for its highest solubility rate and shortest time for dissolution compared with the other plain brands[31]. Brands A2, A3 and A4 are all plain aspirin tablets; various factors such as particle size and shape of the aspirin content, type and/or amount of excipients, method of formulation and compression force employed may influence their dissolution rates [32, 5] The analysis of variance (ANOVA) performed on the percent dissolved in 30 min shows no significant difference ($P>0.05$) among all the brands, they all indicated similar statistical behaviors in their in vitro dissolution profiles.

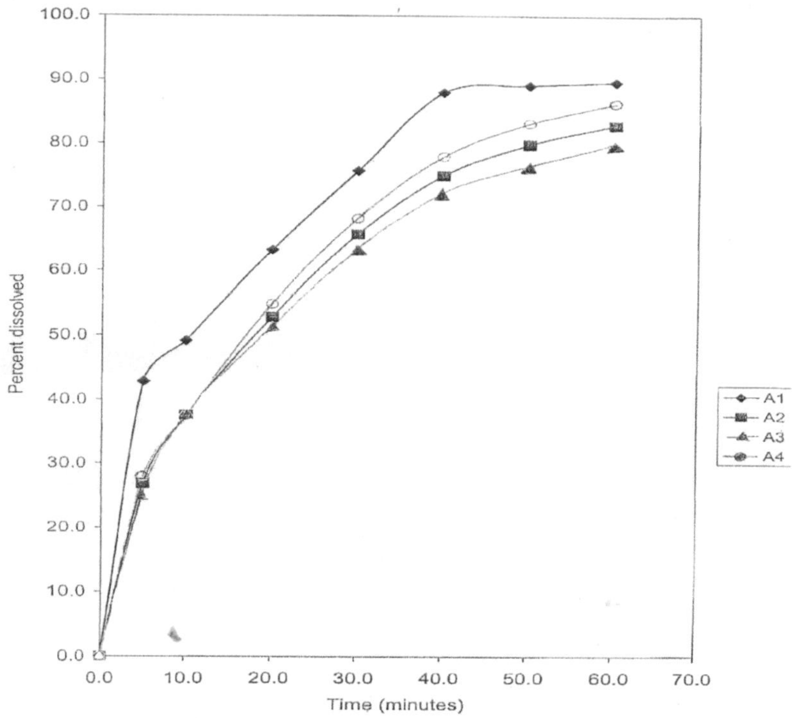

Fig. 1. Percent of actual amount of aspirin dissolved as a function of time for the four different brands.

b. *In vivo* bioavailability

In vivo bioavailability of the same set of aspirin tablets were assessed in eight human volunteers using urinary excretion profiles and various *in vivo* pharmacokinetic parameters such as cumulative amount excreted up to 8 h (E_8), maximum excretion rate $(dE/dt)_{max}$ and time for maximum excretion rate (T_{max}) were calculated using standard methods[30] and are presented in Table 2. The cumulative salicylate excreted and excretion rate profiles of the soluble aspirin and the three plain aspirin tablets are presented in figure 2 and 3 respectively. Pharmacokinetic parameters determined were cumulative amount excreted up to 8h (E_8) and 24h (E_{24}), maximum excretion rate (dE/dt)max and time for maximum excretion rate (T_{max})

Brand	Cumulative amount excreted up to 8h (E_8)	Cumulative amount excreted up to 24 h (E_{24})	Maximum excretion rate $(dE/dt)max$	Time for maximum excretion rate (T_{max})
A1	173.49	290.59	32.76	2.50
A2	165.15	275.68	29.93	3.38
A3	164.36	247.63	29.64	3.50
A4	169.79	281.10	31.36	3.13

Table 2. Pharmacokinetic parameters obtained from urinary excretion analysis of various brands of aspirin.

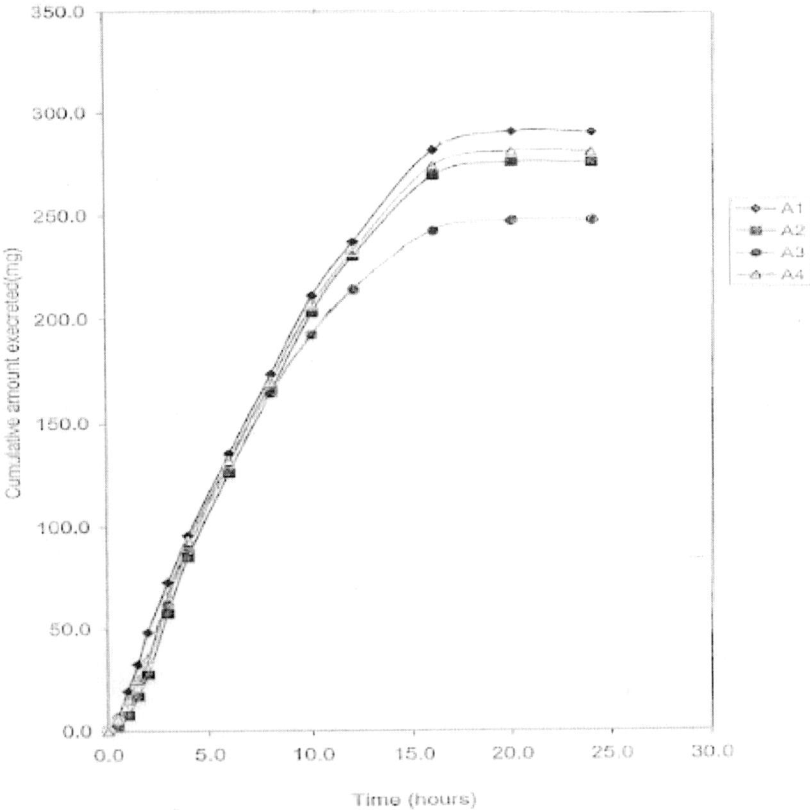

Fig. 2. Cumulative amount of salicylate excreted up to 24 h for the different brands of Aspirin.

The analysis of variance (ANOVA) performed on the pharmacokinetic parameters shows that all the four brands are bioequivalent in terms of (E_8), (E_{24}) and $(dE/dt)_{max}$, but the T_{max} of the three plain brands are inequivalent to the soluble brand A1 which has the fastest time for maximum excretion rate. Figure 3 shows that graphs for A2, A3 and A4 were almost super imposable attesting further to their equivalence. The formulation factors that enhanced the in vitro dissolution of the soluble aspirin are possibly responsible for increase in its in vivo bioavailability, compared to other plain brands, since its dissolution process is the rate limiting step [14, 29].

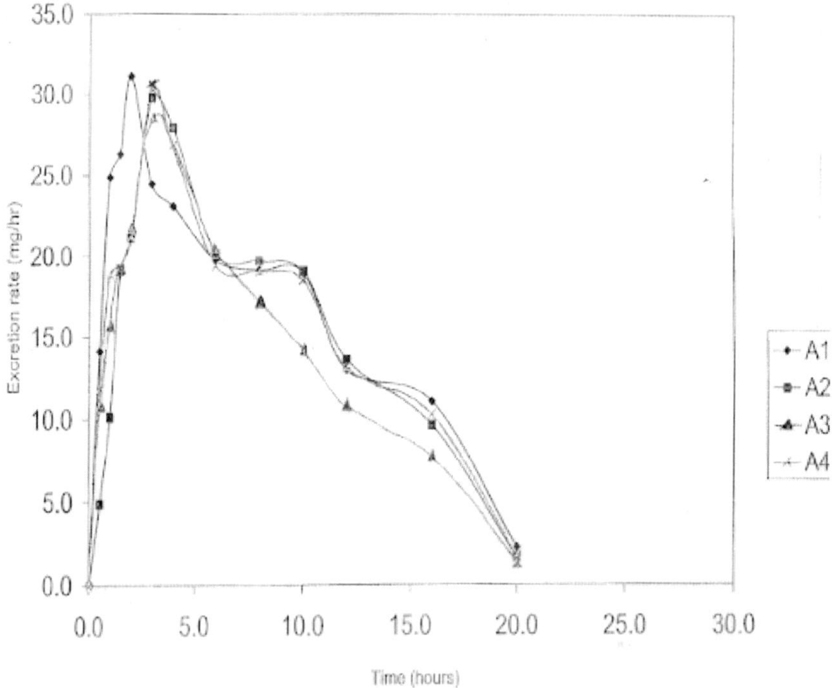

Fig. 3. Excretion rate profiles of the four different brands of Aspirin.

c. *In vitro-in vivo* correlation (IV- IVC)

To establish the relevance of the *in vitro* dissolution performances to the *in vivo* pharmacokinetic parameters of the four aspirin brands, level C IV-IVC was employed. When various dissolution parameters were correlated with various bioavailability parameters, no significant IV-IVC could be established using E_{24} value. However, significant IV-IVC was observed when cumulative amount excreted up to 8 hours (E_8) was employed (Figure 4) with correlation coefficients $r^2 > 0.8$. As shown in Figure 4, good quantitative correlation coefficients were observed between percent dissolved in 30 min and: (a) cumulative amount excreted up to 8 hours (E_8) ($r^2 = 0.9532$, $p < 0.05$), (b) Maximum excretion rate $(dE/dt)_{max}$, $r^2 = 0.9697$, $p < 0.05$) and (c) Time for maximum excretion rate (T_{max}) ($r^2 = 0.9932$, $p < 0.05$), thus the in vitro parameter correlated well with the in vivo parameters. Similarly, from Figure 5, good quantitative correlation coefficients were also observed between dissolution rate constant (k) and T_{max} ($r^2 = 0.9813$,

$p < 0.05$). With regards to E_8 and $(dE/dt)_{max}$, the correlation was not as perfect as that of T_{max}, with correlation coefficients just above 0.8, with exact values of 0.8564 and 0.8879 respectively.

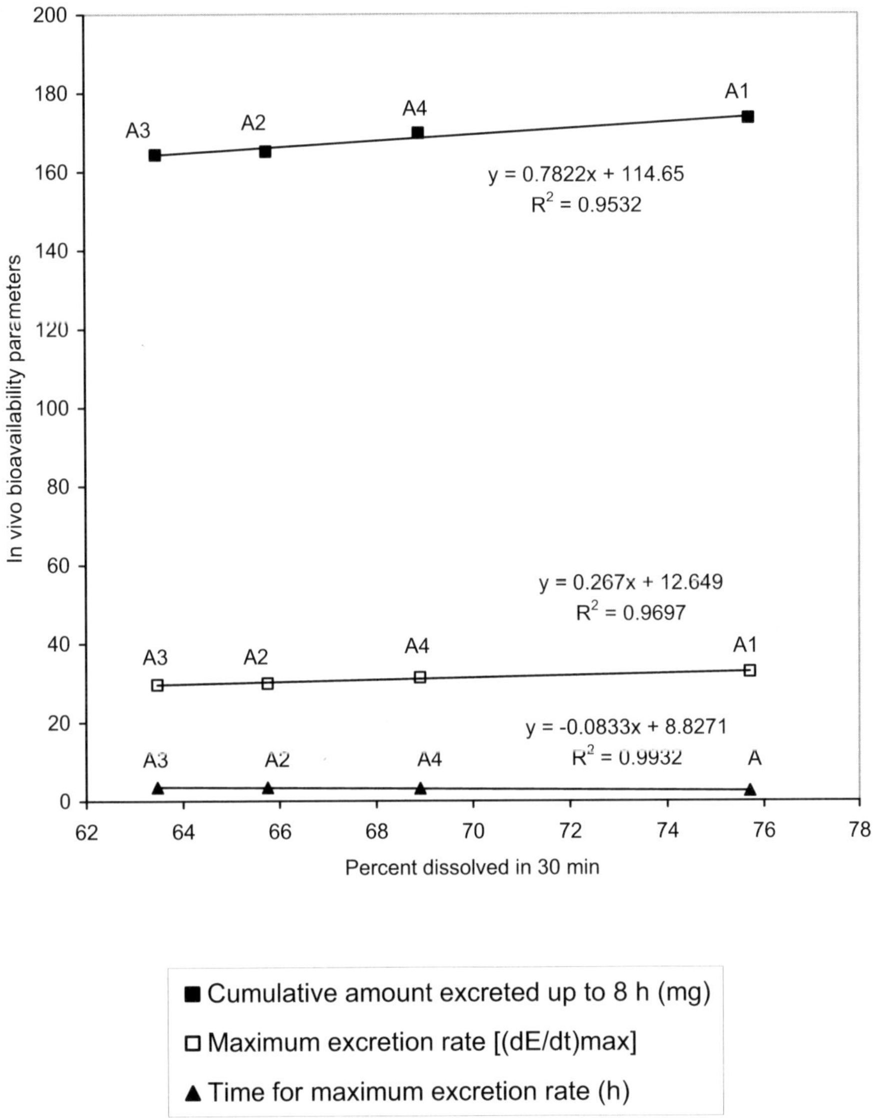

Fig. 4. Correlation of *in vitro* dissolution parameter (percent dissolved in 30 min) with various *in vivo* bioavailability parameters.

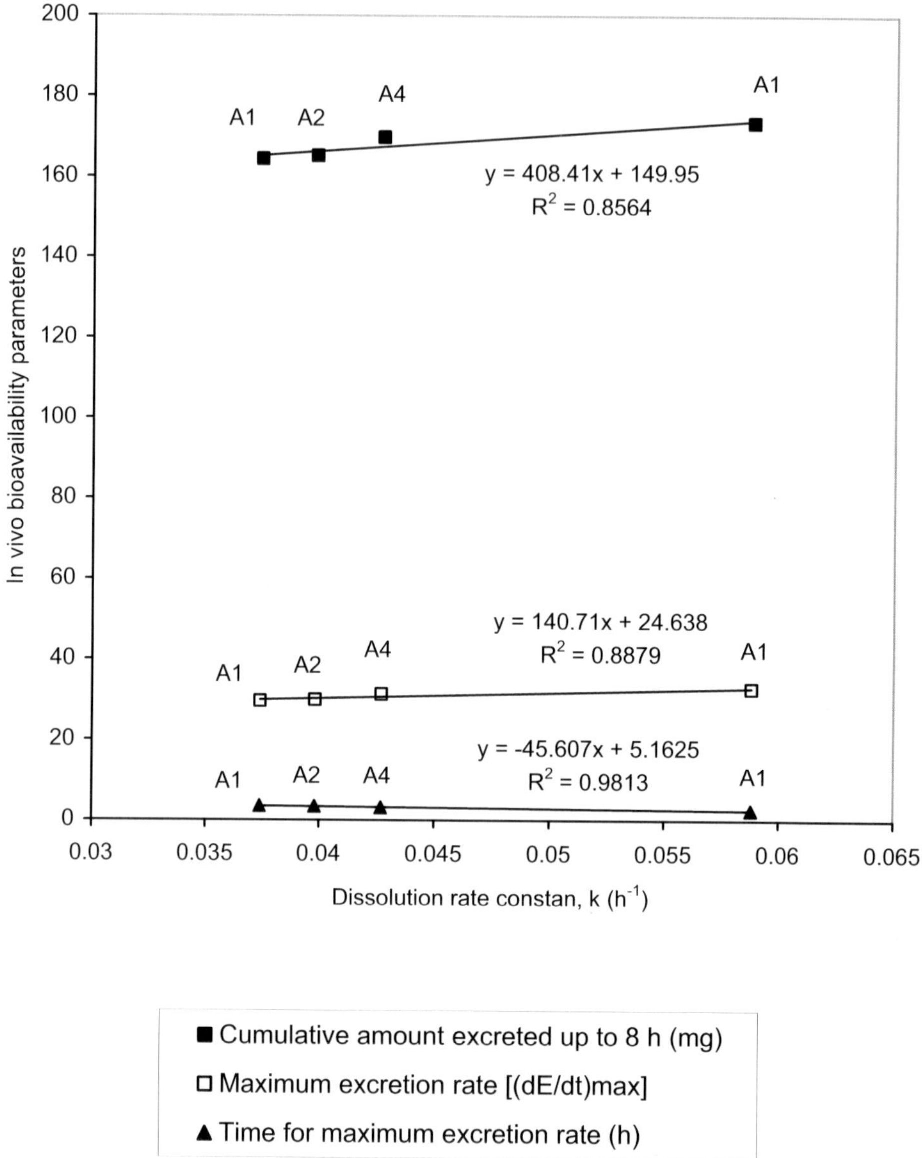

Fig. 5. Correlation of *in vitro* dissolution rate constant with various *in vivo* bioavailability parameters.

Finally, Figure 6 equally shows that good quantitative correlations were established between time for 50% dissolution ($DT_{50\%}$) and (a) E_8 ($r^2 = 0.9041$, $p < 0.05$), (b) $(dE/dt)_{max}$ ($r^2 = 0.9297$, $p < 0.05$) and (c) T_{max} ($r^2 = 0.9954$, $p < 0.05$)

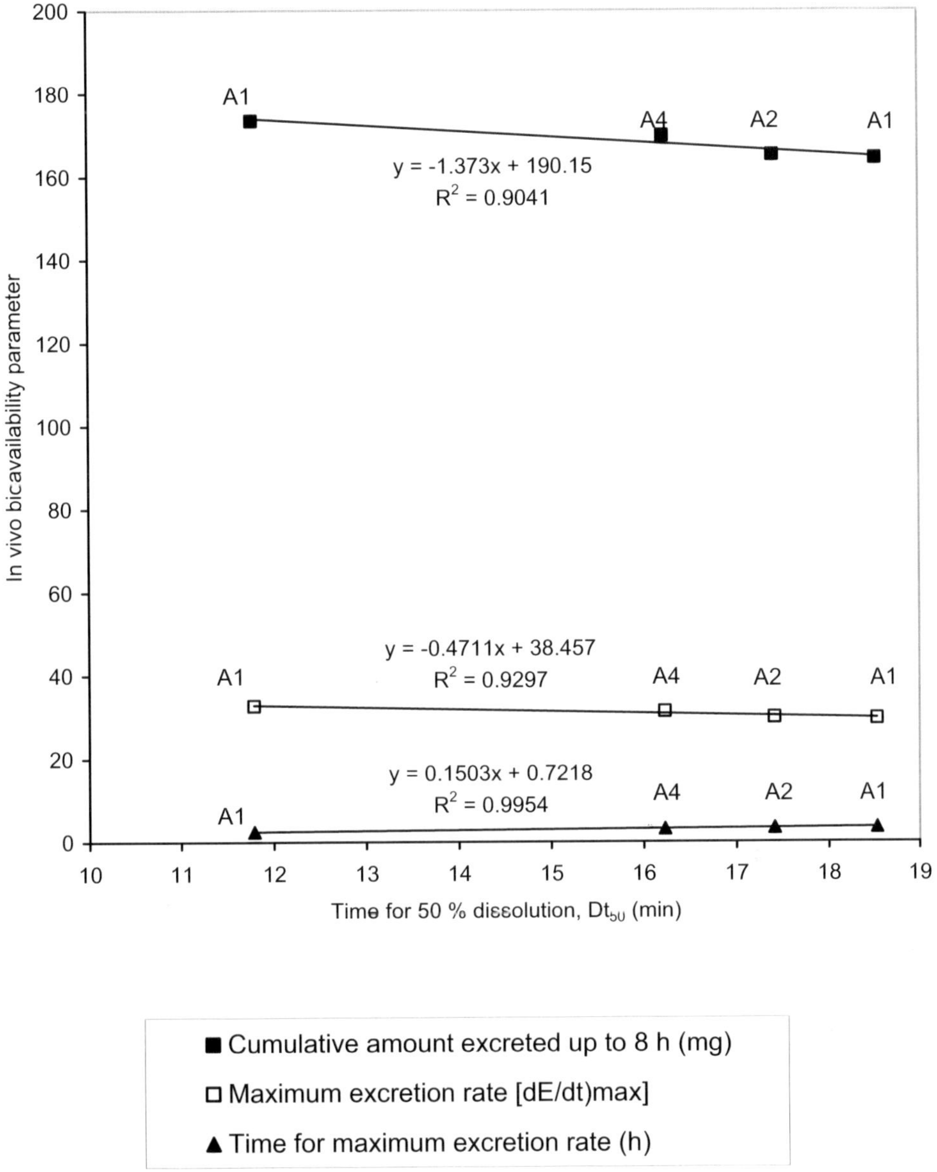

Fig. 6. Correlation of time for 50 % *in vitro* dissolution with various *in vivo* bioavailability parameters.

In all the IV-IVC performed, best correlation was obtained between the in vivo parameter T_{max}, and all the in vitro parameters used for the correlation. The correlation coefficient recorded in each case was higher than others. The significant IV-IVC observed were in agreement with the observations of some workers [12, 25] who carried out their own studies on aspirin in centers outside Nigeria.

2. Summary

Using USPXXI rotating basket dissolution apparatus, soluble brand of aspirin tablet A1 exhibited the highest dissolution profile, when compared to other plain brands of aspirin

ANOVA of pharmacokinetic data obtained from colorimetric assay of urinary salicylate excretion of the four brands of aspirin showed that all the four brands are bioequivalent in terms of (E_8), (E_{24}) and $(dE/dt)_{max}$, but the T_{max} of the three plain brands are not equivalent to the soluble brand A1 which has the fastest time for maximum excretion rate.

Good in vitro-in vivo correlations were established between various dissolution and bioavailability parameters of four commercial brands of aspirin tablets using Level C in vitro-in vivo correlation approach. Therefore, with proper standardization of methods of assessment, in vitro dissolution parameters can be used to predict in vivo bioavailability of these aspirin tablets marketed in Nigeria.

3. References

[1] Smith, R.V. and Stewart, J.T. Introduction in textbook of biopharmaceutical analysis: Philadelphia: Henry Kimpton publisher 1981; pp 3-15

[2] Shargel, L and Yu A.B.C. (3rd edn). Applied Biopharmaceutics and Pharmacokinetics, New Jersey, USA: Appleton and Lange, 1993; pp 599.

[3] Wilfred, O. O., Ogunbona, F. O. and Olaniyi, O. O. Biopharmaceutical Methods. In A. A. Olaniyi (edn). Principles of Drug Quality Assurance and Pharmaceutical Analysis. Ibadan. Mosuro publisher 2000; pp 388 – 429.

[4] Akanni, O.O. Bioequivalence of medicinal products. In A. A. Olaniyi (1st edn). Towards Better Quality Assurance of Drug and Food. Ibadan, Nigeria, Department of Pharmaceutical Chemistry, University of Ibadan, 1993; pp 125 -135.

[5] Olaniyi, A.A., Babalola, C.P., Oladeinde, F.O., and Adegoke, A.O. (9th edn). Towards Better Quality Assurance of Drugs. In Biopharmaceutical methods. Department of Pharmaceutical Chemistry, University of Ibadan, 2001; pp. 7 – 23.

[6] Pernarowski, M. Dissolution methodology. In J.T. Carstensen (edn). Dissolution Technology. Washington, D.C. Academy of Pharmaceutical Sciences, 1975; pp 58

[7] Dakkuri, A., Shah, A. C. Dissolution methodology: An overview. Pharmaceutical Technology, 1982; pp 28 -32

[8] Hardwidge, E., Saparu, A and Laughlin, W. Comparison of operating characteristics of different dissolution test system. Journal of Pharmaceutical Sciences. 1978; 66:1732 - 1735

[9] Mandal, T. K., Chiao, C. S. and Ace, L. N. Evaluation of in vitro-in vivo correlation utilizing a rotating basket paddle dissolution apparatus. Drug Dev. Ind. Pharm. 1995; 21(13):1529-1543

[10] Levy, G. Clinical pharmacokinetics of salicylates: A re-assessment. British Journal of Clinical Pharmacology. 1980; 10: 2855-2860

[11] Joseph, C. (1987). Special problems with biological fluids. In: Analysis of Drug in Biological Fluids (4th Edn.) Florida, CRC Press Inc., 1984; pp. 25 – 48.

[12] Gadalla, M.A.F., Abd El-Hameed, M.H. and Ismail, A.A. *In vivo* evaluation of commercial and formulated conventional aspirin tablets. Drug Dev. Ind. Pharm. 1986; 12(5): 747 – 781.

[13] Quiroga, P. A., Bustillo, P. M. and Volonte, M. G. In vitro dissolution and urinary excretion study of metoclopramide tablets. Biopharmaceutics and Drug Disposition. 1998; 19: 479 - 482

[14] Emami, J. In vitro – In vivo Correlation: From Theory to Applications. J Pharm. Pharmaceut Sci. 2006; 9(2): 169 – 189.

[15] Xiao Hong, M., Michael, J.-T., John, N. Development and evaluation of bio-dissolution systems capable of detecting the food effect on a polysaccharide-based matrix system. J. Control. Release 2003; 93: 309–318.

[16] Leeson, L. J. *In vitro / In vivo* correlations. Drug Inform. J. 1995; 29: 903 – 915.

[17] Shah, V.P., Lesko, L.J. Current challenges and future regulatory directions in *in vitro* dissolution. Drug Inform. J. 1995; 29: 885–891.

[18] Rowland, M., Riegelman, S., Harris, P. A. and Sholkoff, S. D. Absorption kinetics of aspirin in man following oral administration of aqueous solution. Journal of Pharmaceutical Sciences. 1972; 61:379-385

[19] Miaskiewicz, S.L., Shively, C, A. and Vesell, E.S. Sex difference in absorption kinetics of sodium salicylate. Clinical Pharmacology and Therapeutics. 1982; 31: 30-37

[20] Chio, W. L. and Onyemelukwe, I. Simple modified colorimetric method for total salicylate assay in urine after salicylate administration. J. Pharm. Sci.1974; 63(4): 630-632.

[21] Amidon, G. L., Robinson, J. R., and Williams, R. L. (edn.). Scientific Foundations for Regulating Drug Product Quality. American Association of Pharmaceutical Scientists. Alexandria, Virginia: AAPS Press. 1997.

[22] Young, D., Devane, J. G., and Butler, J. (Eds.). *In Vitro - In Vivo* Correlations. New York: Plenum Press. 1997

[23] Wood, R. W., Martis, L., Lin, L. and Bernardo, P. *In vivo* bioavailability of commercial Levothyroxine sodium tablets in the hypothyroid dog model. 1990; 79(2): 124 - 127.

[24] Hussein, Z., and Friedman, M. Release and absorption characteristics of novel theophylline sustained-release formulations: In *vitro/ in vivo* correlation. Pharmaceutical Research. 1990; 7(11): 1167- 1171.

[25] Derendorf, H., Drehsen, G. and Rohdewald, P. *In vitro – in vivo* correlation of salicylate saliva levels and continuous flow cell dissolution rate. Int. J. Pharm. 1983; 15(6): 167 - 175.

[26] Jung, H., Milan, R. C., Girard, M. E., Leon, F., and Montoya, M. A. Bioequivalence study of carbamazepine tablets: *In vitro/In vivo* correlation. International Journal Pharmaceutics. 1997; 152: 37- 44.

[27] Abuzarur-aloul, R., Gjellan, K., Sjound, M., and Graffner, C. Critical dissolution tests of oral systems based on statistically designed experiments. III. *In vitro/in vivo* correlation for multiple-unit capsule of paracetamol based on PLS modeling. Drug Development and Industrial Pharmacy. 1998; 24: 371-383.

[28] Amamar, H. O., and Khalil, R. M. Discrepancy among dissolution rates of commercial tablets as a function of dissolution method. Part 3: In vitro/in vivo correlation of paracetamol tablets. Pharmazie. 1993; 48: 136-139.

[29] Gordon, M.S., Ellis, D.J. and Molony, B. *In vitro* dissolution versus in *vivo* evaluation of four different aspirin products. Drug Dev. Ind. Pharm. 1994; 20(10): 1711 – 1723.

[30] Khan, M. K., Khan, M. F., Khan, H. and Mustafa G. (2009). Bioavailability of Ciprofloxacin tablets in humans and its correlation with the dissolution rate. Pak. J. Pharm. Sci. 2009; 22(3): 329-334.

[31] Serajuddin, A. T. Salt formation to improve drug solubility. Adv. Drug Deliv. Rev. 2007; 59(7) 603-616

[32] Kader, A. and Jalil, R. Formulation factors affecting drug release from poly (lactic acid) (PLA) microcapsule tablets. Drug Dev. Ind. Pharm. 1999; 25(2): 141-151.

Optimal Pharmacokinetics of Cyclosporine and Tacrolimus Based Relationship Among AUC, Trough and Peak Concentration

Hironori Takeuchi
Department of Practical Pharmacy,
Tokyo University of Pharmacy and Life Sciences, Tokyo
Japan

1. Introduction

Calcineurin inhibitors (CNIs) are maintenance immunosuppressive drugs that have been used as the main therapy for organ transplantation for many years. Of the CNIs, cyclosporine (CYA) and tacrolimus (TAC) are used in clinical practice. The CYA binding protein is cyclophilin and that of TAC is FK-binding protein (FKBP), but both drugs have same mechanism of action: the inhibition of interleukin 2 (IL-2) production by binding the binding protein complex to calcineurin (CN). It is thought that the area under the concentration time curve (AUC) for both drugs may be the pharmacokinetic (PK) parameter that is the most associated with clinical effect. However, oral CYA administration gave a blood concentration–time curve with a high CYA peak concentration (C_p), and oral TAC showed a gradual blood concentration–time curve, keeping at the minimum of the therapeutic range; both drugs vary significantly in their pharmacokinetics[1)]. The C_p of CYA has increased since the Neoral® preparation of CYA was used, compared with Sandimmune®, whereas the C_p of TAC decreased since using a sustained release preparation; thus the differences between CYA and TAC are considerable[2)]. Although the optimal pharmacokinetics of both drugs may be similar to those of other drugs with the same mechanism of action, no conclusions have been reached on whether the peak blood concentration, or a specific maintained blood concentration, is required for CNI pharmacokinetics, even if both drugs show identical AUCs. In addition, although CYA and TAC are similar CNI drugs, there are differences in the recommended monitoring points of CYA and TAC; these points are the C_2 level (the blood concentration 2 h after oral administration), which mainly reflects $C_{p,}$ and the trough concentration (C_t)[3-8)], respectively[9-11)]. To solve these problems, it is necessary to consider comprehensively not only AUC, but also C_p, C_t, and time above the minimum effective concentration (%T > MEC). We discuss the optimal pharmacokinetics of CNIs by comparing various aspects of CYA and TAC.

2. Which parameter is the most closely associated with clinical results?

2.1 Cyclosporine

It is a well-known fact that C_t is associated with clinical effect. As when the C_t become higher, the AUC and the Ct $_p$ are consequently higher. it is not surprising that C_t, C_p, and

AUC are all correlated with clinical effect. The question, therefore, is which of these PK parameters is the most associated with clinical effect. It is commonly thought that the AUC of CYA is most closely associated with clinical effect[12,13]. However, it is often difficult to measure $AUC_{0\text{-}12}$ for 12 h after administration in clinical practice. Accordingly $AUC_{0\text{-}4}$ (the area under the concentration time curve at 0–4 h following oral administration) is generally used as an alternative absorption phase to $AUC_{0\text{-}12}$. This earlier blood sampling point that has been used since the introduction of cyclosporine microemulsion preconcentrate (Neoral), in which oral absorption is significantly stabilized[3,14]. Even $AUC_{0\text{-}4}$ requires several blood sampling points, and this causes problems such as increased burden on patients, cost, and medical staff duties. It has therefore been recommended that a single blood sampling point, C_2, be used; this is the sampling point at which the majority of patients show peak level in the absorption phase, and is better correlated with $AUC_{0\text{-}12}$ than C_0[3-8]. It has been reported that $AUC_{0\text{-}4}$ and C_2 are associated with the incidence rate of acute rejection and nephropathy or similar conditions[3,15-19], and a relationship with clinical effects and side effects was demonstrated. Nevertheless, there are several problems relating to the use of C_2 because its determination involves the measurement of absorption values. As it means the change in blood concentration over time is great; there is a possibility that C_2 may vary significantly over a small interval in blood sampling times, in comparison with trough value [20,21], and complicated procedures for outpatients are increased. Given the above, the monitoring of C_2 in routine clinical practice is questionable [22,23], and it has been reported that there is little evidence in which it is useful to monitor C_2[24].

2.2 Tacrolimus

On the other hand, the AUC of TAC, like that of CYA, is commonly considered to be a parameter which is highly associated with clinical effect, despite little evidence for TAC treatment showing clinical effects such as acute rejection[25,26] or side effects such as nephrotoxicity[27]. Therefore, TAC was examined to show which blood sampling point is the best correlated with AUC as CYA. One study reported that C_o is the best correlated with AUC[27], whereas another study suggested that a formula with fewer blood sampling points, and not C_o, is the most closely correlated with AUC (limited sampling strategy) [28-31].

Thus, although the AUC of CNIs is regarded as the PK parameter, which is the most closely associated with clinical effect, its monitoring point is not clear. In addition, it has not been much discussed whether the peak blood concentration, or a specific maintained blood concentration, is required for pharmacokinetics even if both drugs show identical AUC. For the purpose of solving this problem, the authors analyzed the pharmacokinetics of CYA and TAC by comparing AUC, C_p, and C_t parameters, used not as independent parameters but in a new manner, which could indicate the interrelationship between these parameters.

2.3 Comparison between pharmacokinetics of oral cyclosporine and tacrolimus[1]

There has been no study comparing the differences between the blood concentration time curves of CYA and TAC in detail. Therefore, the authors thought that the pharmacokinetics of both drugs could be compared by using the blood concentration (C/D/BW), adjusted for dose per body weight. Although the AUC/(D/BW) of both CYA and TAC, which should show the relative availabilities, was equal, the C_p/(D/BW) of CYA was comparatively higher than that of TAC and, on the other hand, the C_t/(D/BW) of CYA was lower than that of TAC, which illustrated a blood concentration time curve with a sharp peak. On the other hand, the pharmacokinetics of TAC showed that the C_p/(D/BW) of TAC was lower and the C_t/(D/BW) was higher, which illustrated a gently hunched blood concentration time curve, which was similar to the curve for continuous intravenous infusion (Figure 1, Table 1).

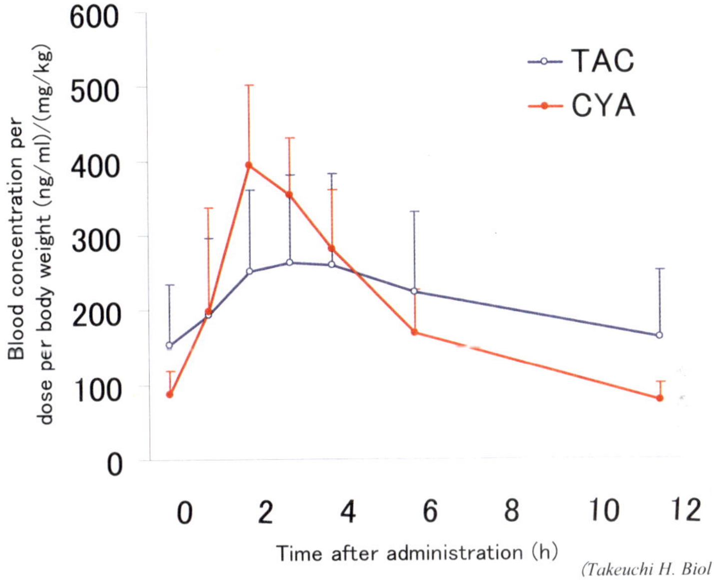

Fig. 1. Comparison of the mean blood concentration-time curves for CYA (n=20) and TAC (n=24)

	CYA (n = 20)	TAC (n = 24)	p value
AUC/D/BW (ng/mL·h)/(mg/kg)	2323±447	2507±1255	N.S.
C_p/C_t	6.00±1.78	1.93±0.43	<0.0001
C_p/D/BW (ng/mL)/(mg/kg)	433.1±90.3	292.6±135.7	<0.005
C_t/D/BW (ng/mL)/(mg/kg)	77.1±23.6	160.0±91.8	<0.005
AUTL/AUC(%)	41.9±6.9	73.4±8.1	<0.0001

(Takeuchi H. Biol Pharm Bull. 2008)

Table 1. Comparison of pharmacokinetic parameters between CYA and TAC

Thus, even if the AUC of both drugs were equal, the pharmacokinetics of the both drugs is totally different, from the viewpoint of the correlation with each peak value and each trough value. We developed AUTL/AUC% (percentage of the area under the trough level in the area under the blood concentration) in order to assess the interrelationship between AUC, C_p, and C_t in comparing CYA and TAC (Figure 2). As a result, the AUTL/AUC% of CYA was as low as 41.9%, and the AUC had a higher percentage of dependence on C_p than on C_t. On the contrary, the AUTL/AUC% of TAC was as high as 73.4%, and the AUC had a higher percentage of dependence on C_t than on C_p (Figure 3).

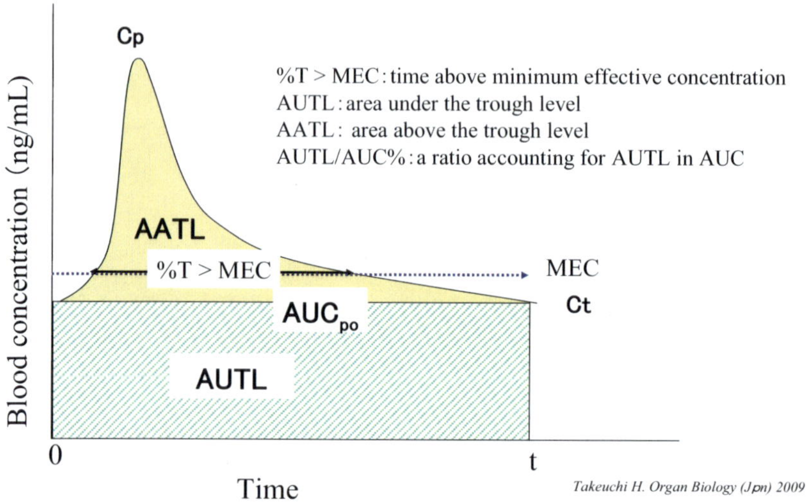

Fig. 2. Blood concentration curve and pharmacokinetic parameters

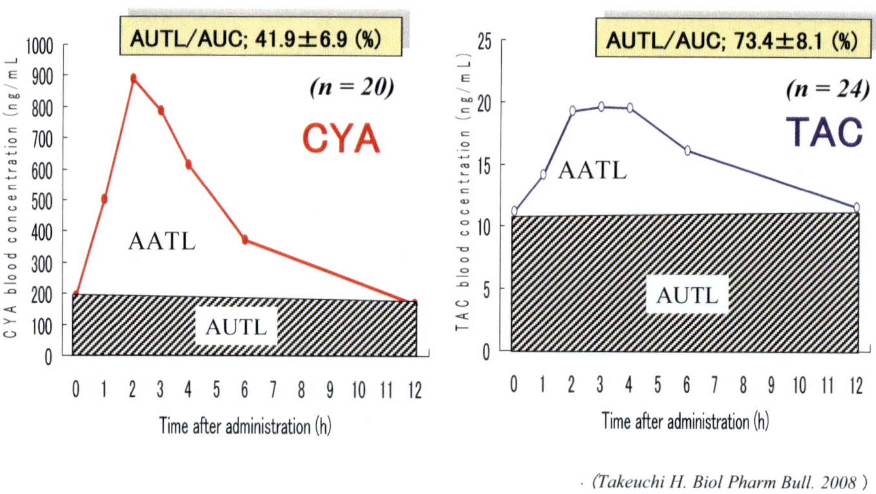

Fig. 3. Comparison of the pharmacokinetic parameters of AUTL/AUC% between CYA and TAC.

To demonstrate these results further, we examined the correlation between the AUC and the area above trough level (AATL) or AUTL, and found that these results were consistent with the theory that CYA had higher correlation with AATL, and TAC had higher correlation with AUTL (Table 2). If AUC is most closely associated with clinical effect, it may be appropriate to monitor C_p and C_t for CYA and TAC, respectively. However, considering that the blood concentration per unit time for C_p changes dramatically, and taking into account the measurement convenience and complexity of the methods, it is thought that TAC to measure Ct is preferable as a drug to perform TDM than CYA to recommend measuring C_2. However, it is thought that Ct as monitoring paint is not a clinical problem, as the measurement of CYA Ct reflects the AUC adequately.

	correlation coefficients (R^2)	
	AUC vs. AUTL	AUC vs. AATL
CYA (n = 20)	0.7110	0.9024
TAC (n = 24)	0.9029	0.7123

Takeuchi H. Organ Biology (Jpn) 2009

Table 2. Comparison of correlation coefficients between AUC and AUTL or AATL in CYA- and TAC-treated recipients

Furthermore, the influences on clinical effect, such as effectiveness or side effects, would be different between pharmacokinetics with a higher peak value, namely with low AUTL/AUC% and pharmacokinetics with a maintained minimum effective concentration, namely with high AUTL/AUC%, such as the blood concentration of continuous intravenous infusion, even if the AUC of both drugs were equal. By illustrating this, as shown in Figure 4, it is possible to see a difference between the pharmacokinetics of A and B, even if both AUCs are equal. The C_{max} of A is lower than that of B but the C_{min} of A is higher than that of B. This relation can be applied to the correlation of CYA and TAC discussed above. In addition, considering PK parameters involved pharmacodynamics (PD) such as the minimum effective concentration (MEC), A may maintain MEC over a certain time (%T > MEC), which is longer than for B, even if the AUCs for both A and B are equal. CNIs may be a drug for which time above MIC (MEC) is associated with drug efficacy, as is the case with antimicrobial agents such as beta-lactam antibiotics, This suggests that the effects of A and B may be different, by the correlation of AUC, C_p, and C_t.

Thus, the examination of clinical effect using only AUC is limited, and therefore, an analysis including the interrelationship between AUC, C_p, C_t, and time is required.

3. Correlations among AUTL/AUC%, effects, side effects, and PK parameters for other drugs practicing TDM

Table 3 shows the results of correlations among the PK parameters, effects, and side effects of current drugs investigated for TDM in the literature. As a result, the blood concentration time curves can be classified into the following categories: a drug group showing a sharp peak curve (AUTL/AUC < 50%, $C_p/C_t > 6$), such as aminoglycoside antibiotics (AGs), and a drug group showing a gentle peak curve (AUTL/AUC% > 60%, $C_{max}/C_{min} < 2$), such as antiarrhythmic drugs, bronchodilators, and anticonvulsant drugs (Figure 5).

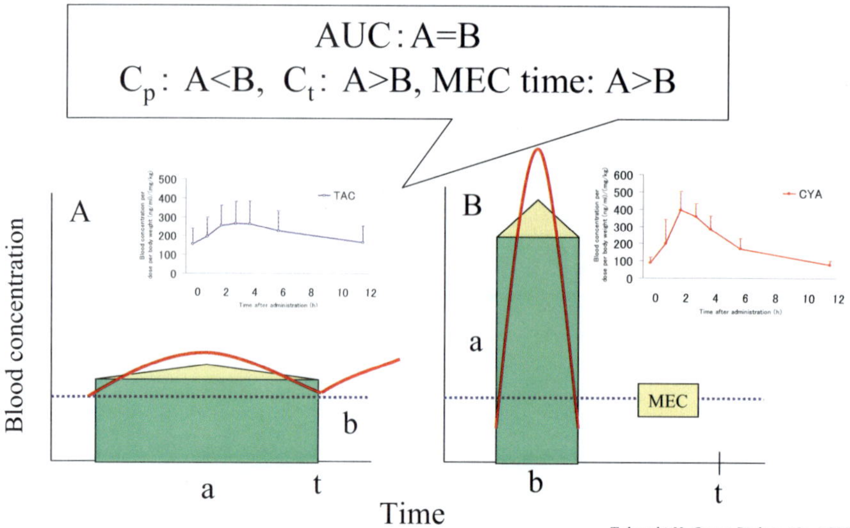

Fig. 4. Pattern diagrams in the case that C_p, C_t, and MEC time are different, even though AUC is the same.

drug	AUTL/AUC%	C_p/C_t	efficacy parameter	side effect parameter
Cyclosporine MEPC*	41.9±6.9	6.0±1.8	AUC_{0-4}、C_2、Ct	AUC_{0-4}, C_2, Ct
Tacrolimus	73.4±8.1	1.9±0.4	C_t	C_t
Amikacin*(injection)	16.5	14.4	Cmax	Ct(Cmax)
Vancomycin*(injection)	29.8	11.1	Ct	Ct(Cmax)
Teicoplanin*(injection)	47.1	6.0	Ct	Ct
Disopyramide	76.8	1.7	C_t maintenance of effective blood concentration	C_t
Procainamide	65.1	1.9		
Mexiletine	71.6	1.8		
Sodium valproate	90.4	1.2		
	75.9	1.7		
Theophylline	90.5	1.3		
	72.4	1.9		
	80.7	1.5		
	77.6	1.5		
	82.7	1.5		

*AUTL/AUC%<50%、Cmax/Cmin>6

Takeuchi H. Organ Biology (Jpn) 2009

Table 3. AUTL/AUC%, C_p/C_t, and parameters of the efficacy and side effect of drugs that are used in therapeutic drug monitoring (TDM)

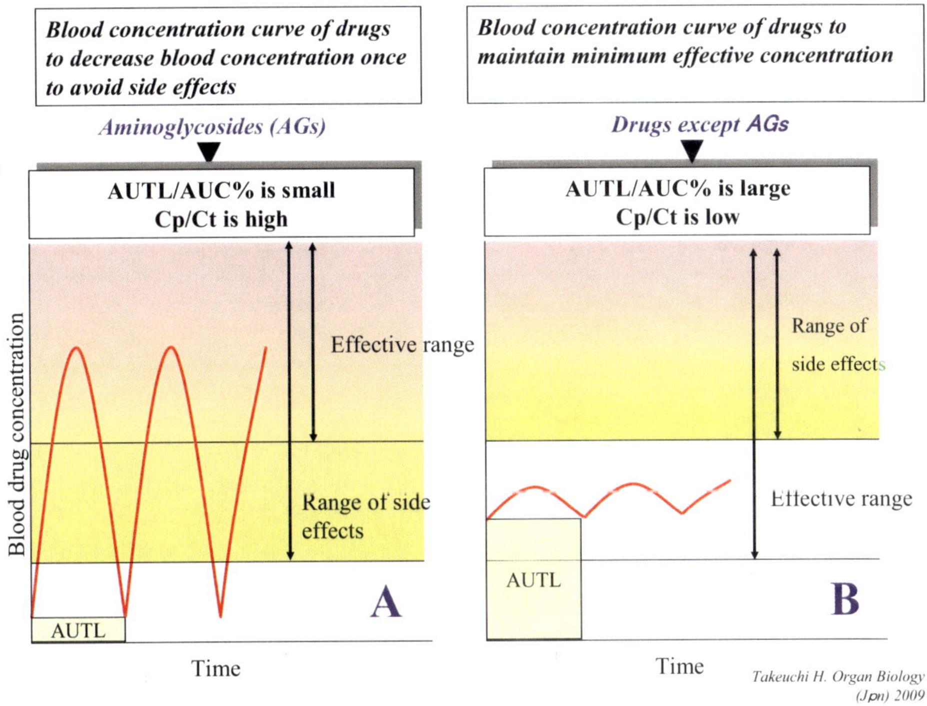

Fig. 5. Two patterns of blood concentration curve based on AUTL/AUC%

All drugs except AGs, glycopeptide antibiotics, and CYA, which required AUTL/AUC% ≥60% and C_p/C_t ≤2 to maintain the therapeutic range, had a gentle blood concentration time curve and the monitoring point was C_t. It is preferred that AGs maintain a concentration to the peak value for as long as possible, but it must be reduced to below a specific blood concentration on a temporary basis to avoid nephrotoxic side effects. Therefore, AUTL/AUC% decreased to a low level and C_p/C_t increased to a high level to show a blood concentration time curve with a sharp peak. Furthermore, AGs have a post-antibiotic effect (PAE), so that it can maintain its effect even if it falls below the therapeutic range.

Furthermore, the pharmacokinetics of AGs and glycopeptide antibiotics relate to administration by injection, and these drugs are not required to control a clinical condition for a long period. Therefore, the results showed that CYA (Neoral) was the only oral drug used for prevention of a long-term pathologic condition that showed a sharp peak curve. Drugs with a sharp peak concentration were the only drugs for which the blood concentration needed to be reduced on a temporary basis to avoid side effects, and there was no drug that needed to be at peak concentration in order to have an effect. However, when the CYA used was switched from Sandimmune to Neoral to increase and stabilize absorption, the absorption rate constant (K_a) became large such that the peak value necessarily increased, and the AUTL/AUC% decreased.

CYA may not require higher peak concentration, if the trough concentration can be higher to keep the AUC, although it is impossible that raising the trough value and decreasing the peak value (to increase the AUTL/AUC%) using the existing CYA formulation, keep the AUC.

4. Optimal pharmacokinetics based on PK/PD analysis

In connection with the preceding paragraph, regarding patients treated with CYA (Neoral), it has been reported that the inhibitory action of CN was in proportion to the blood concentration following administration[32], and that IL-2 was stably suppressed at the peak value rather than the trough value[33]. On the other hand, another report showed that TAC above a certain level continuously had an inhibitory action of CN after administration[34]. It is possible that the differences between the both drugs may contribute to these results (Figure 6). In other words, CYA shows sufficient CN inhibitory action at the peak value, but the data suggests that the CN inhibitory action may be insufficient at the trough value. On the other hand, TAC is at a concentration that shows a certain level of CN inhibitory action throughout all time points, including the trough value, which suggests that it may always show inhibitory action of CN above a certain concentration.

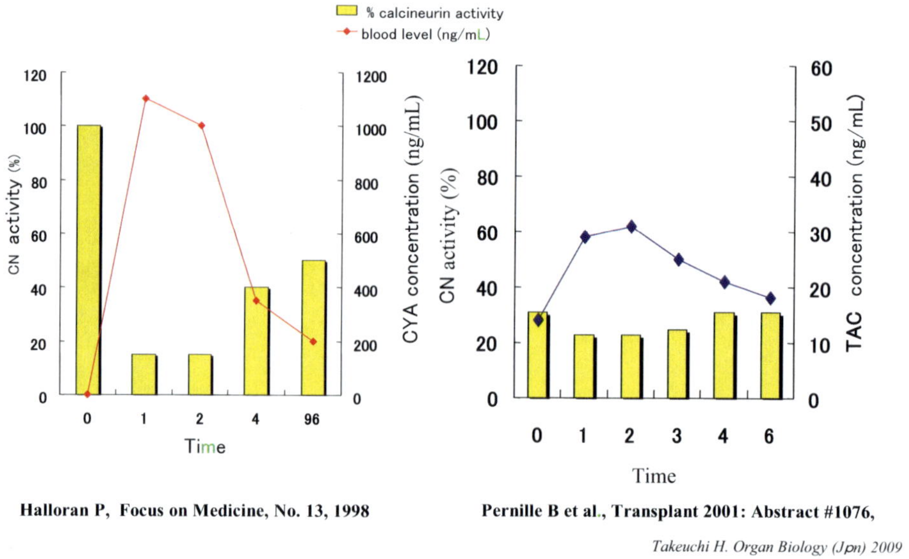

Fig. 6. Relationship between blood concentration and calcineurin activity in CYA and TAC.

The authors analyzed the relationship of the concentration–lymphocyte proliferation rate curves (PD) of CYA and TAC with the target blood concentration (PK) and found that lymphocyte proliferation was completely suppressed at the trough level of TAC. On the other hand, CYA had a low inhibition ratio at the trough value and was more than sufficient inhibited at the peak value, so that there was no need for the concentration to be as high as the peak value in terms of pharmacodynamics; consequently, it was necessary to make the trough value higher (Figure 7).

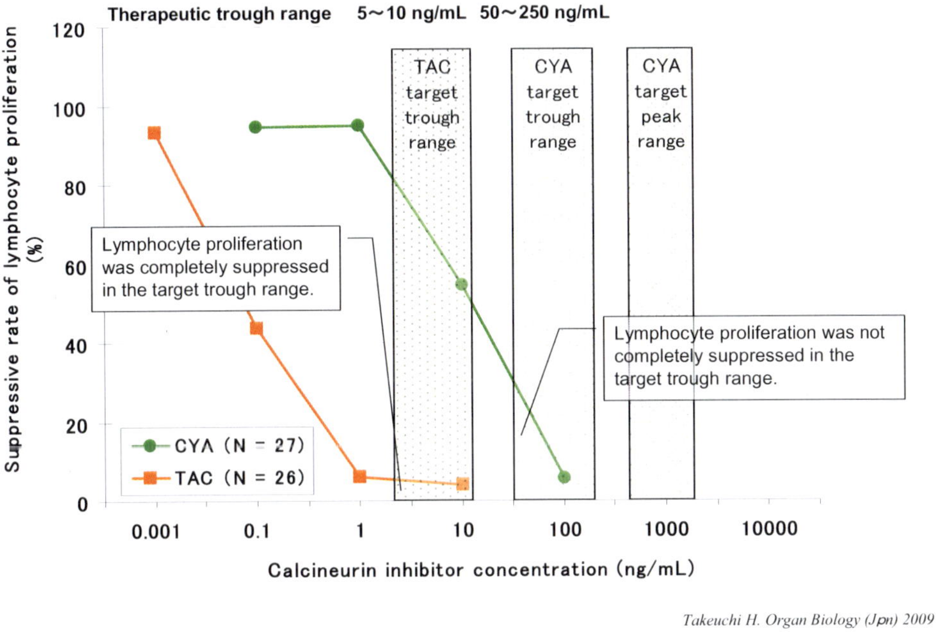

Fig. 7. Relationship between average concentration-lumphocyte proliferation rate curves and target blood concentration of calcineurin inhibitors.

5. Optimal blood concentration for continuous intravenous infusion based on AUC

Currently, intermittent intravenous administration and 24-h continuous intravenous administration can be compared for optimal pharmacokinetics in clinical practice.

For patients undergoing hematopoietic stem cell transplantation, drugs are administered by intravenous injection for relatively long periods, from several weeks to several months, because ingestion is not possible. However, the theoretical optimum targeted blood concentration for continuous infusion has never been clearly determined. If AUC is the parameter most closely associated with clinical effect, it can be considered correct, in theory, to adjust the blood concentration of oral and intravenous administration to the level that achieves the same AUC. We used the AUTL (area under trough level) parameter developed by the authors to calculate the target blood concentration for continuous intravenous infusion from the trough level for oral administration[35,36]. As a result, the target blood concentration for continuous intravenous infusion of TAC (C_{ss}) was 1.4 times that of the C_t because AUTL/AUC% is large. These results were almost close to the blood concentration in the present practice of continuous intravenous infusion. Meanwhile, CYA has a small AUTL/AUC% so that a trough value 2.55 times higher and a considerably high C_{ss} were required in theory (Figure 8).

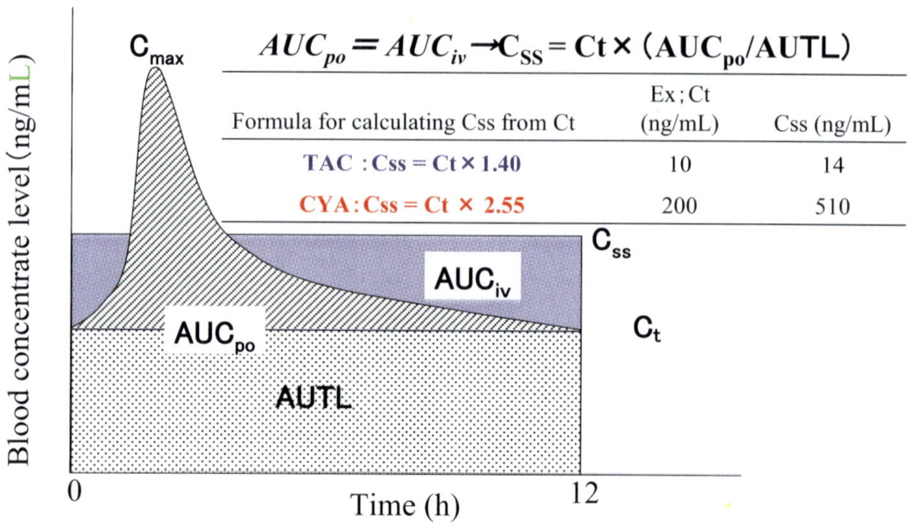

Nakamuka Y, Transplant Proc, 2005

Fig. 8. Formula for calculating C_{ss} from C_t, and the relationship between the AUC of oral administration and continuous intravenous infusion.

In actual hematopoietic stem cell transplantation, it has been reported that continuous intravenous infusion of CYA at 250–400 ng/mL C_{ss}, which is lower than the theoretical value, showed lower nephrotoxicity than intermittent intravenous administration twice a day, and that the incidence rate of acute graft-versus-host disease (GVHD) was high[37]. However, in a study by the same group, comparing a 300 ng/mL C_{ss} group with a 500 ng/mL C_{ss} group, it was reported that the incidence rates of acute and chronic GVHD were significantly lower in the 500 ng/mL group, and there was no difference in side effects, such as nephrotoxicity, between both groups of the trial[38]. In another study by Miller et al. using a C_{ss} of 450–500 ng/mL, similar results on acute GVHD and tolerability were reported[39] and these reports were consistent with the authors' hypothesis. Continuous intravenous infusion is the ultimate method for maintaining a minimum effective concentration (Figure 4-A), and it may be possible for the pharmacokinetics to have no peak if the AUC of CYA can be obtained; in other words, the pharmacokinetics as minimum effective concentration is maintained.

Meanwhile, in many institutions, patients undergoing hematopoietic stem cell transplantation received different dosages, such as 3 mg/kg/day twice a day (3 h continuous infusion) by I.V. infusion, once a day (4 h continuous infusion) by I.V. infusion, once a day (10 h continuous infusion) by I.V. infusion, and 24 h continuous intravenous. However, there are slight differences in the clinical results[40]. Each AUC was almost the same, at around 11,000 ng·h/mL, in all the dosages above, but the results calculated by the authors revealed that each AUTL/AUC% was approximately equal (35-44%) in intermittent administration and it was 100% in continuous intravenous infusion (Figure 9). Moreover, we set various therapeutic ranges to simulate and calculate %T > MEC and found that the values significantly varied depending on MEC (Figure 10). These results suggest that CYA has a wide tolerance of blood concentration in terms of action and side effects, and that all dosages might be clinically equal.

methods of administration	24 h CIV	10 h × 1	3 h × 2	p.o. × 2	4 h × 1
Dose	3 mg/kg/day	3 mg/kg/day	3 mg/kg/day	2-3 × of iv	3 mg/kg/day
Target AUC	11000	11000	11000	11000	11000
Target Ct	458	200	200	192	160
Target Cp	458	800	900	1049	1500
AUTL	11000	4800	4800	4608	3840
AUTL/AUC%	100%	44%	44%	42%	35%

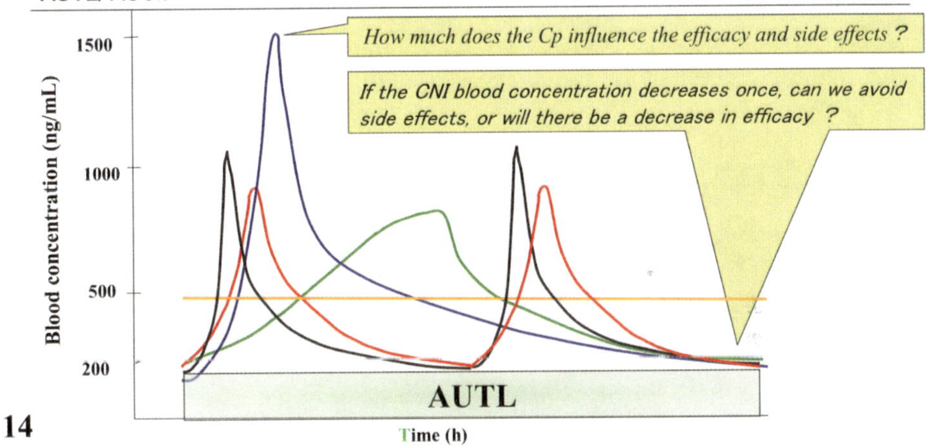

Fig. 9. Comparison of pharmacokinetic parameters among various administration methods of CYA in hematopoietic stem cell transplants.

For TAC, it has already been shown in a clinical trial that numerous side effects, such as nephropathy or neurologic symptoms, are caused by twice daily intermittent intravenous administration. Therefore, the package insert indicates that it should be administered by 24 h continuous intravenous administration, and it is known that continuous intravenous administration is appropriate. It may be because the method for oral use has a large AUTL/AUC% and no high peak, whereas intravenous injection twice a day by high speed drip has a high peak. It is considered that the effect range and the side effect range of TAC may be closer than those of CYA and that pharmacokinetics showing a gentle blood concentration time curve (large AUTL/AUC%) may be suitable.

MEC	24-hCIV	4 h×1	p.o.×2*	3 h×2	10 h×1
300 ng/mL	100%	73%	69%	69%	69%
400 ng/mL	100%	61%	54%	51%	43%
500 ng/mL	100%*	51%	42%	36%	27%

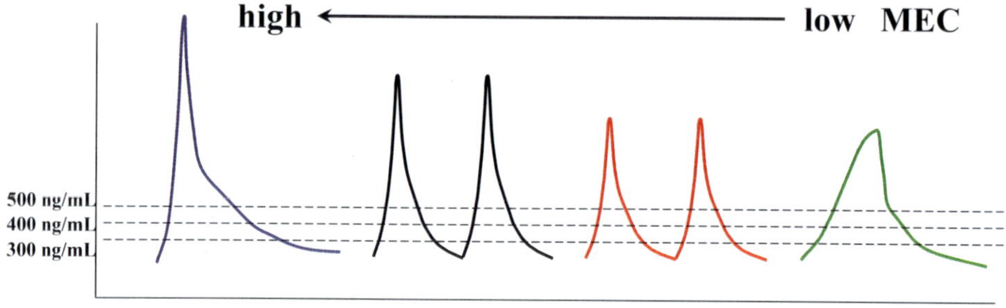

15

Fig. 10. T%>MEC of various CYA administration methods for each MEC in hematopoietic stem cell transplants.

6. Pharmacokinetic differences between morning and evening

In studies monitoring the blood concentration of CYA and TAC for 24 h and comparing the pharmacokinetics of morning and evening, some studies reported that there was no difference in pharmacokinetics between morning and evening[41,42], whereas several other studies reported that there was a difference[43-45]. In the authors' data, the AUC_{0-12}, AUC_{0-4}, C_2, and C_{max} following evening administration were significant lower than those following morning administration both in patients treated with CYA and patients treated with TAC[46,47] (Figure 11). As TAC shows gradual blood concentration-time curve in comparison with CYA, TAC is hardly affected by delayed or reduced absorption in the evening, so that the differences between various PK parameters between morning and evening were smaller in TAC (Table 4). Therefore, a drug such as TAC, which shows pharmacokinetics with a large AUTL/AUC% may have potential benefits because it has little difference in pharmacokinetics between morning and evening. However, a sustained release preparation of TAC administered once a day has been launched and its pharmacokinetics has no peak value in the evening because it is administered only in the morning, but its efficacy is equal to that of a drug administered twice a day. From this fact, it is possible that the pharmacokinetic difference between morning and evening is not a clinical problem.

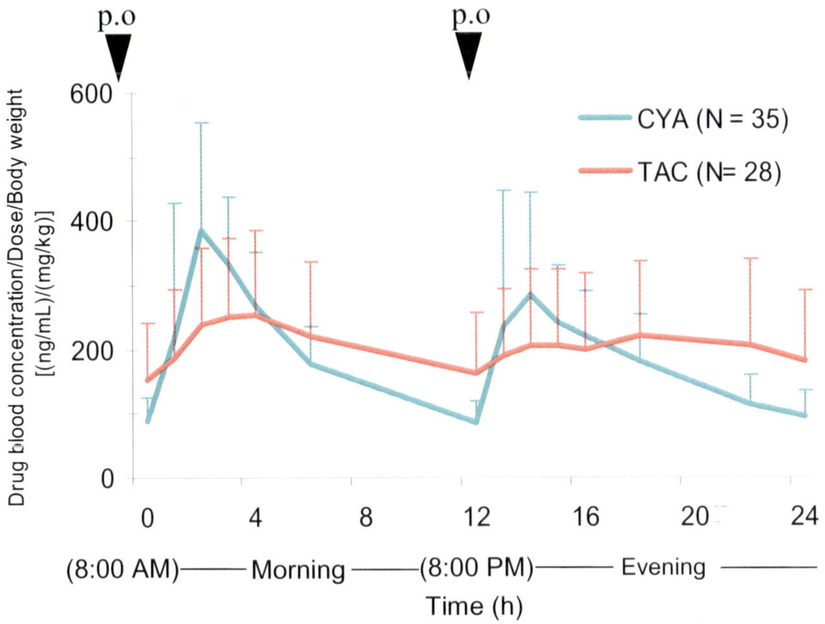

Fig. 11. Comparison of blood concentration-time curves through 24 hours between CYA and TAC.

	TAC(n=12)	CYA(n=10)	P値
AUC_{0-12}(ng·hr/ml)	0.91±0.10	0.77±0.31	0.0073*
AUTL/AUC(%)	1.22±0.18	1.42±0.27	0.0538
AUC_{0-4}(ng·hr/ml)	0.74±0.14	0.56±0.19	0.0144*
C_2(ng/ml)	0.70±0.31	0.51±0.25	0.1382
Cmax(ng/ml)	0.79±0.26	0.55±0.14	0.0161*
Cmin(ng/ml)	1.17±0.21	1.28±0.30	0.3131
Cmax/Cmin	0.71±0.32	0.45±0.16	0.0343*
Tmax(hr)	2.67±1.42	1.63±0.80	0.0287*

Table 4. Comparison of pharmacokinetic parameter ratios of evening to morning administrations between TAC and CYA

7. Calculation of optimal dose and blood trough concentration on switching between CYA and TAC

The authors calculated the optimal dose and the C_t concentration on switching between CYA and TAC, with a comparison of the pharmacokinetics (AUC, C_p, and Ct) of CYA and TAC. AUC/D/BW is equal, but the C_t of TAC is relatively higher than that of CYA as a result of the pharmacokinetic differences; considering this, the dosage ratio is as follows: CYA:TAC = 25:1, and the targeted C_t ratio is as follow: CYA:TAC = 13:1[48,49] (Figure 12). These reduced values were equal to the titer ratio calculated from the IC_{50} value of the PD data.

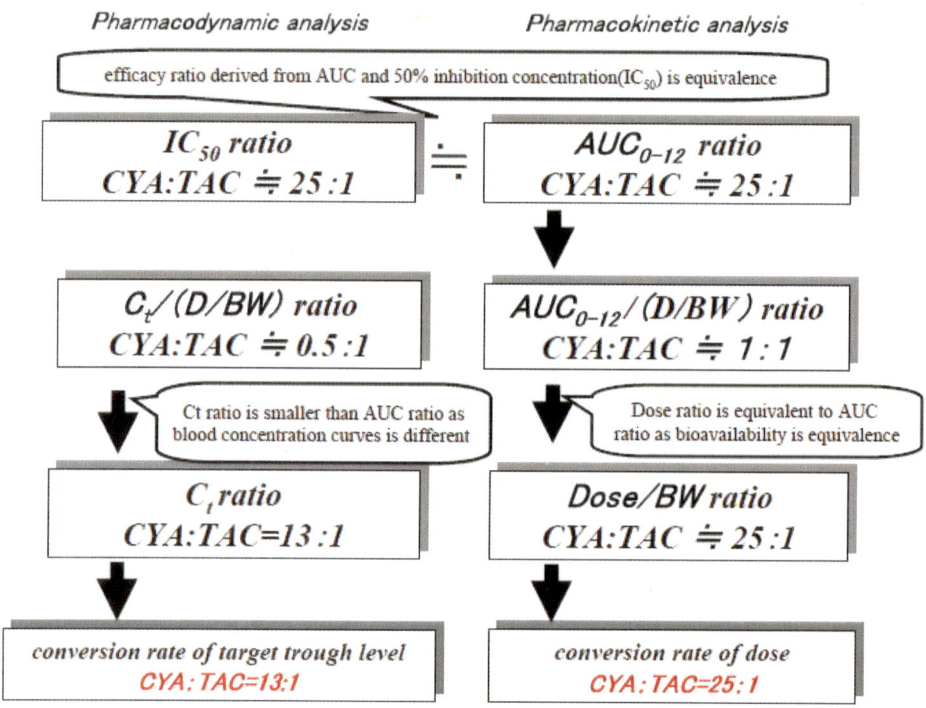

Fig. 12. Conversion rate of dose and target trough level derived from pharmacodynamic and pharmacokinetic analyses.

8. Conclusion

Although both CYA and TAC belong to CNIs and the availabilities (AUC/D/BW) are the same, significant differences in the pharmacokinetics (blood concentration-time curve) of both drugs were found. Given that the AUC is the parameter that is most closely associated with clinical effect, it is optimal to monitor C_p and Ct for oral CYA and TAC, respectively.

However, even if both drugs show identical AUC, the clinical effects, such as effectiveness or side effects, may vary according to differences in the blood concentration time curve based on the relative correlation of C_p and C_t. From the report on inhibitory action of CN and blood concentration[32] and the results of PK/PD analysis, It is also thought that CYA status is shown in Figure 13-A. On this basis, it is supposed that the clinical effect of CYA is slightly lower than that of TAC[50-52]. It is plausible that the C_t of CYA can be reduced on a temporary basis to avoid nephrotoxicity, as is done with AGs (Figure 13-A). Conversely, there is a possibility that C_p is associated with side effects as shown in Figure 13-B. CYA can reduce the C_p (Figure 13-D) and can also keep the AUC in the blood concentration time curve to elevate the C_t. In fact, CYA shows good results by continuous intravenous infusion for hematopoietic stem cell transplantation[38]. However, it has been found that there is a slight difference in the clinical results of the hematopoietic stem cell transplantation[40] (Figure 14). Therefore, CYA has wide tolerance of blood concentration, even if it is administered at various dosages or if it has various blood concentration time curves.

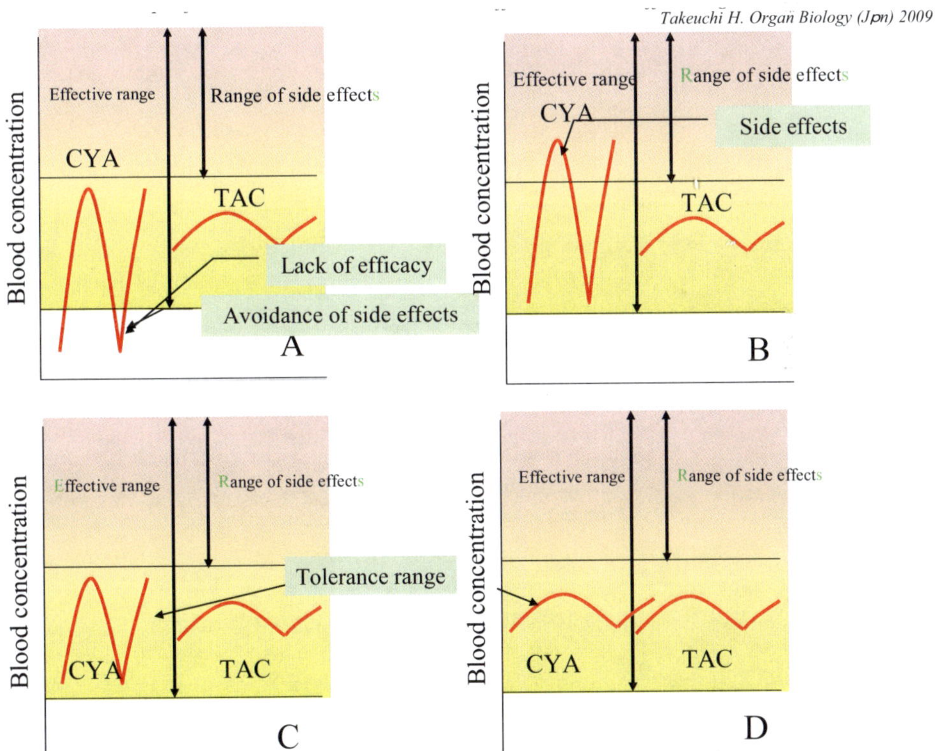

Fig. 13. Various relationships of blood concentration curve and the effective and side effect ranges, when AUCs are equivalent.

CYA and TAC are used equally in clinical practice in terms of the existing therapeutic dose and the AUC, and there are no particular problems (Figure 13-C). On the other hand, it is thought that a gentle (with AUTL/AUC% high) blood concentration time curve is suitable for TAC because its tolerance level is low (Figure 14).

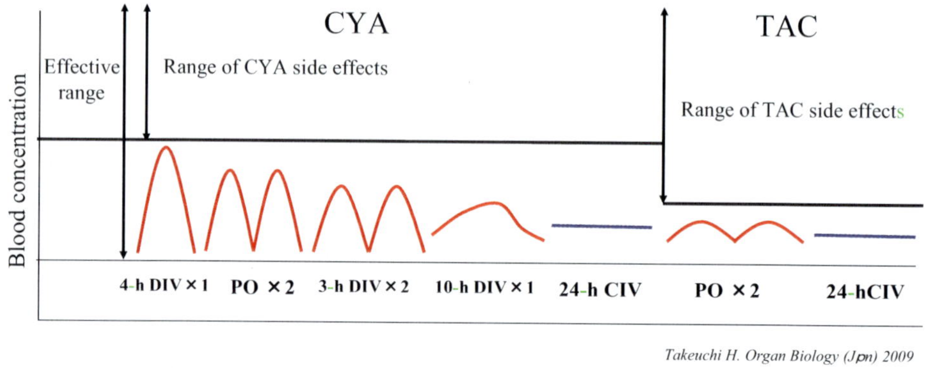

Fig. 14. Difference in range of effective and side effect bllod concentrations between CYA and TAC.

9. References

[1] Takeuchi H, Matsuno N, Senuma K et al. Evidence of different pharmacokinetics including relationship among AUC, peak, and trough levels between cyclosporine and tacrolimus in renal transplant recipients using new pharmacokinetic parameter--why cyclosporine is monitored by C(2) level and tacrolimus by trough level--.Biol Pharm Bull 31:90-94, 2008

[2] Heffron TG, Pescovitz MD, Florman S et al. Once-daily tacrolimus extended-release formulation: 1-year post-conversion in stable pediatric liver transplant recipients. Am J Transplant 7:1609-1615, 2007

[3] .Mahalati K, Belitsky P, Sketris I, West K, Panek R. Neoral monitoring by simplified sparse sampling area under the concentration-time curve. Transplantation 68:55-62, 1999

[4] International Neoral Renal Transplantation Study Group. Cyclosporine microemulsion (Neoral) absorption profiling and sparse-sample predictors during the first 3 months after renal transplantation. Am J Transplant 2:148-156, 2002

[5] Cantarovich M, Barkun J, Besner JG et al. Cyclosporine peak levels provide a better correlation with the area-under-the-curve than trough levels in liver transplant patients treated with neoral. Transplant Proc 30:1462-1463, 1998

[6] Cantarovich M, Barkun JS, Tchervenkov JI, et al. Comparison of neoral dose monitoring with cyclosporine through levels versus 2-hr postdose levels in stable liver transplant patients. Transplantation 6:1621-1627, 1998

[7] Cantarovich M, Besner JG, Barkun JS, et al. Two-hour cyclosporine level determination is the appropriate tool to monitor Neoral therapy. Clin Transplant 12:243-249, 1998

[8] Jaksch P, Kocher A, Neuhauser P, et al. Monitoring C2 level predicts exposure in maintenance lung transplant patients receiving the microemulsion formulation of cyclosporine (Neoral). *J Heart Lung Transplant* 24:1076-1080, 2005

[9] Staatz C, Taylor P, Tett S. Low tacrolimus concentrations and increased risk of early acute rejection in adult renal transplantation. Nephrol Dial Transplant 16:1905–1909, 2001

[10] Böttiger Y, Brattström C, Tydén G, Säwe J, Groth CG. Tacrolimus whole blood concentrations correlate closely to side-effects in renal transplant recipients. Br J Clin Pharmacol 48:445–448, 1999

[11] Venkataramanan R, Shaw LM, Sarkozi L et al. Clinical utility of monitoring tacrolimus blood concentrations in liver transplant patients. J Clin Pharmacol 41:542-551, 2001

[12] Lindholm A, Kahan BD. Influence of cyclosporine pharmacokinetics, trough concentrations, and AUC monitoring on outcome after kidney transplantation. Clin Pharmacol Therapeutics. 54:205-218, 1993

[13] Schroeder TJ, Hariharan S, First MR. Relationship between cyclosporine bioavailability and clinical outcome in renal transplant recipients. Transplant Proc 26:2787-2790, 1994

[14] Johnston A, David O, Cooney G. Pharmacokinetic validation of neoral absorption profiling. Transplant Proc 32: 53S, 2000

[15] Levy GA. Neoral is superior to FK506 in liver transplantation. Transplant Proc 30:1812-1815. 1998

[16] Keown P (on behalf of the Canadian Neoral Study Group). Absorption profiling of cyclosporine microemulsion (Neoral) during the first 2 weeks after renal transplantation. Transplantation 72:1024-1032, 2001

[17] Keown P (on behalf of International Neoral Renal Transplantation Study Group). Randomized, International Study of Cyclosporine Microemulsion Absorption Profiling in Renal Transplantation with Basiliximab Immunoprophylaxis. Am J Transplant 2:157-166,2002:

[18] Mahalati K, Belitsky P, West K, et al. Approaching the therapeutic window for cyclosporine
in kidney transplantation: a prospective study. J Am Soc Nephrol 12:828-833, 2001

[19] Pescovitz MD, Barbeito R; Simulect US01 Study Group. Two-hour post-dose cyclosporine level is a better predictor than trough level of acute rejection of renal allografts. Clin Transplant 16:378-382, 2002

[20] Levy G, Thervet E, Lake J, Uchida K, On behalf of the CONCERT group. Patient management by Neoral C(2) monitoring: An international consensus statement. Transplantation 73:S12-18, 2002

[21] Saint-Marcoux F, Rousseau A, Le Meur Y, et al. Influence of sampling-time error on cyclosporine measurements nominally at 2 hours after administration. Clin Chem 49:813-815, 2003

[22] Campbell SB, Johnson DW. Patient management by cyclosporine C2 monitoring: not enough science yet to justify the practice. Transplantation 75:1917-1918, 2003

[23] Birsan T, Wekerle T, Steininger R, Muhlbacher F. C2 versus C0 cyclosporine monitoring: The end for us. Transplantation 80: 543, 2005

[24] Knight SR, Morris P. The clinical benefits of cyclosporine C2-level monitoring: a systematic review. Transplantation 83:1525-1535, 2007

[25] Kuypers DR, Claes K, Evenepoel P, Maes B, Vanrenterghem Y. Clinical efficacy and toxicity profile of tacrolimus and mycophenolic acid in relation to combined long-term pharmacokinetics in de novo renal allograft recipients. Clin Pharmacol Ther 75:434-447, 2004

[26] Undre NA, VanHooff J, Christiaans M et al. Stevenson P. Low systemic exposure to tacrolimus correlates with acute rejection. Transplant Proc 31:296–298, 1999

[27] Jorgensen K, Povlsen J,Madsen S et al. C2 (2-h) levels are not superior to trough levels as estimates of the area under the curve in tacrolimus-treated renal-transplant patients. Nephrol Dial Transplant 17:1487–1490, 2002

[28] Yolanda A, Leonor P, Carme C et al. Evaluation of a limited sampling strategy to estimate area under the curve of tacrolimus in adult renal transplant patients. Ther Drug Monit 27:431–434, 2005

[29] Wong KM, Shek CC, Chau KF, Li CS. Abbreviated tacrolimus area under the curve monitoring for renal transplant recipients. Am J Kidney Dis 35:660–666, 2000

[30] Mathew BS, Fleming DH, Jeyaseelan V et al. A limited sampling strategy for tacrolimus in renal transplant patients. Br J Clin Pharmacol 66:467-472, 2008

[31] Stolk LML, Van Duijnhoven EM, Christiaans MHL, Van Hooff JP. Trough levels of tacrolimus. Ther Drug Monit 24:573-574, 2002

[32] Halloran PF, Helms LM, Kung L, Noujaim J. The temporal profile of calcineurin inhibition by cyclosporine in vivo. Transplantation 68:1356-1361, 1999

[33] Sindhi R, LaVia MF, Paulling E et al. Stimulated response of peripheral lymphocytes may distinguish cyclosporine effect in renal transplant recipients receiving a cyclosporine+rapamycin regimen. Transplantation 69:432-436, 2000

[34] Pernille B, Nielsn K, Gesualdo MB et al. Blood tacrolimus levels and calcineurin phosphatase activity early after renal transplantation. AST abstract 1076, 2001

[35] Nakamura Y, Takeuchi H, Okuyama K et al. Evaluation of appropriate blood level in continuous intravenous infusion from trough concentrations after oral administration based on area under trough level in tacrolimus and cyclosporine therapy. Transplant Proc 37:1725-1727, 2005

[36] Takeuchi H, Okuyama K, Akashi T et a.l Evaluation of Blood Level in Continuous Intravenous Infusion from Blood Trough Level after Oral Administration Based on

Area Under Trough Level (AUTL) in Tacrolimus and Cyclosporine The Japanese Journal of Therapeutic Drug Monitoring (Jpn) 21:268-272, 2004

[37] Ogawa N, Kanda Y, Matsubara M et al. Increased incidence of acute graft-versus-host disease with the continuous infusion of cyclosporine A compared to twice-daily infusion. Bone Marrow Transplant 33: 549-552, 2004

[38] Oshima K, Kanda Y, Nakasone H et al. Decreased incidence of acute graft-versus-host disease by continuous infusion of cyclosporine with a higher target blood level. Am J Hemato 83:226-232, 2008

[39] Miller KB, Schenkein DP, Comenzo R et al. Adjusted-dose continuous-infusion cyclosporin A to prevent graft-versus-host disease following allogeneic bone marrow transplantation. Ann Hematol 68:15-20, 1994

[40] Furukaw T. overview of therapeutic drug monitoring of cyclosporine in the allogeneic hematopoietic stem cell transplantation Transplantation Now (Jpn) 21 : 608-612, 2008

[41] Milanian I, Ghods AJ, Mahmoudian M et al. Study of circadian variation of cyclosporine pharmacokinetics. Transplant Proc 29:2930-2931, 1997

[42] Kovarik JM, Mueller EA, van Bree JB et al. Within-day consistency in cyclosporine pharmacokinetics from a microemulsion formulation in renal transplant patients. Ther Drug Monit 16:232-237, 1994

[43] Chateauvert N, Cote H. Circadian variations in the pharmacokinetics of a new microemulsion formulation of cyclosporine in cardiac transplant recipients. Pharmacotherapy 18:364-370, 1998

[44] Min DI, Chen HY, Fabrega A et al. Circadian variation of tacrolimus disposition in liver allograft recipients. Transplantation 62:1190-1192, 1996

[45] Park SI, Felipe CR, Pinheiro-Machado PG et al Circadian and time-dependent variability in tacrolimus pharmacokinetics. Fundam Clin Pharmacol 21:191-197, 2007

[46] Takeuchi H, Akashi T, Akashi I et al. Difference of Pharmacokinetics between Morning and Evening Administration in Cyclosporine Microemulsion Formulation -Slower and Lower Absorption in Evening Administration Japanese Journal of Transplantation (Jpn) 38:74-82, 2003

[47] Iwahori T, Takeuchi H, Matsuno N at al. Pharmacokinetic differences between morning and evening administration of cyclosporine and tacrolimus therapy. Transplant Proc 37:1739-1740, 2005

[48] Takeuchi H, Matsuno N, Takeshi Nagaoat al.. Clinical applications of optimal converting values of dose and target trough level in conversion of tacrolimus to cyclosporine as evaluated by pharmacokinetic and pharmacodynamic analysis. Transplantation Now (Jpn) 18:725-728, 2005

[49] Takeuchi H, Okuyama K, Konno O et al. Optimal dose and target trough level in cyclosporine and tacrolimus conversion in renal transplantation as evaluated by lymphocyte drug sensitivity and pharmacokinetic parameters. Transplant Proc 37:1745-1747, 2005

[50] Ekberg H, Tedesco-Silva H, Demirbas A et al. Reduced exposure to calcineurin inhibitors in renal transplantation. N Engl J Med 357;2562-2575, 2007

[51] Margreiter R;European Tacrolimus vs Ciclosporin Microemulsion Renal Transplantation Study Group. Efficacy and safety of tacrolimus compared with ciclosporin microemulsion in renal transplantation: a randomised multicentre study. Lancet 359;741-746, 2002

[52] Webster A, Woodroffe RC, Taylor RS, Chapman JR, Craig JC. Tacrolimus versus ciclosporin as primary immunosuppression for kidney transplant recipients: meta-analysis and meta-regression of randomised trial data. BMJ. 331;810-820, 2005

14

Pharmacokinetic/Pharmacodynamic (PK/PD) Modeling of Anti-Neoplastic Agents

Daniel Lexcen[1], Ahmed Salem[2],
Walid M. El-Khatib[3], Virginia Haynes[4] and Ayman Noreddin[5,*]
[1]*University of Minnesota*
[2]*Abbott Co Ltd.*
[3]*Ain-Shams University*
[4]*Lake Superior College*
[5]*Hampton University*
USA

1. Introduction

Development of tumor resistance to chemotherapeutics is related to inherent tumor variations regarding sensitivity to chemotherapeutics and to sub-optimal dosing regimens, including variation in patient pharmacokinetics that result in suboptimal exposure of tumor cells to anti-neoplastic drugs [1, 2]. The rate and extent of drug efficacy depends on the extent of drug exposure at the tumor site and the time above the effective concentration [3]. *In vitro* models that incorporate these pharmacokinetic and pharmacodynamic (PK/PD) principles to optimize therapeutic response may be considered the method of choice for optimizing dosing schedules before translating data from static assays to animals and clinical trials [4, 5]. The hollow fiber bioreactor was recently used to evaluate pharmacokinetic/pharmacodynamic (PK/PD) effects of gemcitibine in lung and breast cancers and to model HIV treatments [4-6].

2. Hollow fiber bioreactor model

The hollow fiber bioreactor model (Figure 1) is a dynamic system that provides a cell culture with constant flow of fresh medium through a 3D polysulfone cartridge (support for cell growth) with capillary sized passages (cells grow in the extracapillary space), at physiologically relevant flow rates. Automatic programmable pumps accurately regulate dosing of chemotherapeutics into the system.

The hollow fiber cartridge consists of two compartments, the porous capillaries through which medium flows and the extra-capillary space (ECS) that separates the cell culture from the flowing medium. Medium is constantly perfused through the fibers into the ECS, carrying nutrients and infused drugs to the cell culture. Due to the dynamic nature of the

* Corresponding Author

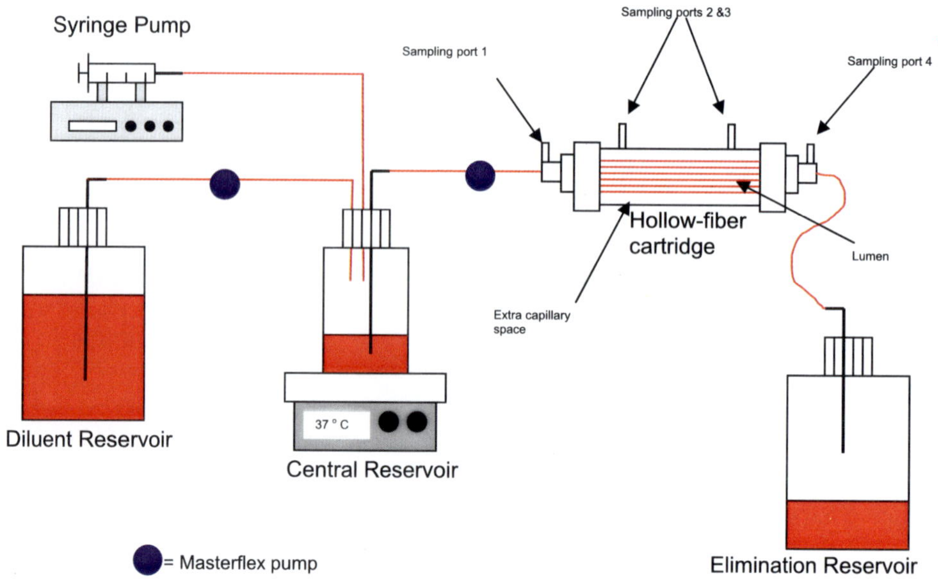

Fig. 1. Schematic of the bioreactor setup

model, cells can be exposed to carefully chosen drug concentrations that simulate patient pharmacokinetics from published clinical data, simulating drug half-life and renal clearance [6]. This change in concentration over time cannot be achieved in static assays. To monitor cell growth and viable counts in undisturbed hollow fiber cultures, we used an assay based on measurement of fluorescence resulting from the reduction of non-fluorescent resazurin to its red fluorescent form (resorufin) by metabolically active cells [7]. The intensity of the fluorescence is proportional to the viable cell count [8]. Achievement of cell cycle arrest, as a surrogate marker of the therapeutic outcome, was measured by flow cytometry. We hypothesized that we could use the proposed dynamic model to accurately simulate (*R*)-roscovitine (ROSC) pharmacodynamics, incorporating pharmacokinetic data. To achieve this, we used the MCF-7 human breast cancer cell line and compared the peak values from two proposed dosing regimens of ROSC to untreated controls.

MCF-7 cells are derived from the pleural effusion of an estrogen receptor positive, human breast adenocarcinoma [9, 10]. Cells were cultured in EMEM, 2mM L-glutamine, 0.1mM non-essential amino acids, 1mM sodium pyruvate, 0.01mg/mL bovine insulin and 10% fetal bovine serum; grown in 5% CO_2 at 37° C and dispersed when confluent with of 0.25% trypsin/0.5mM EDTA. Hollow fiber cartridges were prepared according to manufacturers instructions. To prepare hollow fiber cultures, briefly, trypsinized cells were diluted to 1.67 x 10^6/mL; 3mL were seeded into the ECS of each cartridge. Two cartridges were seeded for each experiment; one for drug treatment and one control. Cartridges were placed on a dual recirculating pump in the incubator at 37°C with 5% CO_2 to circulate fresh sterile medium to each cartridge simultaneously while establishing the cultures.

2.1 Pharmacokinetic simulation for (R)-roscovitine

After 24 hours, cartridges were removed from the recirculating pump, connected to a linear pump system (Masterflex) and a digital syringe pump was used to control the rate of drug infusion (Figure 1). Mathematical pharmacokinetic drug profiles were simulated by adjusting the input of ROSC and medium in the system. Infusion of the drug at peak concentration was followed by simulation of its clearance rate over a 6 hour period. Controls were perfused with drug free medium under the same conditions. Each dosing schedule was performed at least in duplicate.

2.2 PK/PD simulation for the bioreactor

A one compartment model, oral absorption and first order elimination was constructed using STELLA software (isee systems inc., Lebanon, NH). This model simulated pharmacokinetic profiles of peak and trough plasma levels after 800 mg twice daily (BID) and three times daily (TID) dosage regimens using pharmacokinetic parameters from a previously published clinical trial [11]. STELLA simulation provided a profile range of several C_{max} from which to mimic the C_{ss} (steady state concentration) in the bioreactor. To accomplish this infusion, peak and trough concentrations of the C_{ss} range were used to determine the final dose, which represented the population pharmacokinetics and was infused to the central reservoir. Simulated BID peak and trough concentrations were 3167 ng/mL and 808 ng/mL, respectively. Simulated TID peak and trough concentrations were 3893 ng/mL and 1923 ng/mL, respectively. Flow rates for the pumps were determined using the following equation for oral administration:

$$Cl = k_e \bullet V_d \quad (1)$$

$$k_e = \frac{Cl}{V_d} = \frac{\ln(\frac{C_1}{C_2})}{} = \frac{\ln C_1 - \ln C_2}{(t_2 - t_1)} \quad (2)$$

where C_l is clearance of drug and is equal to the rate set on the Masterflex pumps, k_e is the elimination rate constant for ROSC, V_d is central reservoir volume, C_1 is C_{max} from the simulation during the steady state, C_2 is C_{min} from the simulation during the steady state, and t (time) is the experiment duration. The rate of the digital pumps simulated the patient drug clearance.

2.3 LC/MS

To confirm the achievement of peak drug concentrations, samples were collected from the ECS of the hollow fiber cartridge and analyzed by LC/MS. The system included two Shimadzu LC- 20AD pumps, SIL-20AC autosampler, 2010 EV mass spectrometer with cosense module. A BDS Hypersil C18 (30mm x 2.1mm x 3µm) analytical column was used in conjunction with the co-sense system fitted with a Shimadzu MAYI-ODS 10L x 4.6 column. Mobile phase; A (10% ACN/ 90%, 0.1% Formic Acid) v/v and B (80% ACN and 20%, 0.1% Formic Acid) v/v; gradient at 50 % B increasing to 100% B over 1 min and remained isocratic at 100% B for 6 minutes until returning to 50% B. Flow rate was 0.150 ml/min with detection wavelength of 292 nm with an injection volume of 10µL. Mass spectrometry peaks were analyzed using Shimadzu's data analysis program. Peak integrations were compared to a standard curve to obtain the concentrations of ROSC.

2.4 Resazurin assay

Fluorescent conversion of resazurin is directly related to the number of metabolically active cells in culture and serves as a surrogate probe for viable cell count. Medium containing 5% v/v resazurin was added to the hollow fiber system and circulated for 30 minutes for homogenous distribution of resazurin containing medium. System valves were closed and the cartridge incubated 2 hours; 200 µl samples were drawn from medium in the ECS. Fluorescence was measured on a microplate reader (Biotek, Winooski, VT). Resazurin was removed by pumping fresh medium through the system with linear pumps, collecting the resazurin medium as waste. Assays were performed before and after treatment for assessing baseline fluorescence and the effect of drug on cell proliferation. Resazurin has been reported to be cytotoxic at high concentrations and exposure beyond 24 hours [12]. Since cell lines respond differently to resazurin, [13], we conducted a static assay to establish that 5% (v/v) resazurin could be used over at least a 24 hour period without toxicity to the MCF-7 cell line. Cells incubated with resazurin, and untreated controls, were harvested, stained with trypan blue and counted at the conclusion of the experiment. This confirmed that growth and viability were unaffected by resazurin at 5% v/v (unpublished data).

2.5 Flow cytometry

MCF-7 cells were harvested from the hollow fiber cartridge by trypsinization and centrifuged at 300x g for 5 minutes. Supernatant was removed and the pellet resuspended in 0.5ml of PBS-T with 20 µg/mL of RNAse and incubated at 37°C for 30 min. 10µg/ml propidium iodide was added to the cell suspension and incubated at 37°C for 30 min. The stained nuclei (200,000 per sample) were analyzed with a Becton Dickinson FACSCalibur (San Jose, California) flow cytometer using medium flow mode. Cell cycle distribution was analyzed with Modfit LT program (Verity, Maine).

3. Results

Pharmacokinetic simulation of ROSC was used to predict the C_{max} of BID and TID dosing regimens. The predicted bolus dose values for the BID and TID were 3167ng/mL (8.9µM) and 3893ng/mL (10.9µM), respectively. From this data, we modeled a one dose peak profile that we could assess in the *in vitro* hollow fiber model. Actual concentrations of ROSC achieved in the model reached a C_{max} of 2953 ng/mL (8.3µM) for the BID schedule, an accuracy of 93.2% compared to the predicted value. Actual concentration for the TID schedule was 3307ng/mL (9.3µM) as compared to the mathematical profile C_{max} of 3893ng/mL, an accuracy of 85.0%. This level of accuracy for infused drug is consistent with the reports of Kirstein, et al. in their PK/PD studies in the hollow fiber model [5, 6]. To monitor cell proliferation and viability before treatment, without disturbing established cultures, we used the resazurin assay on all cartridges. There was no significant difference in cell proliferation between cartridges before treatment (p=0.86), indicating consistency in seeding the hollow-fiber cartridges. In post-treatment resazurin assays, ROSC treated cartridges had decreased cell proliferation compared to control cartridges. The TID (9.3µM) simulated dose had a 15-20% decrease in growth that was not evident with the BID (8.3 µM) simulated dose (Figure 2). To determine the effect of ROSC on cell cycle, cells were collected by trypsinization from the hollow-fiber cartridge at 24 hours post-treatment and analyzed by flow cytometry. An increase was seen in the proportion of cells in the G1 phase in both the BID and TID treatments compared to the control. Correspondingly, there was a statistically significant decrease of the proportion of S phase cells in both the TID (p=0.004) and BID (p=0.003) doses compared to the control and a statistically significant increase in G2 for BID simulation (Table 1).

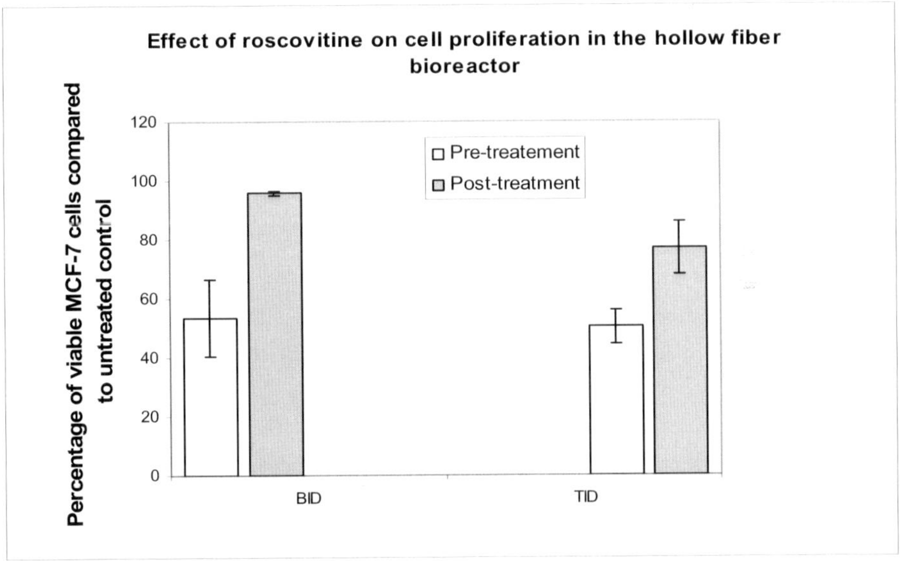

Fig. 2. Evaluation of cell proliferation in undisturbed cultures in the hollow fiber cartridge. Samples were taken for each set of cartridges for each experiment (n=2). A sample was taken from each cartridge before treatment (n=6). ROSC was infused at steady state value and clearance rate was simulated over 6 hours. Sample was taken at 24 hours (18 hours after infusion). Fluorescence was quantified as RFU and all values were normalized to the untreated control (final average value as 100%).

	G1 (%)	S (%)	G2 (%)
Control (n=5)	48.75 ± 3.71	33.93 ± 6.36	17.23 ± 2.68
BID (n=6)	54.51 ± 3.69	23.15 ± 1.89	22.34 ± 1.86
TID (n=5)	59.77 ± 3.86	22.49 ± 1.86	17.72 ± 5.55

n= number of experimental repetitions; BID 800mg twice daily; TID 800mg three times daily.

Table 1. Effect of ROSC dose increase on cell cycle distribution.
MCF-7 cells in each measured phase of growth cycle (G1, S or G2) are expressed as a percentage (± Standard Deviation) of the total number of cells.

4. Discussion

Uncontrolled proliferation is a defining characteristic of tumor cells. This is known to occur through mutation in genes that produce regulatory proteins which modulate cell cycle, such as the Cyclin Dependent Kinases (Cdks) [14-16]. Cdks are highly conserved serine/threonine kinases whose activation depends on formation of a heterodimeric complex with cyclins [17-19]. Thus, Cdks are a promising therapeutic target for cancer treatment [20]. ROSC is a novel Cdk inhibitor that induces cell cycle arrest and apoptosis through multiple intracellular targets in a variety of tumor cell lines. When tested in static *in vitro* assays, IC_{50} values of about 14μM are reported with 24 hours of drug exposure [21-24]. However, dosing schedules of 2500 mg/day over 5 days in 3 week cycles or the reduced dose of 1600mg/day BID for 10 days were recommended based on early human trials [25] and a concomitant Phase one trial that indicated a dose limiting toxicity of 800 mg BID for 7 days. With this dosing schedule, peak plasma levels were achieved in 1-4 hours with elimination by 2-5 hours. The highest plasma concentration achieved clinically was 10μM within a treatment period. There was no tumor response to this dose, although the disease was stabilized over several courses of treatment [11]. To investigate the effect of administration of ROSC as a monotherapy by altering the dosing schedule, we employed a dynamic hollow fiber model in this study. We established our model using STELLA to simulate pharmacokinetic profiles of ROSC derived from clinical data. These profiles were simulated in the *in vitro* hollow fiber model for assessing the effectiveness of two dosing regimens against MCF-7 cells by using flow cytometry to measure cell cycle distribution under each condition. The results revealed increasing numbers of MCF-7 cells accumulating in G1 phase after simulating the BID and TID dosing peaks with ROSC, and indicating a significant difference between TID and the control. Also, BID dosing simulation had a significant increase in G2 arrest ($p<0.05$). This data is consistent with previous studies which indicated arrest of MCF-7 cell proliferation at the G1/S transition and G2/M transition with accumulation in G2. However, Wesierska-Gadek, *et al.* revealed ROSC activity only at the G2/M transition and accumulation of arrested MCF-7 cells only in the G2 phase. The differences may be attributed to differences in their experimental design, as they exposed MCF-7 cells in a static system to 10μM ROSC for 24 hours [26]. In this study, we tested concentrations of ROSC based on human clinical trial values of a maximum value of 10μM over 1-4 hours, with ROSC clearance within 5 hours, which were below the levels tested in static systems [11]. In this case, dose limiting toxicity of the drug precludes achievement of effective plasma concentrations in humans, which is consistent with the clinical trials. Consequently, ROSC is now being tested in combination therapies [27]. In conclusion, this study demonstrated the application of the dynamic hollow fiber model with controlled pharmacokinetic profiles to simulate clinically relevant dosing schedules of ROSC for treatment of breast tumor cells and the use of a resazurin assay for monitoring cell viability of hollow fiber cell cultures. With this methodology, cells can be recovered for further analysis. The applied hollow fiber model in this study can be used for PK/PD assessment of different anti-neoplastic drugs (single and in combination), with different exposure times against many tumor cell lines.

5. References

[1] Donnelly JG. Pharmacogenetics in cancer chemotherapy: balancing toxicity and response. Ther Drug Monit 2004;26:231-5.

[2] Buschbeck M. Strategies to overcome resistance to targeted protein kinase inhibitors in the treatment of cancer. Drugs R 2006;7:73-86.

[3] Levasseur LM, Slocum HK, Rustum YM, Greco WR. Modeling of the time-dependency of in vitro drug cytotoxicity and resistance. Cancer Res 1998;58:5749-61.

[4] Drusano GL, Bilello PA, Symonds WT, et al. Pharmacodynamics of abacavir in an in vitro hollow-fiber model system. Antimicrob Agents Chemother 2002;46:464-70.

[5] Kirstein MN, Brundage RC, Moore MM, et al. Pharmacodynamic characterization of gemcitabine cytotoxicity in an in vitro cell culture bioreactor system. Cancer Chemother Pharmacol 2008;61:291-9.

[6] Kirstein MN, Brundage RC, Elmquist WF, et al. Characterization of an in vitro cell culture bioreactor system to evaluate anti-neoplastic drug regimens. Breast Cancer Res Treat 2006;96:217-25.

[7] Page B, Page M, Noel C. A new fluorometric assay for cytotoxicity measurements *in vitro*. Int J Oncology 1993;3:473-6.

[8] Gloeckner H, Jonuleit T, Lemke HD. Monitoring of cell viability and cell growth in a hollow-fiber bioreactor by use of the dye Alamar Blue. J Immunol Methods 2001;252:131-8.

[9] Brooks SC, Locke ER, Soule HD. Estrogen receptor in a human cell line (MCF-7) from breast carcinoma. J Biol Chem 1973;248:6251-3.

[10] Soule HD, Vazguez J, Long A, Albert S, Brennan M. A human cell line from a pleural effusion derived from a breast carcinoma. J Natl Cancer Inst 1973;51:1409-16.

[11] Benson C, White J, De Bono J, et al. A phase I trial of the selective oral cyclin-dependent kinase inhibitor seliciclib (CYC202; R-Roscovitine), administered twice daily for 7 days every 21 days. Br J Cancer 2007;96:29-37.

[12] Squatrito RC, Connor JP, Buller RE. Comparison of a novel redox dye cell growth assay to the ATP bioluminescence assay. Gynecol Oncol 1995;58:101-5.

[13] Nakayama GR, Caton MC, Nova MP, Parandoosh Z. Assessment of the Alamar Blue assay for cellular growth and viability in vitro. Journal of Immunological Methods 1997;204:205-8.

[14] Malumbres M, Carnero A. Cell cycle deregulation: a common motif of cancer. Prog Cell Cycle Res 2003;5:5-18.

[15] David-Pfeuty T, Nouvian-Dooghe Y, Sirri V, Roussel P, Hernandez-Verdun D. Common and reversible regulation of wild-type p53 function and of ribosomal biogenesis by protein kinases in human cells. Oncogene 2001;20:5951-63.

[16] Bach S, Knockaert M, Reinhardt J, et al. Roscovitine Targets, Protein Kinases and Pyridoxal Kinase. J Biol Chem 2005;280:31208-19.

[17] Whittaker SR, Walton MI, Garrett MD, Workman P. The Cyclin-dependent Kinase Inhibitor CYC202 (R-Roscovitine) Inhibits Retinoblastoma Protein Phosphorylation, Causes Loss of Cyclin D1, and Activates the Mitogen-activated Protein Kinase Pathway. Cancer Res 2004;64:262-72.

[18] Shapiro GI. Cyclin-Dependent Kinase Pathways As Targets for Cancer Treatment. J Clin Oncol 2006;24:1770-83.

[19] Iseki H, Ko TC, Xue XY, Seapan A, Hellmich MR, Townsend CM,Jr. Cyclin-dependent kinase inhibitors block proliferation of human gastric cancer cells. Surgery 1997;122:187,94; discussion 194-5.

[20] Benson C, Kaye S, Workman P, Garrett M, Walton M, de Bono J. Clinical anticancer drug development: targeting the cyclin-dependent kinases. Br J Cancer 2005;92:7-12.

[21] McClue SJ, Blake D, Clarke R, et al. In vitro and in vivo antitumor properties of the cyclin dependent kinase inhibitor CYC202 (R-roscovitine). Int J Cancer 2002;102:463-8.

[22] Węsierska-Gądek J, Hajek SB, Sarg B, Wandl S, Walzi E, Lindner H. Pleiotropic effects of selective CDK inhibitors on human normal and cancer cells. Biochemical Pharmacology 2008;76:1503-14.

[23] Węsierska-Gądek J, Kramer MP, Maurer M. Resveratrol modulates roscovitine-mediated cell cycle arrest of human MCF-7 breast cancer cells. Food and Chemical Toxicology, 2008;46:1327-33.

[24] Wojciechowski J, Horky M, Gueorguieva M, Wesierska-Gadek J. Rapid onset of nucleolar disintegration preceding cell cycle arrest in roscovitine-induced apoptosis of human MCF-7 breast cancer cells. Int J Cancer 2003;106:486-95.

[25] Pierga JY, Fiavre S, Vera K, Laurence V, Delbaldo C, Bekradda M, Armand JP, Gianella-Borradori A, Dieras V, Raymond E: A phase 1 and pharmacokinetic (PK) trial of CYC202, a novel oral cyclin-dependent kinase (CDK) inhibitor, in patients (pts) with advanced solid tumors. Proc am soc clin oncol 2003;22:abstr 840.

[26] Węsierska-Gądek J, Maurer M, Schmid G. Inhibition of farnesyl protein transferase sensitizes human MCF-7 breast cancer cells to roscovitine-mediated cell cycle arrest. J Cell Biochem 2007;102:736-47.

[27] Appleyard MV, O'Neill MA, Murray KE, et al. Seliciclib (CYC202, R-roscovitine) enhances the anti-tumor effect of doxorubicin in vivo in a breast cancer xenograft model. Int J Cancer 2008;124:465-72.

15

Bioavailability of Citrus Polymethoxylated Flavones and Their Biological Role in Metabolic Syndrome and Hyperlipidemia

Malkanthi Evans, Prachi Sharma and Najla Guthrie
KGK Synergize Inc.
Canada

1. Introduction

Flavonoids are a group of polyphenolic compounds ubiquitous in many plants including fruits, vegetables, nuts, seeds, grains, tea and wine (Hollman & Katan, 1999). Flavonoids belong to two classes i) Flavanones and ii) Flavones. The most common flavanones are hesperetin from oranges and naringenin from grapefruit. The most common flavones, also known as polymethoxylated flavones, are tangeretin and nobiletin, present in orange and tangerine peel (Kurowska & Manthey, 2004).

Recently, there has been an increasing interest in the health promoting properties of PMFs, which are known to play an important role in a number of biological functions as well as having anti-cancer (Silalahi, 2002), anti-inflammatory (Lin et al., 2003), and neuroprotective properties (Datla et al., 2001). Previously our team had performed pilot studies to investigate the biological properties of both nobiletin and tangeretin in small-animal and human clinical trials. Results of these studies have shown significant decreases in serum triglycerides, total cholesterol, and low density lipoprotein cholesterol and very low density lipoprotein cholesterol levels (Kurowska & Manthey, 2004; Roza et al., 2007) and increases in glucose tolerance (Li et al., 2006).

Metabolic syndrome is a constellation of medical disorders that substantially increases the risk of individuals developing cardiovascular disease and diabetes. Metabolic syndrome has become increasingly common in Western society with a prevalence of 20-25% in the adult US population (Li et al., 2006). Early identification, prevention and treatment of metabolic syndrome portray a major challenge for the healthcare industry. During recent years, dietary supplements have been reported to be promising in reducing hyperglycemia and lipid disorders in individuals with type II diabetes or with predisposition to type II diabetes or hyperlipidemia. To date, little research has been conducted in investigating dietary supplements for their efficacy as hypolipidemic and antidiabetic therapeutic agents.

Sufficient absorption of a drug or nutrient is important to obtain a successful therapeutic response. Bioavailability of a nutrient is simply the quantity or fraction of the ingested dose that is absorbed. Since oral bioavailability appears to be a limiting factor in the metabolism of citrus flavonoids and polyphenols, future studies are recommended to further investigate the biochemical factors influencing the bioavailibility of polymethoxylated flavones. This chapter focuses on bioavailability of polymethoxylated flavones and presents results from *in vitro, in vivo* and human studies.

2. Polymethoxylated flavones (PMFs)

PMFs are a group of methoxylated phenolic compounds found exclusively in tissues and peels of *Citrus reticulata* (tangerine), *Citrus paradisi* (grapefruit), *Citrus sinensis* (sweet orange), and *Citrus aurantium L.* (sour orange) (Horowitz & Gentili, 1977; Dugo & McHale, 2002). These various citrus species show very high variability in their content of PMFs.

The main reason for the low oral bioavailability of the dietary flavonoids is the extensive conjugation of the free hydroxyl groups (Walle, et al., 2004; Manach & Donovan, 2004; Walle, et al., 2005). PMFs have a benzo-gamma-pyrone skeleton with a carbonyl group at the C-3 position and methoxy groups in different positions on the benzo-gamma-pyrone skeleton (Fig.1). The exclusive feature in the chemical structure of PMFs is the polymethylation of polyhydroxylated flavonoids, one of the major naturally occurring polyphenolic compounds. This results in increased metabolic stability and membrane transport in the intestine and liver, improving oral bioavailability (Walle, 2007).

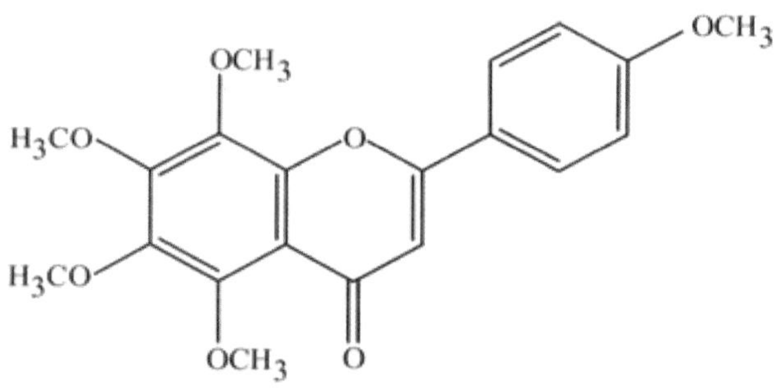

Tangeretin

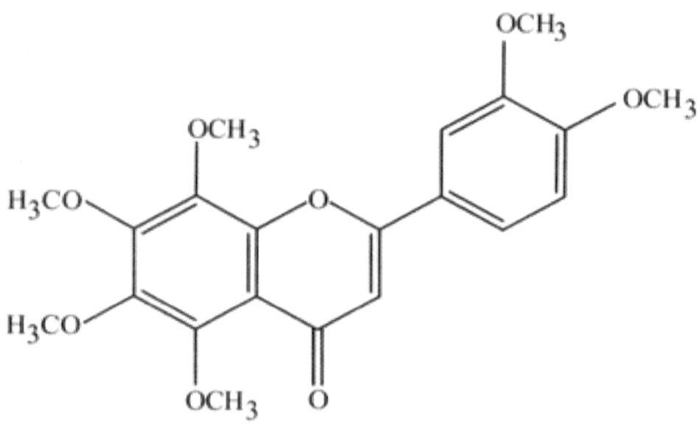

Nobiletin

Fig. 1. Chemical structures of nobiletin and tangeretin (Ishii et al., 2010)

The two most common PMFs are nobiletin and tangeretin. They exhibit distinctive chemical and physical properties in comparison to other plant flavonoids which influence the metabolism and pharmacokinetics of these compounds in animals. Nobiletin (5,6,7,8,3',4'-hexamethoxyflavone) has a molecular formula of $C_{21}H_{22}O_8$. Tangeretin (5,6,7,8,4'-pentamethoxyflavone) has a molecular formula of $C_{20}H_{20}O_7$. The bioavailability of PMFs is considered to be high in comparison to other citrus flavonoids because of the lipophilic nature of the multiple methoxy groups on the PMF structure. The smaller methoxyflavones, sinensetin, eupatorin and rutin, with one to three methoxy groups and without any hydroxyl groups, have been much less studied.

3. Biological role of PMFs

3.1 Metabolic syndrome

Metabolic syndrome refers to a group of risk factors that increase the risk for heart disease and diabetes. The main risk factors of metabolic syndrome include central obesity, insulin resistance, hypertension and cholesterol abnormalities. Obesity contributes to insulin resistance, which has been proposed as the major underlying cause of type II diabetes, dyslipidemia, hypertension, and atherosclerosis (Kopelman, 2000).

Results from previous experimental and clinical studies have suggested that citrus PMFs may improve glycemic control and reduce insulin resistance (Kurowska & Manthey, 2004., Miyata et al., 2011; Li et al., 2006; Judy et al., 2010).

It is known that an increase in the number and size of adipocytes in adipose tissues leads to obesity-related insulin resistance. In a recent study, both nobiletin and tangeretin were found to increase the secretion of adiponectin (insulin-sensitizing factor) and decrease the secretion of MCP-1 (insulin-resistance factor) in 3T3-L1 adipocytes demonstrated by lower intracellular triglyceride levels as compared to vehicle-treated adipocytes. Further, nobiletin also decreased the secretion of resistin, which serves as an insulin-resistance factor (Miyata et al., 2011).

Mulvihill & Huff, 2011, reported on the ability of nobiletin to improve whole-body insulin sensitivity and decrease hepatic gluconeogenesis induced in *Ldlr*$^{-/-}$ mice when fed a high-fat Western type diet. This effect of nobiletin was achieved by both an increase in peripheral glucose disposal and enhanced suppression of hepatic glucose production by insulin (Mulvihill & Huff, 2011). Prevention of insulin resistance, glucose intolerance and adiposity required 0.3% nobiletin suggesting that prevention of obesity and improved glucose tolerance by nobiletin are linked (Mulvihill & Huff, 2011).

Furthermore, in *Ldlr*$^{-/-}$ mice, nobiletin supplementation reduced bodyweight, very low density lipoprotein cholesterol–triglyceride secretion and improved dyslipidemia. A study by Lee et al., 2010 suggested that nobiletin improved hyperglycemia and insulin resistance in obese diabetic *ob/ob* mice by regulating expression of glucose transporter (Glut) 4 levels in the whole plasma membrane, white adipose tissue (WAT) and muscle, and by regulating expression of adipokines in WAT. In addition, a mixture of nobiletin and tangeretin were found to regulate glucose metabolism in hamsters with fructose-induced insulin resistance by modulating adipokines (Li et al., 2006). In this study PMF supplementation also reduced triglyceride content in both the liver and heart and was able to significantly suppress serum tumor necrosis factor-α (TNF-α), interferon-γ (INF-γ), interleukin-1β (IL-1β) and interleukin-6 (IL-6) expression and increased serum adiponectin protein in insulin resistant hamsters. Additionally, in a study in hamsters with insulin resistance induced by feeding 60% fructose, the addition of 1% PMFs improved glucose tolerance, as demonstrated by the reduced area under the curve (AUC) measured after the intra-peritoneal injection of glucose (3g/kg body weight)(Kurowska & Manthey, 2004).

In a recent study, the anti-diabetic potential of Diabetinol®, a dietary supplement consisting of >62% PMF extract from dried fruit and orange peel, composed mainly of nobiletin and tangeretin in a 4:1 ratio, was tested in fructose induced insulin resistant male Syrian golden hamsters. The Diabetinol® treatment group and positive control group were fed a fructose-enriched diet for three weeks to induce hypertriglyceridemia and insulin resistance (Taghibiglou et al., 2000). Hamsters (n=18) were fed regular chow, 60% fructose or a 60% fructose diet + 1% Diabetinol®. At the end of the study (Day 49), hamsters fed 60% fructose + 1% Diabetinol® demonstrated lower blood glucose, total cholesterol and triacylglycerol levels as compared to the fructose-fed animals (Judy et al., 2010).

3.2 Effect of Diabetinol® on symptoms of metabolic syndrome – A human pilot study

3.2.1 Subjects and study design

The objective of the study was to investigate the efficacy of Diabetinol® (2 × 525 mg/day) vs. Placebo (Cellulose, 2 × 525mg/day) in glycemic control and management of risk factors of metabolic syndrome when supplemented for 12 weeks. Nineteen subjects with impaired fasting glucose (IFG) on stable oral medications were presented with a standard oral glucose challenge for the study.

The study was a randomized, double-blind, placebo-controlled study. Subjects included were between ages of 18-75 years and had a body mass index (BMI) 25.0 to 39.9kg/m^2, were weight stable (for 3 months prior to study), had a fasting glucose level between 6.1 and 9.0mmol/L (109.8–162.0mg/dL), and a HbA1c level<7%. Subjects were excluded from participating if they were diabetic and required insulin therapy (Judy et al., 2010).

The study included 5 clinic visits, which occurred at screening, baseline (Day 0), day 28, 56 and 84.

At baseline (randomization visit) and at all other visits anthropometric measurements were recorded, and BMI and waist/hip ratio were calculated. Fasting blood was collected for the determination of glucose, insulin and HbA1c. An oral glucose tolerance test (OGTT), where subjects consumed 100g of a glucose beverage over a 10min period was conducted and blood samples collected at 30, 60, 120, 180 and 240min post glucose consumption for analysis of glucose and insulin. On day 84, prior to the OGTT an additional 10mL of blood was collected for serum chemistry, hematology and for the determination of the lipid profile.

Fasting glucose, insulin, HbA1c and AUC glucose and insulin were compared within group and HbA1c levels between the two groups by Student's t-test. Statistical significance was established at $p<0.05$.

3.2.2 Results

Analysis of subject demographics demonstrated that baseline fasting glucose was not different between groups (Diabetinol® 130.33 ± 3.64 mg/dL and placebo 129.80 ± 8.52mg/dL) but was above acceptable levels (<100mg/dL) and indicated that subjects in both groups had mild hyperglycemia (100–150mg/dL). Baseline HbA1c levels were not significantly different between subjects on placebo and Diabetinol® (6.53 ± 0.22% and 6.39 ± 0.22%, respectively).

At baseline, 28, 56 and 84 days the peak in the plasma glucose curve following the glucose challenge, occurred between 60 and 120min in subjects on Diabetinol® or placebo (Fig. 2 a and 2 b). After supplementation for 56 and 84 days the glucose response curve of subjects on the Diabetinol® group was blunted as compared to the levels in the baseline OGTT curve.

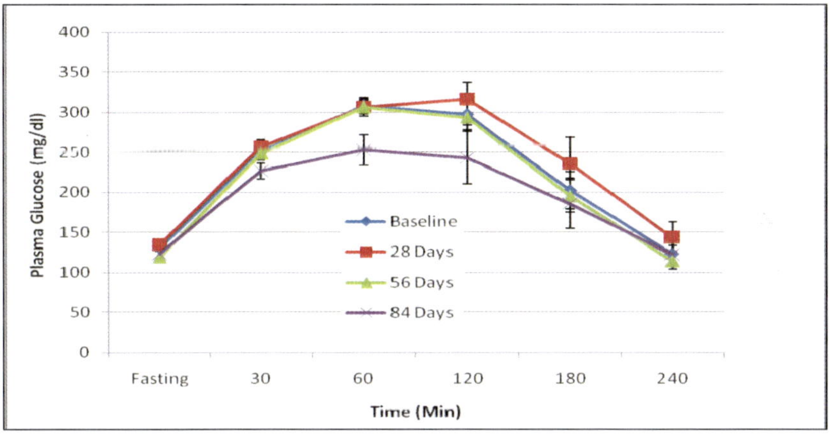

(a)

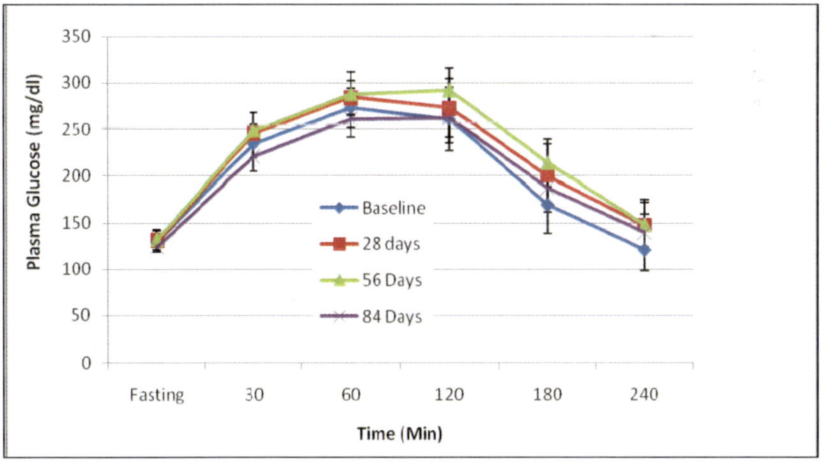

(b)

Fig. 2. Plasma glucose response curves to a standard glucose tolerance test before and after 28, 56 and 84 days of (a) Diabetinol® and (b) placebo supplementation. The plasma response curve at 84 days was significantly different ($p<0.01$) from baseline at 30, 60 and 120min for Diabetinol® by Student's *t*-test. Each data point is represented as mean ± SEM.

Further, after 84 days of supplementation subjects on Diabetinol® demonstrated a significant reduction in plasma glucose at 30, 60 and 120min after the glucose challenge when compared to baseline (Day 0) plasma glucose levels after the OGTT ($p<0.01$). The plasma glucose response curves after a glucose challenge at 28, 56 and 84 days for subjects on the placebo were not significantly different from that of their baseline values (Fig. 2b).

There was no significant difference in mean fasting glucose values at baseline or day 84 between, Diabetinol® (from 130.33 ± 3.64mg/dL at baseline to 123.33 ± 6.70mg/dL) or placebo (129.80 ± 8.52 to 123.90 ± 5.04mg/dL) (Fig. 2a and b).

There was an increase of 9.0mg/dL in mean plasma glucose on day 28 and a reduction of 9.0mg/dL on Day 56, and a significant reduction of 56.0mg/dL ($p<0.01$) on day 84 from baseline in subjects on Diabetinol® compared to those on placebo (data not shown). A mean reduction in AUC of 127mg/dL/h from baseline to day 84 was demonstrated in the Diabetinol® group while there was a 10mg/dL/h increase in subjects in the placebo group.

There was no difference in plasma HbA1c levels between placebo and Diabetinol® groups at baseline, day 28, 56 or 84 (Fig. 3). HbA1c levels are not expected to change for 3-4 months after an intervention. However, in this study after 84days of supplementation decreasing trends in the HbA1c were observed in subjects supplemented with Diabetinol® compared to subjects on placebo. Fasting plasma insulin levels were not significantly different between subjects on placebo and Diabetinol® at baseline, day 28, 56 or 84 and did not change significantly from baseline to day 28, 56 or 84 in the Diabetinol® or placebo groups.

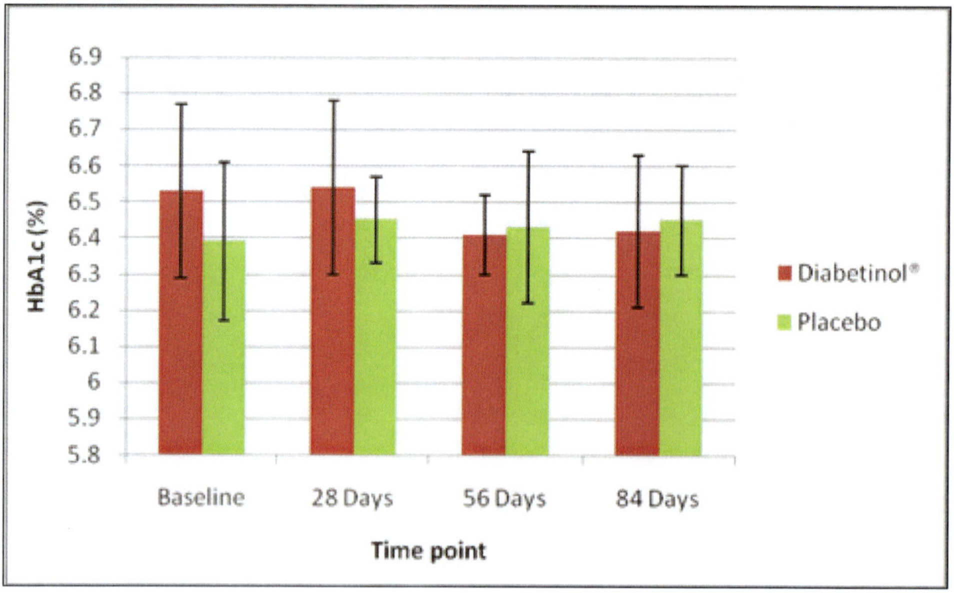

Fig. 3. Plasma HbAlc levels for placebo and Diabetinol® after 28, 56 and 84 days of supplementation. Statistical analysis was determined using Student's *t*-test. Each data point is represented as mean ± SEM.

There were no statistically significant differences between subjects on placebo and Diabetinol® at baseline for total plasma cholesterol, triacylglycerols, low density lipoprotein cholesterol (LDL-C) and high density lipoprotein cholesterol (HDL-C) levels (Fig. 4). This cohort of subjects had lipid levels which were higher than the clinically acceptable range for these parameters. Subjects in the Diabetinol®group demonstrated a 13.29% reduction in total cholesterol ($p<0.01$) and a 22.79% reduction in LDL-C ($p<0.01$) from baseline to 84 days (Fig. 5a). There were no significant changes in the lipid profiles from baseline to day 84 in subjects on placebo (Fig. 5b).

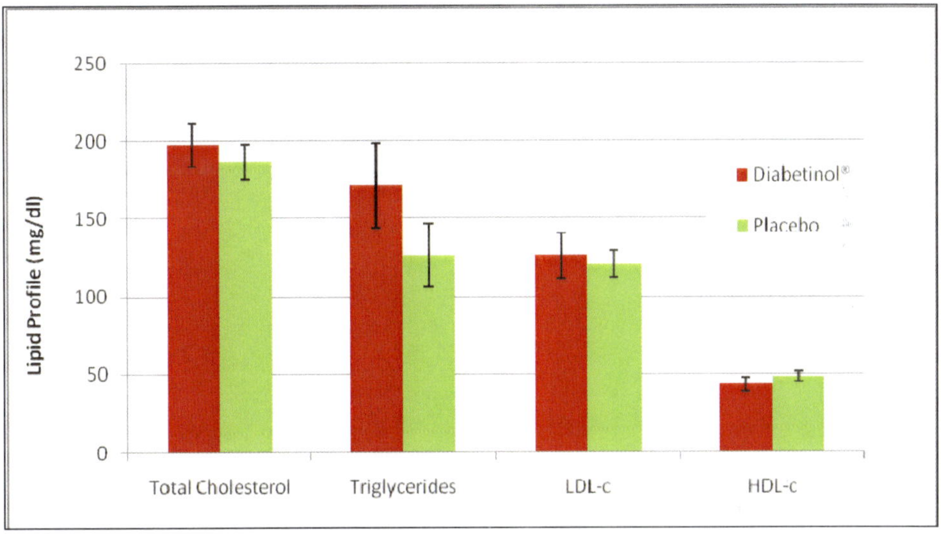

Fig. 4. Baseline (Day 0) plasma lipids for placebo and Diabetinol®. Statistical analysis of plasma lipids were determined using Student's *t*-test. Data points are represented as mean ± SEM.

3.3 Hyperlipidemia

Elevated blood total cholesterol, higher LDL-C and reduced HDL-C are established risk factors of cardiovascular disease. Interest in PMFs has increased in recent years because of strong evidence showing that PMFs might lower total cholesterol, triglycerides, LDL-C and increase HDL-C in a number of *in-vivo* (Kurowska & Manthey, 2004; Li et al., 2006), *in-vitro* (Kurowska & Manthey, 2002; Kurowska et al., 2004) and human studies (Kurowska et al., 2000; Roza et al., 2007).

Previous studies demonstrated that PMFs from citrus, especially tangeretin and nobiletin, produce hypolipidemic responses in cells (Kurowska & Manthey, 2002; Kurowska et al., 2004) and animals (Kurowska & Manthey., 2004), and that they also normalize some metabolic defects associated with experimentally induced insulin resistance (Kurowska & Manthey, 2004).

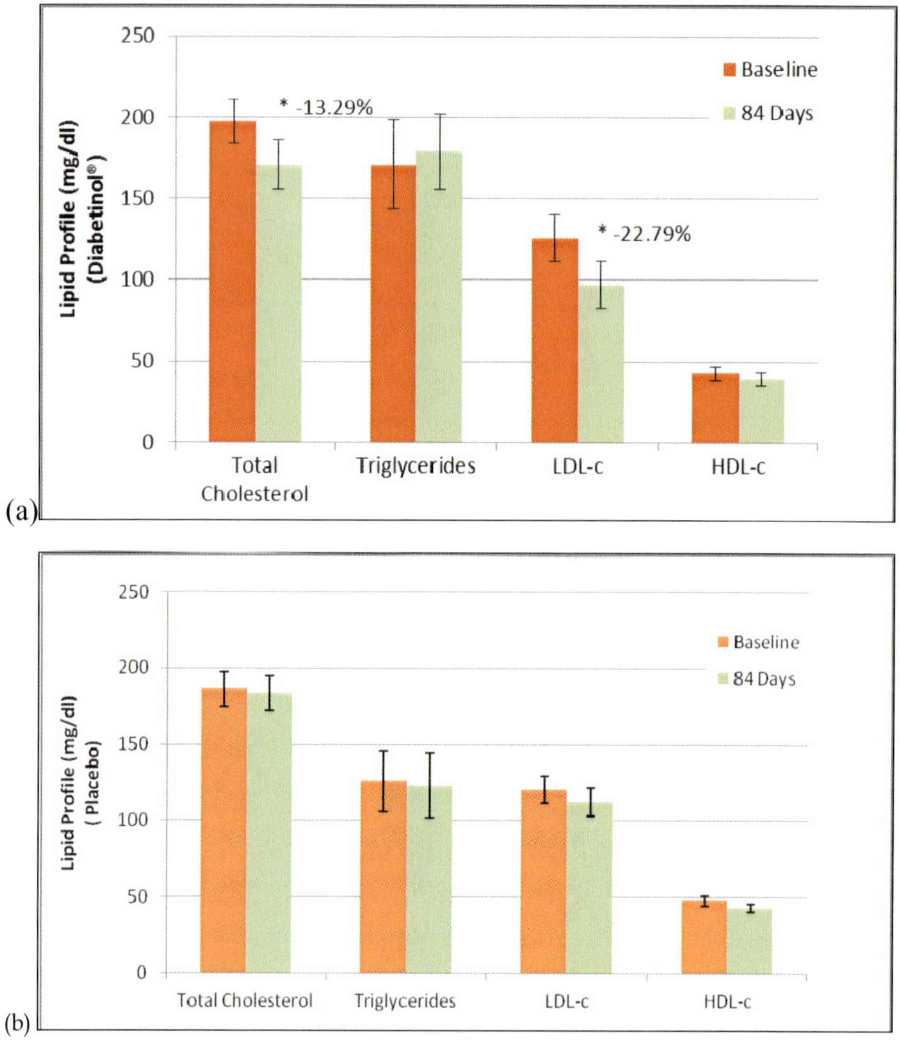

Fig. 5. (a) ∗ Diabetinol® group plasma lipids levels after 84 days of supplementation compared to the baseline (Day 0) levels (b) placebo control group plasma lipids levels after 84 days of supplementation compared to the baseline (Day 0) levels. ∗p<0.01, day 84 values are significantly different from baseline values by Student t-test. Each data point is represented as mean ± SEM.

Cell culture studies, demonstrated that several natural and synthetic PMFs have the ability to inhibit the net secretion of apolipoprotein B (Apo-B) in human liver cell line HepG2 (Kurowska & Manthey, 2002). In HepG2, tangeretin substantially reduced the secretion of Apo-B and the synthesis of triacylglycerols which was associated with the activation of peroxisome proliferator-activated receptor (PPAR). PPAR is the nuclear transcription factor which is known to possess positive regulatory impact on sugar, fatty acids and lipoprotein metabolism (Kurowska et al., 2004). Nobiletin has been reported to inhibit macrophage acetylated LDL metabolism, resulting in the blockage of formation of macrophage foam-cells, which are essential to atherosclerotic plaque formation (Whitman et al., 2005).

Results from animal studies demonstrated that dietary supplementation with 1% tangeretin or 1% PMFs (largely tangeretin and nobiletin) significantly reduced serum total cholesterol, very low density lipoprotein cholesterol and LDL-C (by 19–27 and 32–40%, respectively) and also decreased serum and liver triglycerides in hamsters with diet-induced hypercholesterolemia (Kurowska & Manthey, 2004). Positive effects of PMFs were also reported with respect to adipocytokine production and PPAR in insulin resistant hamsters. The PMF supplementation showed a reversal in metabolic defects including a reduction in insulin level and an improvement in glucose tolerance, thus confirming their antiinflammatory and antidiabetic effects (Li et al., 2006). This action is speculated to occur via the inhibition of the synthesis of core protein Apo-B required for LDL synthesis in the liver (Borradaile et al., 1999).

In human studies, the responses to dietary supplements containing citrus PMFs in subjects with moderate hypercholesterolemia and baseline characteristics consistent with metabolic syndrome, demonstrated that a four week period improved blood lipid profiles without causing any adverse effects (Kurowska et al., 2001). Previously lipid lowering effects were also seen in hypercholesterolemic subjects taking orange juice for four weeks (Kurowska et al., 2000). Consistently, in moderately hypercholesterolemic men, mixtures of nobiletin and tangeretin at a dose of 270 mg/day, in combination with tocotrienols (30 mg/day), reduced plasma LDL-C, Apo-B and triglycerides (Roza et al., 2007). This suggests that PMFs have substantial cholesterol and triacylglycerol lowering potential.

4. The importance of pharmacokinetics studies of PMFs

Pharmacokinetics is the study of the mechanisms of absorption, metabolism and routes of excretion of the metabolites of an administered drug or nutrient. Bioavailability of a nutrient is simply the quantity or fraction of the ingested dose that is absorbed. Pharmacokinetic studies on PMFs are important in identifying the composition of metabolites of administered supplements. They may also help in differentiating different supplements on the market which have different levels and ratios of PMFs (i.e. nobiletin, tangeretin). Additionally, these studies may further provide information regarding absorption and metabolism of different formulations (i.e. soft gel capsule, hard shell capsule etc).

There are multiple challenges in the development of PMFs which must be overcome to increase their bioavailability. For example, PMFs exist as aglycones. The solubility of aglycone forms is low, which may lead to slower dissolution rates in addition to the fact that absorbed aglycones are rapidly conjugated to glucuronides and sulfates in the intestine and liver (Li et al., 2007). Therefore, it is important to perform systematic studies to demonstrate how changes in PMF structures affect solubility and dissolution rates.

Previous studies in hamsters showed, that when they were fed a tangeretin-enriched diet for 35 days, the main PMF metabolites identified in serum, urine and in liver tissue included dihydroxytrimethoxyflavone and monohydroxytetramethoxyflavone glucuronides and aglycones (Kurowska & Manthey, 2004). This demonstrated considerable intestinal absorption of tangeretin based on urinary excretion of several metabolites. However, no unchanged (parental) tangeretin was detected in the circulating plasma (Kurowska & Manthey, 2004).

In a recent study by Manthey et al., 2011, nobiletin and tangeretin were administered to rats by gavage and intraperitoneal (ip) injection. By using high-performance liquid chromatography−electrospray ionization−mass spectrometry (HPLC-ESI-MS), blood serum concentrations of metabolites were monitored. Over 24 hours, two metabolites of tangeretin and eight metabolites of nobiletin were detected with the administered compounds. Results from this study demonstrated that with identical oral doses nearly 10-fold higher absorption of nobiletin occurred in comparison to tangeretin. Further, in the blood serum, maximum levels of glucuronidated metabolites occurred later than nobiletin and tangeretin and occurred at higher concentrations than aglycone metabolites (Manthey et al., 2011). It is also confirmed in previous trials that overall expression of biological actions of nobiletin and tangeretin in animals is due to the biological actions of aglycone metabolites (Eguchi et al., 2007; Li et al., 2007; Lai et al., 2008; Xiao et al., 2009).

Wan & Walle, 2006, demonstrated that the flavonoid chrysin (5,7-dihydroxyflavone) has poor bioavailability, but when two hydroxyl groups in chrysin were methylated, as in 5,7-dimethoxyflavone (5,7-DMF), using cofactors for glucuronidation, sulfation and oxidation, chrysin was rapidly metabolized within 20 minutes of incubation showing no parent compound at the end. In contrast, over the whole 60-min time-course studied, 5,7-DMF was found to be metabolically stable (Wen & Walle, 2006). Further, there is evidence of the role of different cytochrome P450 isozymes, in oxidative demethylation in PMFs metabolism (Koga et al., 2007; Breinholt et al., 2003).

Results from these studies on oral bioavailability thus indicated that the methoxylated flavones have a great advantage over the nonmethylated flavones. Future studies are needed to investigate the biochemical factors influencing the pharmacokinetics of PMFs.

5. Pharmacokinetics of PMFs in Sytrinol®

5.1 Sytrinol®: A proprietary supplement consisting of PMFs and Tocotrienols

Sytrinol® is a proprietary supplement developed by KGK Synergize Inc and consists of PMFs, mainly tangeretin and nobiletin (1:1 v/v) and palm oil tocotrienols. Tocotrienols are a group of dietary constituents, which are analogues of tocopherol (vitamin E), found mainly in palm oil and cereal grains. Tocotrienol-rich fractions from palm oil usually contain tocotrienols α, λ and Δ, as well as 15-40% α-tocopherol (Guthrie & Carroll, 1998). The cholesterol-lowering potential of PMFs and tocotrienols has been investigated in preclinical studies and in clinical trials (Kurowska et al., 2004; Kurowska & Manthey, 2004; Roza et al., 2007).

5.2 Human bioavailability study of three Sytrinol® formulations in healthy subjects

5.2.1 Subjects & study design

The objective of this study was to determine whether PMFs may be detected and quantified in serum obtained from healthy adults after a single dose administration of Sytrinol® capsules (containing 1053 mg of total PMFs). The study compared oral bioavailability of three Sytrinol® formulations in healthy subjects. The endpoints were the determination of various pharmacokinetic parameters, specifically area under the concentration-time curve ($AUC_{0\text{-}48h}$), time at maximum concentration (T_{max}) and maximum serum concentration (C_{max}) for each of tangeretin and nobiletin.

The study was conducted as a randomized crossover trial. Ten healthy subjects, five men and five women, age 23 ± 3 years, were recruited for the study. Prior to the start of the study, subjects had blood drawn for routine tests to confirm eligibility. All subjects were asked to avoid caffeine-containing products 12 h prior to the study and during the study.

Subjects were administered a single dose of the first Sytrinol® product (either Sytrinol® soft gel capsules (Product A), Sytrinol® powder hard shell capsules (Product B) or Sytrinol® hard shell capsules with added lecithin (Product C), containing 1053 mg of PMFs, largely tangeretin and nobiletin (1:1 v/v) and tocotrienols. Standard citrus-free meals (breakfast, lunch and dinner) were provided on each of the days of the multiple blood sampling. Participants took the second PMF product 14 days later and the third product after another 14 day washout period.

Peripheral blood was taken by venipuncture at time 0 (baseline), 0.25, 0.5, 1, 2, 4, 6, 8, 24 and 48 hours after ingestion of Sytrinol® capsules. Quantitation of tangeretin and nobiletin in serum was done by Liquid chromatography/Mass spectrometry (Varian 1200 L LC/MS/MS system equipped with ESI and APCI sources). The identities of these PMFs were verified by comparing fragment ion mass spectra of authentic tangeretin and nobiletin standards.

5.2.2 Results

The serum samples obtained from healthy subjects following oral administration of three different Sytrinol® formulations demonstrated detectable amounts of parental tangeretin and nobiletin. Tangeretin and nobiletin peaks were identified and quantitated in all serum samples collected after administration of Sytrinol® formulations A, B or C.

Results demonstrated that for both tangeretin and nobiletin, the $AUC_{0\text{-}48h}$ and C_{max} values were significantly higher ($P<0.001$) after administration of formulation A than after treatment with products B or C, suggesting greater bioavailability of formulation A vs. B or C (Tables 1 & 2). For all three formulations, the $AUC_{0\text{-}48h}$ values were higher for nobiletin than for tangeretin indicating that nobiletin might be more bioavailable than tangeretin. The time-concentration curves and pharmacokinetic results demonstrated that for both tangeretin and nobiletin, significantly higher $AUC_{0\text{-}48h}$ and C_{max} values were obtained following the administration of formulation A than following the administration of either B or C (Figure 6 & 7). The effects of the Sytrinol® formulations A, B and C on $AUC_{0\text{-}48h}$ and C_{max} of tangeretin and nobiletin derivatives are depicted in Figures 8 & 9. For nobiletin, the $AUC_{0\text{-}48h}$ values were 2.7-3.0 times higher for supplement A than for B or C whereas for tangeretin, the $AUC_{0\text{-}48h}$ values were 1.7-2.3 times higher for A than for B or C. Changes in mean serum concentrations of tangeretin and nobiletin products after a single-dose administration of Sytrinol® A, B or C formulations are shown in Figures 6 and 7. The T_{max} values were not affected by the type of treatment and also were similar for tangeretin and nobiletin peaks (1.3-1.4 h).

	A	B	C	P value
Initial conc. (µg/L)	49.5 ± 10.6	63.5 ± 51.6	28.5 ± 20.8	
$AUC_{0\text{-}48h}$(µg x min/L)	4654.4 ± 1929.3	1538.0 ± 249.3***	1715.0 ± 914.2***	<0.0001
C_{max} (µg /L)	1006.4 ± 555.3	51.8 ± 18.8***	63.7 ± 33.2***	<0.0001
T_{max} (h)	1.4 ± 0.5	1.48 ± 0.8	1.4 ± 0.6	

***A vs. B, C are significantly different (p<0.001) by ANOVA followed by Tukey's test.

Table 1. Pharmacokinetics of serum nobiletin (means ± SD).

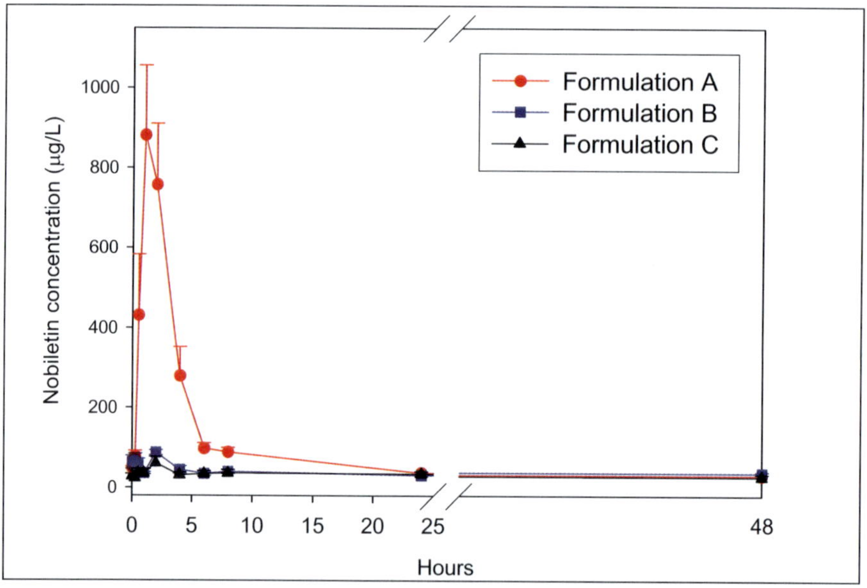

Fig. 6. Changes in serum concentrations of nobiletin after a single dose administration of Sytrinol® formulations A, B and C (1053 mg PMFs per product) (means ± SEM).

Capsules contained both PMFs in equal amounts, however, more nobiletin than tangeretin was generally found in the blood. The differences were particularly striking in blood samples collected after administration of supplements A and B (with the $AUC_{0\text{-}48h}$ ratios of nobiletin to tangeretin 1.85 and 1.42, respectively) but also tended to occur after the administration of C (with the nobiletin to tangeretin ratio 1.14). The results suggest that in healthy human subjects, nobiletin might be more bioavailable than tangeretin. The pharmacokinetic results showed that in healthy human subjects, Sytrinol® product A (Soft Gel) was significantly more bioavailable than the remaining two products, B (hard shell) and C (hard shell + lecithin). Formulation A differed from B and C in respect to $AUC_{0\text{-}48h}$ and C_{max} but not in respect to T_{max}, which was not affected by treatments. Our data also suggest that nobiletin present in Sytrinol® formulations is more bioavailable than tangeretin.

	A	B	C	P value
Initial conc. (µg / L)	31.4 ± 5.7	37.2 ± 25.6	29.9 ± 21.6	
$AUC_{0\text{-}48h}$ (µg x min/L)	2509.6 ± 1092.8	1085.8 ± 198.8**	1499.3 ± 864.0*	0.0041
C_{max} (µg / L)	532.3 ± 335.7	76.4 ± 49.9***	48.0 ± 30.1***	<0.0001
T_{max} (h)	1.3 ± 0.5	1.3 ± 0.8	1.2 ± 0.6	

*A vs. C is p<0.05, **A vs. B is p<0.01,
***A vs. B, C are p<0.001 by ANOVA followed by Tukey's test.

Table 2. Pharmacokinetics of serum tangeretin (means ± SD)

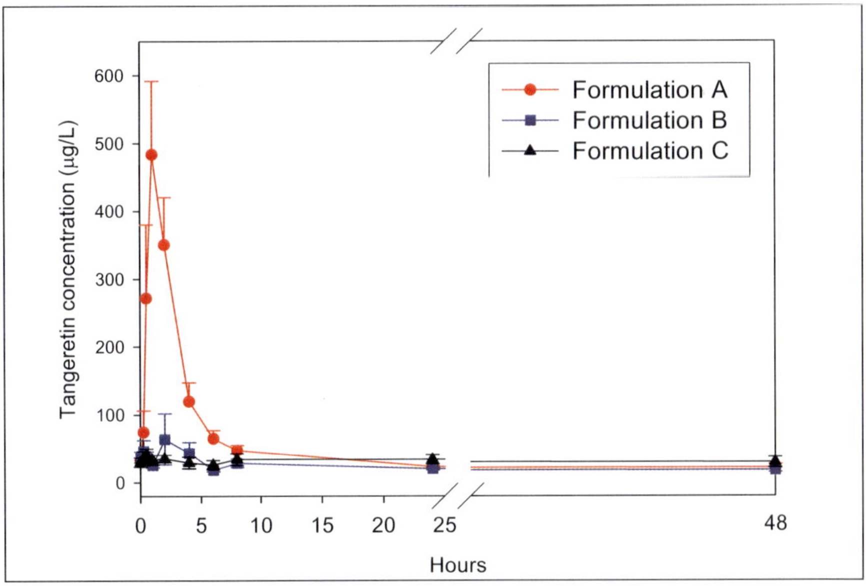

Fig. 7. Changes in serum concentrations of tangeretin after a single-dose administration of Sytrinol® formulations A, B and C (1053 mg PMFs per each dose (means ± SEM).

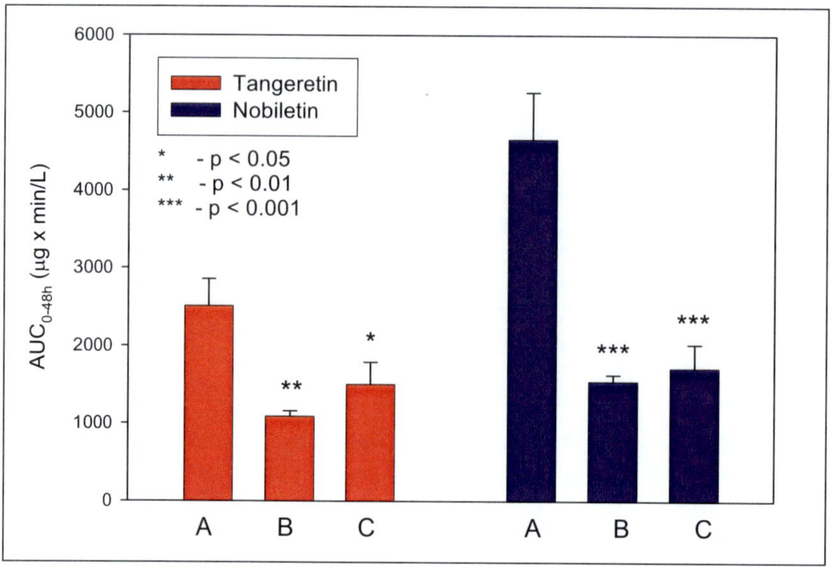

Fig. 8. Effects of Sytrinol® formulations A, B and C on $AUC_{0\text{-}48h}$ of tangeretin and nobiletin (means ± SEM). Values significantly different by ANOVA followed by Tukey's test. *A vs. C is $p<0.05$, **A vs. B is $p<0.01$, ***A vs. B, C are $p<0.001$.

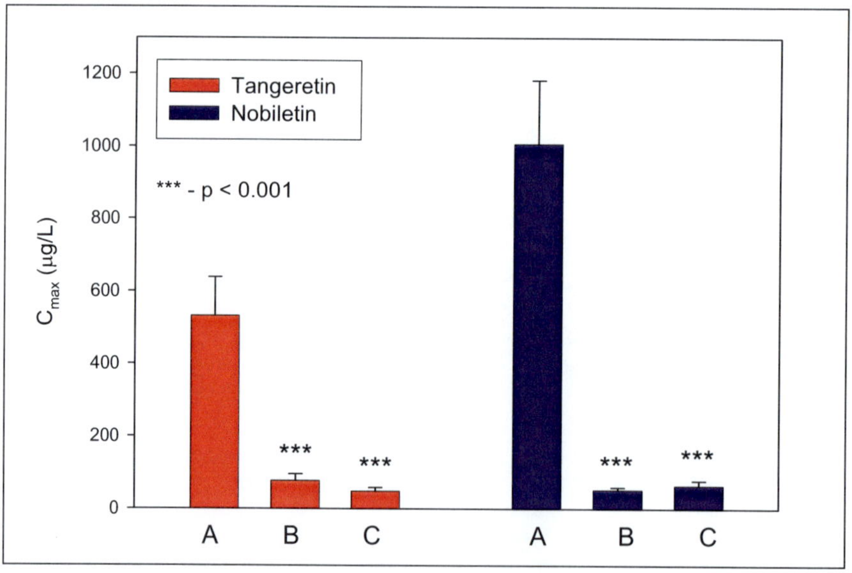

Fig. 9. Effects of Sytrinol® formulations A, B and C on C_{max} of tangeretin and nobiletin (means ± SEM). Values significantly different by ANOVA followed by Tukey's test. ***A vs. B, C are significantly different ($p<0.001$).

6. Conclusion

Bioavailability of a drug or nutrient supplement is largely determined by the properties of the dosage form. Yet, further characterizations of the metabolism and the biochemical factors influencing these compounds' pharmacokinetics are essential, especially as oral bioavailability appears to be a significant limiting factor to the efficacy of these and other citrus PMFs.

Both nobiletin and tangeretin have demonstrated efficacy in metabolic syndrome and hyperlipidemia, but vary in their pharmacokinetic properties. Research has demonstrated that nobiletin has greater bioavailability and efficacy as compared to tangeretin. Diabetinol® was developed with this concept in mind in order to address metabolic syndrome and hyperlipidemia.

The pharmacokinetic profiles of nobiletin and tangeretin were previously based on the detection and quantification of their metabolites. In this chapter we have presented data on the detection of the parental compound nobiletin and tangeretin and suggest that in future research it is important to determine these compounds in human pharmacokinetic studies.

Differences in bioavailability among formulations of a given supplement may have clinical significance; thus, knowing whether nutrient or drug formulations are equivalent is essential in making reasonable conclusions.

7 Acknowledgements

We would like to thank the volunteers of the Sytrinol® and Diabetinol® studies for their willingness and diligence in complying with the protocol. These studies were conducted at KGK Synergize, Inc London, ON, Canada and SIBR Research, Inc., West Bradenton, FL, USA respectively. The results of the Diabetinol® study are published in Judy et al., 2010. The authors would like to thank J. Baisley for his technical expertise.

8. References

Borradaile, N.M., Carroll, K.K., & Kurowska, E.M. (1999) Regulation of HepG2 cell apolipoprotein B metabolism by the citrus flavanones hesperetin and naringenin. *Lipids*, Vol.34, No.6, pp.(591-598), ISSN 0024-4201

Breinholt, V. M., Rasmussen, S. E., Brosen, K., & Friedberg, T. H. (2003) In vitro metabolism of genistein and tangeretin by human and murine cytochrome P450s. *Pharmacol. Toxicol.*, Vol. 93, pp.(14- 22), ISSN 0742-8413

Datla, K. P., Christidou, M., Widmer, W. W., Rooprai, H. K., & Dexter, D. T. (2001) Tissue distribution and neuroprotective effects of citrus flavonoid tangeretin in a rat model of Parkinson's disease. *NeuroReport*, Vol.12, No.17, pp. (3871-3875), ISSN 0959-4965

Dugo, P., & McHale, D. (2002). The oxygen heterocyclic compounds of citrus essential oils. *Citrus. The Genus Citrus*, pp. (355- 390), CRC Press, ISBN 04152-84910

Eguchi, A., Murakami, A., Li, S., Ho, C. T., & Ohigashi, H. (2007) Suppressive effects of demethylated metabolites of nobiletin on phorbol ester-induced expression of scavenger receptor genes in THP-1 human monocytic cells. *Biofactors*, Vol. 31, pp. (107- 116), ISSN 0951-6433

Guthrie, N., Carroll K. K. (1998) Inhibition of mammary cancer by citrus flavonoids. *Adv Exp Med Biol*, Vol. 439, pp.(227-236) Kluwer Academic/ Plenum Publishers ISBN 0-306-48177-4 New York

Hollman, P. C., & Katan, M.B. (1999). Dietary flavonoids: intake, health effects and bioavailability. *Food Chem Toxicol*. Vol. 37, pp. (937-42), ISSN 0278-6915

Horowitz, R. M., & Gentili, B. (1977). Flavonoid constituents of citrus. *Citrus Science and Technology*, Vol. 1, pp.(397– 426), Avi Pub Co. ISBN 10: 087055221X, ISBN 13: 978-0870552212The University of California

Ishii, K., Tanaka, S., Kagami, K., Henmi, K., Toyoda, H., Kaise, T., & Hirano, T. (2010). Effects of naturally occurring polymethyoxyflavonoids on cell growth, p-glycoprotein function, cell cycle, and apoptosis of daunorubicin-resistant T lymphoblastoid leukemia cells. *Cancer Invest*. Vol. 28, No. 3, pp (220-9), ISSN 0735-7907

Judy, W., Stogsdill, W., Judy, D., Judy, J., Sharma, P., Evans, M., & Guthrie, N. (2010) Efficacy of Diabetinol™ on glycemic control in insulin resistant hamsters and subjects with impaired fasting glucose - a pilot study. *J of Fun Foods*, Vol.2, No. 3, pp. (171-178), ISSN 1756-4646

Koga, N., Matsuo, M., Ohta, C., Haraguchi, K., Matsuoka, M., Kato, Y., Ishii, T., Yano, M., & Ohta, H. (2007) Comparative study of nobiletin metabolism with liver microsomes from rats, guinea pigs and hamsters and rat cytochrome P450. *Biol. Pharm. Bull,*. Vol. 30, pp.(2317– 2323), ISSN 1347-5215

Kopelman, P. G. (2000), Obesity as a medical problem. *Nature*, Vol.404, No.6778, pp.(635–643), ISSN 0028-0836

Kurowska, E. M., & Manthey, J. A. (2004). Hypolipodemic effects and absorption of citrus polymethoxylated flavones in hamsters with diet-induced hypercholesterolemia. *J. Agric. Food Chem.*, pp. (2879– 2886), ISSN 0021-8561

Kurowska, E. M., Manthey, J.A., Casaschi A., & Theriault, A.G. (2004) Modulation of HepG2 cell net apolipoprotein B secretion by the citrus polymethoxyflavone, tangeretin. *Lipids*. Vol.39, No.2, pg.(143-51), ISSN 0024-4201

Kurowska, E. M., & Manthey, J. A. (2002) Regulation of lipoprotein metabolism in HepG2 cells by citrus flavonoids. *Adv Exp Med Biol*, Vol. 505, pp.(173-179), Kluwer Academic/ Plenum Publishers ISBN 0-306-48177-4 New York

Kurowska, E. M. (2001) Hypolipidemic activities of tangeretin, a flavonoid from tangerines, invitro and invivo. *FASEB*, Vol.15, pp.(A395) ISSN 0892-6638

Kurowska, E.M., Spence, J. D., Jordan, J., Wetmore, S., Freeman, D.J., Piche, L.A., & Serratore, P. (2000), HDL-cholesterol-raising effect of orange juice in subjects with hypercholesterolemia. *Am J of Clin Nut*, Vol.72, No.5, pp.(1095-1100), ISSN 0002-9165

Lai, C. S., Li, S., Chai, C. Y., Lo, C. Y., Dushenkov, S., Ho, C. T., Pan, M. H., & Wang, Y. J. (2008) Anti-inflammatory and antitumor promotional effects of a novel urinary metabolite, 3',4'-didemethylnobiletin, derived from nobiletin. *Carcinogenesis*, Vol.29, pp (2415– 2424), ISSN 0143-3334

Lee, Y. S., Cha, B. Y., Miyataa, Y., Saitoa, K., Yamakawab, H., Choia, S. S., Yamajuchia, K., Yonezawaa, T., Teruya, T., Nagaia, K., & Wooa, J.T. (2010) Nobiletin improves hyperglycemia and insulin resistance in obese diabetic ob/ob mice. Bichemical Pharmacology, Vol.79, No. 11, pp.(1674-1683), ISSN 0006-2952

Li, R. W., Theriault, A. G., Au, K., Douglas, T. D., Casachi, A., Kurowska, E. M., & Mukherjee, R. (2006). Citrus polymethoxylated flavones improve lipid and glucose homeostasis and modulate adipocytokines in fructose-induced insulin resistant hamsters. *Life Sci.*, Vol 79, pp. (365- 373), ISSN 0024-3205

Li, S., Sang, S., Pan, M. H., Lai, C. S., Lo, C. Y., Yang, C. S., & Ho, C. T. (2007) Anti-inflammatory property of the urinary metabolites of nobiletin in mouse Bioorg. *Med. Chem. Lett.* Vol. 17, pp.(5177- 5181), ISSN

Lin, N., Sato, T., Takayam, Y., Mimaki, Y., Sashida, Y. & Yano, M. (2003) Novel anti-inflammatory actions of nobiletin, a citrus polymethoxy flavonoid, on human synovial fibroblasts and mouse macrophages. *Biochem Pharmacol,* Vol.65, No.12, pp. (2065–2071), ISSN 0006-2952

Manach, C., & Donovan, J. L. (2004) Pharmacokinetics and metabolism of dietary flavonoids in humans. *Free Rad. Res.*, Vol.38, pp.(771 785), ISSN 1071-5762

Manthey, J. A., Cesar, T.B., Jackson, E., & Mertens-Talcott, S. (2011). Pharmacokinetic study of nobiletin and tangeretin in rat serum by high-performance liquid chromatography-electrospray ionization-mass spectrometry. *J Agric Food Chem.* Vol. 59, No. 1, pp. (145-51), ISSN 1520-5118

Miyataa, Y., Tanakaa, H., Shimadaa, A., Satob, T., Itob, A., Yamanouchic, T., & Kosanoa, H., (2011) Regulation of adipocytokine secretion and adipocyte hypertrophy by polymethoxyflavonoids, nobiletin and tangeretin. *Life Sciences,* Vol. 88, No 13-14,ISSN 0024-3205

Mulvihill, E. E., & Huff, M. W. (2011) How can nobeletin prevent obesity? *Expert Review of Endocrinology & Metabolism*, Vol.6, No.4, pp.(501-503), ISSN 1744-6651

Roza, J. M., Xian-Liu, Z., Guthrie, N. (2007). Effect of citrus flavonoids and tocotrienols on serum cholesterol levels in hypercholesterolemic subjects. *Alternative Ther,* Vol 13, pp. (44- 48), ISSN 1078-6791

Silalahi, J. (2002) Anticancer and health protective properties of citrus fruit components. *Asia Pac J Clin Nutr*, Vol.11, No.1, pp.(79–84), ISSN 1440-1647

Taghibiglou, C. (2000) Mechanism of hepatic very low density lipoprotein overproduction in insulin resistance. *Journal of Biological Chemistry.* Vol.275, pp.8416 ISSN 0021-9258

Walle, T. (2007) Methoxylated flavones, a superior cancer chemopreventive flavonoid subclass? *Semin Cancer Biol.*, Vol.17, No.5, pp.(354-62), ISSN1044-579X

Walle, T., Browning, A. M., Steed, L. S., Reed, S. G., & Walle, U. K. (2005) Flavonoid glucosides are hydrolyzed and thus activated in the oral cavity in humans. *J. Nutr.*, Vol.135, pp.(48 52), ISSN 0022-3166

Walle, T., Hsieh, F., DeLegge, M. H., Oatis, J. E. Jr., & Walle, U.K. (2004) High absorption but very low bioavailability of oral resveratrol in humans. *Drug Metab Dispos,* Vol.32, pp.(1377-1382), ISSN 0090-9556

Wen, X., & Walle, T. (2006) Methylated flavonoids have greatly improved intestinal absorption and metabolic stability. *Drug Metab Dispos. Vol.*34, pp.(1786–92), ISSN 0090-9556

Whitman, S.C., Kurowska E.M., Manthey J.A., Daugherty A. (2005) Nobiletin, a citrus flavonoid isolated from tangerines, selectively inhibits class A scavenger receptor-mediated metabolism of acetylated LDL by mouse macrophages. *Atherosclerosis.* Vol.178, No.1, pp.(25-32), ISSN 0021-9150

Xiao, H., Yang, C. S., Li, S., Jin, H., Ho, C. T., & Patel, T. (2009) Monodemethylated polymethoxyflavones from sweet orange (*Citrus sinensis*) peel inhibit growth of human lung cancer cells by apoptosis. *Mol. Nutr. Food Res.*, Vol. 53, pp. (398– 406), ISSN 1613-4125

16

Pharmacokinetic (PK) and Pharmacodynamic Profiles of Artemisinin Derivatives Influence Drug Neurotoxicity in Animals

Qigui Li and Mark Hickman
Division of Experimental Therapeutics
Walter Reed Army Institute of Research,
Silver Spring, MD,
USA

1. Introduction

In the past decade, there have been major advances in our knowledge of severe CNS neurotoxicity in mice, rats, dogs, and rhesus monkeys repeatedly administered the oil-soluble artemisinins (ARTs) of arteether (AE) or artemether (AM), and water-soluble artelinic acid (AL). Studies have shown that those drugs are toxic to the central nervous system and induce neuropathologic changes in these animals (Li & Hickman, 2011). Pharmocokinetic and toxicokinetic studies of model animals administered various artemesinin derivitives through different routes have yielded important information that is relevant and useful in predicting possible neurotoxicity in man, particularly as artemesinin drugs are used more widely for other indications beyond malaria treatment such as cancer therapy.

The fat soluble artemesinin derivitives AE and AM are particularly prone to induce neuropathological damage at low doses. For example, in rats, CNS damage was induced by dosing with AE intramuscularly at a daily dose of 12.5 mg/kg for 7 days , while a daily dose of 6 mg/kg for 28 days was required to induce neuropathological changes in dogs, and dosing of 8 mg/kg daily for 14 days was required to induce similar damage in rhesus monkeys (Brewer et al., 1994a; Classen et al., 1999; Genovese et al., 1995, 1998; Kamchonwongpaisan et al., 1997; Li et al., 2007a; Petras et al., 1997). A similar finding was observed for rats treated with oral AL, which was reported to have similar pathological neurotoxicity following an oral dose at 160 mg/kg daily for 9 days (Si et al., 2007).

Despite extensive studies of AE, AM, and AL neurotoxicity, there is no evidence of neurotoxicity in animals related to another water soluble ART derivative, artesunate (AS), the most widely used ART in humans (Li & Weina, 2010). AS was designed for intravenous injection and, up to now, no neurotoxicity (pathologic or behavioural) has been observed in animals following intravenous administration at any repeated doses up to its maximum tolerated doses (MTD). The MTD of AS has been shown to be 240 mg/kg following intravenous injection daily in rats for 3 days, but no neurotoxicity was detected in these animals (Xie et al., 2005). In another study, intravenous AS in sodium bicarbonate dosed daily for 7 days at 120 mg/kg had no effect on neurotoxicity scores (our unpublished data). A third study of AS treatment in rats administered one intramuscular injection of AS at a high dose of 420 mg/kg did not induce any neuronal necrosis. In addition, dosing of up to 200 mg/kg of

AS orally daily for 5-7 days did not result in neuronal changes or any specific clinical signs (Dayan, 1998), and there was little clinical or neuropathological evidence of neurotoxicity found at high dose levels of over 200 mg/kg/day for 28 days in mice treated with oral AS and dihydroartemisinin (DHA), as well as oral AM (Nontprasert et al., 1998, 2000, 2002).

To date, no systematic toxicity has been reported in humans, despite the use of ART and its derivatives in clinical trials designed with special emphasis to detect changes in neurological indicators such as movement, hearing, vestibular, or cerebral abnormalities (Efferth & Kaina 2010). Although ART agents, mainly the oil-soluble derivatives, have been shown to induce fatal neurotoxicity in animal models, a striking fact in treating patients with the ARTs is the lack of any serious adverse events, despite careful monitoring in several clinical studies. Severe malarial infection, particularly cerebral malaria in multi-drug resistant strains in the developing world, often leaves patients with decreases in neural function. This development has made characterization of potential neurotoxic effects of the ART derivatives very difficult to ascertain, even though these drugs are clinically utilized in ever growing numbers (Karbwang et al., 1994; Van Vugt et al., 2000; Angus et al., 2002). In a study of 3500 patients in Thailand, evidence of serious toxicity was not noticed (Price et al., 1999). From other reports, rare neurologic side effects have been noted in humans receiving ART drugs, however, these findings were difficult to dissect from the effects of malaria infection (Li & Hickman 2011).

Five cases have been reported that suggest episodes of neurotoxicity due to multiple courses of ARTs therapy (Elias et al., 1999; Franco-Paredes et al., 2005; Haq et al., 2009; Miller & Panosian 1997; Panossian et al., 2005). These reports may constitute evidence of a causal association that merits further investigation. The possibility exists that repeated and longer duration administration of ART compounds in malaria endemic areas could result in cumulative neuronal damage, especially since these drugs are often freely available for use in tropical countries. Although the authors reported that the toxicity observed in these five cases is drug related, there is considerable disagreement regarding these putative episodes of neurotoxicity, and the evidence of such a causal association may or may not be only related to ART administration (Gachot et al., 1997; Newton et al., 2005; White et al., 2006).

Several perplexities still continue to vex us with the ARTs. Why is neurotoxicity so easily observed in animal models but not seen in humans getting equal or even higher doses of the drug? Why does this neurotoxicity mostly occur in animals treated with intramuscular AE, AM, and oral AL, but not with AS? Why does neurotoxicity mostly take place with the intramuscular and oral dosing routes, but not in intravenous injections? In this chapter, pharmacokinetic characteristics will be evaluated and discussed that may shed light on some of these questions. Principally, we will discuss:

i. the role of DHA in neurotoxicity and the conversion rates of AM, AE, AL, and AS to DHA;
ii. the role of drug tissue distribution levels in cerebrospinal fluid (CSF) and brain tissue at the onset of neurotoxicity;
iii. the role of drug total exposure levels (AUC and C_{max}) in plasma in neurotoxicity; and
iv. the role of drug half-life in neurotoxicity.

In addition, the drug PK parameters required to induce neurotoxicity in animals after administration of ARTs will be discussed in depth from the available pharmacological literature. We will outline the data that supports the hypothesis that drug accumulation with prolonged exposure time (half-life) demonstrated by PK profiling accompanies the neurological effects shown by Pharmacodynamic (PD) profiling. As will be shown, there is considerable data to support the view that the drug exposure time is a more important marker to determine and predict ART-driven neurotoxicity than other factors.

2. Key PK parameters associated with artemisinin induced neurotoxicity in animals

2.1 The role of DHA in artemisinin-induced neurotoxicity

DHA is obtained by sodium borohydride reduction of ART, an endoperoxide containing sesquiterpene lactone. Through *in vitro* bioassays, DHA has been shown to have similar antimalarial activity to AS and it is 1.4-5.2 fold more active than other ARTs (Li et al., 2007b). AS has also been shown to be 2-4 fold more toxic than other ARTs *in vitro* and *in vivo* (Li et al., 1998a; 2002; Fishwick et al., 1995; McLean & Ward, 1998; Wesche et al., 1994). Due to its poor solubility in water or oils, DHA has only been formulated as an oral preparation and has been used primarily as a semisynthetic compound for derivatization to other oil soluble and water-soluble ARTs. The effectiveness of AS has been attributed to its rapid and extensive hydrolysis to DHA (Li & Weina 2010). The efficacy of AM and AE has also been credited to their conversion to DHA, but their rates of conversion were significantly lower and less complete than in AS (Li et al., 1998b; Navaratnam et al., 2000). AL is a very stable ART agent *in vitro* and *in vivo*, and AL has almost no biotransformation to DHA in animals (Li et al., 1998c; Lin et al., 1987).

Accordingly, evaluating the conversion rates of various ART drugs is very important for assessing the risk of neurotoxicity for the four compounds that are the focus of this chapter. Conversion evaluations of AM, AE, AS, or AL to DHA in laboratory animals are summarized in Table 1. This summary also illustrates the conversion of ART drugs to DHA in humans, which seems to be much more efficient than in animals. When comparing the data from animals and humans treated with AM or AS in various regimens, one difference that is immediately apparent is that the ratios of AUC_{DHA} to AUC_{AM} or AUC_{AS} are significantly higher in humans (0.41-9.71) than in animals (0.04-2.96), suggesting that the human hydrolysis system is more active and complete (Li et al., 2007a).

The conversion rates of the four ART agents to DHA are different in various animal species. The most extensive hydrolysis of AS to DHA has been shown to be in rats and dogs with a DHA/AS ratio in the range of 0.31-2.74, while the ratio of AM or AE conversion to DHA is less than 0.23. In addition, the calculated ratio of AL conversion to DHA in rats and dogs lies in the range of 0.001-0.03, so it appears that DHA is not contributing as much to the effects of neurotoxicity associated with dosing these three drugs (AM, AE, and AL) while it appears to be a much larger contributor to DHA after AS dosing (Table 1). Data derived from pharmacokinetic studies has demonstrated that the AUC of DHA hydrolyzed from AS is in the range of 236–596 ng·h/ml compared to the AUC of DHA hydrolyzed from AM and AE which lies in the range of 29-71 ng·h/ml at the same dose level in rats (Li et al., 1998b). AM and AE treatment has been shown to induce severe neurotoxicity in animals, AS treatment has not been shown to do so (Genovese et al., 2000). Similar results have been observed in dogs, where the AUC of DHA produced from AS was shown to be 1,109 ng·h/ml at a dose of 10 mg/kg with no neurotoxicity symptoms observed (Li et al., 1999a). In comparison, the AUC of DHA derived from AM and AE dosing in dogs is 312 and 181 ng·h/ml, respectively, at a dose of 20 (AM) and 15 (AE) mg/kg, and those treatments have been shown to result in fatal neurotoxicity following intramuscular injection (Classen et al., 1999; Li et al., 2000).

Drugs and administrations	Animals		Humans	
	Rats	Dogs	Volunteers	Malaria Patients
Artemether (AM)				
Intravenous	0.04 (65/1857)	-	-	-
Intramuscular	0.07 (71/1007)	0.14 (312/2240)	0.41 - 1.62	1.06
Oral	0.10 (38/366)	2.96 (5592/1887)	1.12 - 7.69	1.42 - 8.55
Arteether (AE)				
Intravenous	0.04 (29/842)	-	-	-
Intramuscular	0.15 (43/286)	0.23 (181/804)	-	0.16 - 0.19
oral	0.17 (50/298	-	-	-
Artesunate (AS)				
Intravenous	0.64 (474/738)	0.50 (778/1533)	-	2.81 - 8.12
Intramuscular	0.31 (236/773)	0.73 (1109/1521)	-	-
Oral	2.74 (595/217)	0.45 (299/660)	4.29 - 5.36	6.35 - 9.71
Rectal	-	-	2.31	-
Artelinic acid (AL)				
Intravenous	0.01 (63/12706)	0.001 (7/11262)	-	-
Intramuscular	0.01 (44/5023)	0.003 (23/10195)	-	-
Oral	0.03 (62/1650)	0.002 (14/8849)	-	-

DHA = dihydroartemisinin

Table 1. Mean ratios of AUC_{DHA} (an active metabolite) / $AUC_{AM, AE, AS, and AL}$, and the concentration values (ng·h/ml) of $AUC_{DHA}/AUC_{AM, AE, AS, and AL}$ as the conversion evaluation of artemisinin derivatives (AM, AE, AS, and AL) to DHA in animals and humans (Li et al., 2007a)

The maximum tolerated dose (MTD) of intravenous AS has been shown to be 240 mg/kg dosed daily for 3 days (Xie et al., 2005). In this study, animals were sacrificed at 24 hrs (day 1) and 192 hrs (day 8) after the last dose. Histopathological evaluation demonstrated mild renal tubular necrosis in uninfected rats treated with AS at 240 mg/kg, however, fewer pathological lesions (minimal tubular necrosis) were observed in malaria infected rats. The renal injury was reversible in all cases by day 8 after cessation of dosing, and also no neurotoxicity was found after any of the intravenous AS dosing regimens (Li et al., 2007c). The AUC of DHA derived from a dose of AS of 240 mg/kg ranged from 6,984–15,768 ng·h/ml. This AUC can be simulated daily in rats using this regimen according to our previous published study (Li et al., 1998c). Although DHA is 2-4 fold more active and more toxic than other ART derivatives (Fishwick et al., 1995; Li et al., 1998a, 2002; McLean & Ward 1998; Wesche et al., 1994), the high level of DHA generated from AS did not seem to have a key role in the induction of neurotoxicity in these animal studies.

In another comparative PK study of DHA hydrolysis, AL and AS were administered to malaria-infected rats using 3 daily equimolar doses (96 µmoles/kg, which equals 36.7 mg/kg for AS and 40.6 mg/kg for AL) via intravenous administration. The plasma concentration of AS observed was one-third less on day 3 than on day 1, similar to the plasma concentrations of its active metabolite, DHA (Li et al., 2005a). The results were similar for other ART drugs with an auto-induction metabolic profile (van Agtmael et al., 1999; Ashton et al., 1996, 1998; Khanh et al., 1999), but not for AL. The PK parameters of AL were very comparable from day 1 to day 3 at the same molecular doses of AS (40.6 mg/kg daily). AS seems to be the pro-drug of DHA with a DHA/AS ratio of 5.26 (AUC_{DHA} of 13,051 ng·h/ml) compared to the ratio of 0.01 (AUC_{DHA} of 524 ng·h/ml) for DHA/AL. In this study, dosing with the two drugs did not induce any CNS toxicity (Li et al., 2005a), but the general toxicity of AL was 3-fold greater than that of AS in malaria-infected rats (Xie et al., 2005). In conclusion, we believe the conclusions drawn from our data and from other published work support the hypothesis that DHA is not an important factor in induction of neurotoxicity in animals.

2.2 The impact of ARTs distributed in the CNS on neurotoxicity

There are only a few studies of tissue distribution of ART derivatives in the animal brain, and these published studies used a variety of methods that differ significantly. Therefore, there are no comparative published results for quantitative evaluation of the ART drugs distributed in the central nervous system (CNS).

The first quantitative determination study of ARTs in the CNS using the thin-layer chromatography densitometry method found that ART, AM, and AS can cross the blood-brain barrier (BBB) and the blood-placenta barrier in rats (China Cooperative Research Group, 1982). ART has been noted to be more readily detected in the brain after oral administration than after intravenous injection (Niu et al., 1985). By radioimmunoassay, the highest level of AS was found in the rat intestine 10 minutes after intravenous administration, followed by the brain, liver, kidney, and other organs, in decreasing order. After one hour, the AS drug levels dropped significantly but not uniformly in all tissues, with high levels still remaining in the brain, fat, intestine and serum. The highest levels were found in rat brains 5 minutes after intravenous injection (Zhao & Song, 1989). Moderate levels of AM were also found in the heart, lung and skeletal muscles, while AM levels in liver and kidney were low (Jiang et al., 1989).

Using the tissue homogenate method, intramuscular injection of ^{14}C-arteether resulted in higher levels of radioactivity detected 24h after dosing in the intestinal tract, liver, kidneys, and spleen, while lower amounts of drug were found in the brown fat and in the brain . High-performance liquid chromatographic data from this work indicated that three metabolites of arteether, but not arteether itself, could cross the BBB. The calculated apparent concentration in the whole brain was 0.89% of the total radioactivity after intramuscular injection of 25 mg/kg AE (Li et al., 2007a).

Using the whole body autoradiograph method, administration of ^{14}C-AL showed widespread distribution of the radiolabeled drug in rats one hour following dosing. The relative activity of ^{14}C-AL found in various body tissues (as density per unit area) was, from highest to lowest, in the intestinal tract followed by the liver, kidney, bone marrow, spleen, brown fat and salivary glands, heart & testes, and lastly by the brain. At 48 h, the relative activity of ^{14}C-AL found in various body tissues (as density per unit area) was, from highest to lowest, in the intestinal tract, followed by the spleen, kidney, liver, salivary glands, brown fat and bone marrow, testes, and lastly by the brain. The low residual activity found in the brain appeared to be uniformly distributed. Autoradiographic evidence confirmed the presence of ^{14}C-AL in the brain from 1 to 192h. However, the presence of ^{14}C-AL in the brain was at a lower level than the presence of ^{14}C-AL in most other tissues. There was no evidence of a label concentration in any area of the brain that was visible in the whole body sections. Penetration of the BBB by ^{14}C-labelled AL was shown to be very poor. An apparent concentration of 0.1% of total radioactivity/brain was calculated from an intravenous and oral administration of 10 mg/kg AL (Li et al., 2005a).

Another neurotoxic dose range study showed that neuronal damage occurred in all beagle dogs dosed with multiple daily intramuscular treatments of AM at 40 and 80 mg/kg. After dosing with AM at 20 mg/kg administered through multiple daily treatments, minimal neuronal effects were observed in 5 out of 8 dogs. Two hours after the eighth administration (on day 8), only low levels of AM (25, 60, and 71 ng/ml)were found in the cerebrospinal fluid (CSF) after dosing with 20, 40, and 80 mg/kg respectively. AM levels in the CSF were < 10% of the AM observed in the plasma concentration (Classen et al., 1999).

These limited and incomparable data indicates that the oil-soluble derivatives, AE (0.89% of total dose in brain) and AM (10% of plasma level in CSF) appear to possess the ability to cross the BBB more readily than water-soluble ART compounds, like AL (0.1% of total dose in brain). If this is true, then the higher degree of neurotoxicity of AE and AM compared to the neurotoxicity observed after treatment with water soluble forms of artemisinin is easily understood. However, this deduction is not supported by the observation that AS has the ability to easily cross the BBB. The largest fraction of AS has been found in rat brains after intravenous administration by radioimmunoassay (Zhao & Song, 1989). Recent studies found that the levels of ^{14}C-AS in rat brains were more than 2 fold higher in the brain than in plasma, and the AUCs of radioactivity observed in the brain and in plasma were 70.7 μg·h/g and 29.4 μg·h/ml, respectively, by both of quantitative whole-body autoradiography (QWBA) and tissue dissection techniques (LSC) methods (Li et al., 2008). During a 192 hour period, 1.27% of the total radioactivity dose was detected in the rat brain. The half-life of ^{14}C-AS in the brain tissue was 94.2 hours, which is significantly longer than the 63.7 hour half-life observed in the plasma (Li et al., 2006a; Li et al., 2008). These results showed that the resident time of ^{14}C-AS was longer in the brain than in plasma. This may reflect a "sink effect" of DHA uptake transfer by the lipid-rich structures of the brain (Kearney & Aweeka, 1999).

After intravenous AS injection, samples were found in CSF that contained no parent drug which is consistent with the low lipid solubility of the metabolites of AS (Davis et al., 2001). The types of AS metabolites present in the CNS are completely unknown (Li et al., 2005a), and whether these metabolites in the brain are associated with neurotoxicity is also unknown. AS is converted stoichiometrically to DHA and the DHA concentrations observed peak at 5-10 min after dosing in plasma (Batty et al., 1998; Davis et al., 2001). DHA is highly lipid soluble and has a low molecular mass (284 Da), and both of these factors favor penetration of DHA into the CSF (Kearney & Aweeka, 1999). Since DHA is poorly soluble in water, it should be able to cross cell membranes and the BBB. After treatment with AS in patients, however, the parent drug (AS) cannot be detected in the CSF. DHA levels in the CSF after AS treatment increase with time while DHA levels in plasma decrease. These finding suggest a continuing influx but a slower efflux of DHA in which DHA might accumulate in the CSF during frequent AS dosing (Davis et al., 2003; Kearney & Aweeka, 1999).

AS and/or its metabolites have been shown to easily cross the BBB and have higher accumulation in brain tissues when compared to the other ARTs, as described above (Kearney & Aweeka, 1999; Jiang et al., 1989; Li et al., 2005a; Zhao & Song, 1989). After intravenous injection of 120 mg AS in malaria patients, DHA levels in the CSF were shown to increase ranging from 1,100-1,450 ng/ml, which is much higher than the DHA levels observed in plasma which ranged from 104-120 ng/ml (Davis et al., 2003). No neurotoxicity, however, was observed in these studies. Therefore, while the ART agents distribute in brain tissue and CSF, they do not appear to be an important factor in induction of neurotoxicity.

2.3 The role played by the drug exposure level of artemisinins in neurotoxicity

Recognizing the fact that if there is no drug exposure, there is no toxicity leads us to the conclusion that if there is exposure, toxicity can ensue when exposure exceeds a certain level and/or time and that will be dependent on pharmacokinetics and pharmacodynamics.

2.3.1 PK profiles of ARTs in rats

After daily intramuscular injections of AE at a dose of 25 mg/kg for 7 days, accumulation and prolonged exposure of AE in plasma was noted in rats with severe neurotoxicity. This accumulation was shown to be due to slow and prolonged absorption of AE in the muscle injection site (Li et al., 1999b). The absorption of AE from muscle at the injection site was incomplete in the first 48 hours after a single injection. At 24 and 48 hours after dosing, 38% and 22% of the total dose of AE still remained in the injection site, respectively. The amount of AE in muscle rapidly decreased for 1-2 hours and then exhibited a much slower rate of decrease. Half-lives for the fast and slow absorption phases in the muscle were 1.0 hour and 26.3 hours, respectively. It was expected that the remaining dose amount would be absorbed later because an intramuscular total dose of AE with sesame oil should be 100% absorbed in the absence of decomposition or metabolism at the injection site.

The analysis of toxicokinetic (TK) parameters on day 1 of this study was similar to that of the single intramuscular dose. After day 1, however, the kinetic data estimates from days 2-7 showed a notable change in the TK parameter estimated for day 1 (Figure 1, top). The C_{max} of AE (410 ng/ml) on day 7 was found to be three times higher than on day 1 (130 ng/ml). The AUC of AE observed after the intramuscular dose was found to be 4.5-fold higher on day 7 at steady state (4367 ng·h/ml) than on day 1 (905 ng·h/ml) (Table 2). This indicates that the exposure concentration of AE was significantly increased, and the system of excretion and biotransformation in the rats in this study may not have been normal (Rowland & Tozer, 1995). Only a pathophysiological factor could change the slopes of distribution and elimination associated with biotransformation, excretion, and protein or tissue binding (Mayer, 1995; Shargel & Yu, 1993).

Neurotoxic Severity Animal & PK Parameters	**Severe & Death**	**Moderate**	**Minimal**	**Not affected**
Sprague-Dawley Rats	Arteether, IM (Sesame oil) 25 mg/kg x 7	Arteether, IM (1:2 CRM/ saline) 25 mg/kg x 7	Arteether, IM** (Sesame oil) 12.5 mg/kg x 7	Artesunate, IM (5% $NaHCO_3$) 25 mg/kg x 7
$AUC_{1\text{-}7D}$ (μg·h/ml)	16.92 ± 4.04	46.29 ± 2.06	12.31 ± 1.57	8.57 ± 3.34
$C_{max\ Day\ 1}$ (ng/ml)	130 ± 39	1227 ± 171	65 ± 19	3981 ± 992
$C_{max\ Day\ 7}$ (ng/ml)	410 ± 91	1826 ± 118	205 ± 45	2078 ± 416
$t_{1/2\ Day\ 1}$ (hr)	13.74 ± 1.71	6.96 ± 0.93	13.23 ± 1.32	0.43 ± 0.05
$t_{1/2\ Day\ 7}$ (hr)	31.24 ± 4.31	9.06 ± 1.69	22.03 ± 4.83	0.39 ± 0.04
LONEL (ng/ml)	41.32	41.32	41.32	NA
Neuro-exposure time (hr)*	164.3 ± 7.9	103.0 ± 5.3	67.1 ± 5.6	NA
Sprague-Dawley Rats		Artelinic acid Oral (Suspension) 160 mg/kg x 9	Artelinic acid Oral (Suspension) 288 mg/kg x 5	Artelinate IM (5% $NaHCO_3$) 25 mg/kg x 7
$AUC_{1\text{-}7\ or\ 9D}$ (μg·h/ml)		1420 ± 454	1302 ± 905	86.84 ± 5.59
$C_{max\ Day\ 1}$ (ng/ml)		11293 ± 8291	14069 ± 10905	20044 ± 3459
$C_{max\ Day\ 7\ or\ 9}$ (ng/ml)		12230 ± 7139	14341 ± 9339	15585 ± 1476
$t_{1/2\ Day\ 1}$ (hr)		2.84 ± 0.52	3.33 ± 0.25	1.89 ± 0.22
$t_{1/2\ Day\ 7\ or\ 9}$ (hr)		10.68 ± 1.84	3.60 ± 0.25	1.73 ± 0.17
LONEL (ng/ml)		346.26	346.26	NA
Neuro-exposure time (hr)*		186.0 ± 28.0	75.0 ± 12.0	NA
Beagle Dogs	Arteether, IM (Sesame oil) 15 mg/kg x 14	Artemether, IM (Peanut oil) 40 mg/kg x 7	Artemether, IM (Peanut oil) 20 mg/kg x 7	Artelinic acid Oral (Capsules) 25 mg/kg x 14
$AUC_{1\text{-}7,\ 14,\ or\ 28D}$ (μg·h/ml)	24.39 ± 18.04	86.27	32.13	191.14 ± 90.80
$C_{max\ Day\ 1}$ (ng/ml)	90 ± 15	580	190	6279 ± 2995
$C_{max\ Day\ 7,\ 14,or\ 28}$ (ng/ml)	352 ± 203	720	346	7177 ± 6248
$t_{1/2\ Day\ 1}$ (hr)	9.23 ± 1.32	17.24	10.93	1.51 ± 0.16
$t_{1/2\ Day\ 7,\ 14,or\ 28}$ (hr)	21.53 ± 2.08	22.43	20.75	1.94 ± 0.56
LONEL (ng/ml)	40.92	75.69	75.69	346.26
Neuro-exposure time (hr)*	277.6 ± 10.7	147.8	113.2	14.6 ± 1.8
Rhesus monkeys***		Arteether, IM (Sesame oil) 16 mg/kg x 14	Arteether IM** (Sesame oil) 8 mg/kg x 14	
$AUC_{1\text{-}14D}$ (μg·h/ml)		70.96 ± 4.59	31.25 ± 2.61	
$C_{max\ Day\ 1}$ (ng/ml)		63 ± 9	38 ± 5	
$C_{max\ Day\ 14}$ (ng/ml)		1038 ± 622	527 ± 306	
$t_{1/2\ Day\ 1}$ (hr)		22.59 ± 1.55	16.56 ± 1.20	
$t_{1/2\ Day\ 14}$ (hr)		82.09 ± 41.98	50.58 ± 16.77	
LONEL (ng/ml)		193.80	193.80	
Neuro-exposure time (hr)*		307.4	179.5	

*The neuro-exposure times above LONEL concentration were calculated with neurotoxic outcome.
** PK data were simulated from our previous studies.
***The monkey results are from our unpublished data. Neurotoxic severity were graded as minimal = 1-5 neurons affected, moderate = 10-30 neurons affected, and severe = >40 neurons affected.
DHA = Dihydroartemisinin; CRM = cremophore; AUC = area under the curve; IM = intramuscular

Table 2. Drug accumulation, exposure level and neurotoxic exposure time of arteether (AE), Artemether (AM), artesunate (AS) and artelinic acid (AL) at above the lowest observed neurotoxic effect level (LONEL) in rats, dogs, and monkeys concerning with histopathological neurotoxicity after various dose regimens (Li et al., 2007a; Si et al., 2007).

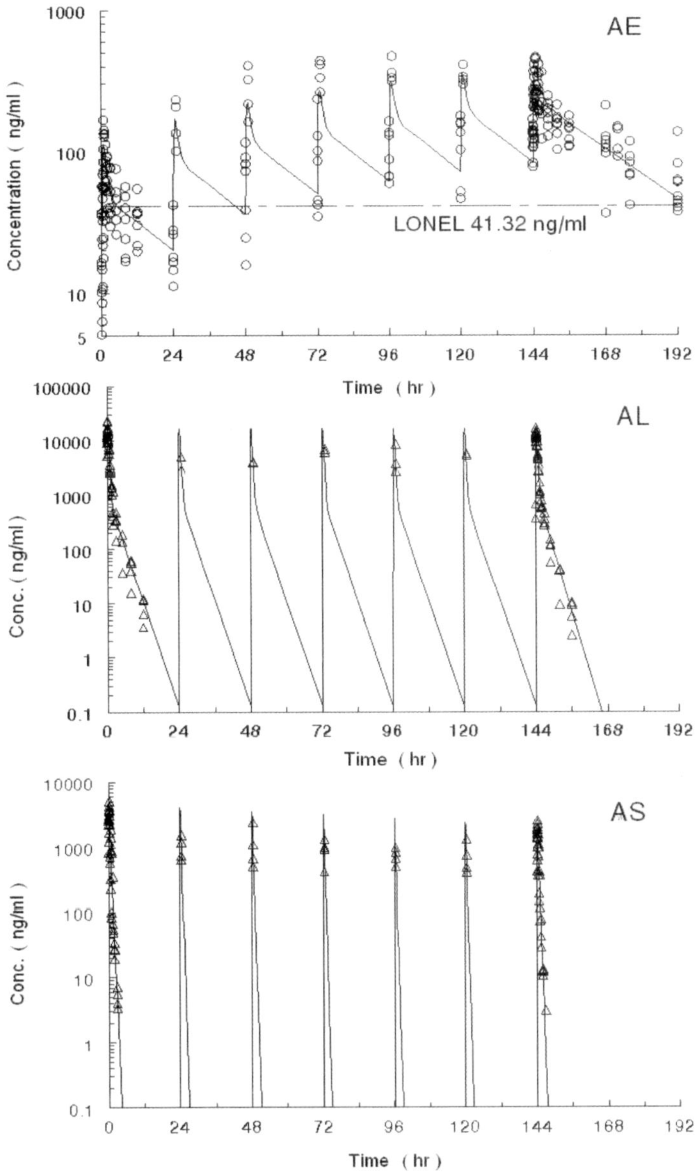

Fig. 1. Pharmacokinetic profiles measured by HPLC-ECD (markers) and computer fitted curves (solid line) of 25 mg/kg of arteether with sesame oil (top, n = 4, Li et al., 2007a). Artelinate (middle) and artesunate (bottom) with 5% $NaHCO_3$/0.9% saline following daily intramuscular injection 25 mg/kg daily for 7 days in male rats. (n = 3, Li et al., 2005b). The lowest observed neurotoxic effect level (LONEL) from AE measurement was estimated at 41.32 ng/ml (dashed line) in male rats.

The drug exposure level shown by the total AUC data observed after a 7 day intramuscular treatment dosing of 25 mg/kg AE was 16.92 μg·h/ml, and this dosing regimen induced severe neurotoxicity and animal death (Li et al., 1999b). Following intramuscular injection, the exposure concentration level of AE in this study was just one-fifth of the total AUC of AL (86.84 μg·h/ml) with the same dosing regimen (Table 2) (Li et al., 2005b). Clinical observation of rats in this experiment treated with AL did not show any indications of neurotoxicity (Figure 1, middle), even after multiple intramuscular injections of high AL doses of 100 mg/kg (our unpublished data). Computer simulation indicated that the total AUC after 7 day treatment with 100 mg/kg AL was 341.88 μg·h/ml, 21 times higher than that of AE treated rats. This result suggests that the 5-21 fold higher exposure concentrations of AL did not seem to be a principal independent factor in causing neurotoxicity (Table 2).

In order to demonstrate that the neurotoxicity of AE is related to drug accumulation in blood as a consequence of slow and prolonged absorption from the intramuscular injection sites, a study was conducted designed to decrease the accumulation and toxicity of AE through the replacement of traditional sesame oil with a cremophore vehicle (Li et al., 2002). When administered at a daily dose of 25 mg/kg for 7 days, the AUC of AE formulated in sesame oil (AESO) was 7.5-fold higher on day 7 (last day of dosing) than on day 1 (first day of dosing), while treatment with AE formulated with cremophore (AECM) resulted in only a 1.8-fold higher AUC. The C_{max} of AECM (1826 ng/ml) on day 7 was found to be only slightly higher than on day 1 (1227 ng/ml).

Although the accumulation of AECM was greatly reduced, its total exposure level (total $AUC_{1\text{-}7D}$ of 46.29 μg·h/ml) was still 2.7-fold higher than AESO (total $AUC_{1\text{-}7D}$ of 16.92 μg·h/ml) due to the higher bioavailability of AECM (74.5%) compared with AESO (20.3%), and the data for this study are shown in Table 2. While the histopathological examinations of the brain demonstrated neurotoxic changes in both groups, the animals in the AESO group showed significantly more severe neurotoxicity than in the AECM group. Brain injury scores in animals treated with AECM were mild to moderate (severity index 2.3 to 3.0), but in animals treated with AESO they were moderate to severe (3.0 to 4.7) on day 7 and day 10, respectively. This study further demonstrates that the toxicity of AE is not dependent on its exposure level in animals.

2.3.2 PK profiles of ARTs in dogs

Daily intramuscular administration of 15 mg/kg AE for 14 days resulted in drug accumulation in the plasma of beagle dogs who also presented clinically with severe neurotoxicity and death (Li et al., 2000). The peak concentration (C_{max}) of AE (352 ng/ml) was found to be four times higher on the last dosing day (day 14) compared to the C_{max} observed on the first dosing day (90 ng/ml). The AUC (7.09 μg·h/ml) of AE observed on the last dosing day was 8.7-fold higher than on the first dosing day (0.81 μg·h/ml), indicating that the exposure concentration of AE had been greatly increased (Figure 2, middle). The total AUC observed during the 14 days of daily intramuscular AE dosing at 15 mg/kg was 24.39 μg·h/ml (Table 2).

Similar accumulation results for AM were reported in dog plasma after daily intramuscular administration of 20, 40, and 80 mg/kg for 7 days (Classen et al., 1999). The PK profiles of AM dosed IM at 20 and 40 mg/kg in beagles is shown in Table 2. The analysis of the toxicokinetic parameters on day 2-7 was changed, with the parameter estimated on day 1. In the dogs treated with 20 mg/kg dosed IM minimal neurotoxicity was observed, and the

C_{max} of AM (346 ng/ml) doubled on day 7 from the C_{max} observed on day 1 (190 ng/ml). The AUC (6.16 µg·h/ml) of AM observed on day 7 was 2.7-fold higher than the AUC of AM observed on day 1 (2.25 µg·h/ml) after IM dosing. Similar results were found in animals treated IM with AM at 40 mg/kg daily for 7 days. The C_{max} of AM (720 ng/ml) on day 7 was much higher than on day 1 (580 ng/ml), and the AUC (12.52 µg·h/ml) doubled on day 7 from the AUC observed on day 1 (6.70 µg·h/ml), indicating that the exposure concentration of AM had been increased (Classen et al., 1999).

In comparison to the dogs treated with intramuscular AE, the total AUCs observed in animals treated with AM dosed IM at 20 mg/kg (32.13 µg·h/ml) and 40 mg/kg (86.27 µg·h/ml) were significantly higher than the AUC observed after dosing with AE at 15 mg/kg (24.39 µg·h/ml) (Classen et al., 1999; Li et al., 1999a). The severity of neurotoxicity observed after dosing with intramuscular AM in dogs, however, was minimal in the 20 mg/kg group and moderate in the 40 mg/kg group. The observed neurotoxicity was much less in AM treated animals than in AE treated dogs who presented with severe neurotoxicity and death. These comparison studies demonstrate that the neurotoxicity of AE and AM is not dependent on plasma concentrations in dogs.

In another comparison study, dogs treated with oral AL showed much higher plasma concentrations. The AUC observed after daily oral dosing with AL for 14 days at 20 mg/kg in a suspension formulation was 231.6 µg·h/ml. The AUC value dropped to 191.1 µg·h/ml in animals dosed with oral AL in a 25 mg/kg capsule formulation given daily for 14 days (Table 2). The dogs in both groups did not show any clinical toxicity (Li et al., 1994). In dogs treated with AL at two different dose regimens the exposure concentrations were 2-9 times higher than in dogs treated with AE and AM. No neurotoxicity was detected in those animals, however, dosed with 20 or 25 mg/kg oral AL daily for 14 days (Noker & Lin, 2000).

The drug exposure levels of these treatments suggest that a much higher total exposure concentration of AL in dogs ($AUC_{1\text{-}14D}$ = 191.14 µg·h/ml) does not correlate with clinical observations of neurotoxicity while the drug exposure levels of AE ($AUC_{1\text{-}14D}$ = 24.39 µg·h/ml) and AM ($AUC_{1\text{-}7D}$ = 32.13 µg·h/ml), correlated well with neurotoxicity at much lower exposure concentrations in dogs (Li et al., 2007a). These results also showed the exposure level of AM at daily dose of 20 and 40 mg/kg ($AUC_{1\text{-}7D}$ = 32.13 and 86.27 µg·h/ml) is higher than the exposure level of AE in dogs ($AUC_{1\text{-}14D}$ = 24.39 µg·h/ml), but the clinical observations of neurotoxicity were less severe in dogs treated with AM than with AE (Table 2). These studies further demonstrate that the toxicity of AE, AM or AL is not dependent on exposure levels in dogs.

2.3.3 PK studies in monkeys

Significant accumulations of AE were shown in the plasma of rhesus monkeys after daily intramuscular administration of AE at 16 mg/kg for 14 days (Figure 2, bottom). The concentration-time profile of AE dosed at 16 mg/kg in monkeys showed that the C_{max} of AE (1038 ng/ml) on day 14 was 19-fold higher than the C_{max} of AE observed on day 1 (63 ± 9 ng/ml). The AUC (53.10 µg·h/ml) of AE observed on the last dosing day was shown to be 60-fold higher than the AUC of AE observed after intramuscular dosing on the first day (0.88 µg·h/ml), indicating that the exposure concentration of AE was greatly increased. The total AUC of AE observed during the entire 14 days of treatment was 70.96 µg·h/ml (Li & Hickman, 2011).

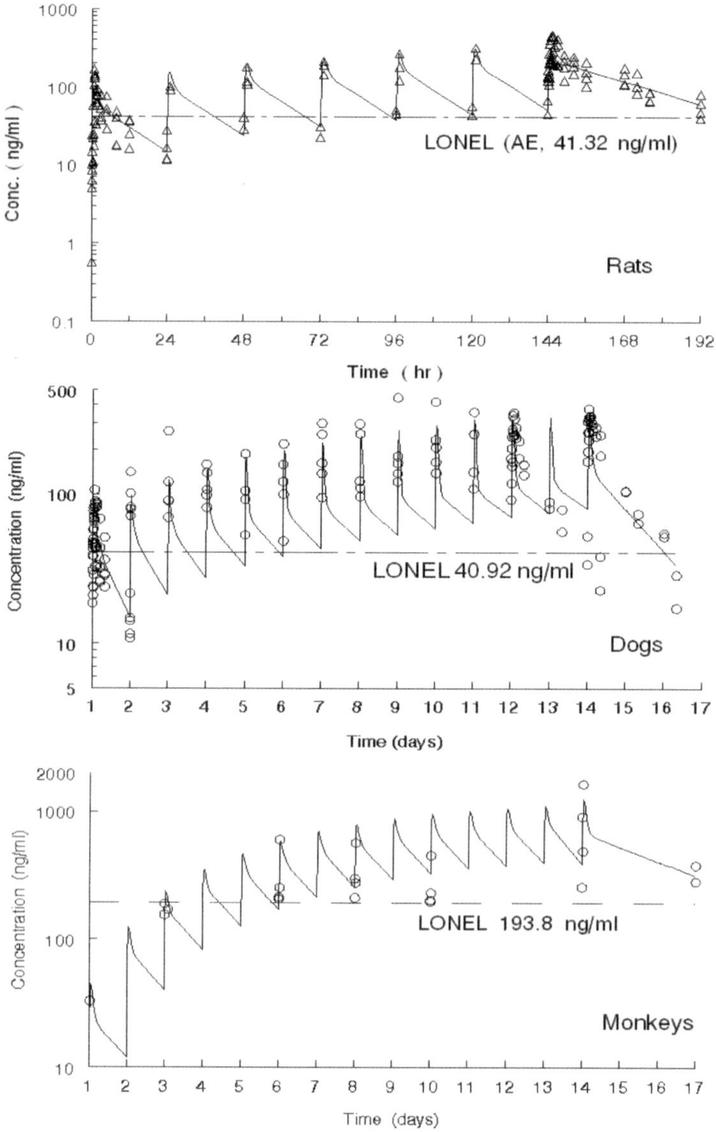

Fig. 2. Pharmacokinetic profiles measured by HPLC-ECD (markers) and computer fitted curves (solid line) of arteether (AE) in sesame oil in rats at daily dose of 12.5 mg/kg for 7 days (top, Li et al., 1999b), in beagle dogs at daily dose of 15 mg/kg for 14 days (middle, Li et al., 2000), and in rhesus monkeys at daily dose of 16 mg/kg for 14 days (bottom, Li & Hickman, 2011). The lowest observed neurotoxic effect level (LONEL, dashed line) from AE measurement was estimated 41.32 ng/ml in rats, 40.92 ng/ml in dogs, and 193.8 ng/ml in rhesus monkeys, respectively.

2.4 The importance of artemisinin drug half-life in neurotoxicity

While the exposure level of ARTs has not been shown to be a major factor involved in the induction of neurotoxicity, the exposure time may play a role in causing neurotoxicity. There are a number of similar reports of exposure investigations in the literature that have obtained the same observations that continued exposure of artemisinins over time (drug exposure time) rather than a high concentration (drug exposure level) over a short time (interval time) substantially contribute to neurotoxicity (Jorgensen, 1980; Rangan et al., 1997; Rozman & Doull 2000).

2.4.1 Half lives of ARTs in rats

The biological half-life of test drugs in blood controls the time exposure of drugs in animals and humans. The biological half-life is the amount of time it takes the body to eliminate one half of the drug initially present. In the animal PK studies with ARTs, the half lives of drugs administered were noted. Rats treated with daily intramuscular injections of AE at 25 mg/kg for 7 days presented with clinical observations of severe neurotoxicity (Li et al., 1999b). The absorption of AE from the muscle at the injection site was incomplete in the first 48 hours after a single injection. The elimination half life of AE in plasma after 7 daily doses was prolonged from 13.74 hours on day 1 to 31.24 hours on day 7, suggesting that the elimination half life of AE had been greatly extended.

To examine the question of whether AE accumulation in blood is due to the slow and prolonged absorption of drug from the intramuscular injection sites, a comparison study was conducted designed to decrease the accumulation of AE through the replacement of the sesame oil formulation with a cremophore vehicle (Li et al., 2002). When administered at a daily dose of AE at 25 mg/kg for 7 days, the half life (13.74 hr) of AE with sesame oil (AESO) on the first dosing day (day 1) showed a 2.5-fold higher half life than AE formulated with cremophore (AECM, 6.96 hr). Similar results were observed on the last dosing day (day 7), and the half life of AE in animals treated with AESO was 31.24 hr, which was 3.3-fold higher than AECM treated rats (9.06 hr) on the same day. Although the new formulation of AE with cremophore greatly increased the absorption rate from the muscles of rats, the half life observed in AECM treated animals was slightly lengthened from 6.96 hr on day 1 to 9.06 hr on day 7, suggesting that the exposure time of AECM was greatly reduced compared to animals treated with AESO. In this comparison, the neurotoxic severity observed was also significantly reduced from severe with death in animals treated with AESO to moderate in animals treated with AECM, and the drug half-lives appear to strongly correlate to clinical observations of neurotoxicity observed in these animals (Li et al., 2002).

No prolonged half lives and neurotoxicity were found in animals treated with intramuscular AL and AS at a dose of 25 mg/kg per day for 7 days, which closely follows the conditions of the experiments conducted in the previously mentioned AE study (Li et al., 1999b; Li et al., 2005b). The half-lives of AL and AS, both of which are water soluble, were very short ranging from 0.39 to 1.89 hr (Table 2), which is significantly shorter than the half life observed after dosing with AE intramuscularly. In addition, the half lives of AL and AS were not prolonged when comparing the half life observed on day 7 to the half life observed on day 1 post-injection (Figure 1, middle & bottom), suggesting that drug accumulation was not observed in those animals treated with repeated intramuscular doses of AL and AS. This result suggests that the significantly shorter half-lives of AL and AS compared to the half-life of AE seem to be an important element in avoiding clinical neurotoxicity. In other words, treatment of animals with intramuscular AL and AS is one means by which these animals avoided neurotoxic risk.

After changing the administration route from intravenous and intramuscular to intragastric, AL showed moderate neurotoxicity in rats treated with 160 mg/kg daily in 9 multiple doses for 9 days but not in animals dosed with 288 mg/kg every other day in 5 multiple doses for 9 days (Si et al., 2007). The elimination t½ of AL in plasma after oral dosing at 160 mg/kg daily for 9 days doses was prolonged from 2.84 hrs on day 1 to 10.68 hrs on day 9, suggesting that the elimination half life of AL had been greatly extended (Figure 4, middle). A slight increase of the half life, however, from 3.33 hrs on day 1 to 3.60 hrs on day 9 was noted in the rats treated with 288 mg/kg every other day in 5 multiple doses for 9 days (Figure 4, bottom). The neurotoxic severity of AL changed from moderate in the group treated with an oral daily dose of 160 mg/kg for 9 days to minimal in the group treated orally with AL every other day at a dose of 288 mg/kg for 9 days. These results indicate a correlation between observed clinical symptoms of neuropathology in rats and prolonged AL half lives in the animals dosed daily. The data further suggest that if the drug half life were shortened it might be possible to reduce the neurotoxic risk in animals treated with ARTs (Li et al., 2006b).

2.4.2 Half lives of ARTs in dogs

Beagle dogs treated with multiple daily intramuscular doses of AE at 15 mg/kg for 14 days developed severe neurotoxicity with death (Li et al., 2000). Similar to what was observed in the rat AE PK studies; the dogs demonstrated prolonged AE half-lives and drug accumulation. (Figure 2, middle). In this study, the most striking data observed was the elimination t½ of AE during the two weeks of daily dosing. The half life was prolonged from 9.23 hrs on the first dosing day (day 1) to 21.53 hrs on the last dosing day (day 14), suggesting that the exposure time of AE had been extended by two-fold (Table 2). In addition, half life extensions s were also reported in dog plasma after daily AM intramuscular administration of 20, 40, and 80 mg/kg dissolved in peanut oil for 7 days (Classen et al., 1999). The concentration-time profile of AM dosed at 20 and 40 mg/kg in beagles is shown in Table 2 and Figure 4. The elimination t½ of AM dosed at 20 mg/kg after 7 days daily dosing was prolonged from 10.93 hours on day 1 to 20.75 hours on day 7, suggesting that the exposure time of AM had been significantly increased. Similar results were found in animals treated with AM dosed intramuscularly at 40 mg/kg. Daily AM dosing for 7 days did not result in severe neurotoxicity, unlike the 14 day treatment with AE where severe neurotoxicity and death were noted. The difference in dosing time from 7 days to 14 days is the most likely factor related to this difference in clinical outcomes (Classen et al., 1999).

The minimal AE dose of multiple intramuscular injections which induced neuropathological findings was 6 mg/kg for 28 days in dogs (Brewer et al., 1994b; Davidson, 1994; Dayan, 1998). Through PK simulation of data from our dogs treated with intramuscular AE, the elimination half-lives of AE were found to be slightly prolonged from 8.22 hrs on day 1 to 10.45 hrs on day 28 with no significant difference. The neurotoxicity findings were also significantly reduced when comparing different compound dosing groups and treatment durations. Severe neurotoxicity was observed in dogs treated with AE at 15 mg/kg daily for 14 days, and minimal toxicity in animals treated with AE at 6 mg/kg daily dose for 28 days (Table 2). When compared to the drug half-lives of AE and AM, much shorter half lives were found in dogs treated with AL orally at 25 mg/kg daily for 14 days. The half lives of AL in dogs were 1.51 hrs on day 1 and 1.94 hrs on day 14 after oral capsule administration. The half life of AL observed was much shorter and no prolonged elimination half lives were found after oral daily dosing for 14 days. No neurotoxicity was observed in any of the AL treated animals (Noker & Lin, 2000). These studies further demonstrate that the neurotoxicity in beagles following AE, AM or AL administration is likely dependent on the half life of drug.

These studies strongly support the findings that neurotoxicity is half life (exposure time) dependent in the animals regardless of drug formulations and administration routes. As a result, the half lives of ARTs in animals are critical elements in the induction of neurotoxicity (Li et al., 2006b). Other pharmacokinetic parameters, such as drug distribution in the brain, toxicity of DHA, the active metabolite of ARTs or drug exposure level, tend to be of minor importance.

2.4.3 Half lives of ARTs in monkeys

AE dissolved in sesame oil formulation showed high plasma concentrations in rhesus monkeys after daily intramuscular administrations of AE at 16 mg/kg for 14 days (Li & Hickman, 2011). The concentration-time profile of monkeys dosed with AE at 16 mg/kg showed the C_{max} of AE (1038 ng/ml) on day 14 was 19 fold higher than on day 1 (63 ng/ml). The half lives of intramuscular AE were 22.59 hrs on day 1 and 82.09 hrs on day 14 after daily multiple dose regimens. Accordingly, the half life of AE was significantly prolonged from the first dosing day to the last dosing day after intramuscular AE administrations. The monkey showed moderate neurotoxicity after this intramuscular AE dosing regimen (Petras et al., 1997, 2000).

Since AE-induced brainstem neuropathology in monkeys has been shown to occur at a minimal dose of 8 mg/kg dosed daily for 14 days, we chose to simulate the main AE PK parameters on day1 and day 14 from our own rhesus PK data (Table 2). We noted a drug half life of 50.28 hrs on day 14 which was extended from 16.56 hrs on day 1 in monkeys treated with multiple doses of 8 mg/kg. This half life value is still shorter than the 82.09 hrs half life observed in animals treated with multiple intramuscular doses of AE at 16 mg/kg. The former dose induced minimal neurotoxicity, and the latter doses produced moderate toxicity in monkeys. Therefore, the AE half lives in monkeys appear to also have an important impact on the induction of neurotoxicity.

In conclusion, the data on ART half lives in animals supports the hypothesis that induction of neurotoxicity is much more dependent on the exposure time than other PK parameters. The summary data illustrates that the water-soluble ARTs, AL and AS, have very short half lives of 0.39-1.94 hrs in animals without any neurotoxic observations with the exception of oral AL dosed in rats at a very high dose of 160 mg/kg daily for 9 days. High dose AL treatment resulted in a significantly prolonged drug half life on day 9, the animals showed moderate neurotoxicity, and this treatment was also associated with GI toxicity. In rats or dogs treated with the oil-soluble ARTs, AE and AM, the drug half-lives were significantly extended due to slow absorption from the site of the intramuscular injection. Those animals presented with a moderate to severe neurotoxicity and some died. It is notable that the drug half-lives (9.23 - 82.09 hrs) in animals treated with AE and AM were extremely extended compared to the half lives observed after AL and AS treatment. Although we lacked a full set of PK data after AE dosing in monkeys, we noted several PK results in different animals that showed the half lives on day 14 after intramuscular AE was dosed at 16 mg/kg daily were much longer than those observed in rats and dogs.

In addition, the monkeys dosed with AE for 14 days showed moderate neurotoxicity, suggesting that monkeys appear less sensitive to AE-induced neurotoxicity than rats and dogs which showed severe neurotoxicity and death when dosed with AE for 14 days. We conclude, from the dose amounts of ARTs used in various experiments to induce neurotoxicity, that the rank order of ARTs in terms of toxic potency is AE first followed by AM, AL, and lastly by AS. There is a strong correlation between the drug half-lives and the severity of neurotoxicity observed after treatment which supports the hypothesis that the drug exposure time during treatment plays a very important role in the induction of neurotoxicity.

3. Blood accumulation of ARTs leads to prolonged half-lives

The studies described thus far support the hypothesis that neurotoxicity induced by ARTs is highly dependent on the half-lives of these drugs. These studies also show that the ART drug half-life is due to the accumulation of ART drugs in the plasma following multiple doses of AE and AM administered intramuscularly and AL administered orally. In accordance with the published literatures and our research experience, ARTs (QHS, AS, AM, and DHA) elicit auto-induction of a drug metabolism pathway during multiple oral treatments in malaria patients and healthy subjects (van Agtmael et al., 1999; Ashton et al., 1996 and 1998; Khanh et al., 1999: Li et al., 2004; Park et al., 1998). The C_{max} and AUC values of these patients were markedly reduced from one-third to one-seventh on the last dose day compared with the first dosing day. The decrease in drug exposure levels during treatment is not disease-related, since the PK parameters of ART drugs in treated patients is similar to that reported in healthy subjects. Similar time-dependent declines were also found in animals treated with intravenous AS (Figure 3, top, Li et al., 2005a), intramuscular AS (Figure 3, middle, Li et al., 2007a), and oral AM (Figure 3, bottom, Classen et al., 1999). This data leads to pertinent questions: if all ART drugs have a pathway of metabolism auto-induction, why do drugs accumulate in animals treated with AE and AM after multiple intramuscular doses and with AL after repeated oral dosing?

3.1 Cause of AM and AE accumulation after intramuscular injection

PK data from various animal studies have shown that AE and AM will accumulate in the plasma of rats (Li et al., 1999b), beagle dogs (Classen et al., 1999), rhesus monkeys (Li et al., 2007a), and humans (Kager et al., 1994) following multiple intramuscular injections. Data collected from rat studies showed that the accumulation of AE in the plasma is due to a slow and prolonged absorption from the injection sites. The elimination $t^{1/2}$ of AE after 7 daily doses at 25 mg/kg was prolonged from 13.7 hr on the first dosing day to 31.2 hr on the last dosing day (Li et al., 1999b) (Fig. 1, top). AE accumulation was also observed in beagle dogs with severe neurotoxicity and death after daily intramuscular administration of AE at 15 mg/kg for 14 days (Li et al., 2006b). The elimination $t^{1/2}$ of AE after dosing the dogs for 14 days was prolonged from 9.23 hr on day 1 to 21.53 hr on day 14 (Fig. 2, middle).

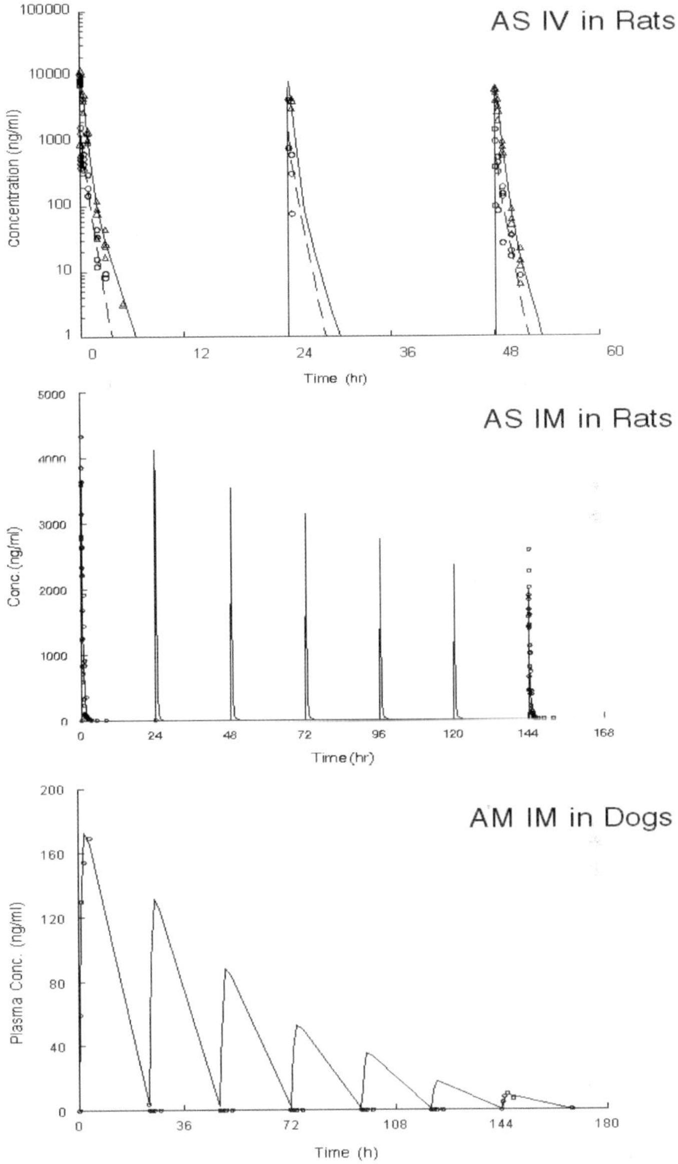

Fig. 3. Auto-induction metabolic profiles measured by HPLC-ECD (markers) and computer fitted curves of 36.7 mg/kg of intravenous artesunate (AS, top, dashed line), and its active metabolite DHA (top, solid line) once daily for 3 days (Li et al., 2005a). Study of 25 mg/kg of intramuscular AS (middle) was dosed daily for 7 days in rats (Li et al., 2007a). Another PK profiles after oral dose at 600 mg/kg of AM (bottom) daily for 7 days in beagle dogs (Classen et al., 1999).

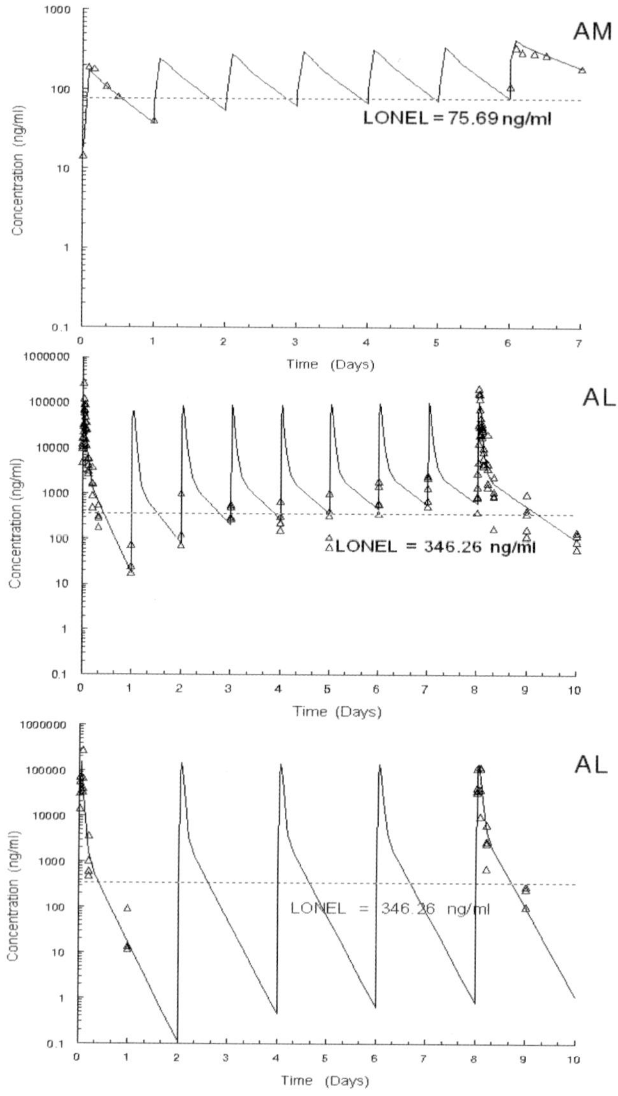

Fig. 4. Pharmacokinetic profiles measured by HPLC-ECD (markers) and computer fitted curves (solid line) of intramuscular artemether (AM) in peanut oil at 20 mg/kg daily for 7 days in beagle dogs (top, Classen et al., 1999). Oral artelinic acid (AL) in suspension at 160 mg/kg daily for 9 dosages (middle, n = 5) and oral AL at 288 mg/kg every other daily for 5 dosages in rats (bottom, n = 4, Si et al., 2007). The two regimens of AL have the same total dose with 1440 mg/kg and same treatment period for 9 days. The lowest observed neurotoxic effect level (LONEL) was defined as the plasma level of 75.69 ng/ml of AM in dogs and 346.26 ng/ml of AL in rats, at which anorectic and neuropathological toxicities were noted in daily dosing cohort.

Similar accumulation results for AM were reported in dog plasma after daily intramuscular administration of AM at 20, 40, and 80 mg/kg for 7 days (Classen et al., 1999). The analysis of TK parameters on day 2-7 was significantly different when compared to the parameters estimated on day 1. The elimination t½ of AM at 20 mg/kg after 7 daily doses increased from 10.93 hr on the first day of dosing day to 20.75 hr on the last day of dosing (Table 2; Figure 4, top), suggesting that the exposure time of AM had greatly increased. In addition, accumulation of AE was shown in the plasma of rhesus monkeys after daily intramuscular administration of AE at 16 mg/kg for 14 doses (Fig. 2, bottom). The elimination t½ of AE after 14 daily doses increased from 22.59 hr on day 1 to 82.09 hr on day 14 (Li et al., 2006b).

The intramuscular administration of AM and AE was associated with slow absorption because the drugs were dissolved in sesame oil or peanut oil that, when injected, formed a depot from which the drug was slowly released (Kager et al., 1994: Li et al., 2004). The slow elimination of AE was recently demonstrated in a rat study, which also found significant accumulation of AE in the plasma from injection sites (Li et al., 1999b). The results of a rat study conducted by daily intramuscular injections of AE at 25 mg/kg in sesame oil for 7 days confirmed and extended the results of earlier studies (Li et al., 1998b) by demonstrating that the absorption of AE from the injection site of the muscle was incomplete. This study also indicated that up to 38% of the total single dose of AE remained in the injection site for 24 hr after dosing, and 22% of the total single dose still remained in the muscle 48 hr after dosing. Following 7 days of daily intramuscular injections of AE (25 mg/kg), 91.4% of a single dose (25 mg/kg/day) was still left in the muscles from the injection sites 24 hr after the last dose (Li et al., 1999b).

Date*	Findings	Sesame oil control	AE	AM	Student** T-Test
Day 7	fascial inflammation, pseudocysts, muscle necrosis, & hemorrhage	1.75 ± 0.43	3.17 ± 0.37	2.50 ± 0.50	P = 0.0019
Day 10	fascial inflammation, pseudocysts, & hemorrhage	1.50 ± 0.50	3.00 ± 0.58	2.00 ± 0.0	P = 0.0045

Finding severity were grading as 0 = no significant lesions, 1 = minimal, 2 = mild, 3 = moderate, 4 = marked, and 5 = severe. *Day 7 and 10 are one day after last treatment of daily dose for 7 and 10 days. The date is given the dosing day as day 0. **The t-test was conducted between animals treated both with AE and AM in sesame oil.

Table 3. Muscle injury severity in the injection site areas following repeated arteether (AE) and artemether (AM) injection with vehicle sesame oil by multiple daily intramuscular dosing at 25 mg/kg for 7 days (n = 3) in rats (Li & Hickman, 2011).

Our histopathological data demonstrated that the cytotoxicity induced by AE in muscle cells occurred at the injection site. The severity of the damage observed after dosing was graded where no significant lesion detected was scored as 0; subacute to minimal damage and mild inflammation was scored as 1-2; damage along the connective tissue and between major skeletal muscle bundles showing subacute to chronic inflammation was scored as 2-3;

inflammation observed rarely extending into or between muscle fibers was scored as 3-4; prominent muscle damage with coagulative necrosis surrounded by a reparative response of fibroplasia, fibrosis, skeletal muscle regeneration, and muscle atrophy was scored as 4-5. The distribution of damage observed involves major muscle bundles and occurred in linear tracts, suggesting the damage may have been the result of a direct effect of the injected drug and/or vehicle on the muscle. Overall, the rats in the 7-day group (24 hr after last treatment) had more severe lesions than those in the 10-day group (96 hr after last dosing), and animals treated with AE had significantly more severe lesions than those treated with AM. The results showed that the chronic inflammation of the muscle located at the site of AE injection is more severe (moderate severity 3.00-3.17) than the inflammation noted at the AM injection site (mild severity 2.00-2.50)(Table 3). The inflammation of muscles induced by AE and AM injection may, therefore, be a factor prolonging the absorption of drugs from the muscles (Li & Hickman, 2011).

3.2 Cause of AL accumulation after intragastric administration

Oral administration of AL has also been shown to result in gastrointestinal toxicity that is associated with delayed gastric emptying. Similar findings of gastrointestinal toxicity were observed in rats treated intramuscularly with other ARTs (Li et al., 1998a). Rats treated with AL at a daily oral dose of 160 mg/kg for 9 days showed moderate neurotoxicity during treatment which was associated with prolonged absorption of AL in the stomach. Comparison of the day 1 and day 9 results revealed that the PK parameters were very different. A significantly longer (3.82-fold) elimination half-life was noted on day 9 (10.68 hr) in comparison to that observed on day 1 (2.84 hr), and this prolonged elimination results in drug accumulation (Figure 4, middle). The mean AUC of AL was higher on day 9, the last dosing day, (168.01 μg·h/ml) than the AUC observed on day 1, the first dosing day (128.38 μg·h/ml). Furthermore, progressive delays in gastric emptying and drug accretion were only found in rats treated with oral AL at 160 mg/kg. These results imply that the observations of delayed gastric emptying in turn results in AL accumulation, and the mean half-life of AL was correspondingly extended on the last dosing day compared to day 1 (Si et al., 2007).

This report of drug accumulation is illustrated in rats dosed daily with 160 mg/kg of AL orally for 9 days. These rats showed moderate neurotoxicity due to prolonged oral absorption in the stomach. This reservoir is similar to the depot effect seen with the oil-soluble ARTs (AM and AE) at intramuscular injection sites. The stomach contents of rats dosed orally with AL at 160 mg/kg daily for 9 days were examined at 8 and 24 hr after dosing at different time points during the study. On days 3, 5, 7, and 9, we detected 0, 46.52, 178.59, and 486.21 μg of AL/g in the stomach contents at 8 hr after the last dose. The increasing amount of AL observed remaining in the stomach over the course of dosing showed that gastric emptying was inhibited. The inhibition of gastric emptying progressed from mild inhibition seen on day 5 to severe inhibition observed on day 9. The inhibition of gastric emptying persisted even at 24 hr post dosing. At twenty-four hr post dosing on days 5, 7, and 9, we observed 5.74, 25.50, and 29.11 μg of AL/g, respectively, in the stomach contents. Similar anorectic toxicity was also reported in animals treated with AM, AE and DHA (Li et al., 1998a). It is postulated that this decrease in GI motility could result from a decrease in vagal tone as a consequence of a decline in sympathetic outflow (Hull & Maher 1990; Si et al., 2007).

4. Lowest observed neurotoxic effect level (LONEL) as a neurotoxic indicator

The body of literature cited supports the hypothesis that drug accumulation extends the drug exposure time, which we believe is a major causative factor in ART-induced neurotoxicity (Li et al., 2006b). The current methodology for assessing the no observed adverse effect level (NOAEL) involves identifying the highest concentration or dose administered that does not cause a statistically significant or biologically significant response to treatment in comparison to the control group. The lowest observed neurotoxic effect level (LONEL) represents the minimal plasma concentration associate with the lowest dose that is found to cause a neurologically and/or statistically significant response to treatment in comparison to the control group. Therefore, determining the neurotoxic exposure time (drug exposure time spent above the LONEL) is critical, and the LONEL should also be determined before evaluating the drug neurotoxic exposure time for each drug in various animals.

4.1 Neurotoxicity induced by intramuscular AE and oral AL in rats

A minimal daily dose of AE at 6.25 mg/kg for 7 days was estimated as a no observed neurotoxic effect dose (NONED), which was defined by AE dosing that did not result in histopathological findings in rats (Genovese et al., 1998). Significant changes of neuropathology in brain stem nuclei, however, were observed in a group of rats treated with AE at 12.5 mg/kg for 7 days. These results demonstrate that AE-induced brainstem neuropathology in rats can occur at the relatively high dose of 12.5 mg/kg for 7 days. The lowest plasma concentration of AE in rats was shown to be 41.32 ng/ml following intramuscular dosing of AE at 12.5 mg/kg in previous studies (Li et al., 1999b and 2002). Based on the NONED value of 6.25 mg/kg obtained in previous studies, it was possible to correctly identify the minimal neurotoxic effect level at 41.32 ng per ml, which has thus been defined as a LONEL in rat plasma (Figure 2, top). Administration above this concentration with a certain exposure time should result in neuropathological effects (Dayan 1998; van Agtmael et al., 1999; Brewer et al., 1994b).

In a PK simulation, 7 multiple AE treatments at a dose of 12.5 mg/kg were administered intramuscularly in rats (Li et al., 2002). The exposure time of 67.1 hr in plasma was estimated as the minimum time spent above the LONEL concentration of 41.32 ng/ml that was sufficient to induce positive neurotoxicity (Figure 2, top). After histological examination this estimate of 67.1 hours of AE dosing above LONEL to induce brainstem injury was confirmed by histopathological examination (Genovese et al., 1998) (Table 2). This finding confirmed the estimated LONEL (41.32 ng/ml) for AE in rats after dosing at 12.5 mg/kg for 7 days to induce neurotoxicity based on 100% positive findings of neuropathology (Fig. 2, top) (Li et al., 1999b & 2002).

Recently, AL was shown to induce moderate neurotoxicity after treatment with 160 mg/kg daily for 9 days confirmed by histopathology, and a minimal neuronal degeneration was observed following 5 doses of AL at 288 mg/kg every other day in rats. Although the total dose (1440 mg/kg) and duration (9 days) were identical (Si et al., 2007), different neurotoxic results were observed. This observation could be due to a prolonged exposure time in the 160 mg/kg group in comparison to the shorter time spent above the LONEL in the

288 mg/kg group (Table 2). Based on the minimal inhibition of gastric emptying on day 5 and histopathological data obtained from animals treated with oral AL daily for 9 days, the LONEL was calculated as 346.26 ng/ml in this study (Figure 4, middle). This data demonstrates that AL induced moderate brainstem injury in rats at a severity of 3.25 during a neurotoxic exposure time of 186.0 hr at daily doses of 160 mg/kg, and AL induced minimal brainstem injury in rats at a severity of 1.17 during a neurotoxic exposure time of 75.0 hr at a daily dose of 288 mg/kg dosed every other day. The reduction of the neurotoxic exposure time from 186.0 hrs to 75.0 hrs correlates well with the reduction of neurotoxicity observed between the two doses regimens.

This study also showed that the LONEL value (346.26 ng/ml) following oral AL administration in rats is approximately 8-fold higher than the LONEL observed after dosing with intramuscular AE (41.32 ng/ml). A tissue distribution study was also conducted comparing the intramuscular injection of ^{14}C-AE to intravenous administration of ^{14}C-AL in rats. The results of this study showed 0.89% total radioactivity in the brain after ^{14}C-AE administration while the administration of ^{14}C-AL in rats showed 0.1% of total radioactivity in the brain (Li et al., 2005a). This result suggests that ^{14}C-labelled AL seems to be less capable of penetrating through the blood-brain barrier than ^{14}C-AE.

4.2 Neurotoxicity induced by intramuscular AE and AM in dogs

Davidson (1994) showed that a daily dose of AE at 3 mg/kg for 28 days is a NONED that does not cause clinical neurotoxicity or pathology in beagles. AE-induced brainstem neuropathology in dogs has been detected after administration of a dose as low as 5 mg/kg/day as shown by Brewer (1994a, 1994b, 1998), 6.25 mg/kg observed by Dayan (1998), and 6.75 mg/kg dosed daily for 28 days observed by Davidson (1994). Based on these three findings, the calculated average of the minimal dose necessary to produce neurotoxicity by histopathology in dogs is 6 mg/kg daily for 28 days. The minimal plasma concentration of AE with a dose of 6.0 mg/kg daily for 28 days has been estimated at 40.92 ng/ml, and this value could, therefore, be defined as a LONEL in plasma. The LONEL of 40.92 ng/ml should be the first "at risk" level for causing neurotoxicity in dogs at a daily dose of 6 mg/kg for 28 days (Li et al., 2006b). As a result, the LONEL for toxicity of AE in dogs was estimated based on all positive findings of neuropathology in these animal studies.

A TK simulation of 28 repeated AE treatments at 6 mg/kg dosed intramuscularly in beagles was conducted, and an exposure time of 103.7 hr in plasma was estimated as a minimum time above the LONEL (40.92 ng/ml) to induce positive neurotoxicity, which was confirmed by histopathological examination (Brewer et al., 1994b; Davidson 1994; Dayan 1998) (Table 2). The result demonstrated that AE-induced brainstem injury in dogs occurred during a minimal period of 103.7 hr with plasma exposure of AE above this LONEL. Therefore, the LONEL for neurotoxicity of AE was simulated based on 100% positive findings of neuropathology at a daily dose of 6 mg/kg for 28 days in beagles (Li et al., 2006b and 2007a).

Classen (1999) showed that a minimal daily dose of AM at 20 mg/kg given for 7 days caused a minimal clinical neurotoxicity or pathology in beagles. The minimal plasma concentration of AM achieved after a dose of 20 mg/kg given daily for 7 days has been estimated at 75.69 ng/ml, and this value could, therefore, be defined as a LONEL in dog plasma. The LONEL of 75.69 ng/ml should be the first "at risk" level for causing neurotoxicity in dogs at a daily dose of 20 mg/kg for 7 days (Figure 4, top). As a result, the LONEL for toxicity of AM in dogs was estimated based on all positive findings of neuropathology in these animals (5 out of 8 dogs). PK analyses of 7 repeated AM treatments of beagles at 20 and 40 mg/kg dosed intramuscularly were conducted, and exposure times of 153 and 188 hrs, respectively, were estimated as a minimum time above the LONEL (75.69 ng/ml) to induce neurotoxicity, which was confirmed by histopathological examination (Table 2). The results of this study showed that AM-induced brainstem injury occurred during a minimal period over 153 hrs at drug plasma level above this LONEL. It is to be noted that the LONEL of AM (75.69 ng/ml) has been shown to be much higher than that of AE in beagles (40.92 ng/ml), suggesting that AE may have a higher potential for neurotoxicity than AM.

4.3 Neurotoxicity induced by intramuscular AE in monkeys

Since AE-induced brainstem neuropathology in rhesus monkeys occurred at a minimal dose of 8 mg/kg dosed daily for 14 days (Petras et al., 1997, 2000), the LONEL of AE was estimated to be 193.8 ng/ml. This estimate is based on our TK analysis conducted by dosing monkeys with AE at 16 mg/kg dosed daily for 14 days which should, based on a number of repeat dosing studies, result in evidence of AE-induced neurotoxicity (Petras et al., 1997; Li et al., 2006b, 2007a). By conducting TK simulations of 14 repeated AE treatments of monkeys dosed intramuscularly at 8 mg/kg, a neurotoxic exposure time of 179.5 hr in plasma was calculated as the minimum time spent above the LONEL (193.8 ng/ml) required to induce pathological neurotoxicity (Figure 2, bottom). The results of this study showed that AE-induced brainstem injury occurred during a minimal duration of 179.5 hr spent above the LONEL of AE (Li et al., 2006b, 2007a). The data also showed that the LONEL value of 193.8 ng/ml in rhesus monkeys is 4-fold higher than that of rats (41.32 ng/ml) and dogs (40.92 ng/ml), indicating that rats and dogs appear to be more vulnerable than rhesus monkeys to neurotoxic ART-induced toxicity.

5. TK/TD analysis of artemisinin-induced neurotoxicity

To determine the relationship between drug exposure time (toxicokinetics, TK) and neurotoxic effects (toxicodynamics, TD) after administration of ARTs in varying dose and time regimens, we calculated the time required for the drug plasma concentration to reach a neurotoxic level above the LONEL. Although the LONEL is a minimum observed neurotoxic effect level, a certain exposure time was required to be necessary to determine the neurotoxic effects in our previous studies where ARTs were shown to produce neurotoxicity. This process gave us an initial estimate of drug LONEL and exposure times and allowed us to correlate these data with observed histopathology or neurotoxic effects from ARTs tested in various regimens in different animal species. For the evaluation of toxicity, if the recovery (consisting of adaptation, repair and reversibility) half-life of an organism is longer than the half-life of the causative agent in the organism, then TD would become the rate-determining or rate-limiting step, and the organism would survive. If the

TK half-life of the compound is longer than the recovery half-life, then TK will be a rate-determining or rate limiting step. In this scenario, the TK exposure time would be identical to a TD exposure time, and the organism might die. Therefore, neurotoxicity induced by ARTs in animals may be determined through either TD or TK/TD processes.

5.1 Exposure time with neurotoxic effects of AE and AL in SD rats

A neurotoxicity study was conducted to compare AE in two vehicles, sesame oil and cremophore (Li et al., 2002). The authors calculated the neurotoxic exposure time in rats of AE in sesame oil to be 164.3 hrs after dosing over the LONEL (41.32 ng/ml) during treatment with 25 mg/kg AE dosed intramuscularly daily for 7 days (Figure 1, top). The total neurotoxic exposure time of AE in a formulation of 1:2 cremophore/saline at the same dose regimen was 103.0 hrs. The exposure time for AE in a cremophore formulation was over one-third less than the exposure time observed with AE in sesame oil. Neurotoxicity outcomes in these rats were reduced from severe to moderate. After simulating the TK data on daily dosing at 12.5 mg/kg for 7 days (Li et al., 2007a), the drug exposure time spent over the LONEL was only 67.1 h, and the severity of neuropathological toxicity was further reduced to a minimum (Genovese et al., 1998), demonstrating that drug exposure time plays a key role that correlates with the development of neurotoxicity (Figure 2, top).

In a further study, the neurotoxic exposure time (drug exposure time spent over the LONEL at 346.26 ng/ml) for oral AL was shown to be 186 hr which defines the exposure period threshold to achieve neurotoxicity (Fig. 4, middle). These results indicated a correlation between the neuropathology observed in rats and a prolonged AL exposure time. In this study, the AL exposure time was related to an accumulation of drug in plasma likely resulting from delayed gastric emptying, which, in turn, was hypothesized to induce prolonged absorption of the drug from the stomach (Si et al., 2007). When rats were treated intermittently with 5 doses of AL at 288 mg/kg every other day for 9 days, neuronal degeneration was minimal until day 7 after the last treatment (Table 2). The minimal exposure time required to induce neurotoxicity in these animals was calculated to be 75 hr (Fig. 4, bottom). The data, therefore, supports the hypothesis that shortening the drug exposure time above LONEL level may reduce the risk of neurotoxicity.

The LONEL cannot be estimated for intramuscular AL and AS dosed in rats daily at 25 mg/kg for 7 days because no neurotoxicity (pathological or/and behavioral neurotoxicity) was detected in those animals. PK data showed that drug accumulation in the plasma was not observed in these animals. The lack of AL and AS drug accumulation is likely due to their rapid elimination and short half-lives with clear and long time intermissions between each dosing without drug exposure (Figure 1, middle and bottom). Confirmation of the hypothesis that the short drug exposure times of AL and AS after intramuscular injection do not induce neurotoxicity (Table 2) is a very relevant finding as animals treated with AL and AS intramuscularly would likely avoid the risk of neurotoxic outcome due to a reduction of drug exposure times. This result suggests that the shorter exposure times of AL and AS without drug exposure at LONEL appears to be a major contributing factor for avoiding clinical neurotoxicity.

5.2 Exposure time with neurotoxic effects of AE, AM and AL in dogs

Drug accumulation was also observed in the plasma of beagles after daily intramuscular administration of AE at 15 mg/kg for 14 days (Li et al., 2006). The mean concentration-time profile of AE in beagles obtained from this experiment is shown in Fig. 2 (middle). The most significant data observed were found to involve different parameters of the AUC and the drug half-lives. The elimination t½ of AE was prolonged from 9.23 hr on the first dosing day to 21.53 hr on the last dosing day, suggesting that the exposure time of AE had nearly doubled. Also, the LONEL of AE (40.92 ng/ml) in beagles was first reached in that study on day 6-7 (Li et al., 2006b). At this time, the food intake of these animals decreased by 70%, and the QT interval also increased by more than 25%. We believe, based on the TK data analysis, that day 6-7 is the earliest time possible to induce minimal neurotoxicity in beagles, which also showed GI toxicity, following high level AE dosing. The exposure time of AE in this 14 day study which induced severe neurotoxicity and death involved daily intramuscular injections of 15 mg/kg AE in dogs was estimated to be at concentrations above the LONEL (40.92 ng/ml), and the exposure period was calculated to be 277.6 (Table 2).

Although AM and AE are both oil-soluble ARTs, there are differences in the TK and TD profiles of these two drugs: 1) AM injection has been shown to result in less local inflammatory toxicity at the muscle injection site than AE formulated with the same sesame oil vehicle; 2) AM has been shown to have a significantly higher absorption rate (C_{max}) from intramuscular injection sites than AE; 3) AM has been shown to have much higher drug exposure levels (total AUC) than AE which likely results in much less drug accumulation; and 4) AM has been shown to have a LONEL that is almost two fold higher (75.69 ng/ml) than AE (41.32 ng/ml) in beagles. Although the multiple dose levels of AM employed in this study were higher than those used for AE (Table 2), the AM dosing period of 7 days was half that of the 14 day AE dosing period. Therefore, the LONEL data for AM and AE would suggest that the predicted neurotoxic exposure time for AM (113.2 - 147.8 hrs) required to induce neurotoxicity should be significantly shorter than the neurotoxic exposure time for AE (277.6 hrs) required to induce neurotoxicity. Correspondingly, the clinical observations of animals dosed with AM showed a lower degree of neurotoxicity than dogs treated with AE intramuscularly (Table 2). This finding supports the hypothesis that intramuscular AM treatment is less prone to induce neurotoxicity in animals than intramuscular AE.

The neurotoxic exposure time spent above the LONEL after oral AL dosing (346.26 ng/ml) in dogs was calculated to be 17.9 hr for a suspension formulation of AL (Li et al., 2005b) and 14.6 hr for a capsule formulation of AL both dosed at 25 mg/kg daily for 14 days (Table 2). Similar to intramuscular administration, animals treated with oral AL did not show any evidence of induction of neurotoxicity due to the shorter drug exposure times above the LONEL. The drug exposure times observed for AL were much shorter than the neurotoxic exposure time above the LONEL of 75.0 h, which is required to induce a minimal pathological neurotoxicity in rats (Table 2).

5.3 Exposure time with neurotoxic effects of AE in rhesus monkeys

Substantial plasma accumulation of AE was shown in the plasma of rhesus monkeys after daily intramuscular administration of AE at 16 mg/kg for 14 days (Fig. 2, bottom). Based on the minimal injury observed to the neuronal tissues in the monkeys treated with 8 mg/kg daily for 14 days, it was possible to correctly identify 193.8 ng/ml as the LONEL (Li & Hickman, 2011). The neurotoxic exposure period of AE was calculated as 307.4 hr in this study following daily intramuscular injection of 16 mg/kg for 14 days in monkeys with moderate neurotoxicity (Petras et al., 1997 and 2000) (Table 2). This calculation was based on the estimated exposure time of AE above the LONEL concentration (193.8 ng/ml). The rhesus monkeys treated with intramuscular AE at 8 mg/kg daily for 14 days showed that the drug exposure time spent above LONEL with minimal pathological toxicity was estimated at 179.5 hr, which was shorter than the exposure time (307.4 hr) from a previous study following daily intramuscular administration of AE at 16 mg/kg for 14 days (Li et al., 2006b). The longer neurotoxic exposure time is likely the key factor involved in the induction of neurotoxicity in rhesus monkeys (Li et al., 2007a).

6. Neurotoxic consideration of ARTs in antimalarial and anticancer treatments

Though no animal model exists capable of completely mimicking ARTs-induced neurotoxicity, the comparison of monkeys to humans is the closest that can be achieved. With animal experiments, only certain aspects of the whole complex TK/TD environment can be analyzed. In order to achieve the best prediction of neurotoxicity based on TK/TD parameters, the choice of animals and experimental design requires careful consideration to represent the conditions existing in humans in as suitable a model as possible. The more the model deviates from human TK/TD conditions, the less likely the prediction will be relevant. Today more information is available on the TK/TD properties of ARTs in animals. This body of literature will provide data on the neurotoxic doses of ARTs and on their non-neurotoxic doses relevant to man.

Studies with laboratory animals have demonstrated fatal neurotoxicity associated with intramuscular administration of AM and AE or oral administration of AL. These effects suggest that the exposure time of ARTs was extended in these studies due to the accumulation of drug in the bloodstream, and this accumulation, in turn, resulted in neurotoxicity. In our previous studies, the drug exposure time with a neurotoxic outcome (neurotoxic exposure time) was evaluated as a predictor of neurotoxicity *in vivo* (Li & Hickman, 2011). The neurotoxic exposure time represents a total time spent above the lowest observed neurotoxic effect levels (LONEL) in plasma. The effects of ARTs do vary in different animal species. For example, the dose of AE required to induce minimal neurotoxicity requires a 2-3 fold longer exposure time in rhesus monkeys (179.5 hr) than in rats (67.1 hr) and dogs (103.7 hr) when using a daily dose of 6-12.5 mg/kg for 7-28 days. This finding suggests that the safe drug dosing of LONEL duration in monkeys should be longer than 7.0 days (> 168 hrs) under this exposure.

In addition, the effects of ARTs vary from compound to compound. For example the LONEL for intramuscular AM required to induce neurotoxicity (75.69 ng/ml) is twice as high as the LONEL for intramuscular AE required to induce neurotoxicity (40.92 ng/ml). Oral AL treatment required a LONEL to induce neurotoxicity (346.26 ng/ml) that is 4-fold higher than the LONEL of AM required to induce neurotoxicity (75.69 ng/ml) and 8-fold higher than the LONEL of AE (40.92 ng/ml), required to induce neurotoxicity. A determination of LONEL for oral and injectable AS was not possible because no neurotoxicity was observed in animals treated with various AS dose regimens, suggesting that water-soluble ARTs (AS and AL) appear to be much safer than oil-soluble ARTs.

The various animal species treated with different ARTs clearly show the different neurotoxic effects associated with corresponding exposure times. The current marketed drugs for ART therapy are based on oral administration of drug and combination therapies to malaria patients. Oral administration results in lower peak concentrations and shorter exposure times which is less likely to induce neurotoxicity than intramuscular ARTs. Since more than 99% of malaria patients have been treated with oral ARTs or intravenous AS, this may be the reason for the lack of neurotoxicity observed in malaria patients. When relating the animal and human neurotoxicity of ARTs, the different neurotoxic exposure times may possibly provide a greater margin of safety in humans. The current clinical dose regimens of three-day ART combined therapies (ACTs) for uncomplicated cases of malaria, and the dose regimens recommended for intravenous AS treatments for severe malaria, which include a few days of a loading dose, may be too short of a drug exposure time to induce neurotoxicity in humans. Also, with regard to acute toxicity, humans appear to be less sensitive than animals (Geyer et al., 1990; Kimbrough 1990), and humans have much better repair capabilities than animals to respond to such toxicity (Culotta & Koshland 1994).

Although the water-soluble ARTs, like AS, appear to be much safer, further study is needed when employing ARTs as anticancer agents (Li & Hickman, 2011). At high concentrations, ARTs appear to be active against cancer *in vivo*. The use of ARTs at high concentrations or for long drug exposure times, however, has substantial risk of inducing severe toxicities, such as the neurotoxic effects we have described here. Animal studies have shown that high concentrations of AS and DHA can induce embryotoxicity, and longer exposure times have been shown to be associated with fatal neurotoxicity (Li et al., 2007a). To provide maximum benefit and minimal risk of toxicity, ARTs should be combined with other anticancer agents to increase the efficacy of cancer drugs, enhance the survival rate of patients with cancer, and prolong the time to progression (Zhang et al., 2008). The diversity in targets of ARTs supports the possibility that these compounds could be used in combination with other agents, which mimics the current strategy promoted by the WHO as policy recommendations on the use of ARTs for malaria therapy (WHO 2006).

7. Conclusion

Studies with laboratory animals have demonstrated neurotoxicity following administration of some intramuscular doses of oil-soluble AM and AE, or intragastric treatment of water-soluble AL. The various PK studies of ARTs conducted using numerous animal models show that the drug exposure time appears to be a more important factor than other PK parameters measured for inducing neurotoxicity. There are significant differences in neurotoxicity observed when comparing the effects of ARTs on rats, dogs and monkeys suggesting that the exposure time required inducing neurotoxicity after dosing with ARTs is likely to be longer in humans. Extensive TK/TD analyses of neurotoxicity after ART treatment of rats, dogs, and monkeys have provided a wealth of data which can be used to predict the neurotoxic exposure time of ARTs in humans. Based on the dose amounts of ARTs used in various experiments to induce neurotoxicity we would rank the ARTs in terms of toxic potential with AE being the most toxic followed in order by AM, AL, and lastly by AS. There is a strong correlation between the drug half-lives of ARTs and the severity of neurotoxicity observed after treatment which supports the hypothesis that the drug exposure time during treatment plays a very important role in the induction of neurotoxicity.

In the this chapter, the lowest observed neurotoxic effect level (LONEL) represents the minimal plasma concentration associated with the lowest dose that is found to cause a neurologically and/or statistically significant response to treatment in comparison to the control group. Based on the determination of the LONEL in various animal species for ARTs, the neurotoxic exposure time (drug exposure time spent above the LONEL) was evaluated. Our analysis of this data leads us to the prediction that the safe dosing duration of AE or AM in humans should be longer than 7 days (> 168 hr), and the safe dosing duration of AS therapy is likely much longer than that. Accordingly, the 3-5 days dosing duration currently used in antimalarial therapy of ARTs should be quite safe. Neurotoxicity may be caused in humans, however, treated with inappropriate dose regimens, and therefore, evaluation of the sustained drug exposure times appears to be the critical factor to assess and prevent neurotoxicity. Advances in our knowledge of ART-induced neurotoxicity can help refine the treatment regimens used as therapies for malaria and cancer with ART-based combination therapy and injectable AS products to avoid drug accumulation and reduce the risk of toxicity.

8. Acknowledgments

This report was supported by the United States Army Research and Materiel Command. The opinions or assertions contained herein are the private views of the author and are not to be construed as official, or as reflecting true views of the Department of the Army or the Department of Defense.

9. References

van Agtmael, M.A., Cheng-Qi, S., Qing, J.X., Mull, R., van Boxtel, C.J. (1999) Multiple dose pharmacokinetics of artemether in Chinese patients with uncomplicated falciparum malaria. Int. J. Antimicrob Agents. 12, 151-158.

Angus, B.J., Thaiaporn, I., Chanthapadith, K., Suputtamongkol, Y., White, N.J. (2002) Oral artesunate dose-response relationship in acute falciparum malaria. Antimicrob Agents Chemother. 46, 778-782.

Ashton, M., Sy, N.D., Gordi, T., Hai, T.N., Thach, D.C., Huong, N.V., Johansson, M., Coeng, L.D. (1996) Evidence for time-dependence artemisinin kinetics in adults with uncomplicated malaria. Pharm Pharmacol Lett. 6, 127-130.

Ashton, M., Hai, T.N., Sy, N.D., Huong, D.X., Van Huong, N., Nieu, N.T., Cong, L.D. (1998) Artemisinin pharmacokinetics is time-dependent during repeated oral administration in healthy male adults. Drug Metab Dispos. 26, 25-27.

Batty, K.T., Thu, L.T., Davis, T.M., Ilett, K.F., Mai, T.X., Hung, N.C., Tien, N.P., Powell, S.M., Thien, H.V., Binh, T.Q., Kim, N.V. (1998) A pharmacokinetic and pharmacodynamic study of intravenous vs oral artesunate in uncomplicated falciparum malaria. Br. J. Clin. Pharmacol. 45, 123-129.

Brewer, T.G., Grate, S.J., Peggins, J.O., Weina, P.J., Petras, J.M., Levine, B.S., Heiffer, M.H., Schuster, B.G. (1994a) Fatal neurotoxicity of arteether and artemether. Am. J. Trop. Med. Hyg. 51, 251-259.

Brewer, T.G., Peggins, J.O., Grate, S.J., Petras, J.M., Levine, B.S., Weina, P.J., Swearengen, J., Heiffer, M.H., Schuster, B.G. (1994b) Neurotoxicity in animals due to arteether and artemether. Trans. R Soc. Trop. Med. Hyg. 88 (Suppl, 1), S33-36.

Brewer, T.G., Genovese, R.F., Newman, D.B., Li, Q.G., 1998. Factors relating to neurotoxicity of artemisinin antimalarial drugs "listening to arteether". Med. Trop. (Mars). 58(3 Suppl), 22-27.

China Cooperative Research Group on Qinghaosu and Its Derivatives as Antimalarials. (1982) Metabolism and pharmacokinetics of qinghaosu and its derivatives. J. Trad. Chin. Med, 2, 25-30.

Classen, W., Altmann, B., Gretener, P., Souppart, C., Skelton-Stroud, P., Krinke, G. (1999) Differential effects of orally versus parenterally administered qinghaosu derivatives artemether in dogs. Exp. Toxicol. Pathol. 51, 507-516.

Culotta, E., Koshland, D.E Jr. (1994) DNA repair works it works its way to the top. Science. 266(5193), 1926-1929.

Davis, T.M., Phuong, H.L., Ilett, K.F., Hung, N.C., Batty, K.T., Phuong, V.D., Powell, S.M., Thien, H.V., Binh, T.Q. (2001) Pharmacokinetics and pharmacodynamics of intravenous artesunate in severe falciparum malaria. Antimicrob Agents Chemother. 45, 181-186.

Davis, T.M., Binh, T.Q., Ilett, K.F., Batty, K.T., Phuong, H.L., Chiswell, G.M., Phuong, V.D., Agus, C. (2003) Penetration of dihydroartemisinin into cerebrospinal fluid after administration of intravenous artesunate in severe falciparum malaria. Antimicrob Agents Chemother. 47, 368-370.

Davidson, D.E. (1994) Role of arteether in the treatment of malaria and plans for further development. Trans. R Soc. Trop. Med. Hyg. 88 Suppl, 1, S51-52.

Dayan, A.D. (1998) Neurotoxicity and artemisinin compounds do the observations in animals justify limitation of clinical use? Med Trop (Mars). 58(3 Suppl), 32-37.

Efferth, T., Kaina, B. (2010) Toxicity of the antimalarial artemisinin and its derivatives. Crit. Rev. Toxicol. 16, 1-17.

Elias, Z., Bonnet, E., Marchou, B., Massip, P. (1999) Neurotoxicity of artemisinin: possible counseling and treatment of side effects. Clin. Infect. Dis. 28, 1330-1331.

Fishwick , J., McLean, W.G., Edwards, G., Ward, S.A. (1995) The toxicity of artemisinin and related compounds on neuronal and glial cells in culture. Chem. Biol. Interact. 96, 263-271.

Franco-Paredes, C., Dismukes, R., Nicolls, D., Kozarsky, P.E. (2005) Neurotoxicity due to antimalarial therapy associated with misdiagnosis of malaria. Clin. Infect. Dis. 40, 1710-1711.

Gachot, B., Eliaszewicz, M., Dupont, B. (1997) Artesunate and cerebellar dysfunction in falciparum malaria. N. Engl. J. Med. 337, 792-793.

Genovese, R.F., Petras, J.M., Brewer, T.G. (1995) Arteether neurotoxicity in the absence of deficits in behavioural performance in rats. Ann. Trop. Med. Parasitol. 89, 447-449.

Genovese, R.F., Newman, D.B., Li, Q.G., Peggins, J.O., Brewer, T.G. (1998) Dose-dependent brainstem neuropathology following repeated arteether administration in rats. Brain Res. Bull. 45, 199-202.

Genovese, R.F., Newman, D.B., Brewer, T.G. (2000) Behavioral and neural toxicity of the artemisinin antimalarial, arteether, but not artesunate and artelinate, in rats. Pharmacol. Biochem. Behav. 67, 37-44.

Geyer, H.J., Scheuntert, I., Rapp, K., Kettrup, A., Korte, F., Greim, H., Rozman, K. (1990) Correlation between acute toxicity of 2,3,7,8-tetrachlorodibenzo-p-dioxin (TCDD) and total body fat content in mammals. Toxicology 65, 97-107.

Haq, M.Z., Mishra, B.R., Goyal, N., Sinha, V.K. (2009) alpha/beta-Arteether-induced mania in a predisposed adolescent. Gen. Hosp. Psychiatry. 31, 391-393.

Hull, K.M., Maher, T.J. (1990) L-Tyrosine potentiates the anorexia induced by mixed-acting sympathomimetic drugs in hyperphagic rats. J. Pharmacol. Exp. Ther. 255, 403-409.

Jiang, J.R., Zou, C.D. Shu, H.L., Zeng, Y.L. (1989) Assessment of absorption and distribution of artemether in rats using a thin layer chromatography scanning technique. Zhongguo Yao Li Xue Bao. 10, 431-434.

Jorgensen, R.J. (1980) Dictyocaulus viviparous: Migration in agar of larvae subjected to a variety of physicochemical exposure. Exp Parasit. 49, 106-115.

Kager, P.A., Schultz, M.J., .Zijlstra, E.E., van Berg, B., van Boxtel, Ch.J. (1994) Arteether administration in humans: preliminary studies of pharmacokinetics, safety and tolerance. Trans. R. Soc. Trop. Med. Hyg. 88 (Suppl 1), S53-54.

Kamchonwongpaisan, S., McKeever, P., Hossler, P., Ziffer, H., Meshnick, S.R. (1997) Artemisinin neurotoxicity: Neuropathology in rats and mechanistic studies in vitro. Am. J. Trop. Med. Hyg. 56, 7-12.

Karbwang, J., Na-Bangchang, K., Wattanakoon, Y., Thanavibul, A., Harinasuta, T. (1994) Artemether 5 versus 7 day regimen for severe falciparum malaria. Southeast Asian J Trop. Med. Public Health. 25, 702-706.

Kearney, B.P., Aweeka, F.T. (1999) The penetration of anti-infectives into the central nervous system. Neurol Clin. 17, 883-900.

Khanh, N.X., de Vries, P.J., Ha, L.D., van Boxtel, C.J., Koopmans, R., Kager, P.A. (1999) Declining concentrations of dihydroartemisinin in plasma during 5-day oral treatment with artesunate for falciparum malaria. Antimicrob Agents Chemother. 43, 690-692.

Kimbrough, R.D. (1990) How toxic is 2,3,7,8-tetrachlorodibenzodioxin to humans? J. Toxicol. Environ. Health. 30, 261-271.

Li, Q., Peggens, J.O., Brown, L.D., Brewer, T.G. (1994) Pharmacokinetics and hydrolysis of sodium artelinate in dogs. AM. J. Trop. Med. Hyg. 51, 260.

Li, Q., Peggins, J.O. (1998a) Anorectic toxicity of dihydroartemisinin, arteether and artemether in rats following multiple intramuscular doses. Int. J. Toxicol. 17, 663-676.

Li, Q., Peggins, J.O., Fleckenstein, L.L., Masonic, K., Heiffer, M.H., Brewer, T.G. (1998b) The pharmacokinetics and bioavailability of dihydroartemisinin, arteether, artemether, artesunic acid and artelinic acid in rats. J. Pharm. Pharmacol. 50, 173-182.

Li, Q., Peggins, J.O., Lin, A.J., Masonic, K., Trotman, K.M., Brewer, T.G. (1998c) Pharmacology and toxicology of artelinic acid: Preclinical investigation on pharmacokinetics, metabolism, protein and RBC binding, acute and anorectic toxicities. Trans. R. Soc. Trop. Med. Hyg. 92, 332-340.

Li, Q. Carpenter, C., Trotman, C., Kathcart, A.K., Donahue, R., Milhous, W.K. (1999a) Pharmacokinetic comparison of artesunate and dihydroartemisinin in beagle dogs. Am. J. Trol. Med. Hyg. 61, 274.

Li, Q., Brueckner, R.P., Peggins, J.O., Trotman, K.M., Brewer, T.G. (1999b) Arteether toxicokinetics and pharmacokinetics in rats after 25 mg/kg/day single and multiple doses. Eur. J. Drug Metab. Pharmacokinet. 24, 213-223.

Li, Q., Bossone, C.A., Ohrt, C., Chung, H., Harris, D., Harre, J., Lee, P., Kathcart, A.K., Brueckner, R.P. (2000) Early signs and biomarkers of neurotoxicity: toxicokinetic and toxicodynamic evaluation following 15-mg/kg arteether daily intramuscular injections for two weeks in beagle dogs. Am. J. Trol. Med. Hyg. 62, 142.

Li, Q., Mog, S.R., Si, Y.Z., Kyle, D.E., Gettayacamin, M., Milhous, W.K. (2002) Neurotoxicity and efficacy of arteether related to its exposure times and exposure levels in rodents. Am. J. Trop. Med. Hyg. 66, 516-525.

Li, Q., Lugt, C.B., Looareesuwan, S., Krudsood, S., Wilairatana, P., Vannaphan, S., Chalearmrult, K., Milhous, W.K. (2004) Pharmacokinetic investigation on the therapeutic potential of artemotil (beta-arteether) in Thai patients with severe Plasmodium falciparum malaria. Am. J. Trop. Med. Hyg. 71, 723-731.

Li, Q., Xie, L.H., Si, Y., Wong, E., Upadhyay, R., Yanez, D., Weina, P.J. (2005a) Toxicokinetics and hydrolysis of artelinate and artesunate in malaria-infected rats. Int. J. Toxicol. 24, 241-250.

Li, Q., Milhous, W.K., Weina, P.J. (2005b) Regimen strategy to decrease artemisinin agents related failure and recrudescence in severe and complicated malaria treatment. Medicine and Health in the Tropics (Marseille-France) Abstract Book 2005, 131.

Li, Q., Xie, L.H., Haeberle, A., Zhang, J., Weina, P. (2006a) The evaluation of radiolabeled artesunate on tissue distribution in rats and protein binding in humans. Am. J. Trop. Med. Hyg. 75, 817-826.

Li, Q., Milhous, W.K., Weina, P.J. (2006b) Fatal neurotoxicity of the artemisinin derivatives is related to drug pharmacokinetic profiles in animals. Curr. Topics Toxicol, 3, 1-16.

Li, Q., Milhous, W.K., Weina, P.J. (2007a) Antimalarial in Malaria Therapy. 1st edition. Nova Science Publishers Inc, New York, pp. 1-133.

Li, Q., Gerena, L., Xie, L.H., Zhang, J., Kyle, D.E., Milhous, W.K. (2007b) Development and validation of flow cytometric measurement for parasitemia in cultures of P. falciparum vitally stained with YOYO-1. Cytometry Part A. 71A, 297-307.

Li, Q., Xie, L.H., Johnson, T.O., Si, Y.Z., Haeberle, A.S., Weina, P.J. (2007c) Toxicity evaluation of artesunate and artelinate in Plasmodium berghei-infected and uninfected rats. Trans. R. Soc. Trop. Med. Hyg. 101, 104-112.

Li, Q., Xie, L., Zhang, J., Weina, P.J. (2008) The distribution pattern of intravenous [^{14}C] artesunate in rat tissues by quantitative whole-body autoradiography and tissue dissection techniques. J Pharm Biomed Anal. 48, 876-884.

Li, Q., Weina, P., (2010) Artesunate: the best drug in the treatments of severe and complicated malaria. Pharmaceuticals. 3, 2322-2332.

Li, Q., Hickman, M. (2011) Toxicokinetic and toxicodynamic (TK/TD) evaluation to determine and predict neurotoxicity of artemisinins. Toxicology. 279, 1-9.

Lin, A.J., Klayman, D.L., Milhous, W.K. (1987) Antimalarial activity of new water-soluble dihydroartemisinin derivatives. J. Med. Chem. 30, 2147-2150.

Mayer, P.R. (1995) Absorption, metabolism, and other factors that influence drug exposure in toxicology studies. Toxicol. Pathol. 23, 165-169.

McLean, W.G., Ward, S.A. (1998) In vitro neurotoxicity of artemisinin derivatives. Med. Trop. (Mars). 58(3 Suppl), 28-31.

Miller, L.G., Panosian, C.B. (1997) Ataxia and slurred speech after artesunate treatment for falciparum malaria. N. Engl. J. Med. 336, 1328.

Navaratnam, V., Mansor, S.M., Sit, N.W., Grace, J., Li, Q., Olliaro, P. (2000) Pharmacokinetics of artemisinin-type compounds. Clin. Pharmacokinet. 39, 255-270.

Newton, P.N., Day, N.P., White, N.J. (2005) Misattribution of central nervous system dysfunction to artesunate. Clin. Infect. Dis. 41, 1687-1688.

Niu, X.Y., Ho, L.Y., Ren, Z.H., Song, Z.Y. (1985) Metabolic fate of Qinghaosu in rats; a new TLC densitometric method for its determination in biological material. Eur. J. Drug Metab. Pharmacokinet. 1985, 10, 55-59.

Noker, P., Lin, T.T. (2000) Toxicity dose range study of 14 days oral administration of artelinic acid in dogs. Contract Research Reports, Southern Research Institute, Birmingham, USA (Contract Report, our unpublished data)

Nontprasert, A., Nosten-Bertrand, M., Pukrittayakamee, S., Vanijanonta, S., Angus, B.J., White, N.J. (1998) Assessment of neurotoxicity of parenteral artemisinin derivatives in mice. Am. J. Trop. Med. Hyg. 59, 519-522.

Nontprasert, A., Pukrittayakamee, S., Nosten-Bertrand, M., Vanijanonta, S., White, N.J. (2000) Studies of neurotoxicity of oral artemisinin derivatives in mice. Am. J. Trop. Med. Hyg. 62, 409-412.

Nontprasert, A., Pukrittayakamee, S., Prakongpan, S., Supanaranond, W., Looareesuwan, S., White, N. (2002) Assessment of neurotoxicity of oral dihydroartemisinin in mice. Trans. R. Soc. Trop. Med. Hyg. 96, 99-101.

Panossian, L.A., Garga, N.I., Pelletierm D. (2005) Toxic brainstem encephalopathy after artemisinin treatment for breast cancer. Ann. Neurol. 58, 812-813.

Park, B.K., O'Neill, P.N., Maggs, J.L., Pirmohamed, M. (1998) Safety assessment of peroxide antimalarials: clinical and chemical perspectives. Br. J. Clin. Pharmacol. 46, 521-529.

Petras, J.M., Kyle, D.E., Ngampochjana, M., Young, G.D., Bauman, R.A., Webster, H.K., Corcoran, J.D., Peggins, J.O., Vane, M.A., Brewer, T.G. (1997) Arteether: Risks of two-week administration in macaca mulatta. Am. J. Trop. Med. Hyg. 57, 390-396.

Petras, J.M., Young, G.D., Bauman, R.A., Kyle, D.E., Gettayacamin, M., Webster, H.K., Corcoran, K.D., Peggins, J.O., Vane, M.A., Brewer, T.G. (2000) Arteether-induced brain injury in Macaca mulatta. I. The precerebellar nuclei: the lateral reticular nuclei, paramedian reticular nuclei, and perihypoglossal nuclei. Anat. Embryol. (Berl). 201, 383-397.

Price, R., van Vugt., M., Phaipun, L., Luxemburger, C., Simpson, J., McGready, R., ter Kuile, F., Kham, A., Chongsuphajaisiddhi, T., White, N.J., Nosten, F. (1999) Adverse effects in patients with acute falciparum malaria treated with artemisinin derivatives. Am. J. Trop. Med. Hyg. 60, 547-555.

Rangan, U., Hedli, C., Gallo, M., Lioy, P., Snyder, R. (1997) Exposure and risk assessment with respect to contaminated soil: Significance of biomarkers and bioavailability. Int. J. Toxicol. 16, 419-432.

Rowland, M., Tozer, T.N. (1995) Clinical Pharmacokinetics: Concepts and applications, Malcolm Rowland and Thomas N. Tozer (Ed.), Willianms & Wilkins, Baltimore, USA, pp. 83.

Rozman, K.K., Doull, J. (2000) Dose and time as variable of toxicity. Toxicology 144, 169-178.

Shargel, L., Yu, A.B.C. (1993) Applied Biopharmaceutics and Pharmacokinetics, Leon Shargel and Andrew B.C (Ed.), YU. Appleton & Lange, Norwalk, CN, pp. 353.

Si, Y., Li, Q., Xie, L., Bennett, K., Weina, P.J., Mog, S., Johnson, T.O. (2007) Neurotoxicity and toxicokinetics of artelinic acid following repeated oral administration in rats. Int. J. Toxicol. 26, 401-410.

Van Vugt, M., Angus, B.J., Price, R.N., Mann, C., Simpson, J.A., Poletto, C., Htoo, S.E., Looareesuwan, S., White, N.J., Nosten, F. (2000) A case-control auditory evaluation of patients treated with artemisinin derivatives for multidrug-resistant Plasmodium falciparum malaria. Am. J. Trop. Med. Hyg. 62, 65-69.

Wesche, D.L., DeCoster, M.A., Tortella, F.C., Brewer, T.G. (1994) Neurotoxicity of artemisinin analogs in vitro. Antimicrob Agents Chemother. 38, 1813-1819.

White, N.J., Ashley, E.A., Nosten, F. (2006) Toxic brainstem encephalopathy after artemisinin treatment for breast cancer. Ann. Neurol. 59, 725-726.

WHO. (2006) Assessment of the safety of artemisinin compounds in pregnancy. In The Special Pro–gramme for Research and Training Diseases (TDR) and The Global Malaria Programme of the World Health Organization; World Health Organization: Geneva, Switzerland.

Xie, L. H., Johnson, T. O., Weina, P. J., Si, Y. Z., Haeberte, A., Upadhyay, R., Wong, E., Li Q.G. (2005) Risk Assessment and Therapeutic Indices of Artesunate and Artelinate in Plasmodium berghei-infected Rats. Int. J. Toxicol. 24, 251-264.

Zhang, Z.Y., Yu, S.Q., Miao, L.Y., Huang, X.Y., Zhang, X.P., Zhu, Y.P., Xia, X.H., Li, D.Q. (2008)Artesunate combined with vinorelbine plus cisplatin in treatment of advanced non-small cell lung cancer: a randomized controlled trial. Zhong Xi Yi Jie He Xue Bao. 6, 134-138.

Zhao, K.C., Song, Z.Y. (1989) Distribution and excretion of artesunate in rats. Proc. Chin. Acad. Med. Sci. Peking Union Med. Coll. 4, 186-188.

17

Role of Aldehyde Oxidase and Xanthine Oxidase in the Metabolism of Purine-Related Drugs

Mohammad-Reza Rashidi and Roghiyeh Pashaei-Asl
Research Center for Pharmaceutical Nanotechnology, Tabriz University of Medical Sciences, Tabriz, Iran

1. Introduction

Purines are natural compounds that are found in all of the body's cells. They are the most widely distributed kind of N-heterocyclic substances in nature. Purines provide part of the chemical structure of some important co-enzymes and the genes of plants and animals. These compounds also participate in membrane signal transduction, translation and protein synthesis and in the form of purine nucleosides act as neurotransmitters in a variety of tissues. Purine base is also present in the structure of some important drugs such as 6-mercaptopurine (6-MP) and azathioprine (AZT). In addition, it can be found as a nucleobase in some synthetic nucleoside analogues with various pharmacological effects including antiviral and antitumor properties and numerous nucleoside analogues and their prodrugs were developed for cancer chemotherapy, treatment of patients with infections of human immunodeficiency virus (HIV) and infections caused by herpes and hepatitis viruses.

Different enzymes can participate in the metabolism of a drug and alter its function. Aldehyde oxidase (EC 1.2.3.1: aldehyde: oxygen oxidoreductase, AO), and xanthine oxidase (EC 1.17.3.2: xanthine: oxygen oxidoreductase, XO) which are collectively referred as "molybdenum hydroxylases", are two important cytosolic enzymes that are widely distributed throughout the animal kingdom. They are involved in the metabolism of an extensive range of exogenous and endogenous compounds with physiological, pharmacological and toxicological relevance (Beedham, 2010; Rashidi & Nazemiyeh, 2010). The reactions catalyzed by AO and XO usually involve a nucleophilic attack at an electron-deficient carbon atom adjacent to a ring nitrogen atom in N-heterocyclic compounds or found within an aldehyde group. Therefore, purines as N-heterocyclic compounds can act as a substrate for both AO and XO (Hall & Krenitsky, 1986; Krenitsky et al, 1972, 1986; Rashidi et al., 1997, 2007). In spite of having many physicochemical properties in common, AO and XO have different substrate specificities and product regiospecificities. In addition, pronounced species variation is present in the levels of molybdenum hydroxylases activity, in particular in that of AO (Alfaro et al., 2009; Jones et al., 1987; Krenitsky et al., 1984; Rashidi et al., 1997). Therefore, a metabolic pathway mediated by AO or XO could be completely different. This will be more pronounced for those compounds that have several sites for oxidation by these two oxidative enzymes. Purine nucleus has three sites that could be oxidized by molybdenum hydroxylases. It would be difficult, thus, to predict which metabolite will be produced from a purine-based drug by AO or XO, and the recognition of AO and XO contribution in the metabolism of this group of drugs will be a subject for scientific studies. This review highlights the involvement of AO and XO in the metabolism of important purine related drugs focusing on recent studies.

1.1 Biological and pharmacological importance of purines

Purines are an important group of nitrogen-containing compounds that are present in all forms of plant and animal life and play a vital role in biological processes. They serve as the source of cellular energy in ATP and together with pyrimidine, are the building blocks of DNA and RNA. Purines also participate in the structure of the co-enzymes (e.g. NAD^+, $NADP^+$ and FAD) and they are involved in membrane signal transduction, translation and protein synthesis (GTP, cAMP, cGMP, RNA). Over the last decades, a great deal of attention has been focused on the extracellular functions of purine nucleosides as neurotransmitters in a variety of tissues and different types of specific membrane purinergic receptors have been recognized (Di Iorio et al., 1998; Ralevic, 2009).

Purine nucleus is also present in the structure of some important drugs such as 6-thioguanine (6-TG), 6-MP and AZT. In addition, it can be found as a nucleobase in some synthetic nucleoside analogues which are structurally similar to natural nucleosides. Many nucleoside analogues have antiviral and antitumor properties. During the last decades, numerous nucleoside analogues and their prodrugs were developed for cancer chemotherapy, treatment of patients with infections of human immunodeficiency virus (HIV) and infections caused by herpes and hepatitis viruses (Li et al., 2008). In spite of having excellent pharmacological activity, they often suffer from a poor oral bioavailability due to low intestinal absorption. Therefore, intense research efforts have been focused on developing nucleoside analogues prodrugs, mainly in the acyclic form, to improve oral absorption (Li et al., 2008).

1.2 Chemistry of purine

In 1776, uric acid was isolated in a pure form from urinary calculi (stones), although the identification of its structure was not made until about 100 years later. It was this event that later was commemorated in the generic name, "purine" (from purum uricum) for the heterocyclic system (Hitchings, 1978). Xanthine and hypoxanthine were recognized as other members of the system in 1838 and 1850 respectively (Hitchings, 1978). In 1889, the term "nucleic acid" was introduced by Altmann and general methods for isolation of nucleic acids from various sources were developed by this investigator (Hurst, 1980). Then, purines and pyrimidines were discovered in nucleic acids and isolated from calf thymus nucleic acid in 1894 (Hurst, 1980).

The purine nucleus consists of fused pyrimidine and imidazole rings having the numbering system shown in Fig. 1 it is an aromatic compound with -deficient ring system; therefore, all its carbon atoms are susceptible towards nucleophilic attack and are deactivated towards electrophilic attack. Because of the electron-attracting character of the C=N moiety, the 2-, 6- and 8-sites favor nucleophilic attack, although the 8-position would be expected to be less electron deficient than the two other sites due to the electron-releasing character of the -NH- moiety present in imidazole ring. The calculated electron densities of the various sites in purine are given in Figure 1. Purine is a weak base with an overall pKa = 2.3 (Joule, 1995). According to ^{13}C NMR studies all three protonated forms are present in solution but it is suggested that the predominant cation is formed by N^1 protonation (Joule, 1995). Purine is also a weak acid with a pKa of 8.9 (Joule, 1995).

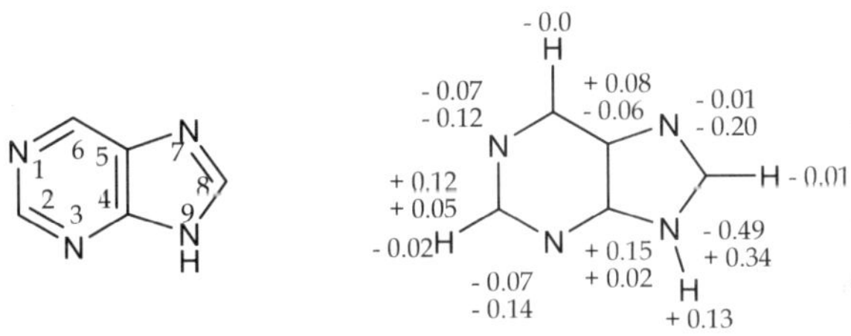

Fig. 1. The numbering system and electron densities of purine. Upper and lower numbers in (b) are - and -charges respectively (Shaw, 1984)

1.3 Purines as substrates for aldehyde oxidase and xanthine oxidase

Different enzymes can participate in the metabolism of a drug either through conversion of a prodrug to an active form or elimination of a drug via its metabolic pathway. AO and XO as two drug metabolizing enzymes can utilize purines as their substrates (Hall & Krenitsky, 1986; Krenitsky et al, 1972, 1986; Rashidi et al., 1997, 2007). They have many properties in common; both enzymes are large homodimeric proteins with a molecular mass of ~ 300,000 Da, composed of two identical subunits. Each subunit contains one atom of molybdenum, one molecule of enzyme-bound flavin adenine dinucleotide (FAD) and two iron–sulfur (2Fe–2S) centers. In spite of these similarities and the existence of an overlap in substrate utilization between AO and XO, they have different substrate specificities and product regiospecificities. As it was mentioned before, molybdenum hydroxylases can catalyze the oxidation of a wide range of aldehydes and N-heterocyclic compounds (Beedham, 2010; Rashidi & Nazemiyeh, 2010). Purines are among those N-heterocyclic compounds that may be oxidized by AO and XO either as a prodrug converted to its active form (Krenitsky et al., 1984; Rashidi et al., 1997) or during their catabolic pathways (Rashidi et al., 2007). However, the manner of oxidation by these two enzymes could be different from one compound to another.

1.4 Metabolism of endogenous purines

Purine metabolism in man may be divided into four interfacing compartments which are illustrated in Fig. 2 (Palella & Fox, 1991).

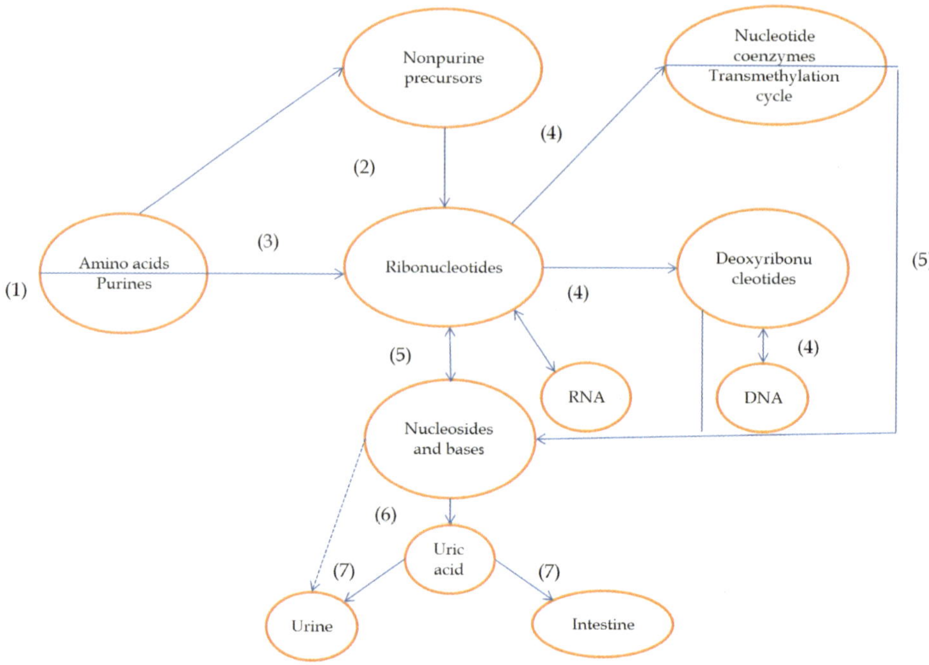

Fig. 2. Overview of purine metabolism in man (Palella & Fox, 1991)

a. De novo purine synthesis: The biosynthetic pathway through which non-purine precursors are combined to form the purine ring is referred to as de novo purine synthesis. These non-purine precursors are provided through dietary intake of amino acids (1). The first reaction in this synthetic process is the formation of 5phosphoribosyl--1-pyrophosphate which is finally converted to inosine-5′-monophosphate (IMP) in a ten step pathway (2).
b. Nucleotide interconversion: Once IMP is formed it may be metabolized to other purine ribonucleotides such as AMP and GMP by interconversion pathways (3).
c. Salvage of performed purine bases: These ribonucleotides may be converted to diphosphate and triphosphate forms which serve as essential substrates for variety of pathways (4), or to be broken down to purine bases or nucleosides (5).
d. Degradation: As a final step in human purine metabolism, nucleosides and purine bases are metabolised to uric acid (6) which is excreted primarily in urine with small amounts excreted into intestine thereby bacterial uricolysis occurs (7). The conversion of hypoxanthine to xanthine and xanthine to uric acid is catalyzed by XO.

2. Purine-related drugs and their metabolism by molybdenum hydroxylases

2.1 Thiopurines: 6-mercaptopurine, azathioprine and 6-thioguanine

Thipurines, 6-MP, AZT and 6-TG, are the analogues of purine nucleosides that serve as the backbone of current childhood acute leukemia treatment. They have also been effective immunosuppressive agents for the past half a century and remain the immunosuppressive of choice for Crohn's disease (Ansari et al., 2008; Fotoohi et al., 2010). In the early 1940s, the first studies on purine analogues as antimetabolites were begun by Hitchings and his group in which 8-azaguanine and 2,6-diaminopurine were found to possess marked anticancer activity in experimental tumors (Elion et al., 1951). Subsequently, 6-MP was synthesized by Elion and Hutchins in 1951 and found to have a high order of activity against human leukemia (Elion et al., 1952); it was successfully employed in the treatment of leukemia in man in 1953. This discovery was an important point in the development of antineoplastic and immunosuppressive agents. In 1958, the immunosuppressive activity of 6-MP in rabbits was demonstrated by Schwartz et al. (1958). Shortly, 6- (1-methyl-4-nitro-5-imidazolyl) thiopurine, AZT, was synthesized by the Hitchings–Elion laboratory and shown that this analogue of 6-MP acts as a pro-drug and is reduced non-enzymatically in body to 6-MP which is converted by sensitive neoplasms to the active form 6-thioinosinate by hypoxanthine-guanine phosphoribosyl-transferase (Van Scoik et al., 1985). AZT has a higher therapeutic index than 6-MP (Van Scoik et al., 1985). AZT has more potent immunosuppressive effect than 6-MP and is preferred drug to prevent or delay graft rejection and treat rheumatoid arthritis (Chabner et al., 2001). 6-MP together with methotrexate are the drugs of choice in the treatment of childhood acute lymphocytic leukemia, especially in those cases where prolonged duration of remission is required (Knoester et al., 1993; Van Scoik et al., 1985); however, this thiopurine is not effective for the treatment of chronic lymphocytic leukemia, Hodgkings disease or other lymphomas/carcinomas (Rider, 2008).

Although thiopurines have been used for over 50 years, many aspects of their complex pharmacology and metabolism remain unclear. However, it has been suggested that (Zimm et al., 1984; Chabner et al., 2001) in the cell, 6-MP is converted first to thioinosinic acid, by hypoxanthine-guanine phosphoribosyl-transferase which is then metabolized to thioguanine ribonucleotide and deoxyribonucleotide; incorporation of these compounds into RNA and DNA results in the antitumour effect of the drug. In addition, thioinosinic acid can be methylated to 6-methylthioinosinate which like thioinosinic acid is able to inhibit glutamine-5-phosphoribosylpyrophosphate amidotransferase, the first enzyme unique to the de novo pathway for purine ribonucleotide synthesis.

The oral bioavailibility of 6-MP in man is low and highly variable (Knoester et al., 1993; Meerten et al., 1995), however, this is the usual rout of administration. The mechanism for this variability is not fully known but it may be due to a combination of differences in the rate of absorption, distribution, elimination and first-pass metabolism of drug (Knoester et al., 1993). After intravenous injection, 6-MP undergoes rapid cellular uptake, hepatic metabolism, and renal excretion. Approximately 50% of an administered dose of the drug is excreted in the urine within 24 hours, with 22% eliminated as unchanged drug (Rider, 2008).

6-MP, after administration, may enter into either anabolic or catabolic metabolic pathways (Lennard et al., 1991; Van Scoik et al., 1985). The anabolic pathway is responsible for conversion of 6-MP to its active form, whereas the drug is degraded to inactive forms in the catabolic pathway via two major inactivation routes (Fig. 3). One is thiol methylation, which is catalyzed by the enzyme thiopurine S-methyltransferase, to form the inactive metabolite methyl-6-mercaptopurine. The second route is thought to involve the initial oxidation of 6-MP to 8-oxo-6-MP followed by conversion to 6-thiouric acid (Elion, 1967; Van Scoik et al.,

1985). However, Zimm et al., (1984) have identified 6-thioxanthine in the urine samples of some patients who received 6-MP by intravenous infusion which may indicate that 6-MP is converted to 6-thiouric acid via 6-thioxanthine. The oxidative inactivation of 6-MP has been attributed to XO activity in intestinal mucosa and liver. The Km value for the oxidation of 6-MP by calf liver and bovine milk xanthine oxidase (BMXO) is 20-30 μM (Chalmers et al., 1969; Krenitsky et al., 1972). 6-MP is also a substrate for rabbit liver AO with a reported Km of 1.6 mM (Hall & Krenitsky, 1986). The second catabolic pathway for 6-MP is methylation of the sulphur atom catalyzed by thiopurine methyltransferase. 6-Methylmercaptopurine then undergoes oxidation at position 8 catalyzed by XO and/or AO (Van Scoik et al., 1985); the difference in metabolite profile between oral and intravenous administration may be indicative of the significant role of AO in 8-hydroxylation (Beedham, 2002). These metabolic pathways are illustrated in Fig. 3.

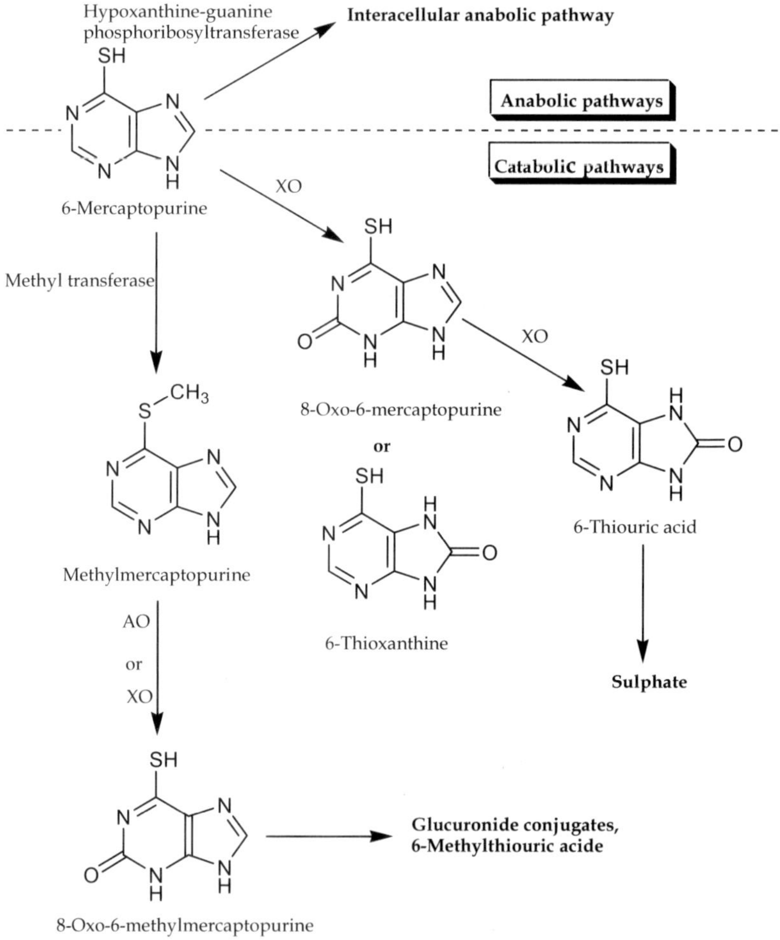

Fig. 3. Proposed metabolic pathways for 6-mercaptopurine (6-MP) (Van Scoik et al., 1985; Zimm et al., 1984). AO: aldehyde oxidase, XO: xanthine oxidase

Although 6-thiouric acid has been detected as the major metabolite of 6-MP after oral administration of drug (Elion, 1967; Van Scoik et al., 1985; Zimm et al., 1984), there is no direct evidence in the involvement of molybdenum hydroxylases in these oxidative reactions and the results obtained from in vitro studies are controversial. 8-Oxo-6-MP (Elion, 1967; VanScoik et al., 1985), 6-methylmercapto-8-hydoxypurine (Keuzenkamp-Jansen et al., 1996) and 6-thioxanthine (Zimm et al., 1984), all have been suggested to be the intermediate in the conversion of 6-MP to 6-thiouric acid. Recently, Rashidi et al. (2007) have demonstrated that 6- MP is more likely oxidized to 6-thiouric acid via 6-thioxanthine rather than 8-oxo-6-MP. The first step which is the rate limiting step is catalyzed solely by XO, whereas both XO and AO are involved in the oxidation of 6-thiouric acid to 6-thiouric acid (Fig. 4).

$$\text{6-Mercaptopurine} \xrightarrow{\text{XO}} \text{6-Thioxanthine} \xrightarrow[\text{Very fast}]{\text{XO \& AO}} \text{6-Thiouric acid}$$

Fig. 4. Proposed metabolic pathway for the oxidation of 6-mercaptopurine by partially purified guinea pig liver fractions (Rashidi et al., 2007). AO: aldehyde oxidase, XO: xanthine oxidase

The metabolism of 6-TG is very similar to that of 6-MP, however, there is a clinically important difference between catabolic pathway of these two thiopurines (Fig. 5). Unlike 6-MP which is first metabolized to 6-thioxanthine by XO and then 6-thiouric acid by both XO and AO (Rashidi et al., 2007), 6-TG must first be metabolized by guanine deaminase (guanase) to 6-thioxanthine, which is then metabolized to 6- thiouric acid (Evans & Relling, 1994; Hogarth et al., 2008). As guanase is not as abundant as XO, more of 6-TG is directly activated to thioguanine nucleotides without oxidation to the inactive metabolite, 6-thiouric acid (Hogarth et al., 2008). This could be a reason for some clinical findings (Lennard et al., 1993) indicating that in children with acute lymphoblastic leukemia, significantly higher concentrations of thioguanine nucleotides are achieved with oral 6-TG therapy compared with oral 6-MP therapy (Evans & Relling, 1994).

In addition, taking into account the important role of XO in the catabolic pathway of 6-MP, co-administration of 6-MP and XO inhibitors such as allopurinol can lead to severe forms of mercaptopurine toxicity and dosage modification of the drug is necessary, whereas in the case of 6-TG dosage modification is not warranted, because the first step of drug inactivation is not catalyzed by XO (Hande & Garrow, 1996).

AO is also involved in the metabolism of 6-TG (Fig. 5). According to Kitchen et al. (1999), 6-TG can be oxidized to 8-hydroxythioguanine by AO. 8-Hydroxythioguanine has been found to be the predominant circulating metabolite in patients receiving continuous i.v. infusion of thioguanine and is likely generated by the action of AO (Kitchen et al., 1999).

AZT can also undergo two different metabolic routes. In the first route, AZT is extensively converted to 6-MP which is then metabolized as in Fig. 6. In the second route, AZT may be directly oxidized to 8-oxo-azathioprine, catalyzed by AO. Cleavage of 8-oxo-azathioprine by glutathione or other nucleophilic compounds gives 8-oxo-6-mercaptopurine which may then be oxidized to 6-thiouric acid by XO (Fig. 6).

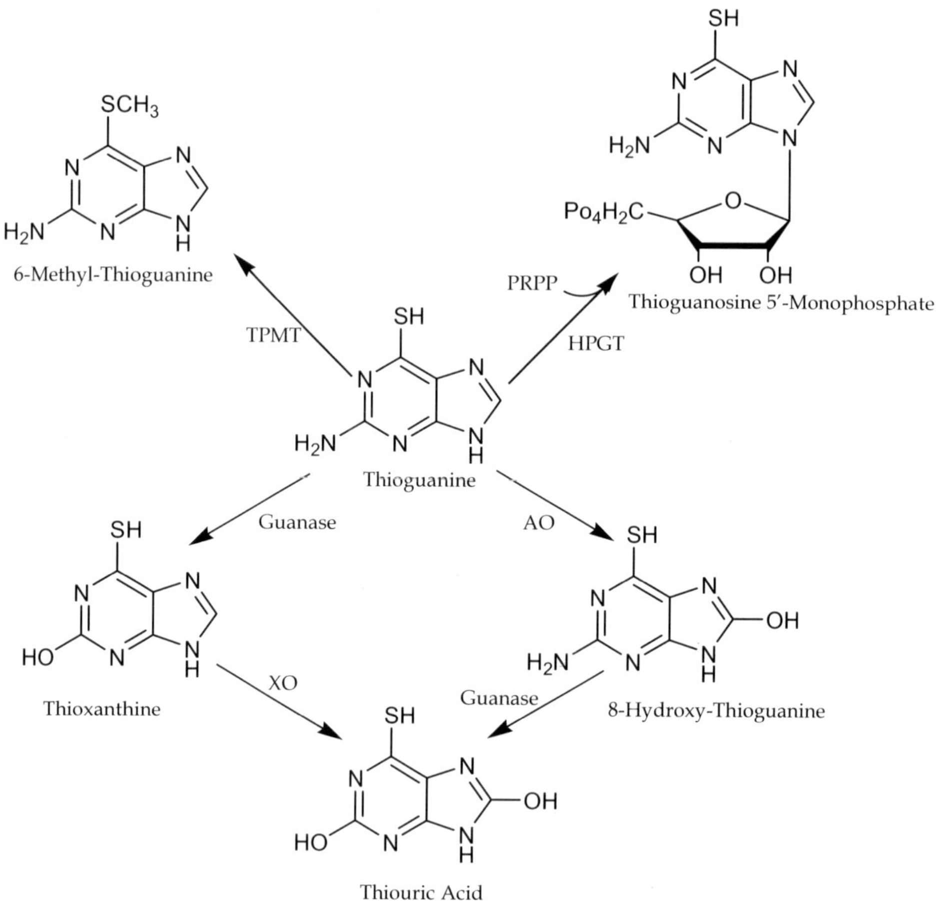

Fig. 5. Metabolic pathways of 6-TG. PRPP: phosphoribosyl pyrophosphate, HPGT: hypoxanthine-guanine phosphoribosyl transferase, TPMT: thioguanosine monophosphate, AO: aldehyde oxidase, XO: xanthine oxidase (from: Kitchen et al., 1999)

The Km value for the oxidation of azathioprine by rabbit liver AO is 80 μM (Chalmers et al., 1969), whereas azathioprine is very poor substrate for XO such that kinetic constants have been measured competitively against the oxidation of 6-methylaminopurine catalyzed by human liver XO (K_i = 340 μM) (Krenitsky et al., 1986). Therefore, it is likely that AZT is oxidized by AO in vivo if the drug comes in contact with the enzyme (Chalmers et al., 1969). It is estimated that the effects of XO and AO activity leaves only about 16% of the total dose of 6-MP available for systemic distribution (Fotoohi et al., 2010).

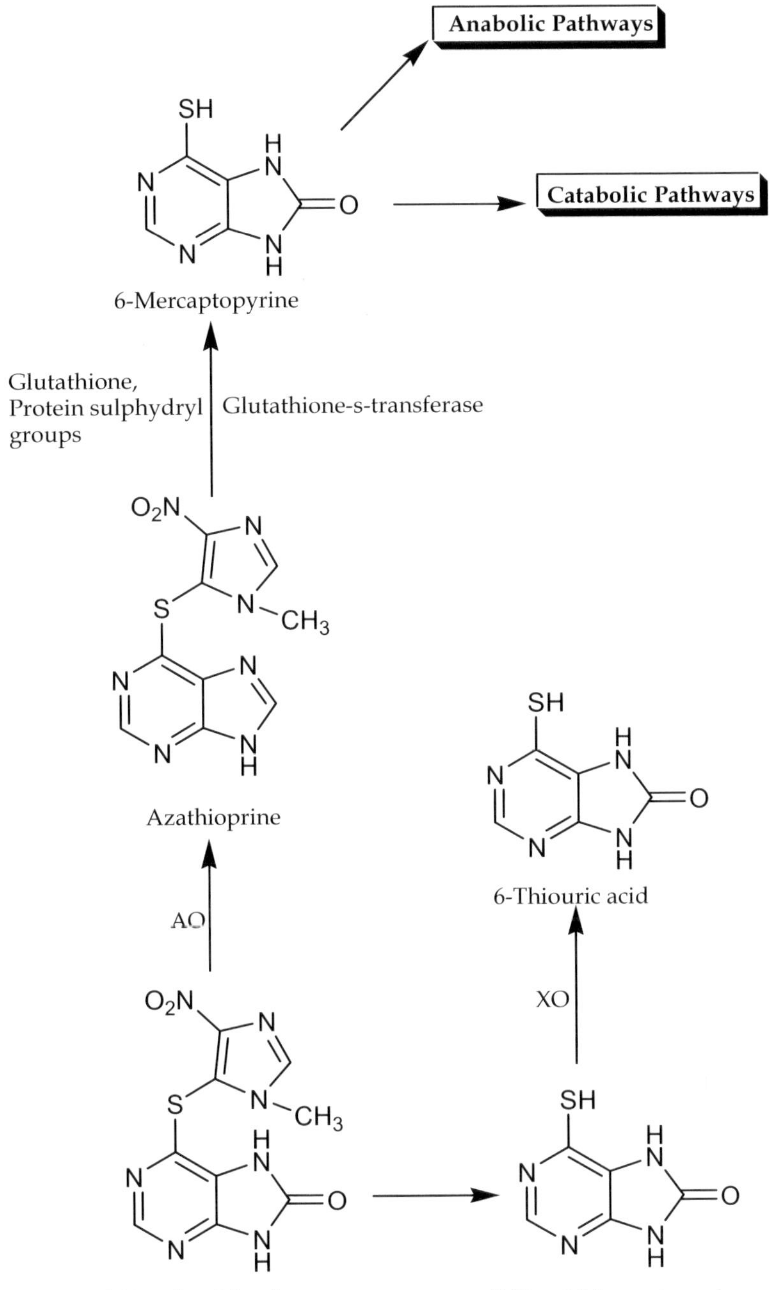

Fig. 6. The metabolic pathways for azathioprine (Van Scoik et al., 1985). AO: aldehyde oxidase, XO: xanthine oxidase

2.2 Famciclovir

Famciclovir 2-[2-(2-Amino-9H-purin-9-yl) ethyl]-1,3-propanediol diacetate (ester) is a synthetic guanine derivative which is metabolized to the potent antiviral compound penciclovir. Penciclovir is active against herpes simplex virus (HSV) types 1 and 2, varicella zoster virus (VZV), Epstein-Barr virus (EBV), and hepatitis B (Perry & Wagstaff, 1995).

The mechanism of action of penciclovir is similar to that of aciclovir. Both drugs are selectively phosphorylated in virus-infected cells to a monophosphate ester by thymidine kinase, followed by further phosphorylation to a triphosphate ester which inhibits virus DNA polymerases (Vere Hodge & Cheng, 1993). However, the concentration of triphosphate ester of penciclovir within infected cells is higher than that of aciclovir and it has a more prolonged intracellular half-life in cells infected with HSV (10-20 hours) and VZV (7-14 hours) compared to aciclovir triphosphate (1 hour) (Perry & Wagstaff, 1995; Vere Hodge & Cheng, 1993). Like aciclovir, penciclovir has very low oral bioavailibility, but its prodrug, famciclovir, is absorbed rapidly and extensively after oral administration, and little or no parent compound can be detected in plasma or urine (Mondal, 2008). The absolute bioavailability of penciclovir is about 77% (Pue & Benet, 1993), which is about four times higher than that of aciclovir (Murray, 1995).

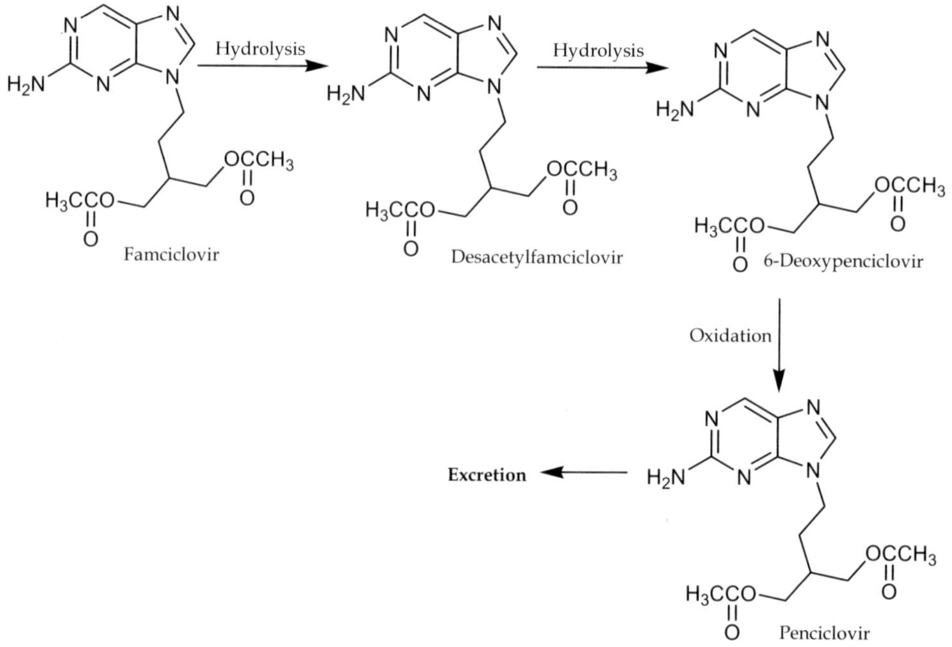

Fig. 7. The major metabolic pathway of famciclovir in man (Vere Hodge et al., 1989)

Metabolism of famciclovir involves sequential hydrolysis of both acetyl groups to give 6-deoxypenciclovir which can be oxidized to penciclovir (Fig. 7); however, both in vivo and in vitro studies have also shown that penciclovir is the major metabolite of famciclovir metabolism (Pue & Benet, 1993; Pue et al., 1994; Rashidi et al., 1997). Although the oxidative step was initially attributed to XO, on the basis of studies performed with 6-deoxyaciclovir and a structural similarity between 6-deoxypenciclovir and guanine which is a substrate of XO (Harrell et al., 1993; Krenitsky et al., 1984; Vere Hodge et al., 1989), later studies demonstrated that AO is the major enzyme in oxidative conversion of famciclovir to penciclovir (Clarke et al., 1995; Rashidi et al., 1997).

According to Rashidi et al. (1997), both famciclovir and 6-deoxypenciclovir are predominantly oxidized at carbon 6 by human, guinea pig and rat hepatic AO, whereas the major metabolites with rabbit enzyme are 8-oxo- and 6-oxo-derivatives with the former metabolite having higher contribution. 6-Deoxypenciclovir is oxidized only at the 6-position by rat liver and BMXO. Famciclovir is a better substrate than 6-deoxypenciclovir for hepatic AO from all species tested (Table 1). The oxidation rate of both compounds is comparable with probe substrates of AO such as phenanthridine and phthalazine (Rashidi et al., 1997).

Enzyme fraction	6-Deoxypenciclovir			Famciclovir		
	K_m (mM)	V_{max} (nmol/mg/min)	V_{max}/K_m (ml/min/mg)	K_m (mM)	V_{max} (nmol/mg/min)	V_{max}/K_m (ml/min/mg)
Human Liver AO (N = 1-2)	0.42	16	0.038	0.15	61	0.407
Guinea pig liver AO (N = 3-5)	0.41± 0.01[a]	209±38	0.510	0.17±0.01	439±48	2.582
Rabbit liver AO (N = 2)	0.44	114	0.259		ND[b]	
AO-Active rat enzyme (N = 3)[a]	0.37±0.05	26±6	0.070	0.08±0.02	41±10	0.506
AO-Deficient rat enzyme (N = 3)[a]	0.26±0.01	4±2	0.015		NR[c]	
BMXO (N = 2)	0.90	155	0.172		NR	

[a] Mean±SD
[b] ND: Not determined
[c] NR: No reaction

Table 1. Kinetic parameters for 6-oxo-metabolite formation by partially purified guinea pig, human, rabbit, rat liver aldehyde oxidase (AO) and bovine milk xanthine oxidase (BMXO) determined by HPLC (Rashidi et al 1997)

Although 6-deoxypenciclovir is oxidized very slowly by rat liver XO and BMXO, famciclovir did not serve as a substrate for either enzyme. In Figures 8-10, the metabolic pathways of famciclovir with different enzyme fractions have been illustrated.

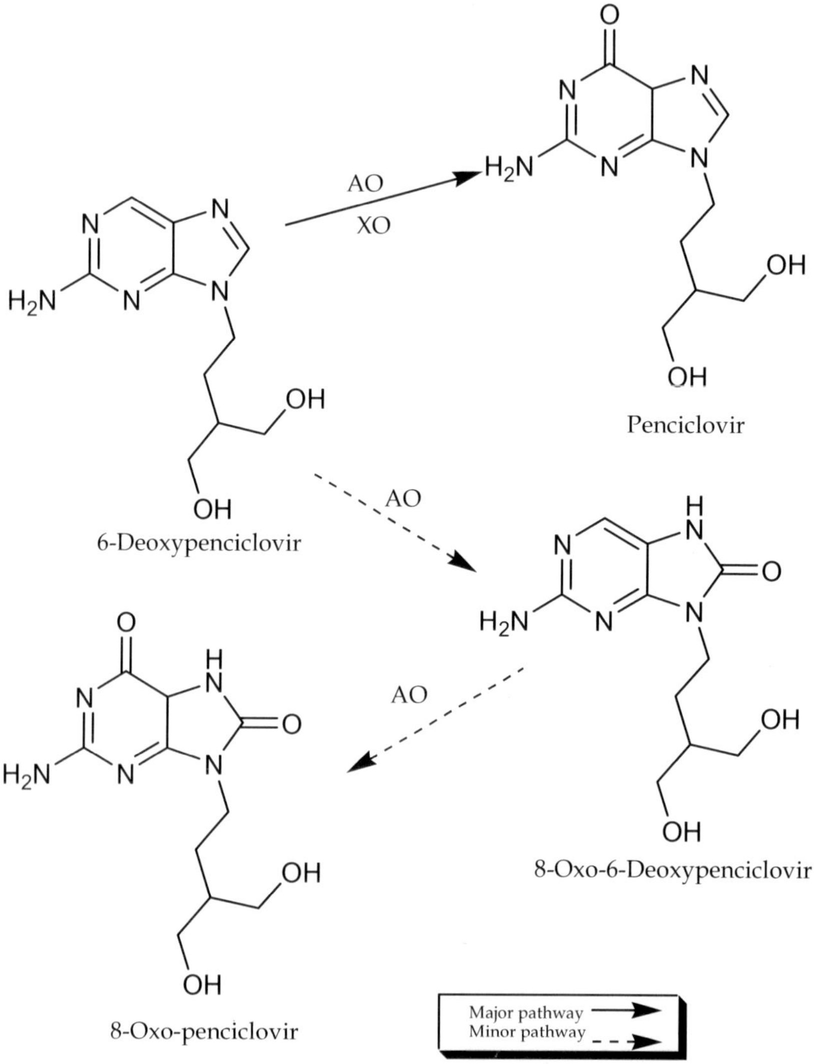

Fig. 8. The oxidative metabolic pathways of 6-deoxypenciclovir catalyzed by partially purified guinea pig, aldehyde oxidase-active rat and human liver fractions (Rashidi, 1996; Rashidi et al., 1997). AO: aldehyde oxidase, XO: xanthine oxidase

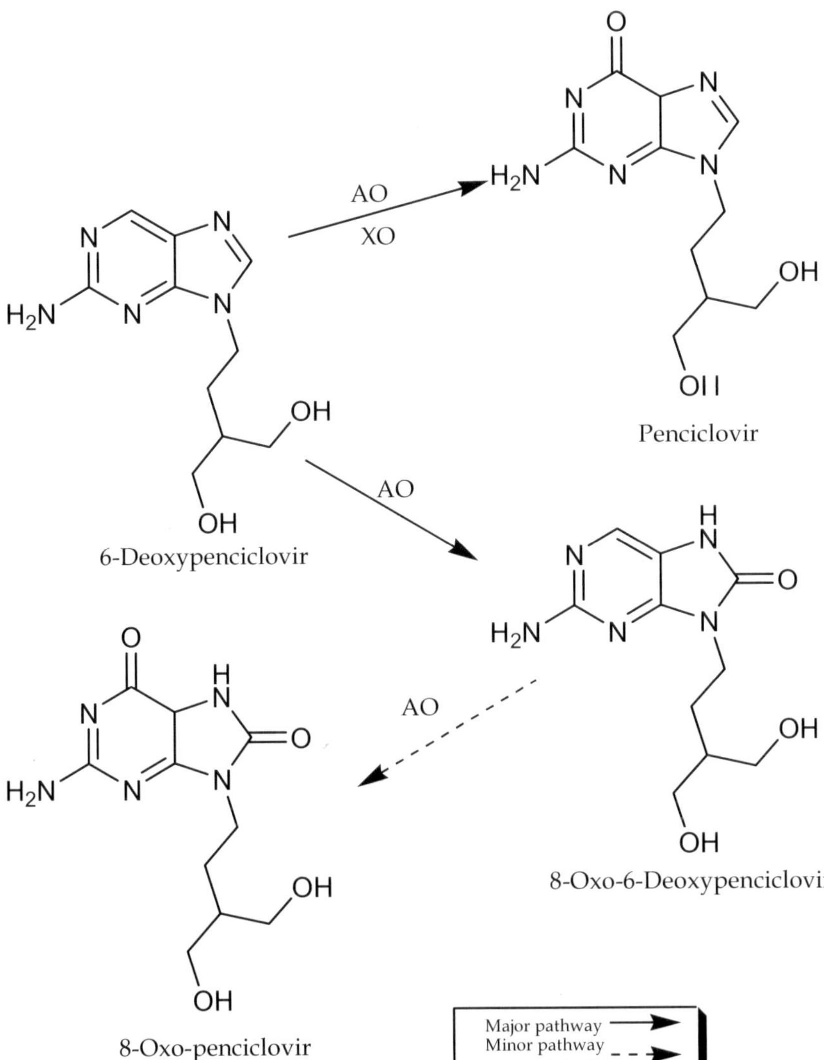

Fig. 9. The oxidative metabolic pathways of 6-deoxypenciclovir catalyzed by partially purified rabbit liver fractions (Rashidi, 1996; Rashidi et al., 1997). AO: aldehyde oxidase, XO: xanthine oxidase

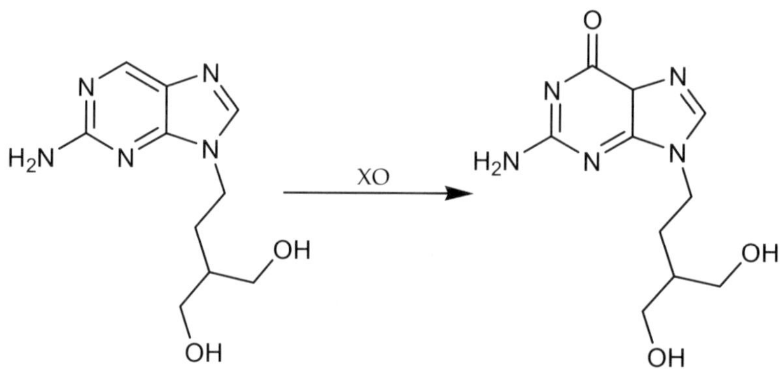

6-Deoxypenciclovir Penciclovir

Fig. 10. The oxidative metabolic pathways of 6-deoxypenciclovir catalyzed by partially purified aldehyde oxidase-deficient rat liver fractions (Rashidi, 1996). XO: xanthine oxidase

2.3 Ganciclovir

Ganciclovir is an acyclic nucleoside analog of 2′-deoxyguanosine from which the 2′ carbon has been deleted. It is used for the treatment of cytomegalovirus (CMV) infections, most commonly retinitis, colitis, and esophagitis, in immunocompromised patients and is administered to transplant patients at risk for CMV retinitis (Mondal, 2008; Physician's Desk Reference, 2000).

Ganciclovir is much more effective than aciclovir against CMV and HSV (De Clercq & Field, 2006; Noble & Faulds, 1998), although it has greater potential toxicity (Crumpacker, 1996). It is more easily phosphorylated in CMV infected cells than aciclovir and its triphosphate has a 5-fold higher affinity for CMV DNA polymerase than aciclovir triphosphate (Krogsgaard-Larsen, 1992). Ganciclovir is also active against VZV and EBV; however, it causes neutropenia and its clinical use is restricted to the treatment of CMV infections in immunocompromised patients (Krogsgaard-Larsen, 1992).

Like aciclovir, the absorption of ganciclovir following oral administration is low. Its absolute bioavailability after oral administration of 1000 mg of ganciclovir capsules three times a day was approximately 8.5% (Anderson et al., 1995). To overcome this problem, in accordance with the prodrug approaches, various analogues of ganciclovir were synthesized. One of the strategies used was the synthesis of C-6 deoxy 2-aminopurine prodrugs of ganciclovir. Significant success with this strategy had been achieved previously by aciclovir. The dipivalate ester of 6-deoxyganciclovir was one of the prodrugs of ganciclovir that was produced using this strategy (Krasny et al., 1995). The dipivalate ester was introduced to increase lipophilicity of the molecule. Because of chemical similarity of aciclovir and ganciclovir, it was also expected that the 6-deoxy prodrug would be converted to gannciclovir. According to preclinical studies in rats, a 7-fold enhancement in oral bioavailability of the compound was observed and the prodrug was rapidly converted to ganciclovir and 6-deoxy ganciclovir in vivo; however, the 6-deoxy ganciclovir was not oxidized to ganciclovir by XO. Rat liver sometimes has insufficient XO activity and the results obtained from this animal model cannot be extrapolated to human, in particular with nucleobase antiviral agents (Rashidi et al., 1997). Therefore, the involvement of AO or XO in conversion of 6-deoxyganciclovir produced from its dipivalate ester analogue to ganciclovir cannot be ruled out and further studies may be required.

The other example of the use of prodrug approach to increase the oral bioavailability of ganciclovir is HOE 602, the bis-isopropyl ether of 6-deoxy ganciclovir. HOE 602 is a nucleobase analog of ganciclovir with high therapeutic efficacy against HSV and MCMV infections in mice (Winkler et al., 1990). Pharmacokinetic studies in mice and rhesus monkeys indicated that this prodrug is converted to ganciclovir via a three-step pathway (Fig. 11) and yields a 4 to 21-fold increase in exposure after oral administration in monkeys compared to an equivalent oral dose of ganciclovir (Winkler et al., 1990). The first step, oxidation of the 6-aminopurine moiety to guanine, is mediated by XO (Winkler et al., 1990). However, no further studies of HOE 602 have been published (Li et al., 2008).

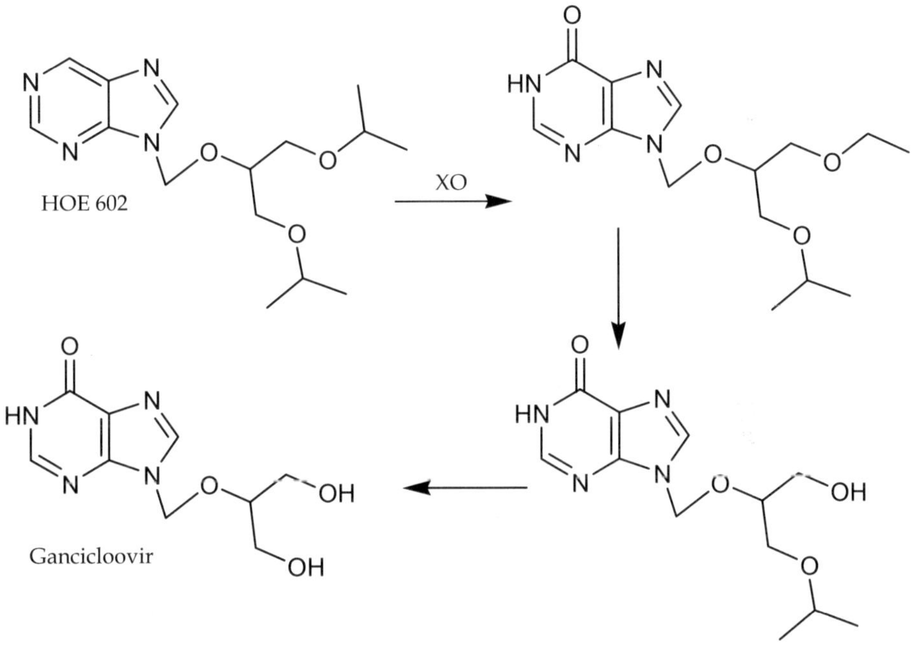

Fig. 11. Conversion of HOE 602 prodrug to ganciclovir (Winkler et al., 1990). XO: xanthine oxidase

Valganciclovir, a valine ester of ganciclovir, is another example of prodrug approach to overcome the poor oral absorption of ganciclovir (Maag, 2002). Following oral administration of valganciclovir in human, the absolute bioavailability of ganciclovir could be 10-fold higher than that from oral ganciclovir (Jung & Dorr, 1999; Pescovitz et al., 2000). According to these studies, no significant amount of the prodrug was detected in plasma which may be indicative of rapid and complete hydrolysis of valganciclovir to ganciclovir in vivo (Li et al., 2008).

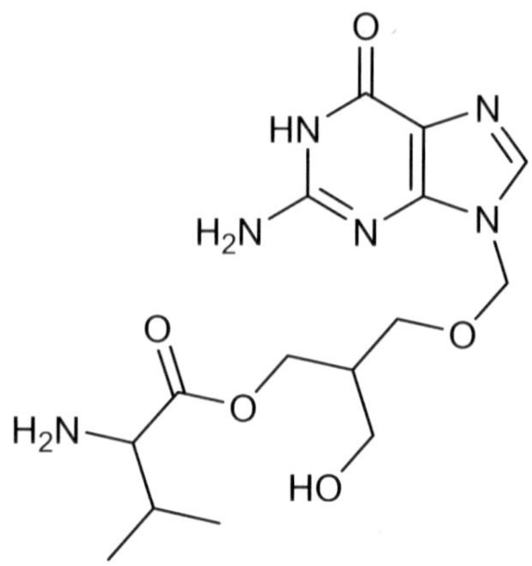

Valganciclovir

Conversion of valganciclovir to ganciclovir is a hydrolytic reaction and therefore is not dependent to molybdenum hydroxylases. However, C-8 carbon in both valganciclovir and ganciclovir, like other purine-based antiviral agents such as 6-deoxypenciclovir and aciclovir, is susceptible for oxidation by these oxidative enzymes which is subject for further studies. Interestingly, according to Krasny et al. (1995), after oral administration of dipivalate ester of 6-deoxyganciclovir to cynomolgus monkey, but not rat, the 8-hydroxy analogs of ganciclovir and 6-doxyganciclovir are also detected alongside of other metabolites.

2.4 Aciclovir and valaciclovir

Acyclovir, 9-[(2-hydroxy ethoxy) methyl] guanine is a guanosine analogue antiviral agent that has a high therapeutic index. It was the first specific antiviral drug described in the early 1980s (Dollery, 1999) and then the spectrum compound of the first aciclovir were boarded to vital therapies for DNA virus and retrovirus infections (Field & De Clercq 2004; De Clercq & Holy, 2005). Aciclovir is initially phosphorylated to a monophosphate derivative by a virus-specific thymidine kinase, and not by the thymidine kinase of uninfected cells (Rajalakshmi et al., 2010) and then to a triphosphate which inhibits competitively DNA synthesis in the infected cells. Phosphorylation does not occur in healthy cells which accounts for its strong selectivity of action (Clercq & Holy, 2005). Consequently, the amount of aciclovir triphosphate formed in the virally infected cells is 40-100 times greater than that in normal uninfected cells (Rajalakshmi et al., 2010). Aciclovir is a potent and selective inhibitor of herpes virus DNA replication. It acts as a substrate for the enzyme viral DNA polymerase in competition with normal deoxy adenosine triphosphate and results in complete and irreversible inhibition of herpes virus DNA polymerase and viral DNA chain termination (Rajalakshmi et al., 2010).

Clinically, aciclovir has been found effective against all types of HSV and VZV but not against other species of viruses (Hirsch & Schooley, 1983). In spite of its effective antiviral activity, aciclovir has some important limitations. Firstly, it is significantly less effective against VZV than against HSV (Safrin & Phan, 1993) (Easterbrook & Wood, 1994). Furthermore, some cases of HSV and VZV isolates resistant to aciclovir have been reported(Safrin & Phan, 1993) (Easterbrook & Wood, 1994). In addition, aciclovir has relatively low (15-20%) and unpredictable oral bioavilability (Easterbrook & Wood, 1994) (de Miranda & Blum, 1983) resulting in the need for frequent high doses or intravenous therapy in conditions where high plasma aciclovir levels are necessary to inhibit less sensitive viruses as in like VZV (de Miranda & Burnette, 1994; Safrin & Phan, 1993).

Consequently, many attempts have been made to improve aciclovir efficiency when given orally in humans or to find new successors to aciclovir. Development of a prodrug of aciclovir with a better absorption from the gastrointestinal tract and then conversion in vivo to aciclovir has been one of the most common strategies used to achieve this goal (Burnette, T.C. & de Miranda 1994; Hay CM, Reichman 2008; Krenitsky et al., 1984).

One such prodrug is 6-deoxyaciclovir or desciclovir, 2-amino-9-[2-hydroxyethoxy) methyl]-9H-purine. 6-Deoxyciclovir is an analog of aciclovir which is 18 times more water soluble than aciclovir (Krenitsky et al., 1984) The prodrug is extensively absorbed following oral administration to healthy volunteers and converted to aciclovir *in vivo* by the XO; however, XO cannot further oxidize aciclovir (Fig. 12) (Krenitsky et al., 1984). On the other hand, aciclovir is hydroxylated at C-8 by AO, but this enzymatic reaction is a minor metabolic pathway in patients (Beedham, 1997).

Although 6-deoxyaciclovir has been reported as XO-activated prodrugs (Krenitsky et al., 1984; Jones et al., 1987), the compound is a better substrate for AO than XO (Table 2). Like 6-deoxypenciclovir, 6-deoxyaciclovir is oxidized to 8-oxo-metabolite as the major metabolite by rabbit liver AO (Fig. 13) and its Vmax/Km value is 57-fold higher than that of BMXO (Krenitsky et al., 1984). It has been reported that allopurinol was less effective in inhibition of 6-deoxyaciclovir oxidation to aciclovir in isolated perfused Sprague-Dawley rat livers (Jones et al., 1987) whose liver AO is very variable. The ratio of 8-oxo-metabolite to 6-oxo-metabolite (aciclovir) from the oxidation of 6-deoxyaciclovir by rabbit liver AO is 95 to 5 (Krenitsky et al., 1984). Although the bioavailability of 6-deoxyaciclovir was improved, further development of the prodrug was terminated due to the chronic toxicity problems highlighted in animal studies (de Miranda P & Burnette, 1994).

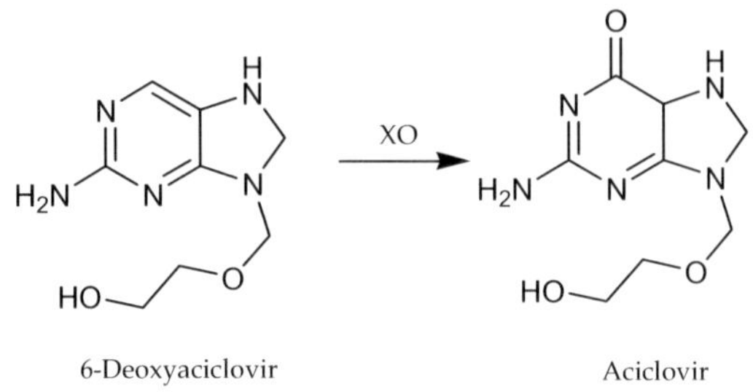

Fig. 12. 6-Deoxyaciclovir as a prodrug of aciclovir is activated by xanthine oxidase (XO) (Krenitsky et al., 1984)

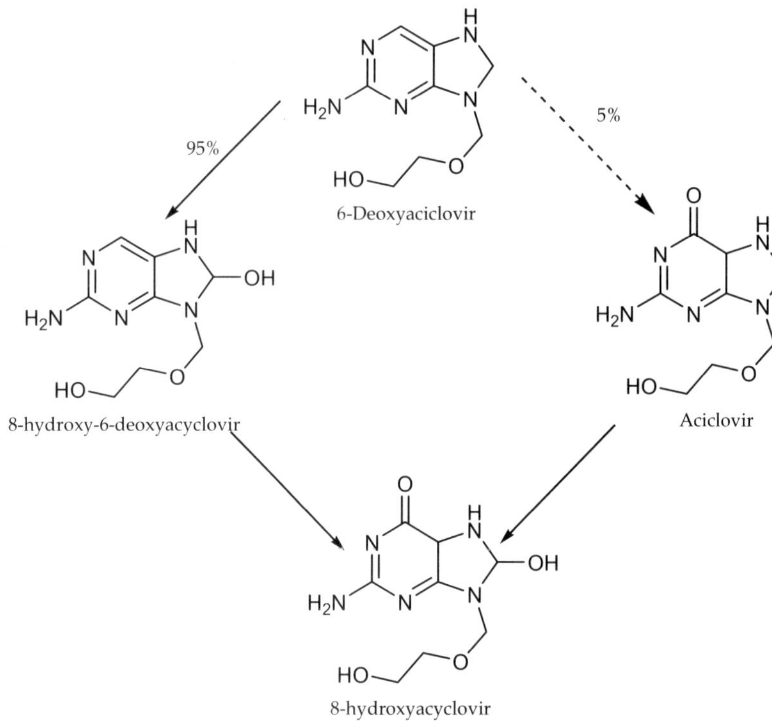

Fig. 13. Metabolism and inactivation of 6-deoxyaciclovir by rabbit liver aldehyde oxidase (Krenitsky et al., 1984)

AO converts 6- Deoxyaciclovir to 8-hydroxy-6-deoxyaciclovir and aciclovir with the ratio of 95 to 5 respectively, and both of them are turned more oxidase to 8-hydroxyaiclovir (Krenitsky et al., 1984).

Valaciclovir, 2-[2-amino-1, 6-dihydro-6-oxo-9H-purin-9-yl-methoxy] ethyl valinate hydrochloride, is another oral prodrug of aciclovir with an oral bioavailibility of higher than that of acyclovir (Burnette, T.C. & de Miranda 1994; Hay CM & Reichman, 2008). Valaciclovir is well absorbed following oral administration and is rapidly converted to aciclovir by hydrolysis of the valyl ester during first pass intestinal and/or hepatic metabolism (Burnette, T.C. & de Miranda, 1994; de Miranda, P. & Burnette, 1994). Therefore, the mechanism of action and spectrum of activity of valaciclovir are the same as that of acyclovir (Rajalakshmi et al., 2010).

2.5 Carbovir

Carbovir is a carbocyclic guanosine derivative with a potent and selective inhibitory effect on HIV-1 replication (Vince et al., 1988). As its oral bioavailability is low (Huang et al., 1991), its prodrug, 6-deoxycarbovir was synthesized in attempt to increase its oral absorption. The chemical structure of 6-deoxycarbovir is very similar to that of 6-deoxypenciclovir and 6-deoxyaciclovir. Like 6-deoxyaciclovir, 6-deoxycarbovir has been reported as XO-activated prodrug (Vince et al., 1995), but it is also a better substrate for AO than XO (Table 2). 6-Deoxycarbovir is oxidized at C-8 position and 8-hydroxy-6-deoxycarbovir is the main metabolite produced from incubation of 6-deoxycarbovir with rabbit liver AO, but with guinea pig liver AO, 6-hydroxylation is the major metabolic pathway and carbovir is produced as almost the only oxidative metabolite.

8-Hydroxy-6-deoxyaciclovir lacks appreciable activity against herpes simplex type I *in vitro* (Krenitsky et al., 1984). As substitution at carbon 8 generally results in loss of antiviral activity (Beedham, 1997), 8-hydrox-6-deoxycarbovir is expected to be dvoid of antiviral activity. It is likely that AO from other sources like guinea pig liver, which is a better animal model for human liver AO (Rashidi, 1996), acts as the main enzyme in oxidative conversion of 6-deoxyaciclovir to aciclovir as it is the case with 6-deoxypenciclovir and 6-deoxycarbovir. The assay of 6-deoxyaciclovir oxidation by hepatic AO from species such as guinea pig and human and pharmacokinetics of 6-deoxyaciclovir following administration of the compound should be subject to further studies.

	6-Deoxypenciclovir		6-Deoxycarbovir		6-Deoxyaciclovir	
Enzyme fraction	**Km (mM)**	**6-oxo-metabolite / 8-oxo-metabolite**	**Km (mM)**	**6-oxo-metabolite / 8-oxo-metabolite**	**Km (mM)**	**6-oxo-metabolite / 8-oxo-metabolite**
Guinea pig	0.41	27	0.40	100	ND	ND
Rabbit	0.44	0.9	0.11	0.3	0.06	0.05
Rat liver XO	0.26	a	0.22	a	ND	ND
BMXO	0.90	a	ND	ND	0.9	a

a: 6-Oxo-metabolite was the only metabolite produced.
ND: Not determined

Table 2. The Km value for the formation of 6-oxo-metabolite and the ratio of 6-oxo- to 8-oxo-metabolite for the oxidation of 6-deoxypenciclovir, 6-deoxycarbovir and 6-deoxyaciclovir catalyzed by guinea pig, rabbit, rat liver xanthine oxidase (XO) and bovine milk xanthine oxidase (BMXO) (Krenitsky et al., 1984; Rashidi 1996; Rashidi et al., 1997).

2.6 Vidarabine

Vidarabine (9-β-D-Arabinosyladenine, adenine arabinoside, Ara-A, Vira-A), a marine-derived drug has been shown to have antitumor activity. However, it has become more notable for its antiviral activity with a high therapeutic index (Hansel et al., 2004; Hirsch & Schooley, 1983). In the 1964, the first study on the antiviral activity of vidarabine was explained by Private de Grilhe and De Rudder (Private de Grilhe & De Rudder, 1964). Following, Whiley described vidarabine activity in the treatment of herpes encephalitis and the other herpes infection in newborns (Field & De Clerq, 2004). Vidarabine possess significant activity against infections caused by herpes viruses, pox viruses, rhabdoviruses, hepadnaviruses, the vaccinia virus, VZV, and some RNA tumor viruses. Although vidarabine is supplanted by acyclovir and other analogs for most applications, it is still used as an alternative therapy for acyclovir-resistant HSV and VZV infections (Gentry et al., 2008).

However, vidarabine is extensively deaminated in the body by adenosine deaminase (ADA) to 9-β-D-arabinofuranosylhypoxanthine (hypoxanthine arabinoside) that has less antiviral activity than vidarabine, which is a major limitation in its clinical use (Shen et al., 2009; Shope et al., 1983; Sloan et al., 1977). Inhibition of ADA by co-administration of modified purine analogues with vidarabine, such as deoxycoformacine, can improve the therapeutic effect of vidarabine (Bryson et al., 1974, 1976). In addition, vidarabine has limited lipid solubility which the low delivery from cell membrane and very low solubility in water (about 0.47 mg/ml), therefore, the large fluid volumes is needed for intravenous administration (Baker et al., 1978; Hirsch & Schooley, 1983; Whitley et al., 1980).

Vidarabine is a nucleoside analog; therefore, it has to be phosphorylated and to be active. It is phosphorylated to its monophosphate, di- and triphosphate nucleotides which during the synthetic (S) phase inhibit DNA polymerase and strongly in the virus such as herpes, vaccinia and varicella zoster viruses than in the host cells (Dicioccio & Srivastava, 1977; Doering et al., 1966; Rose & Jacob, 1978; Shipman et al., 1976). As well, vidarabine is integrated into RNA in virus and inhibit RNA polyadenylation reaction (Rose & Jacob, 1978).

In mammalian cell, vidarabine is rapidly converted by ADA to hypoxanthine arabinoside which has less antiviral activity than vidarabine. Hypoxanthine arabinoside is the major metabolite of vidarabine is excreted renally and biotransformed by XO to xanthine arabinoside (Fig. 14) (Connor et al., 1975; Friedman & Grasela, 1981; Hirsch & Schooley, 1983; Shen et al., 2009). Allopurinol as an inhibitor of XO can interfere with the metabolism of vidarabine and, therefore, co-administration of allopurinol with vidarabine should be avoided or used with caution (Woster, 2007). The role of AO in this metabolic pathway, in particular oxidation of xanthine arabinoside at C-8, has not been investigated and could be a subject for future studies.

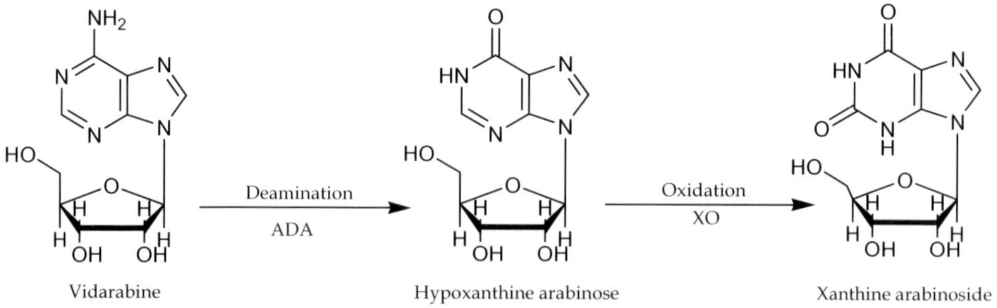

Fig. 14. The biotransformation of vidarabine in mammalian cells. Vidarabine is converted to hypoxanthine arabinoside through deamination by adenosine deaminase (ADA), followed by oxidation to xanthine arabinoside by xanthine oxidase (XO) (Connor et al., 1975; Friedman & Grasela, 1981; Gannon et al., 1984; Shen et al., 2009).

2.7 Theophylline

Theophylline (1,3-dimethylxanthine) is a methylxanthine which is widely distributed in nature. It is widely used as a bronchodilator agent for the treatment of various asthmatic and pulmonary conditions under a variety of brand names and is one of the most widely prescribed drugs for the treatment of airway diseases worldwide (Barnes, 2003). Theophylline acts as an effective drug in clinical trials against air way narrowing and prevents wheezing, cough, shortness of breath and difficulty breathing which is caused by asthma and different lung disease. It is also helpful in patient with chronic obstructive pulmonary disease (COPD) including chronic bronchitis and emphysema which opens air way lung to make breach easer (Aronson et al., 1992; Pauwel, 1987; Vielhaber & Kavuru, 2001).

Theophylline is metabolized in the human liver through N-1 or N-3 demethylation followed by hydroxylation at C-8 producing three main products including 3-methylxanthine (3MX), 1-methyluric acid (1MU) and 1,3-dimethyluric acid (1,3DMU) (Fig. 15) (Brikett et al., 1983; Lu et al., 2003; Yao et al., 2001). It is thought that cytochrome P450 1A2 (CYP1A2) is the most important enzyme involved in the catalysis of these reactions (HR et al., 1995; Tjia et al., 1996). Cytochrome P450 2E1 (CYP2E1) can also mediate C-8 hydroxylation but its contribution in this reaction is low (HR et al., 1995; Tjia et al., 1996).

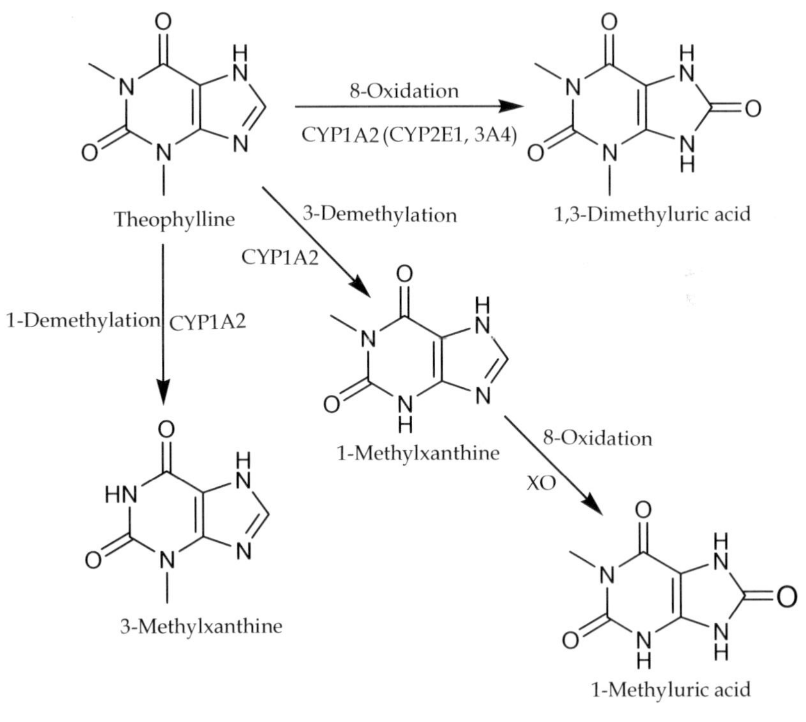

Fig. 15. The biotransformation of theophylline through CYP450 family and xanthine oxidase (Brikett et al., 1983; HR et al 1995; Lu et al., 2003; Tjia, et al 1996; Yao et al., 2001). CYP1A2: Cytochrome P450 1A2, CYP2E1: Cytochrome P450 2E1, XO: Xanthine Oxidase

1-Methyluric acid is the secondary metabolic pathway of theophylline. It is produced following a rapid oxidation from 1-methylxanthin by XO (Fig. 15) (Brikett et al., 1983). In contrast to the other methylxanthines, 1-methylxanthin is a good substrate for XO (Bergmann & Dikstein, 1956; Krenitsky et al., 1972; Lohmann & Miech, 1976) and used as a XO activity index for plasma concentration of oxypurinal in man (Graham et al., 1996). The involvement of XO in the metabolism of theophylline has also been used for the construction of amperometric enzyme electrodes to quantitative measurement of theophylline (Stredansky et al., 2000). Allopurinal as a potent inhibitor of XO activity decreases the formation of 1-methyleuric acid from the 1-methylxanthine in theophylline oxidation (Brikett et al., 1983; German DC, 1986).

3. Conclusion

Drug metabolism is one of the important factors that may play a major role in drug development and toxicity. AO and XO are two molybdenum-containing enzymes that are involved in the metabolism of an extensive range of aldehydes and N-heterocyclic aromatic compounds (Beedham, 1997; Rashidi & Nazemiyeh, 2010). Although the importance of molybdenum hydroxylases in drug metabolism has usually been overshadowed by that of CYP450 as the most important drug metabolizing enzyme system, we will witness a significant increase in the importance of XO and AO in drug metabolism over the next decade (Alfaro et al 2009; Obach et al., 2004). Purines as N-heterocyclic compounds, thus, can serve as substrate for AO and XO and the importance of molybdenum hydroxylases in the metabolism of purines and also the development of purine related prodrugs has been demonstrated by several authors (Clarke et al., 1995; Kitchen et al., 1999; Krenitsky et al., 1984; Rashidi et al., 1997, 2007; Van Scoik et al., 1985).

The reaction catalyzed by AO and XO involves a nucleophilic attack on an electron-deficient *sp*2-hybridized carbon atom adjacent to a ring nitrogen atom in N-heterocyclic compounds. Therefore, nitrogen-containing aromatic compounds including purines can act as appropriate substrates for XO and AO. Purine nucleus contains several nitrogen atoms and is sequentially oxidized at three different positions; in a substituted purine analogue, any of these sites could be attacked by AO and XO with varying affinities and/or rates (Beedham, 2010).

On the other hand, significant interspecies variations exist in both the number and activity of both AO and XO, in particular the former enzyme (Alfaro et al., 2009; Jones et al., 1987; Krenitsky et al., 1984; Rashidi et al., 1997). Therefore, not only it is difficult to predict which metabolite will be produced from a purine-based drug by AO or XO, but also it would be a hard task to recognize which of these two enzymes has a dominant contribution in the metabolic pathway. In addition, it would be difficult to find a suitable animal model and extrapolate the results obtained from the animal studies to man.

As it was shown in the previous sections, there are several purine related drugs or prodrugs that are metabolized by AO and/or XO; however, the manner of the oxidation sites could be completely different for these two enzymes. For example, famciclovir and 6-

deoxycarbovir are converted to their corresponding active agent by AO with purine oxidation occurs at carbon 6. But, rabbit liver enzyme acts differently and attacks mainly at carbon 8 of the purine nucleus. In contrast to AO, XO has a little contribution to the activation of these purine analogues. Not surprisingly, Krenitsky et al. (Krenitsky et al., 1972,1984) has shown that the oxidation occurs at carbons 6 and 8 with XO and rabbit liver AO, respectively. 6-Deoxyaciclovir which is also a purine-based prodrug is oxidized at the 6-position by XO, whereas rabbit enzyme oxidizes 6-deoxyaciclovir to 8-oxo-6-deoxyaciclovir (Krenitsky et al., 1984). However, it has been found that (Iyer, 1992; Rashidi et al., 1997) rabbit liver AO differs to the enzyme from other species in oxidizing carbon 8 of 2-NH_2-9-substituted purines instead of the 6-position. Therefore, it is more likely that 6-deoxyaciclovir is predominantly oxidized to aciclovir by AO from human, guinea pig or rat livers which are subject for further studies. This could be case for other purine related drugs that their metabolism has been attributed to XO. Conducting comparative studies, the like of which has been carried out with famciclovir (Rashidi et al., 1997), would be of great value in elucidating the contribution of AO and XO in the metabolism of these purine-based agents. In these studies, the selection of an appropriate animal model for human AO would be a problem because of the different substrate specificity of enzyme from each species.

4. References

Alfaro, J.F.; Joswig-Jones, C.A.; Ouyang, W.; Nichols, J.; Crouch, G.J.; & Jones, J.P. (2009). Purification and mechanism of human aldehyde oxidase expressed in Escherichia coli. *Drug Metab Dispos,* 37(12): 2393-2398.

Anderson, R.D.; Griffy, K.G.; Jung, D.; Dorr, A.; Hulse, J.D.; & Smith, R.B. (1995). Ganciclovir absolute bioavailability and steady-state pharmacokinetics after oral administration of two 3000-mg/d dosing regimens in human immunodeficiency virus- and cytomegalovirus-seropositive patients. *Clin Ther,* 17(3):425-432.

Ansari, A.; Aslam, Z.; De Sica, A.; Smith, M.; Gilshenan, K.; Fairbanks, L.; Marinaki, A.; Sanderson, J.; & Duley, J. (2008). Influence of xanthine oxidase on thiopurine metabolism in Crohn's disease. *Aliment Pharmacol Ther,* 28(6):749-757.

Aronson. J.K.; Hardman, M.; Reynolds D.J. (1992). "ABC of monitoring drug therapy. Theophylline." *BMJ,* 305(6865):1355-1358.

Baker, D.C.; Haskell, T.H.; & Putt, S.R. (1978). Prodrugs of 9-beta-D-arabinofuranosyladenine. 1. Synthesis and evaluation of some 5'-(O-acyl) derivatives. *J Med Chem,* 21(12): 1218-1221.

Beedham, C. (1997). The role of non-P450 enzymes in drug oxidation, *Pharm World Sci,* 19(6):255-263.

Beedham, C. (2010). Xanthine Oxidoreductase and Aldehyde Oxidase, *Comprehensive Toxicology,* Chapter 4.10, 185-205.

Beedham, C. (2002). Molybdenum hydroxylase, In: *Enzyme systems that methabolize drugs and other xenobiotics,* C. Ioannides (Ed.), John Wiley & Sons Ltd., pp 147-187.

Bergmann, F.; & Dikstein, S. (1956). Studies on uric acid and related compounds. III. Observations on the specificity of mammalian xanthine oxidases. *J Biol Chem,* 223(2):765-780.

Birkett, D.J.; Miners, J.O.; & Attwood, J. (1983). Secondary metabolism of theophylline biotransformation products in man--route of formation of 1-methyluric acid. Br J Clin Pharmacol, 15(1): 117-119.

Bryson, Y.; Connor, J.D.; Sweetman, L.; Carey, S.; Stuckey, M.A.; Buchanan, R. (1974). Determination of plaque inhibitory activity of adenine arabinoside (9-beta-D-arabinofuranosyladenine) for herpesviruses using an adenosine deaminase inhibitor. *Antimicrob Agents Chemother,* 6(1): 98-101.

Bryson, Y.J.; & Connor, J.D. (1976). In vitro susceptibility of varicella zoster virus to adenine arabinoside and hypoxanthine arabinoside. *Antimicrob Agents Chemother,* 9(3): 540-543.

Burnette, T.C.; & de Miranda, P. (1994). Metabolic disposition of the acyclovir prodrug valaciclovir in the rat. *Drug Metab Dispos,* 22(1):60–64.

Chalmers, A.H.; Knight, P.R.; & Atkinson, M.R. (1969). 6-thiopurines as substrates and inhibitors of purine oxidases: a pathway for conversion of azathioprine into 6-thiouric acid without release of 6-mercaptopurine. *Aust J Exp Biol Med Sci,* 47(2):263-273.

Clarke, S.E.; Harrell, A.W.; & Chenery, R.J. (1995). Role of aldehyde oxidase in the in vitro conversion of famciclovir to penciclovir in human liver. *Drug Metab Dispos,* 23(2):251-254.

Chabner, B.A.; Ryan, B.P.; Paz-Ares, L.; Garcia-Carbonero, R.; & Calabresi, P. (2001). Antineoplastic Agents. In *Goodman and Gilman's The Pharmacological Basis of Therapeutics,* 10th ed. J.G.; Hardman, L.E.; Limbird, A.; Gilman, (Eds.), New York: McGraw-Hill. pp. 1389-1459.

Connor, J.D.; Sweetman, L.; Carey, S.; Stuckey, M.A.; & Buchanan, R. (1975). Susceptibility in vitro of several large DNA viruses to the antiviral activity of adenine arabinoside and its metabolite, hypoxanthine arabinoside: relation to human pharmacology. In: *Adenine arabinoside: an antiviral agent. D.;* Pavan-Langston, R.A.; Buchanan, C.A.; Alford, (Eds.), New York: Raven Press, 177-196.

Crumpacker, C.S. (1996). Ganciclovir. *N Engl J Med,* 335(10):721-729.

De Clercq, E.; & Field, H.J. (2006). Antiviral prodrugs-the development of successful prodrug strategies for antiviral chemotherapy. *Br J Pharmacol,* 147(1):1-11.

Di Iorio, P.; Ballerini, P.; Caciagli, F.; & Ciccarelli, R. (1998). Purinoceptor-mediated modulation of purine and neurotransmitter release from nervous tissue. *Pharmacol Res,* 37(3):169-178.

De Clercq, E.; & Holy, A. (2005). Acyclic nucleoside phosphonates: a key class of antiviral drugs. *Nat Re Drug Discov,* 4(11): 928-940.

De Miranda, P.; & Blum, M.R. (1983). Pharmacokinetics of acyclovir after intravenous and oral administration. *J Antimicrob Chemother,* 12 Suppl B:29-37.

De Miranda, P.; & Burnette, T.C. (1994). Metabolic fate and pharmacokinetics of the acyclovir prodrug valaciclovir in cynomolgus monkeys. *Drug Metab Dispos,* 22(1): 55-59.

Dicioccio, R.A.; & Srivastava, B.I. (1977). Kinetics of inhibition of deoxynucleotide-polymerizing enzyme activities from normal and leukemic human cells by 9-beta-D-arabinofuranosyladenine 5'-triphosphate and 1-beta-D-arabinofuranosylcytosine 5'-triphosphate. *Eur J Biochem,* 79(2): 411-418.

Dollery, C. (1999). *Therapeutic drugs.* 2nd ed. Edinburgh: Churchill Livingstone; p. A39-A44.

Doering, A.; Keller, J.; & Cohen, S.S. (1966). Some effects of D-arabinosyl nucleosides on polymer syntheses in mouse fibroblasts. *Cancer Res,* 26(12): 2444-2450.

Easterbrook, P.; & Wood, M.J. (1994). Successors to acyclovir. *J Antimicrob Chemother,* 34(3): 307-311.

Elion, G.B. (1967). Symposium on immunosuppressive drugs. Biochemistry and pharmacology of purine analogues. *Fed Proc,* 26(3): 898-904.

Elion, G.B.; Burgi, E.; & Hitchings,G.H. (1952). Studies on Condensed Pyrimidine Systems. IX. The Synthesis of Some 6-Substituted Purines. *J Am Chem Soc,* 74:411-414.

Elion, G.B.; Hitchings G.H.; & Vander Werff, H. (1951). Antagonists of nucleic acid derivatives. VI. Purines. *J Biol Chem,* 192(2): 505 518.

Evans, W.E.; & Relling, M.V. (1994). Mercaptopurine vs thioguanine for the treatment of acute leukemia. *Leuk Res,* 18(11): 811-814.

Field, H.; & De Clercq, E. (2004). Antiviral drugs-a short history of their discovery and development. *Microbiol Today, 31,*58–61.

Fotoohi, A.K.; Coulthard, S.A.; & Albertioni, F. (2010). Thiopurines: factors influencing toxicity and response. *Biochem Pharmacol,* 79(9):1211-1220.

Friedman, H.M. (1981). Adenine arabinoside and allopurinol--possible adverse drug interaction. *N Engl J Med,* 304(7):423.

Gentry, B.G.; Shen, W.; Breitenbach, J.M.; Hilfinger, J.; & Drach, J.C. (2008). Vidarabine Prodrugs as Potential Inhibitors of Adenosine Deaminase. *Antiviral Res,* 78(2): A56.

German, D.C.; & Holmes, E.W. (1986). Hyperuricaemia and gout. *Med Clinics of North Am,* 70: 419-436.

Hall, W.W.; & Krenitsky, T.A. (1986). Aldehyde oxidase from rabbit liver: specificity toward purines and their analogs. *Arch Biochem Biophys,* 251(1):36-46.

Hande, K.R.; & Garrow, G.C. (1996). Purine antimetabolites. In: *Cancer Chemotherapy and Biotherapy: Principles and Practice,* B.A; Chabner, & D.L. Longo, (Eds.), Lippincott-Raven Publishers, Philadelphia, pp 235–252.

Graham, S.; Day, R.O.; Wong, H.; McLachlan, A.J.; Bergendal, L.; Miners, J.O.; & Birkett, D.J. (1996). Pharmacodynamics of oxypurinol after administration of allopurinol to healthy subjects. *Br J Clin Pharmacol,* 41(4):299-304.

Hansel, T.T.; Tennant, R.C.; Tan, A.J.; Higgins, L.A.; Neighbour, H.; Erin, E.M.; & Barnes, P.J. (2004). Theophylline: mechanism of action and use in asthma and chronic obstructive pulmonary disease. *Drugs Today (Barc),* 40(1): 55-69.

Harrell, A.W.; Wheeler, S.M.; Pennick, M.; Clarke, S.; & Chenery, R.J. (1993). Evidence that famciclovir (BRL 42810) and its associated metabolites do not inhibit the 6 beta-hydroxylation of testosterone in human liver microsomes. *Drug Metab Dispos,* 21(1):18-23.

Hay, C.M.; & Reichman, R.C. (2008). Antiviral Drugs. In: *Fitzpatrick`s Dermatology in General Medicine*. K.; Wolff, L.A.; Goldsmith, S.I.; Katz, B.A.; Gilchrest, A.S.; Paller, D.J.; & Leffel, (Eds.), 7th ed. New York: McGraw-Hill; P. 2203-2211.

Hirsch, M. S. and R. T. Schooley (1983). Drug therapy. Treatment of herpesvirus infections. *N Engl J Med*, 309(16):963-970.

Huang, S.H.; Remmel, R.P.; & Zimmerrman, C.L. (1991). The bioavailability and nonlinear clearance of (-)-carbovir in the rat. *Pharm Res*, 8:739-743.

Hirsch, M.S.; & Schooley, R.T. (1983). Drug therapy. Treatment of herpesvirus infections. *N Engl J Med*, 309(16):963-970.

Hitchings, G.H. (1978). Uric acid: chemistry and synthesis. In: *Uric Acid*, W.N.; Kelley, & I.M.; Weiner (Eds.), Berlin, Heidelberg and New York, Springer-Verlag, pp:1-20. Berlin, Heidelberg, pp. 1-20. ISBN: 3540086110, 9783540086116.New York.

Hurst, D.T. (1980). *An Introduction to the Chemistry and Biochemistry of Pyrimidines, Purines and Pteridines*, John Wiley & Sons.

Hogarth, L.A.; Redfern, C.P.; Teodoridis, J.M.; Hall, A.G.; Anderson, H.; Case, M.C.; & Coulthard, S.A. (2008). The effect of thiopurine drugs on DNA methylation in relation to TPMT expression. *Biochem Pharmacol*, 76(8):1024-1035.

Iyer, K.R. (1992). Evaluation and metabolism of (−)-6-deoxycarbovir as a prodrug for (-)- carbovir. *Dissertation Abst Inter*, 53:1313-B.

Jones, D.B., Rustgi V.K., Kornhauser D.M., Woods A., Quinn R., Hoofnagle J.H., & Jones A. (1987). The disposition of 6-deoxyacyclovir: a xanthine oxidase-activated prodrug of acyclovir in the isolated perfused rat liver. *Hepatology*, 7:345–348.

Joule, J.A., Mills, K.; & Smith, G.F. (1995). *Heterocyclic Chemistry*, 3th Edition, Chapman & Hall, pp. 409-433.

Jung, D.; & Dorr, A. (1999). Single-dose pharmacokinetics of valganciclovir in HIV- and CMV seropositive subjects. *J Clin Pharmacol*, 39(8):800-804.

Keuzenkamp-Jansen, C.W.; van Baal, J.M.; De Abreu, R.A.; de Jong, J.G.; Zuiderent, R.; & Trijbels, J.M. (1996). Detection and identification of 6-methylmercapto-8-hydoxypurine, a major metabolite of 6-mercaptopurine, in plasma during intravenous administration. *Clin Chem*, 42(3):380-386.

Kitchen, B.J.; Moser, A.; Lowe, E.; Balis, F.M.; Widemann, B.; Anderson, L.; Strong, J.; Blaney, S.M.; Berg, S.L.; O'Brien, M.; & Adamson, P.C. (1999). Thioguanine administered as a continuous intravenous infusion to pediatric patients is metabolized to the novel metabolite 8-hydroxy-thioguanine. *J Pharmacol Exp Ther*, 291(2):870-874.

Knoester, P.D.; Underberg, W.J.; & Beijnen, J.H. (1993). Clinical pharmacokinetics and pharmacodynamics of anticancer agents in pediatric patients (review). *Anticancer Res*, 13(5C):1795-1808.

Krenitsky, T.A.; Hall, W.W.; de Miranda, P.; Beauchamp, L.M.; Schaeffer, H.J.; & Whiteman, P.D. (1984). 6-Deoxyacyclovir: a xanthine oxidase-activated prodrug of acyclovir. *Proc Natl Acad Sci USA*, 81(10):3209-3213.

Krenitsky, T.A.; Neil, S.M.; Elion, G.B.; & Hitchings, G.H. (1972). A comparison of the specificities of xanthine oxidase and aldehyde oxidase. *Arch Biochem Biophys*, 150(2):585-599.

Krenitsky, T.A.; Spector, T.; & Hall, W.W. (1986). Xanthine oxidase from human liver: purification and characterization. *Arch Biochem Biophys*, 247(1):108-119.

Krogsgaard-Larsen, P. (992). *A Textbook of Drug Design and Development*, Harwood Academic Publishers, pp. 577-605.

Krasny, H.C.; Beauchamp, L.; Krenitsky, T.A.; & De Miranda, P. (1995). Metabolism and pharmacokinetics of a double prodrug of ganciclovir in the rat and monkey. *Drug Metab Dispos*, 23:1242–1247.

Lennard, L., Hale, J.P.; & Lilleyman, J.S. (1991). *Proceedings of the BPS*, 659P.

Lennard, L.; Davies, H.A.; & Lilleyman, J.S. (1993). Is 6-thioguanine more appropriate than 6-mercaptopurine for children with acute lymphoblastic leukaemia? *Br J Cancer*, 68(1):186-190.

Li, F.; Maag, H.; & Alfredson, T. (2008). Prodrugs of nucleoside analogues for improved oralabsorption and tissue targeting. *J Pharm Sci*, 97(3):1109-1134.

Lohmann, S.M.; & Miech, R.P. (1976). Theophylline metabolism by the rat liver microsomal system. *J Pharmacol Exp Ther*, 196(1):213-225.

Lu, P., M. L. Schrag, Slaughter, D.E.; Raab, C.E.; Shou, M.; & Rodrigues, A.D. (2003). Mechanism-based inhibition of human liver microsomal cytochrome P450 1A2 by zileuton, a 5-lipoxygenase inhibitor. *Drug Metab Dispos*, 31(11): 1352-1360.

Maag, H. (2002). Ganciclovir pro-drugs: Synthesis and pre-clinical development of valganciclovir (Valcyte™). *AAPS Annual Meeting, November 13, Toronto, Canada.*

Murray, A.B. (1995). Valaciclovir: an improvement over acyclovir for the treatment of zoster. *Antiviral Chem Chemother*, 6, 34–38.

Mondal, D. (1995). Ganciclovir. *xPharm: The Comprehensive Pharmacology Reference, 1-5.*

Meerten, E., Verweij, J.; & Schellens, J.H.M. (1995). Antineoplastic agents: drug interactions of clinical significance. *Drug Safety*, 12: 168–182.

Noble, S.; & Faulds, D. (1998). Ganciclovir. An update of its use in the prevention of cytomegalovirus infection and disease in transplant recipients. *Drugs*, 56(1):115-146.

Obase, Y.; Shimoda, T.; Kawano, T.; Saeki, S.; Tomari, S.Y.; Mitsuta-Izaki, K.; Matsuse, H.; Kinoshita, M.; & Kohno, S. (2003). Polymorphisms in the CYP1A2 gene and theophylline metabolism in patients with asthma. *Clin Pharmacol Ther* 73(5):468-474.

Palella, T.D., & Fox, I.H. (1991). Purine and Pyrimidine Metabolism, In: *Encyclopedia of Human Biology*, R.; Dulbecco, (Ed.), Vol. 6, Academic Press, pp. 387-398.

Pauwels, R. (1987). The effects of theophylline on airway inflammation. *Chest*, 92(1 Suppl): 32S-37S.

Physician's Desk Reference 2000. *Physicians' Desk Reference*, Edition 54. , Medical Economics company, Montvale, New Jersey.

Perry, C.M., & Wagstaff, A.J. (1995). Famciclovir. A review of its pharmacological properties and therapeutic efficacy in herpesvirus infections. *Drugs* 50(2):396-415.

Pescovitz, M.D., Rabkin, J.; Merion, R.M.; Paya, C.V.; Pirsch, J.; Freeman, R.B.; O'Grady, J.; Robinson, C.; To, Z.; Wren, K.; Banken, L.; Buhles, W.; & Brown, F. (2000).

Valganciclovir results in improved oral absorption of ganciclovir in liver transplant recipients. *Antimicrob Agents Chemother*, 44(10):2811-2815.

Privat de Garilhe, M., & De Rudder, J. (1964). Effect of 2 arabinose nucleoside on the multiplication of herpes viruse and vairus and vaccine in cell culture. *C R Hebd Seances Acad Sci*, 259: 2725-2728.

Pue, M.A., & Benet, L .Z. (1993). Pharmacokinetics of famciclovir in man. *Antiviral Chem. Chemother*, 4(Suppl. 1), 47–55.

Pue, M.A.; Pratt, S.K.; Fairless, A.J.; Fowles, S.; Laroche, J.; Georgiou, P.; & Prince, W. (1994). Linear pharmacokinetics of penciclovir following administration of single oral doses of famciclovir 125, 250, 500 and 750 mg to healthy volunteers. *J Antimicrob Chemother*, 33(1):119-127

Ralevic, V. (2009). Purines as neurotransmitters and neuromodulators in blood vessels. *Curr Vasc Pharmacol*, 7(1):3-14.

Rajalakshmi, R.; Kumari, R.; & Thappa, D.M. (2010). Acyclovir versus valacyclovir. *Indian J Dermatol Venereol Leprol*, 76(4):439-444.

Rashidi, M.R. (1996). In vitro oxidation of purins by hepatic molybdenum hydroylases. Ph.D. Thesis, University of Bradford, UK.

Rashidi, M.R.; Smith, J.A.; Clarke, S.E.; & Beedham, C. (1997). In vitro oxidation of famciclovir and 6-deoxypenciclovir by aldehyde oxidase from human, guinea pig, rabbit, and rat liver. *Drug Metab Dispos*, 25(7):805-813.

Rashidi, M.R.; Beedham, C.; Smith, J.S.; & Davaran, S. (2007). In vitro study of 6-mercaptopurine oxidation catalysed by aldehyde oxidase and xanthine oxidase. *Drug Metab Pharmacokinet*, 22(4):299-306.

Rashidi, M.R.; & Nazemiyeh, H. (2010). Inhibitory effects of flavonoids on molybdenum hydroxylases activity. *Expert Opin Drug Metab Toxicol*, 6(2):133-152.

Rider, B.J. (2008). Mercaptopurine, *xPharm: The Comprehensive Pharmacology Reference*, 1-4.

Rose, K. M.; & Jacob, S. T. (1978). Selective inhibition of RNA polyadenylation by Ara-ATP in vitro: a possible mechanism for antiviral action of Ara-A. *Biochem Biophys Res Commun*, 81(4): 1418-1424.

Safrin, S. & Phan, L. (1993). In vitro activity of penciclovir against clinical isolates of acyclovir-resistant and foscarnet-resistant herpes simplex virus. *Antimicrob Agents Chemother*, 37(10): 2241-2243.

Schwartz, R.; Stack, J.; & Dameshek, W. (1958). Effect of 6-mercaptopurine on antibody production. *Proc Soc Exp Biol Med*, 99(1):164-167.

Shaw, G. (1984). *In: Comprehensive Heterocyclic Chemistry* (Ed. K.T. Potts), Vol. 5, *Pergamon Press*, pp. 499-605.

Shen, W.; Kim, J.S.; Kish, P.E.; Zhang, J.; Mitchell, S.; Gentry, B.G.; Breitenbach, J.M.; Drach, J.C.; & Hilfinger, J. (2009). Design and synthesis of vidarabine prodrugs as antiviral agents. *Bioorg Med Chem Lett*, 19(3):792-796 .

Shipman, C.,Jr., Smith S.H.; Carlson, R.H.; & Drach, J.C. (1976). Antiviral activity of arabinosyladenine and arabinosylhypoxanthine in herpes simplex virus-infected KB cells: selective inhibition of viral deoxyribonucleic acid synthesis in synchronized suspension cultures. *Antimicrob Agents Chemother*, 9(1): 120-7.

Stredansky, M.; Pizzariello, A.; Miertus, S.; & Svorc, J. (2000). Selective and Sensitive Biosensor for Theophylline Based on Xanthine Oxidase Electrode, Anal. *Biochem*, 285, 225–229.

Tjia, J.F., Colbert, J.; Back, D.J. (1996). Theophylline metabolism in human liver microsomes: inhibition studies. *J Pharmacol Exp Ther*, 276(3): 912-917.

Van Scoik, K.G.; Johnson, C.A.; & Porter, W.R. (1985). The pharmacology and metabolism of the thiopurine drugs 6-mercaptopurine and azathioprine. *Drug Metab Rev*, 16(1-2):157-174.

Vere Hodge, R.A.; Sutton, D.; Boyd, M.R.; Harnden, M.R.; & Jarvest, R.L. (1989). Selection of an oral prodrug (BRL 42810; famciclovir) for the antiherpesvirus agent BRL 39123 [9-(4-hydroxy-3-hydroxymethylbut-l-yl)guanine; penciclovir]. *Antimicrob Agents Chemother*, 33(10):1765-1773.

Vere Hodge, R. A.; & Cheng, Y.C. (1993). The mode of action of penciclovir. *Antiviral Chem. Chemother*, 4(Suppl. 1), 13–24.

Vielhaber, M. M.; & Kavuru, M. (2001). Should we still be using theophylline to treat asthma? *Cleve Clin J Med*, 68(8): 681.

Vince, R.; Hua, M.; Brownell, J.; Daluge, S.; Lee, F.; Shannon, W.M.; Lavell, G.C.; Qualls, J.; Weislow, O.S.; Kiser, R.; Canonico, P.G.; Schultz, R.H.; Narayanan, V.L.; Mayo, J.G.; Shoemaker, R.H.; & Boyd, M.R. (1988). Potent and selective activity of a new carbocyclic nucleotide analogue (carbovir; NSC 614846) against human immunodeficiency virus in vitro. *Biochem Biophys Res Comm*,156:1046-53.

Vince, R.; Brownell, J.; & Beers, S.A. (1995). 6-Deoxycarbovir: a xanthine oxidase activated prodrug of carbovir, Nucleosides Nucleotides, 14, 39-44.

Whitley, R.J.; Tucker, B.C.; Kinkel, A.W.; Barton, N.H.; Pass, R.F.; Whelchel, J.D.; Cobbs, C.G.; Diethelm, A.G.; & Buchanan, R.A. (1980). Pharmacology, tolerance, and antiviral activity of vidarabine monophosphate in humans. *Antimicrob Agents Chemother*, 18(5):709-715.

Whitley, R.J.; Nahmias, A.J.; Soong, S.J.; Galasso, G.G.; Fleming, C.L.; & Alford, C.A. (1980). Vidarabine therapy of neonatal herpes simplex virus infection. *Pediatrics*. 66(4):495-501.

Whitley, R.; Alford, C.; Hess, F.; & Buchanan, R. (1980). Vidarabine: a preliminary review of its pharmacological properties and therapeutic use. *Drugs*. 20(4):267-282.

Woster, P.M. (2007). Antiviral agents and protease inhibitors, In: *Foy's principles of medicinal chemistry*, W.O. Foye, T.L. Lemke, D.A. Williams (Eds.), Lippincott, Williams & Wilkins, p. 1213.

Winkler, I.; Winkelmann, E.; Scholl, T.; Rosner, M.; Jahne, G.; & Helsberg, M. (1990). Antiviral activity and pharmacokinetics of HOE 602, an acyclic nucleoside, in animal models. *Antiviral Res*, 14(2):61-73.

Yao, C.; Kunze, K.L.; Kharasch, E.D.; Wang, Y.; Trager, W.F.; Ragueneau, I.; & Levy, R.H. (2001). Fluvoxamine-theophylline interaction: gap between in vitro and in vivo inhibition constants toward cytochrome P4501A2. *Clin Pharmacol Ther*, 70(5): 415-24.

Zimm, S.; Grygiel, J.J.; Strong, J.M.; Monks, T.J.; & Poplack, D.G. (1984). Identification of 6-mercaptopurine riboside in patients receiving 6-mercaptopurine as a prolonged intravenous infusion. *Biochem Pharmacol*, 33(24):4089-4092.

18

One Step Closer to the Target: Intracellular Pharmacokinetics of Gemcitabine

Matthew Links and Peter Galettis
St. George Cancer Pharmacology and Therapeutic Group, University of New South Wales
St. George Clinical School, South Eastern Illawarrawa Area Health Service
Australia

1. Introduction

Drug dosing is based on the premise that the amount of drug given influences the toxicity and response. The premise of pharmacokinetics is that it is not the amount of drug given, but the amount the patient is exposed to, that determines drug effect. Measurements of drug exposure are usually performed by determining the concentration in serum or plasma. This accounts for variability in drug clearance in determining the patient's exposure. This has resulted in such dosing strategies as carboplatin dosing based on creatinine clearance, therapeutic dose monitoring of methotrexate and pharmacogenetically modified dosing for irinotecan.

However it is well recognised that the plasma is not the compartment that is most relevant in determining tissue effects. For example for the antibiotic azithromycin the organ concentrations in the site of infection, such as lung are the critical feature in determining drug effect for pneumonia (Olsen et al., 1996; Schentag & Ballow, 1991). This argument has been extended to cancer anti-metabolites (Shewach & Lawrence, 2003).

The situation in the treatment of a patient with cancer is even more complex. Tumours occur in an organ of interest such as the lung, or brain and liver. Regional concentrations in these organs are important variables (Reid, et al 1990; Breedveld et al., 2005). However tumours also create their own microenvironment with alterations in blood supply, interstitial pressure and local secretion of growth factors and cytokines (Liotta & Kohn, 2001; Wiig, et al, 2010). The drug concentration of interest is the concentration at the tumour site. Differences in tissue PK (C. Presant et al., 1990) and inter-tumoural and intra-tumoural PK are additional considerations (Zamboni et al., 2002). Therefore variation in the pharmacokinetics of plasma is only one source of variation between patients.

The reason why plasma is sampled is, of course because it is easily accessible. There are limited possibilities for repeated tumour biopsies, although this has been done (Eisbruch et al., 2001) and although there are some techniques for sampling closer to the tumour such as microdialysis (Jain, 1987), nuclear magnetic resonance spectroscopy (Müller et al., 1997) and positron emission tomography (Gupta et al 2002) these have had limited application. Nevertheless it is important to recognise the limitations of plasma and aim for sampling closer to the target where possible.

A special case is that of intra-cellularly activated drugs. The most important class of these drugs in oncology are the nucleoside analogues such as ara-C, fludarabine and gemcitabine. In this situation the drug administered is a pro-drug, which is activated intracellularly. Because the enzymatic pathways required for drug activation are well characterised there is therefore an excellent opportunity to move the consideration of drug pharmacokinetics one step closer to the target, by considering intra-cellular pharmacokinetics.

The pharmacogenetics of gemcitabine are summarized with a curated bibliography at PharmGKB. The reader is also referred to previous reviews for more detailed reports (Danesi et al., 2009; Galmirini et al., 2001; Nakano et al., 2007; Veltkamp et al., 2008). The purpose of this chapter is to bring together the data on pharmacokinetics, pharmacogentics, pharmacodynamics and associated models to provide a worked example of the potential for integrating this information and the utility and limitation of moving one step closer to the target.

2. Gemcitabine background

Gemcitabine (GEM) is a deoxcytidine analogue (2',2'-Difluorodeoxycytidine) which mimics the normal actions of the pyrimidine nucleoside deoxycytidine in its transport, phosphorylation to the tri-phosphate and then incorporation into DNA. Its structure is shown in Figure 1. However during DNA synthesis only one further base can be added then the DNA polymerase is unable to pass the altered base and DNA chain termination results. This causes an S-phase specific cell cycle arrest and programmed cell death (P. Huang, et al, 1991).

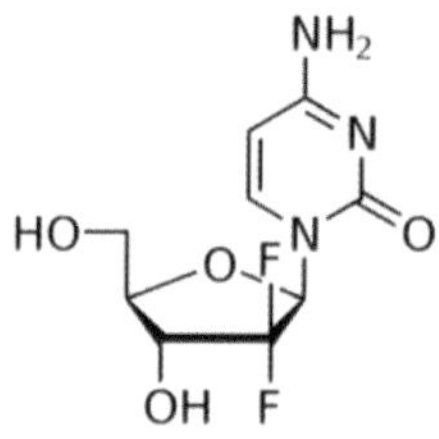

Fig. 1. Chemical structure of Gemcitabine (Creative commons license Wikimedia commons)

The enzymes responsible for each step of these processes are well characterised and variation in their activity are potential causes of variation in the response to GEM. Details on each gene of interest are provided on the entrez-gene link provided. Understanding which steps are causes of variation in toxicity and response and how to model the effects of multiple variables are key issues in understanding this variation. This requires understanding the relationship between the pharmacokinetics of GEM in the plasma and the intracellular activity of gemcitabine triphosphate (GEM-TP). The pathway of GEM activation and inactivation is illustrated in Figure 2.

The importance of understanding this is underlined by the fact that GEM is a commonly used drug in a wide range of important cancer types including non-small cell lung, breast, pancreatico-biliary and bladder.

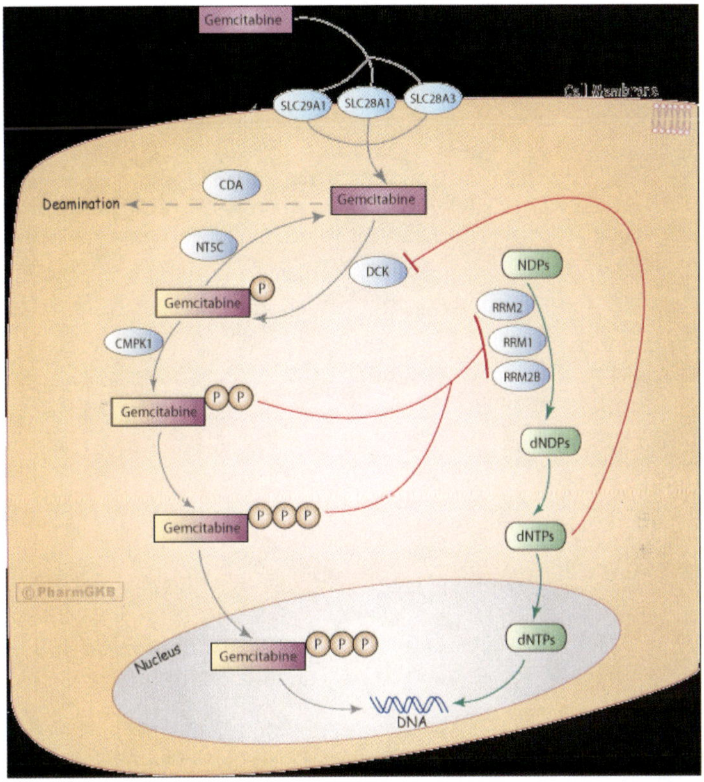

Fig. 2. Gemcitabine pathway (copyright PharmGKB, permission has been given by PharmGKB and Stanford University)

2.1 Uptake

The first step in activation is an active process of transport into the cell. The main mechanism of uptake is via hENT1 (SLC289A1) (Mackey et al., 1998) although a smaller portion is carried via other transporters SLC28A1 and SLC28A3 (Graham et al., 2000).

2.2 Phosphorlyation

Intracellular retention requires phsophorylation via the kinases, deoxyctidine kinase (*DCK*) and *CMPK1*. The rate- limiting step in this process is DCK. Phosphorlyation promotes intracellular retention and allows incorporation of GEM-TP into DNA.

2.3 Inactivation

The major route of inactivation is via deamination via Cytidine deaminase(CDA). *CDA* is ubiquitously expressed and converts GEM to difluorodeoxyuridine (dFdU). dFdU has low level activity and is water soluble and excreted almost entirely by renal excretion. A minor route of deactivation is through dephosphorylation of GEM-TP via 5'Nucleotidase (Dumontet et al., 1999).

2.4 Self- potentiation

One of the remarkable aspects of GEM pharmacology is that it has multiple mechanisms of self-potentiation (W Plunkett et al, 1996). The most important mechanism is that GEM-TP and GEM-DP block the salvage pathway of nucleotide synthesis through inhibition of Ribonucleotide reductase. This has the effect of reducing the pool of nucleotides that are competing with GEM-TP for incorporation and thereby increasing GEM-TP incorporation into DNA. Ribonucelotide reductase is composed of 2 subunits RRM1 and RRM2. The importance of this pathway is underlined by the data that variation in RRM1 is a critical determinant of GEM response (see later).

A second mechanism of self-potentiation occurs via inhibition by GEM of dCMP deaminase, which results in a reduced catabolism for GEM-TP (Heinemann et al., 1992) and a third mechanism of self-potentiation is that the main metabolite of GEM, dFdU (Hodge, et al,, 2011) increases GEM-TP accumulation in a time dependent manner.

3. Pharmacogenetics of GEM

There is considerable inter-patient variability in gemcitabine accumulation and there are polymorphisms described in many of the genes involved in transport, activation and inactivation. Data on pharmacogenetics for key drugs is agregated on the PharmGKB wesite (http://www.pharmgkb.org) and gemcitabine is included in this collection. An excellent review has been published by Wong et al (2009).

3.1 Understanding the significance of polymorphisms

Understanding the significance of a polymorphism will depend upon its changes in structure, functional significance and the frequency of variation. Non coding SNP's can be associated by chance, by linkage disequilibrium or potentially through influences on , alternate splicing, microRNA binding or DNA morphology. Changes in the promoter region can lead to variation in expression. The significance depends more fundamentally on the impact that the coded protein has on function. There are two issues here -how much does each gene product impact on function and how much of human variation is accountable by variation in this gene.

For example there are 23 snp's in the gene SLC28A3 in the dbnsnp database http://www.ncbi.nlm.nih.gov/SNP/snp_ref.cgi?locusId=64078 . Of these most are very infrequent with the heterozygozity rate of 15 loci are > 1% and only 6 are > 5%. Of the six most frequent SNP's, 3 are synonymous. These considerations are complicated by the issue that infrequent polymorphisms with major effects on function can have severe consequences.

Understanding the functional importance of a hapoltype or SNP ultimately requires demonstration of an effect on toxicity or efficacy. Pharmacokinetics however plays a crucial intermediate role in mediating pre-target variation. An association between a genetic variation and pharmacokinetics of the drug greatly increases the pre-test probability that functional differences will be found that are not related to chance.

3.2 CDA

A summary of SNP's in CDA is found in the geneview of the dbDNP database.

In European populations CDA:79A>C (K27Q) where the C allele is seen with a frequency of 0.36. Patients with a copy of the variant allele have reduced clearance and increased haematological toxicity. In Japanese patients this SNP is uncommon but a less common variant G208A has been associated with markedly reduced clearance and increased toxicity. The comparison between the two SNP's shows the importance of both common variations (in contribution to interpatient variability) and uncommon but functionally very important variants in contributing to toxicity "outliers".

3.3 RRM1

A summary of SNP's in RRM1 is found in the gene view of the dbSNP database. RRM1 is of particular interest because there is strong data to support the influence of mRNA protein expression on survival in patients with NSCLC treated with gemcitabine (Ceppi et al., 2006)(Rosell et al., 2004). The data supporting a relationship between RRM1 polymorphisms is not as strong. There are two relatively common polymorphism in the European population c.2223A>G and 2464G>A with minor allele frequencies of 0.5 and 0.16 respectively. The 2464G>A has been shown to be associated with GEM sensitivity in vitro (Kwon et al., 2006)and haplotype is associated with response (but not survival) in patients with NSCLC treated with GEM (Kim et al., 2008). A small study suggested a relationship between -37C>A and progression free survival (PFS) (S. Dong et al., 2010).

3.4 hENT1

In patients with pancreatic cancer treated with gemcitabine hENT1 transcript levels were associated with survival (Giovannetti et al., 2006). However identified polymorphisms are infrequent (SNP:Geneview) and 201A>G has been identified with increased neutropenia (Tanaka et al., 2010). Sugiyama found no relationship with gemcitabine pharmacokinetics (Sugiyama et al., 2001)

Polymorphisms of other potentially important genes such as other transporters and DCK have not yet been shown to have clinical importance.

3.5 Haplotypes

There is a growing view that polymorphism in single genes are unlikely to be informative and that more relevant information is likely to come from sets of informative genes (haplotypes)(Kalow, 2006) or more complex genetic variations (Lee & Morton, 2008). Because of linkage disequilibrium, some combinations will occur more frequently than others and it is therefore possible to map the most common gene combinations and test their significance.

This approach has been taken with CDA in the Japanese population where one haplotype (of various CDA SNP's) termed *3 was associated with reduced clearance of gemcitabine and increased toxicity (Sugiyama et al., January 2010).

Tanaka et al have taken a comprehensive approach (Tanaka et al., 2010; Okazaki et al, 2010). They first screened 17 polymorphisms in relevant (CDA, *dCK, RRM1, hCNT2, hCNT3,* and *hENT1*) genes in a sample of 149 patients with pancreatic cancer receiving chemo-radiation and identified polymorphisms with significant associations for toxicity or trends for effects on survival. None of the SNP's singly was associated significantly with survival.

They then went on to examine the relationship between SNP's and identified that two or three SNPs each of the *dCK, RRM1, hCNT2, hCNT3,* and *hENT1* (IVS12-201A>G and IVS2-549T>C) genes were in linkage disequilibrium ($|D'|>0.5$, $P < 0.01$). This enabled identification of relevant haplotypes.

They next examined relationships between haplotypes and overall survival (OS). The *CDA* C111T and A-79C TA haplotype was significantly associated with increased risk and the *hENT1* A-201G, T-549C, and C913T ACT haplotype was significantly associated with reduced risk of death compared with the most common haplotype of each gene respectively ($P < 0.05$).

They were also able to examine the effects of gene dose by comparing outcomes according to the number of poor risk genotypes. Patients carrying 0 to 1 ($n = 43$), 2 to 3 ($n = 77$) or 4 to 6 ($n = 30$) variant alleles had a Median Survival time T of 31.5, 21.4, and 17.5 mo, respectively.

This work shows the need to consider multiple significant genes in determining significance and the added power this analysis brings. However as discussed below there are fundamental limitations to the SNP approach, that relate to the relationship between genotype and phenotype.

3.6 Considering the influence of transcription and translation

One of the limitations of focusing on genetic polymorphisms as causes of functional variation is the potential influence of gene silencing (Meister & Tuschl, 2004) transcriptional (Goth-Goldstein et al, 2000) and post transcriptional regulation on protein expression (Cress & Seto, 2000). DNA sequence is only one determinant of ultimate function. Genes can be silenced by methylation or acetylation, alternate splicing of gene transcripts can lead to differences in function and allelic imbalance can lead to increased expression. Environmental influences on transcription such as inhibition or induction by drugs or endogenous messages are critical. One way of accounting for these variations is to concentrate on measurement of phenotype rather than genotype (Mahgoub et al, 1977).

With CDA phenotype has been assessed ex vivo by incubation of mononuclear cells, plasma or red cell extracts with pyrimidine analogues and measurement of deamination.

Similarly a furthers study found phenotype as assessed by in vitro deamination correlated with toxicity whereas specific polymorphisms did not (Ciccolini et al., 2010; Mercier et al, 2007)

4. Challenges in measurement of intracellular PK

There are a number of challenges in the measurement of both GEM and the intracellular metabolite GEM-TP. The first of these is related to the fact that CDA is present in plasma, therefore every blood collection tubes requires the presence of tetrahydrouridine (THU) to inhibit CDA. If THU is not included all of the GEM will be converted to dFdU its inactive metabolite in plasma before it can even enter the cell to be converted to the active metabolite GEM-TP. The next challenge is the fact that white cells cannot be stored frozen without the loss of triphosphates, therefore the triphosphates need to be extracted from leucocytes before any of the sample is frozen. This is not a complex processes but does require time and some experience is necessary thus can not easily be performed by a nurse that generally collects the blood samples and adds to the complexity of the studies and probably the main reason why more intracellular measurements are not routinely conducted. The amount of leucocytes present in an individual blood sample is highly variable and can be effected markedly when patients are on chemotherapy. While the analysis of GEM and dFdU in plasma are relatively straight forward and can be quality controlled and give reliable results, the same cannot be said about the assay used to measure GEM-TP. This involves the use of an ion exchange column and high concentrations of salt to remove the triphosphate from the column. This makes the assay difficult to convert to more sensitive LCMS assays. It is not easy to quality control this assay which could lead to varying data being reported by different laboratoties.

5. Pharmacokinetics and dose optimisation

The pharmacokinetics of plasma Gemcitabine and its main metabolite have been described in multiple studies. The findings of the original phase 1 remain typical (JL Abbruzzese, et al., 1991). 77% of Gemcitabine was metabolised to dFdU and excreted in the urine in the first 24hrs dFdU clearance was proportional to creatinine clearance. The clearance of Gemcitabine in the plasma was rapid with a T1/2 of 8 mins. The clearance of GEM was independent of dose. The pharmacokinetics of GEM in some representative studies are shown in Table 1.

	Clearance (L/h/m²)	T1/2 min	AUC(μM*min)	Vss (L)	CMax(μM)
Soo et al., 2006					
Arm A (n29) FDR	164.0±64.0	18.2±4.2	1,346 ±1113	65 ± 37	21 ± 17
Arm B (n=29) 30 min	181.6±74.5	17.1±3.1	1,432 ±529	75 ±41	41 ± 14
Tempero, et al., 2003					
FDR					26 ± 6
Standard (higher dose)					100 ± 19
Grimison, et al 2007					
FDR n=31			1279±629		19± 6
Standard n=30			1642 ± 796		50± 18

Table 1. Representative Plasma Pharmacokinetic Data

The major clinical determinants of clearance are size and gender. The influence of size has been demonstrated through a correlation with BSA, which justifies the use of BSA to adjust dose. The influence of gender has been more variable although some studies show reduced clearance in women.

There is much less data on the pharmacokinetics of GEM-TP. Data from some representative studies are shown in Table 2. In the early development of Gemcitabine it was identified that exposed cells demonstrate saturable accumulation of the Triphosphate. This correlates with the biochemistry of accumulation and retention being limited by intracellular conversion to the Triphosphate by DCK. In phase 1 studies this translated to a saturation of Gemcitabine accumulation in mononuclear cells with increasing dose. This is accompanied by a change in the pattern of elimination with monophasic elimination at low concentrations and biphasic elimination described after the threshold has been reached.

	Clearance ($L/h/m^2$)	AUC(µM*min)	CMax(µM)
Soo et al., 2006			
Arm A (n29) FDR	5.2±2.0	35 079±18 216	174 ± 77
Arm B (n=29) 30 min	7.0±2.61	32 249±11 267	225 ± 74
(Tempero, et al., 2003)			
FDR			398
Standard (higher dose)			188
(Grimison, et al 2007)			
FDR n=31		2600 ± 2483	
Standard n=30		1833± 1833	

Table 2. Representative Intracellular Pharmacokinetic Data

The clinical correlate of this finding is that accumulation can be maximised by prolonging infusion time and indeed this is the case. Based on accumulation in leukemic blasts a target concentration and rate of administration was determined to maximise accumulation. There are several problems with this process. The target concentration and optimal rate of infusion has not been determined in solid tumours, where the kinetics are known to be different. Secondly the "optimum" rate of administration does not take into account inter-individual variation. Differential expression of DCK between tumours and normal tissue and between individuals would be expected to determine different optimum rates of administration.

The rationale for prolonged dosing received a major boost when a randomised phase 2 study demonstrated proof of principle that in a clinically relevant scenario (pancreatic cancer) prolonged infusion at a rate of 10 mg/m2/min (compared to a standard 30 min infusion) was associated with not only increased accumulation of GEM-TP, but with a trend for increased survival. This lead to a proliferation of similar studies in other tumour types confirming the pharmacokinetic finding but underpowered to demonstrate survival differences. Unfortunately a large phase 3 study, in pancreatic cancer, demonstrated that the pharmacological advantage obtained failed to translate into a significant survival advantage.

The challenges in optimising accumulation of Gemcitabine have been highlighted by data from our group showing an increase in Gemcitabine accumulation between week 1 and 2 with weekly administration (Grimison, et al., 2007). This suggests auto induction of Gemcitabine accumulation. In *vivo* modelling suggests this is a generic response to DNA damaging agents (Metharom, et al, 2010). The significance of this increase is not certain, with one study showing a non significant increase (de Lange et al., 2005), but it potentially complicates strategies to achieve a target intracellular concentration if the target changes over time.

We have furthered examined potential explanations for the discordance between the pharmacological advantage seen previously and the negative phase 3 study. Analysis of SNP's from our study has suggested that the pharmacological advantage of prolonged dose rate Gemcitabine is restricted to patients with the variant allele of c.CDA79A>C (Metharom et al., 2011). If this finding is confirmed, then the phase 3 study would have been underpowered to detect a survival difference in this population and consideration of the optimum dosing schedule may require individualisation according to genotype.

5.1 Pharmacokinetic/Pharmacodynamic relationships

The availability of pharmacokinetic data for both the prodrug and the active intracellular metabolite leads to the possibility of exploring differences in the ability of these parameters to predict drug effects of toxicity and efficacy.

There is data that demonstrates correlations between the concentration of Gemcitabine at the end of the infusion and haematological toxicity, however the relationship is weak. There is very limited data exploring the relationship between the pharmacokinetics of intracellular GEM-TP and toxicity. No relationship was seen in combination with Carboplatin (Soo et al., 2006) In our data GEM-TP cMax correlate with AUC and was used for pharmacodynamic correlations. Modelling GEM-TP concentrations to % reduction in white cells improved the fit of the model although the relationship remained modest (r^2 = 0.3739) (Grimison et al., 2007). This provides proof of concept that moving from the plasma to intracellular compartment did improve predictive ability, but that the proportion of variance related to pharmacodynamic variability and the relationship of the sampled compartment to the compartment of interest will determine the utility of this approach.

The relationship of pharmacokinetics to tumour response is much more difficult to assess as tumour Reponses are heterogeneous and seen in a minority of patients treated with Gemcitabine. This then requires PK sampling in large populations of patients, which is unattractive to designers of clinical trials and enrolled patients. As a result there are no large-scale studies correlating clinical benefit, response or survival endpoints with PK parameters. Reported pharmacokinetic/pharmacodynamic relationships are summarised in Table 3.

Treatment	Tumour	n	variable	Finding
Carboplatin and FDR GEM (Wang et al., 2007)	NSCLC	21	% reduction WBC and GEM-CMax	R2= 0.4575
			% reduction plat and GEM CMax	R2= 0.5671
Paclitaxel GEM (Fogli et al., 2001)			% reduction plat and GEM CMax	
High dose GEM and autologous stem cells (Bengala, et al., 2005)	pancreas	23	Mononuclear CDA activity and expression	Low activity /expression associated with response
Gemcitabine and RT (Eisbruch et al., 2001)	Head and neck	29		Poor correlation between dose and tumour concentration

Table 3. Pharmacokinetic/Pharmacodynamic relationships

6. Population models of Gemcitabine PK

6.1 Population PK models

Pharmacokinetic models are a mathematical shorthand way of describing PK data. In the most common approach to estimation of pharmacokinetic parameters, data from an *individual* is used to fit to a model and calculate variables such as clearance. Individual estimates of clearance then describe the population. In the population pharmacokinetic approach the data from the whole *population* is used to develop the model parameters and calculate variables, like clearance. The population approach is more complicated and requires more computing and human resources but has several advantages including the handling of sparse data. It is well positioned to include other co-variates in the model development such as clinical parameters (age, BSA, measure of renal or hepatic function) as well as novel laboratory measures. In both cases the model "compartments" are mathematical constructs rather than physiological compartments. Population PK modelling does lend itself to conforming the model to physiological compartments, which may also be sampled, such as plasma or an intracellular compartment. For a review of population PK modelling of anticancer agents the readers is referred to the review by Zandvliet et al. (2008).

6.2 Population PK models for Gemcitabine

There are 3 reported population pharmacokinetic models for plasma Gemcitabine and dFdU and one model that includes GEM-TP. Each GEM model fits for a 2 compartment model with a presumed peripheral and central compartment. Jiang et al derived our model from 94 patients with various malignancy treated on PK studies. Sugiyama et al derived a model from a population of 250 Japanese patients included in previous PK studies. Zhang et al derived their model from the data from original phase 1 studies. The model parameters for all three models are summarised in Table 4.

Study	Compartments	CL L/min	VC (l)	VP	RV
STG	2	2.7 (31%)	15 (39%)		40
Sugiyama *		1.24	12.6	9.54	
Zhang	2	NR	NR	NR	
Pham	2	5.1	2.96	47.6	35

CL=clearance; VC= volume central compartment VP = volume peripheral compartment and RV = residual variation
*calculated assuming a BSA of 1.78, Cr=100mg/dL age 62.67 and median values for male and female

Table 4. Parameters from Gemcitabine Population Pk Models.

The models allow some significant observations. Significant covariates included in the final version of all models include BSA, age and sex. This confirms univariate observations from individual PK data. The inclusion of BSA is an important observation given the debate over whether clinical doses should be adjusted for BSA for anticancer drugs.

The models also allow evaluation of potential drug interactions with co-administered drugs. The Jiang model compared the impact of co-administered of oxaliplatin with a 35-45% decrease in the Vc for dFdU.

The patients in the Sugiyama paper were administered a variety of partner drugs and this allowed evaluation of potential interactions. They were able to demonstrate a 20% increase in the clearance of GEM following S1, a potentially clinically relevant observation. The speculative mechanism is an increase in hENT1 expression. This demonstrates the relevance of considering intracellular pharmacokinetics because an increase in clearance into the intracellular compartment (which is greater in tumours) has a different implication to an increase in clearance due to increased excretion. A summary of findings of each model for significant covariates is given in Table 5.

Author	n	Examined	Significant	Comments
Sugiyama	248	(BSA), weight, age and sex and co-administered drugs, cisplatin, carboplatin, fluorouracil, S-1, vinorelbine	Including BSA improved modelling of clearance S-1 significantly increased CL	Age and sex did not significantly affect the CL and V1 of Gemcitabine.
Zhang	353	age, sex,(BSA), type of cancer, renal function, rate, and duration of infusion, plasma CDA activity	BSA on Clpc, Vpc,and Vpp,gen-der on Clpc and Vpc,ageon Clpc, and duration of infusion on Vpp.	Note plasma CDA not significant
Tham	56	age, body size, (KPS), stage, creatinine clearance, sex, race, and Smoking history.	Weight and height	No improvement with allometric scaling; fat content can be ignored when using size variable. The influence of sex disappeared when considering lean body mass

Table 5. Co-variates examined versus included in GEM models

6.3 GEM Pop PK including pharmacogenetic variables

The Sugiyama model also investigated the influence of several pharmacogenetic variants in the Japanese population. They had previously reported a variant CDA 208G>A (associated with the*3 haplotype) with a minor allele frequency of 0.022 in the Japanese population as associated with increased toxicity in homozygous patients (Sugiyama, et al., 2009).

They investigated the role of this other polymorphisms in CDA, DCK and hent1 (SLC29A1) and evaluated included the following found common polymorphism in the base model CDA A79>C variant (allele frequency 0.208); -31delC (0.44); 2 polymorphisms in the hENT 1 gene-3797A>G (0.398) and -3268_-3249del AGGCTCGCGAGCGGAGGTGC (0.398). The significance of the final model was driven by CDA*3 , although -31delc and CDA A79>C also contributed. The significance of the *2 haplotype in the absence of *3 (as is seen in Caucasians) is not clear from their model.

One interesting piece of data relating pharmacogenetic and PK comes from a very simple study where the deamination rate of red cell extracts was measured and correlated with genotype (Giovannetti et al., June xx 2008). Mean enzymatic activity was significantly lower in patients carrying the CDA Lys27Lys than in patients with the Lys27Gln or Gln27Gln protein. This highlights the potential of measuring activity in accessible targets (such as ex-vivo plasma) to model phenotype, and explores phenotype-genotype correlations.

6.4 Population PK including intracellular GEM-TP

Zhang et al were able to extend the population model to include estimation of GEM-TP. They used the existing plasma GEM model and added an extra compartment (the intracellular compartment). GEM-TP concentrations were explained by a simple Michaelis-Menten formula. No additional parameters were investigated and the Km was fixed at the median value and the infusion rate was fixed at 10mg/m2/min.

(Tham et al., 2008) also derived a population PK model with intracellular compartment by adding an extra compartment to the Gemcitabine plasma 2 compartment model. They concluded, in comparison, that the GEM-TP was equally as well explained by a linear model, and therefore saturable metabolism did not occur. Interpretation of their data is complicated because it appears that fixed dose rate and standard dose rate Gemcitabine data has been lumped together despite previous data that saturation only occurs with the standard dose rate regimen.

The disparity in interpretations also highlights the assumptions brought to bear in selecting pharmacokinetic models. Tham et al have selected the most parsimonious model and concluded that there was no evidence to support a saturable model; Zhang et al have fitted a Michaelis-Menten model based on previous data and found that it describes their data adequately. This reflects a basic debate about whether science is assumption free. Karl Popper has eloquently argued that all science is based on assumptions. Rejecting the saturable PK model on the basis of lack of improvement in the objective variable should not be taken to mean that saturable metabolism does not occur, just that in this data set the model did not improve performance.

6.5 Physiological modelling

A very sophisticated approach has been taken by (Battaglia & Parker, 2011) they have constructed an intracellular accumulation model based on existing plasma PK models. They have created a physiological based model of Gemcitabine intracellular accumulation with initial estimates based on cell line measurements. They have modelled each of the parameters as first order but the overall model produces saturable metabolism due to the interactions built in. The model includes a variable for the dose rate and includes such physiologic processes as self- potentiation and cell cycle specificity, and diffusion through the interstitial space into solid tumours.

This work demonstrates the potential of combining measurement of clinically relevant compartments with an understanding of the biology involved. One application of such models is that it can be used to drive clinical trial design to determine the optimum conditions for maximising tumour exposure under a variety of circumstances. This can potentially lead to more efficient clinical trial design.

6.6 Modelling of response

The relationship of pharmacokinetics to response is much more difficult to assess as tumour reponses are heterogeneous and seen in a minority of patients treated with Gemcitabine. This then requires PK sampling in large populations' of patients, which is unattractive to designers of clinical trials and to enrolled patients. There is however one very interesting attempt to do this in the literature. Data from a randomised phase 2 study of fixed dose versus standard dose rate administration of Gemcitabine was used to provide PK data and measurements of individual tumours. The pharmacokinetic parameters were estimated from the previously derived 4 compartment population model. The tumour effect compartment was then modelled according to a delayed exposure to estimate tumour exposure. The inhibitory effect of drug exposure on tumour growth was then modelled (from the change in size of the tumour) by a Gompterzian tumour growth model. The impact of drug exposure on tumour inhibition was then tested by Emax, or sigmoid Emax, models with exposure estimated by either dose or estimated AUC. In the final model using Intra-cellular GEM-TP AUC did not improve the fit over using Gemcitabine dose. Interestingly the dose response variability of 146% was much greater than the interpatient variability in Gemcitabine clearance, suggesting that a target concentration approach would not be helpful in dose individualisation.

This work represents a "heroic" attempt to take the PK/PD modelling to its logical extreme, however the interpretation of the observation that intra-cellular GEM-TP did not improve the -prediction of response should be coloured by a realisation of the limitation of the model. Firstly the PK model, the tumour growth model and the final PK/PD model are all based on data from a relatively small number of patients. Secondly the measurements that they are based upon e.g. GEM-TP and tumour size -have relatively large errors. Thirdly the three inter-related models are all based on the assumptions outlined in the paper. Many of these are unlikely to be true, such as the independence of Gemcitabine and Carboplatin. Finally the significance of the observation that a particular co-variate does not improve the fit of the model does depend on the overall fit of the model. Obviously a very poor model will not be sensitive to variations in the inputs chosen; it will perform equally well - or equally poorly. In this regard the overall model has very wide confidence interval the median tumour size at 12 weeks is approximately 4cm with a 95% confidence interval of 2.5-12cm, clinically very significant differences. The relevance of the Gomptzerian model is also in question as it is now very clear that a major part of the benefit of cytotoxic therapy relates to the achievement of prolonged stable disease and tumour dormancy rather than tumour response. Nevertheless this work is a very exciting demonstration of the possibilities of incorporating tumour response into well understood pharmacokinetic models.

6.7 Discussion

These data demonstrate some of the possible applications of a population PK approach. The limitations of each model also demonstrate the potential of using models, which are one step closer to the source.

The Sugiyama model is a very exciting step towards the incorporation of pharmacogenetic data to inform model development. Any pharmacogenetic model will be constrained by the population it is developed in hence the dominant effect of the *3 mutation, which is extremely infrequent in the Caucasian population, may obscure the effects of other polymorphisms in other populations.

The major step towards developing a physiologically based model would be to apply the polymorphisms to the model in a physiologically informed way. CDA is going to be the main determinant of plasma clearance, so its incorporation into the elimination from the central or peripheral compartment is most relevant. However DCK and hENT1 are determinants of uptake into the intracellular compartment. The greatest potential then would be to model them as variants of the transfer into the intracellular compartment.

A further step towards more informative models would be to use preclinical data to inform initial model parameters for variables such as the relationship between GEM-TP accumulation and drug concentration.

7. Discussion and future directions

Gemcitabine provides a model for the study of intracellular pharmacokinetics as a way of moving one step closer to the target. The improved correlation of GEM-TP pharmacokinetics with pharmacodynamic endpoints such as dose reduction or leukocyte nadir is proof of principle that this provides important additional information. Given the accessible nature of this compartment it is difficult to see why correlative studies should continue to pursue plasma pharmacokinetics as an endpoint.

However the data presented also demonstrates the limitations of intracellular-pharmacokinetics. The tissue sampled in this literature is leucocytes, which are presumed to be a surrogate marker of normal tissue and or tumour uptake. The correlation with other normal tissues is the less problematical assumption, as the genotype is the same. It is worth considering in what ways leucocytes are different from other target tissues such as bone marrow progenitor cells.

Firstly the regulation and expression of genes is tissue specific with upregulation of DCK and CDA in tumour tissue (Spasokoukotskaja et al., 1995; van der Wilt et al., 2003). Lack of correlation between genotype and phenotype is an issue with highly regulated genes such as CYP450, which are induced and inhibited by drugs and environmental exposures (Shiran et al., 2003). Secondly issues around tissue penetration into compartments such as the CSF, brain, etc are highly relevant for tumour metastases. Finally the tumour microenvironment is one that provides multiple barriers to drug access such as tumour hypoperfusion, increased interstitial pressure (Willett et al., 2004) and stromal reactions around tumours(Minchinton & Tannock, 2006). There is some evidence that these factors are critical in determining intratumoral and intertumoural heterogeneity in drug exposure (Zamboni et al., 2002; C. A. Presant et al., 1994).

Even given these limitations there are still a number of significant opportunities associated with the ability to measure pharmacokinetics in the intracellular compartment. The first is the ability to assess the clinical significance of availability in genes of known importance. As summarised above there are a great number of potential sources of variability in intracellular Gemcitabine uptake. However the source of human variability in uptake is an empirical question. Early pharmacogenetic evidence already suggests that this may be population specific (Fukunaga et al., 2004). Measurement of intracellular pharmacokinetics allows questions to be asked regarding correlation between variation in genes such as CDA and intracellular uptake. The time taken to perform studies with surrogate makers such as intracellular uptake is much shorter than those requiring clinical endpoints such as survival. This allows prioritisation of potential markers for prospective validation.

A second possibility for the utility of intracellular pharmacokinetics is in the development of strategies for therapeutic dose monitoring. Moving closer to the target increases the possibility of developing an effective TDM strategy. However data from pharmacodynamic modelling suggest the greater part of interpatient variability comes from pharmacodynamic variables suggesting limited value from pharmacokinetic monitoring (Tham et al., 2008). Related to this is a third possibility of pharmacogenetically derived dosing where known polymorphisms in genes of interest affects the dose or scheduling of the drug administered (Ciccolini et al, 2011).

A significant challenge relates to application of pharmacogenetic strategies where drugs are given in combinations. This requires a clear understanding of the effects of the drugs on each other, for example the effect of DNA damaging agents on Gemcitabine accumulation (Metharom et al, 2010) and the conditions under which drugs act synergistically (Luk et al, 2011).

Optimising the dosing of Gemcitabine according to a rational understanding of an individual patients threshold for saturation of GEM-TP is a rational strategy for reducing toxicity and improving efficacy.

A conventional strategy for optimising dose is to build upon a population pharmacokinetic model where clinical or laboratory variables of interest are correlated with clinical outcomes. The next step with such a model would be to incorporate pharmacogenetic variables of interest such as measurement of CDA genotype of phenotype. Determining the coefficients by which the impact of such variables can be adjusted will require very large clinical studies. Intracellular PK measurements offer the possibility of providing initial estimates of such variables from smaller correlative studies both in vivo and in-vitro. The advantage over other scenarios such as liver oxidation or glucuronidation is that the genes are measurable and the pharmacokinetic intermediate is assessable. This is an important area of inquiry to lead us to a goal of a pharmacogenetically guided individualised dosing strategy.

These strategies are of course complimentary to those aimed at measuring drug distribution directly in tissues of interest by the use of tracer radio-pharmaceuticals, microdialysis, NMR or PET. The common theme is that facilitating the contribution of pharmacokinetics to optimising drug administration in oncology requires us to move closer and closer to the target of interest. A variety of techniques to measure intracellular uptake as well as tissue penetration and access to the tumour microenvironment are likely to be required to minimise the effect of drug variability on the response to anticancer treatments. Combining mesurement of more relevant compartments with physiologic modelling and incorporation of pharmacogenetic variation, raises a real possibility of predicting drug response in a way that realises the hopes of individualised medicine.

8. Appendix

Background information on Single Nucleotide Polymorphisms

Finding information

The NCI maintains a database of polymorphism (dbSNP) [1]

Nomenclature

Polymorphisms can be referred to by their unique identifier (rs number) but are preferably described at the DNA level[2] for example

Rs2072671 describes the polymorphism CDA c.79A>C

- which occurs in the CDA gene:
- where the c stands for coding sequence;
- 79 is the first nucleotide affected;
- and the nucleotide A is substitute for C.

This results in a protein change described as p.K27Q where the p stands for protein and the K and Q are exchanged at the 27th amino acid position. Nomenclature for haplotypes becomes more complicated. Because of the sometime complicated nomenclature for complex polymorphisms or haplotypes they are usually given nicknames e.g. *1, *2 etc.

9. References

Abbruzzese, JL, Grunewald, R., Weeks, E., Gravel, D., Adams, T., Nowak, B., Mineishi, S., et al. (1991). A phase I clinical, plasma, and cellular pharmacology study of gemcitabine. *Journal of Clinical Oncology*, *9*(3), 491 -498.

Battaglia, M. A., & Parker, R. S. (2011). Pharmacokinetic/pharmacodynamic modelling of intracellular gemcitabine triphosphate accumulation: translating in vitro to in vivo. *IET Systems Biology*, *5*(1), 34. doi:10.1049/iet-syb.2009.0073

Bengala, C., Guarneri, V., Giovannetti, E, Lencioni, M., Fontana, E., Mey, V, Fontana, A., et al. (2005). Prolonged fixed dose rate infusion of gemcitabine with autologous haemopoietic support in advanced pancreatic adenocarcinoma. *Br J Cancer*, *93*(1), 35-40.

Breedveld, P., Pluim, D., Cipriani, G., Wielinga, P., van Tellingen, O., Schinkel, A. H., & Schellens, J. H. M. (2005). The Effect of Bcrp1 (Abcg2) on the In vivo Pharmacokinetics and Brain Penetration of Imatinib Mesylate (Gleevec): Implications for the Use of Breast Cancer Resistance Protein and P-Glycoprotein Inhibitors to Enable the Brain Penetration of Imatinib in Patients. *Cancer Research*, *65*(7), 2577 -2582. doi:10.1158/0008-5472.CAN-04-2416

Ceppi, P., Volante, M., Novello, S., Rapa, I., Danenberg, K., Danenberg, P., Cambieri, A., et al. (2006). ERCC1 and RRM1 gene expressions but not EGFR are predictive of shorter survival in advanced non-small-cell lung cancer treated with cisplatin and gemcitabine. *Annals of Oncology*, *17*(12), 1818 -1825. doi:10.1093/annonc/mdl300

Ciccolini, J., Dahan, L., André, N., Evrard, A., Duluc, M., Blesius, A., Yang, C., et al. (2010). Cytidine Deaminase Residual Activity in Serum Is a Predictive Marker of Early

Severe Toxicities in Adults After Gemcitabine-Based Chemotherapies. *Journal of Clinical Oncology, 28*(1), 160 -165. doi:10.1200/JCO.2009.24.4491

Ciccolini, J., Mercier, C., Dahan, L., & André, N. (2011). Integrating pharmacogenetics into gemcitabine dosing-time for a change? *Nature Reviews. Clinical Oncology, 8*(7), 439-444. doi:10.1038/nrclinonc.2011.1

Cress, W. D., & Seto, E. (2000). Histone deacetylases, transcriptional control, and cancer. *Journal of Cellular Physiology, 184*(1), 1-16. doi:10.1002/(SICI)1097-4652(200007)184:1<1::AID-JCP1>3.0.CO;2-7

Danesi, Romano, Altavilla, G., Giovannetti, Elisa, & Rosell, Raffael. (2009). Pharmacogenomics of gemcitabine in non-small-cell lung cancer and other solid tumors. *Pharmacogenomics, 10*(1), 69-80. doi:10.2217/14622416.10.1.69

Dong, S., Guo, A.-L., Chen, Z.-H., Wang, Z., Zhang, X.-C., Huang, Y., Xie, Z., et al. (2010). RRM1 single nucleotide polymorphism -37C→A correlates with progression-free survival in NSCLC patients after gemcitabine-based chemotherapy. *Journal of Hematology & Oncology, 3*(1), 10. doi:10.1186/1756-8722-3-10

Dumontet, C., Fabianowska-Majewska, K., Mantincic, D., Callet Bauchu, E., Tigaud, I., Gandhi, V., Lepoivre, M., et al. (1999). Common resistance mechanisms to deoxynucleoside analogues in variants of the human erythroleukaemic line K562. *British Journal of Haematology, 106*(1), 78-85.

Eisbruch, A., Shewach, D. S., Bradford, C. R., Littles, J. F., Teknos, T. N., Chepeha, D. B., Marentette, L. J., et al. (2001). Radiation Concurrent With Gemcitabine for Locally Advanced Head and Neck Cancer: A Phase I Trial and Intracellular Drug Incorporation Study. *Journal of Clinical Oncology, 19*(3), 792 -799.

Fogli, S., Danesi, R., De Braud, F., De Pas, T., Curigliano, G., Giovannetti, E., & Tacca, M. D. (2001). Drug distribution and pharmacokinetic/pharmacodynamic relationship of paclitaxel and gemcitabine in patients with non-small-cell lung cancer. *Annals of Oncology, 12*(11), 1553 -1559.

Fukunaga, A. K., Marsh, S., Murry, D. J., Hurley, T. D., & McLeod, H. L. (2004). Identification and analysis of single-nucleotide polymorphisms in the gemcitabine pharmacologic pathway. *The Pharmacogenomics Journal, 4*(5), 307-314. doi:10.1038/sj.tpj.6500259

Galmarini, C. M., Mackey, J. R., & Dumontet, C. (2001). Nucleoside analogues: mechanisms of drug resistance and reversal strategies. *Leukemia: Official Journal of the Leukemia Society of America, Leukemia Research Fund, U.K, 15*(6), 875-890.

Giovannetti, E., Laan, A. C., Vasile, E., Tibaldi, C., Nannizzi, S., Ricciardi, S., Falcone, A., Danesi, R., & Peters, G. J. (June xx 2008). Correlation between cytidine deaminase genotype and gemcitabine deamination in blood samples (pp. 720-725). Retrieved from http://www.ncbi.nlm.nih.gov/pubmed/18600531?ordinalpos=2&itool=EntrezSystem2.PEntrez.Pubmed.Pubmed_ResultsPanel.Pubmed_DefaultReportPanel.Pubmed_RVDocSum

Giovannetti, Elisa, Del Tacca, Mario, Mey, Valentina, Funel, N., Nannizzi, Sara, Ricci, Sergio, Orlandini, C., et al. (2006). Transcription Analysis of Human Equilibrative Nucleoside Transporter-1 Predicts Survival in Pancreas Cancer Patients Treated with Gemcitabine. *Cancer Research, 66*(7), 3928 -3935. doi:10.1158/0008-5472.CAN-05-4203

Goth-Goldstein, R., Stampfer, M. R., Erdmann, C. A., & Russell, M. (2000). Interindividual variation in CYP1A1 expression in breast tissue and the role of genetic polymorphism. *Carcinogenesis, 21*(11), 2119 -2122. doi:10.1093/carcin/21.11.2119

Graham, K. A., Leithoff, J., Coe, I. R., Mowles, D., Mackey, J. R., Young, J. D., & Cass, C. E. (2000). Differential transport of cytosine-containing nucleosides by recombinant human concentrative nucleoside transporter protein hCNT1. *Nucleosides, Nucleotides & Nucleic Acids, 19*(1-2), 415-434. doi:10.1080/15257770008033018

Grimison, P., Galettis, P., Manners, S., Jelinek, M., Metharom, E., de Souza, P. L., Liauw, W., et al. (2007). Randomized crossover study evaluating the effect of gemcitabine infusion dose rate: evidence of auto-induction of gemcitabine accumulation. *Journal of Clinical Oncology: Official Journal of the American Society of Clinical Oncology, 25*(36), 5704-5709. doi:10.1200/JCO.2007.10.7078

Gupta, N., Price, P. M., & Aboagye, E. O. (2002). PET for in vivo pharmacokinetic and pharmacodynamic measurements. *European Journal of Cancer, 38*(16), 2094-2107. doi:16/S0959-8049(02)00413-6

Heinemann, V., Xu, Y.-Z., Chubb, Sherri, Sen, A., Hertel, Larry W., Grindey, Gerald B., & Plunkett, William. (1992). Cellular Elimination of 2′,2′-Difluorodeoxycytidine 5′-Triphosphate: A Mechanism of Self-Potentiation. *Cancer Research, 52*(3), 533 -539.

Hodge, L. S., Taub, M. E., & Tracy, T. S. (2011). Effect of its deaminated metabolite, 2′,2′-difluorodeoxyuridine, on the transport and toxicity of gemcitabine in HeLa cells. *Biochemical Pharmacology, 81*(7), 950-956. doi:10.1016/j.bcp.2011.01.016

Huang, P., Chubb, S, Hertel, L W, Grindey, G B, & Plunkett, W. (1991). Action of 2′,2′-difluorodeoxycytidine on DNA synthesis. *Cancer Research, 51*(22), 6110-6117.

Jain, R. K. (1987). Transport of Molecules in the Tumor Interstitium: A Review. *Cancer Research, 47*(12), 3039 -3051.

Joerger, M., Burgers, J. A., Baas, P., Doodeman, V. D., Smits, P. H. M., Jansen, R. S., Vainchtein, L. D., et al. (2011). Gene polymorphisms, pharmacokinetics, and hematological toxicity in advanced non-small-cell lung cancer patients receiving cisplatin/gemcitabine. *Cancer Chemotherapy and Pharmacology*. doi:10.1007/s00280-011-1670-4

Kalow, W. (2006). Pharmacogenetics and pharmacogenomics: origin, status, and the hope for personalized medicine. *Pharmacogenomics J, 6*(3), 162-165.

Kim, S.-O., Jeong, J.-Y., Kim, M.-R., Cho, H.-J., Ju, J.-Y., Kwon, Y.-S., Oh, I.-J., et al. (May 15 2008). Efficacy of gemcitabine in patients with non-small cell lung cancer according to promoter polymorphisms of the ribonucleotide reductase M1 gene (pp. 3083-3088). Retrieved from http://www.ncbi.nlm.nih.gov/pubmed/18483375?ordinalpos=11&itool=EntrezSystem2.PEntrez.Pubmed.Pubmed_ResultsPanel.Pubmed_DefaultReportPanel.Pubmed_RVDocSum

Kwon, W. S., Rha, S. Y., Choi, Y. H., Lee, J. O., Park, K. H., Jung, J. J., Kim, T. S., et al. (June xx 2006). Ribonucleotide reductase M1 (RRM1) 2464G>A polymorphism shows an association with gemcitabine chemosensitivity in cancer cell lines (pp. 429-438). Retrieved from http://www.ncbi.nlm.nih.gov/pubmed/16708051

de Lange, S. M., van der Born, K., Kroep, J. R., Jensen, H. A., Pfeiffer, P., Cleverly, A., van Groeningen, C. J., et al. (2005). No evidence of gemcitabine accumulation during weekly administration. *European Journal of Clinical Pharmacology, 61*(11), 843-849. doi:10.1007/s00228-005-0033-7

Lee, C., & Morton, C. C. (2008). Structural genomic variation and personalized medicine. *The New England Journal of Medicine, 358*(7), 740-741. doi:10.1056/NEJMcibr0708452

Liotta, L. A., & Kohn, E. C. (2001). The microenvironment of the tumour-host interface. *Nature, 411*(6835), 375-379. doi:10.1038/35077241

Luk, P. P., Galettis, P., & Links, M. (2011). ERK phosphorylation predicts synergism between gemcitabine and the epidermal growth factor receptor inhibitor AG1478. *Lung Cancer (Amsterdam, Netherlands), 73*(3), 274-282. doi:10.1016/j.lungcan.2010.12.016

Mackey, J. R., Mani, R. S., Selner, M., Mowles, D., Young, J. D., Belt, J. A., Crawford, C. R., et al. (1998). Functional nucleoside transporters are required for gemcitabine influx and manifestation of toxicity in cancer cell lines. *Cancer Research, 58*(19), 4349-4357.

Mahgoub, A., Dring, L. G., Idle, J. R., Lancaster, R., & Smith, R. L. (1977). POLYMORPHIC HYDROXYLATION OF DEBRISOQUINE IN MAN. *The Lancet, 310*(8038), 584-586. doi:16/S0140-6736(77)91430-1

Maring, J. G., Wachters, F. M., Slijfer, M., Maurer, J. M., Boezen, H. M., Uges, D. R. A., de Vries, E. G. E., et al. (2010). Pharmacokinetics of gemcitabine in non-small-cell lung cancer patients: impact of the 79A>C cytidine deaminase polymorphism. *European Journal of Clinical Pharmacology, 66*(6), 611-617. doi:10.1007/s00228-010-0799-0

Meister, G., & Tuschl, T. (2004). Mechanisms of gene silencing by double-stranded RNA. *Nature, 431*(7006), 343-349. doi:10.1038/nature02873

Mercier, C., Evrard, A., & Ciccolini, J. (2007). Genotype-based methods for anticipating gemcitabine-related severe toxicities may lead to false-negative results. *Journal of Clinical Oncology: Official Journal of the American Society of Clinical Oncology, 25*(30), 4855; author reply 4855-4856. doi:10.1200/JCO.2007.13.3918

Metharom, E., Galettis, P., Manners, S., & Links, M. (2010). Modulation of gemcitabine accumulation by DNA-damaging agents: mechanisms and specificity in an in vitro model. *Anticancer Res, 30*(9), 3669-3673.

Metharom, E., Galettis, P., Manners, S., Jelinek, M., Liauw, W., de Souza, P. L., Hoskins, J. M., et al. (2011). The pharmacological advantage of prolonged dose rate gemcitabine is restricted to patients with variant alleles of cytidine deaminase c.79A>C. *Asia Pac J Clin Oncol, 7*(1), 65-74. doi:10.1111/j.1743-7563.2010.01354.x

Minchinton, A. I., & Tannock, I. F. (2006). Drug penetration in solid tumours. *Nat Rev Cancer, 6*(8), 583-592. doi:10.1038/nrc1893

Müller, M., Mader, R. M., Steiner, B., Steger, G. G., Jansen, B., Gnant, M., Helbich, T., et al. (1997). 5-Fluorouracil Kinetics in the Interstitial Tumor Space: Clinical Response in Breast Cancer Patients. *Cancer Research, 57*(13), 2598 -2601.

Nakano, Y., Tanno, S., Koizumi, K., Nishikawa, T., Nakamura, K., Minoguchi, M., Izawa, T., et al. (February 12 2007). Gemcitabine chemoresistance and molecular markers associated with gemcitabine transport and metabolism in human pancreatic cancer cells (pp. 457-463). Retrieved from http://www.ncbi.nlm.nih.gov/pubmed/17224927?ordinalpos=47&itool=EntrezSystem2.PEntrez.Pubmed.Pubmed_ResultsPanel.Pubmed_DefaultReportPanel.Pubmed_RVDocSum

Okazaki, T., Javle, M., Tanaka, M., Abbruzzese, J. L., & Li, D. (2010). Single nucleotide polymorphisms of gemcitabine metabolic genes and pancreatic cancer survival and drug toxicity. *Clinical Cancer Research: An Official Journal of the American Association for Cancer Research, 16*(1), 320-329. doi:10.1158/1078-0432.CCR-09-1555

Olsen, K., San Pedro, G., Gann, L., Gubbins, P., Halinski, D., & Campbell, G. (1996). Intrapulmonary pharmacokinetics of azithromycin in healthy volunteers given five oral doses. *Antimicrob. Agents Chemother., 40*(11), 2582-2585. doi:<p></p>

Plunkett, W, Huang, P., Searcy, C. E., & Gandhi, V. (1996). Gemcitabine: preclinical pharmacology and mechanisms of action. *Seminars in Oncology, 23*(5 Suppl 10), 3-15.

Presant, C. A., Wolf, W., Waluch, V., Wiseman, C., Kennedy, P., Blayney, D., Waluch, V., et al. (1994). Association of intratumoral pharmacokinetics of fluorouracil with clinical response. *The Lancet, 343*(8907), 1184-1187. doi:16/S0140-6736(94)92399-X

Presant, C., Wolf, W., Albright, M., Servis, K., Ring, R., Atkinson, D., Ong, R., et al. (1990). Human tumor fluorouracil trapping: clinical correlations of in vivo 19F nuclear magnetic resonance spectroscopy pharmacokinetics. *Journal of Clinical Oncology, 8*(11), 1868 -1873.

Recommendations for the description of sequence variants. (2011, January). . Human Genome Variation Society. Retrieved from http://www.hgvs.org/mutnomen/recs.html

Reid, J. M., Pendergrass, T. W., Krailo, M. D., Hammond, G. D., & Ames, M. M. (1990). Plasma Pharmacokinetics and Cerebrospinal Fluid Concentrations of Idarubicin and Idarubicinol in Pediatric Leukemia Patients: A Childrens Cancer Study Group Report. *Cancer Research, 50*(20), 6525 -6528.

Rosell, Rafael, Danenberg, K. D., Alberola, V., Bepler, G., Sanchez, J. J., Camps, C., Provencio, M., et al. (2004). Ribonucleotide Reductase Messenger RNA Expression and Survival in Gemcitabine/Cisplatin-Treated Advanced Non-Small Cell Lung Cancer Patients. *Clinical Cancer Research, 10*(4), 1318 -1325. doi:10.1158/1078-0432.CCR-03-0156

Schentag, J. J., & Ballow, C. H. (1991). Tissue-directed pharmacokinetics. *The American Journal of Medicine, 91*(3, Supplement 1), S5-S11. doi:16/0002-9343(91)90394-D

Sherry, S. T., Ward, M. H., Kholodov, M., Baker, J., Phan, L., Smigielski, E. M., & Sirotkin, K. (2001). dbSNP: the NCBI database of genetic variation. *Nucleic Acids Research, 29*(1), 308-311.

Shewach, D. S., & Lawrence, T. S. (2003). It's what's inside that counts. *Journal of Clinical Oncology: Official Journal of the American Society of Clinical Oncology, 21*(18), 3383-3384. doi:10.1200/JCO.2003.05.081

Shiran, M. R., Chowdry, J., Rostami-Hodjegan, A., Ellis, S. W., Lennard, M. S., Iqbal, M. Z., Lagundoye, O., et al. (2003). A discordance between cytochrome P450 2D6 genotype and phenotype in patients undergoing methadone maintenance treatment. *British Journal of Clinical Pharmacology, 56*(2), 220-224. doi:10.1046/j.1365-2125.2003.01851.x

Soo, R A, Wang, L Z, Tham, L S, Yong, W P, Boyer, M., Lim, H. L., Lee, H S, et al. (2006). A multicentre randomised phase II study of carboplatin in combination with gemcitabine at standard rate or fixed dose rate infusion in patients with advanced stage non-small-cell lung cancer. *Annals of Oncology: Official Journal of the European Society for Medical Oncology / ESMO, 17*(7), 1128-1133. doi:10.1093/annonc/mdl084

Soo, Ross A., Wang, Ling Zhi, Ng, S. S., Chong, P. Y., Yong, Wei Peng, Lee, Soo Chin, Liu, J. J., et al. (2009). Distribution of gemcitabine pathway genotypes in ethnic Asians and their association with outcome in non-small cell lung cancer patients. *Lung Cancer, 63*(1), 121-127. doi:16/j.lungcan.2008.04.010

Spasokoukotskaja, T., Arnér, E. S., Brosjö, O., Gunvén, P., Juliusson, G., Liliemark, J., & Eriksson, S. (1995). Expression of deoxycytidine kinase and phosphorylation of 2-chlorodeoxyadenosine in human normal and tumour cells and tissues. *European Journal of Cancer (Oxford, England: 1990), 31A*(2), 202-208.

Sugiyama, E., Kaniwa, N., Kim, S.-R., Kikura-Hanajiri, R., Hasegawa, R., Maekawa, K., Saito, Y., et al. (January 2010). Pharmacokinetics of gemcitabine in Japanese cancer patients: the impact of a cytidine deaminase polymorphism (pp. 32-42). Retrieved from http://www.ncbi.nlm.nih.gov/pubmed/17194903?ordinalpos=15&itool=EntrezSystem2.PEntrez.Pubmed.Pubmed_ResultsPanel.Pubmed_DefaultReportPanel.Pubmed_RVDocSum

Sugiyama, E., Lee, S.-J., Lee, S. S., Kim, W.-Y., Kim, S.-R., Tohkin, M., Hasegawa, R., et al. (2009). Ethnic differences of two non-synonymous single nucleotide polymorphisms in CDA gene. *Drug Metabolism and Pharmacokinetics, 24*(6), 553-556.

Tanaka, M., Javle, M., Dong, X., Eng, C., Abbruzzese, J. L., & Li, D. (2010). Gemcitabine metabolic and transporter gene polymorphisms are associated with drug toxicity and efficacy in patients with locally advanced pancreatic cancer. *Cancer, 116*(22), 5325-5335. doi:10.1002/cncr.25282

Tempero, M., Plunkett, William, Ruiz Van Haperen, V., Hainsworth, J., Hochster, H., Lenzi, R., & Abbruzzese, James. (2003). Randomized phase II comparison of dose-intense gemcitabine: thirty-minute infusion and fixed dose rate infusion in patients with pancreatic adenocarcinoma. *Journal of Clinical Oncology: Official Journal of the American Society of Clinical Oncology, 21*(18), 3402-3408. doi:10.1200/JCO.2003.09.140

Tham, L.-S., Wang, L.-Z., Soo, Ross A, Lee, H.-S., Lee, S.-C., Goh, B.-C., & Holford, N. H. G. (2008). Does saturable formation of gemcitabine triphosphate occur in patients? *Cancer Chemotherapy and Pharmacology, 63*(1), 55-64. doi:10.1007/s00280-008-0707-9

Tham, L.-S., Wang, Lingzhi, Soo, Ross A., Lee, S.-C., Lee, H.-S., Yong, W.-P., Goh, B.-C., et al. (2008). A Pharmacodynamic Model for the Time Course of Tumor Shrinkage by Gemcitabine + Carboplatin in Non–Small Cell Lung Cancer Patients. *Clinical Cancer Research, 14*(13), 4213 -4218. doi:10.1158/1078-0432.CCR-07-4754

Veltkamp, S. A., Pluim, D., van Eijndhoven, M. A. J., Bolijn, M. J., Ong, F. H. G., Govindarajan, R., Unadkat, J. D., et al. (2008). New insights into the pharmacology and cytotoxicity of gemcitabine and 2′,2′-difluorodeoxyuridine. *Molecular Cancer Therapeutics, 7*(8), 2415-2425. doi:10.1158/1535-7163.MCT-08-0137

Wang, Linrun, Wu, X., Huang, M., Cai, J., Xu, N., & Liu, J. (2007). The efficacy and relationship between peak concentration and toxicity profile of fixed-dose-rate gemcitabine plus carboplatin in patients with advanced non-small-cell lung cancer. *Cancer Chemotherapy and Pharmacology, 60*(2), 211-218. doi:10.1007/s00280-006-0363-x

Wiig, H., Tenstad, O., Iversen, P. O., Kalluri, R., & Bjerkvig, R. (2010). Interstitial fluid: the overlooked component of the tumor microenvironment? *Fibrogenesis & Tissue Repair, 3*, 12. doi:10.1186/1755-1536-3-12

Willett, C. G., Boucher, Y., di Tomaso, E., Duda, D. G., Munn, L. L., Tong, R. T., Chung, D. C., et al. (2004). Direct evidence that the VEGF-specific antibody bevacizumab has antivascular effects in human rectal cancer. *Nat Med*, *10*(2), 145-147. doi:10.1038/nm988

van der Wilt, C. L., Kroep, J. R., Loves, W. J. P., Rots, M. G., Van Groeningen, C. J., Kaspers, G. J., & Peters, G. J. (2003). Expression of deoxycytidine kinase in leukaemic cells compared with solid tumour cell lines, liver metastases and normal liver. *European Journal of Cancer*, *39*(5), 691-697. doi:16/S0959-8049(02)00813-4

Wong, A., Soo, Ross A, Yong, W.-P., & Innocenti, F. (2009). Clinical pharmacology and pharmacogenetics of gemcitabine. *Drug Metabolism Reviews*, *41*(2), 77-88. doi:10.1080/03602530902741828

Zamboni, W. C., Gervais, A. C., Egorin, M. J., Schellens, J. H. M., Hamburger, D. R., Delauter, B. J., Grim, A., et al. (2002). Inter- and Intratumoral Disposition of Platinum in Solid Tumors after Administration of Cisplatin. *Clinical Cancer Research*, *8*(9), 2992 -2999.

Zandvliet, A. S., Schellens, J. H. M., Beijnen, J. H., & Huitema, Alwin D.R. (2008). Population Pharmacokinetics and Pharmacodynamics for Treatment Optimization in Clinical Oncology. *Clinical Pharmacokinetics*, *47*(8), 487-513.

Permissions

The contributors of this book come from diverse backgrounds, making this book a truly international effort. This book will bring forth new frontiers with its revolutionizing research information and detailed analysis of the nascent developments around the world.

We would like to thank Ayman Noreddin MS, PhD, RPh, for lending his expertise to make the book truly unique. He has played a crucial role in the development of this book. Without his invaluable contribution this book wouldn't have been possible. He has made vital efforts to compile up to date information on the varied aspects of this subject to make this book a valuable addition to the collection of many professionals and students.

This book was conceptualized with the vision of imparting up-to-date information and advanced data in this field. To ensure the same, a matchless editorial board was set up. Every individual on the board went through rigorous rounds of assessment to prove their worth. After which they invested a large part of their time researching and compiling the most relevant data for our readers. Conferences and sessions were held from time to time between the editorial board and the contributing authors to present the data in the most comprehensible form. The editorial team has worked tirelessly to provide valuable and valid information to help people across the globe.

Every chapter published in this book has been scrutinized by our experts. Their significance has been extensively debated. The topics covered herein carry significant findings which will fuel the growth of the discipline. They may even be implemented as practical applications or may be referred to as a beginning point for another development. Chapters in this book were first published by InTech; hereby published with permission under the Creative Commons Attribution License or equivalent.

The editorial board has been involved in producing this book since its inception. They have spent rigorous hours researching and exploring the diverse topics which have resulted in the successful publishing of this book. They have passed on their knowledge of decades through this book. To expedite this challenging task, the publisher supported the team at every step. A small team of assistant editors was also appointed to further simplify the editing procedure and attain best results for the readers.

Our editorial team has been hand-picked from every corner of the world. Their multi-ethnicity adds dynamic inputs to the discussions which result in innovative outcomes. These outcomes are then further discussed with the researchers and contributors who give their valuable feedback and opinion regarding the same. The feedback is then collaborated with the researches and they are edited in a comprehensive manner to aid the understanding of the subject.

Apart from the editorial board, the designing team has also invested a significant amount of their time in understanding the subject and creating the most relevant covers. They scrutinized every image to scout for the most suitable representation of the subject and create an appropriate cover for the book.

The publishing team has been involved in this book since its early stages. They were actively engaged in every process, be it collecting the data, connecting with the contributors or procuring relevant information. The team has been an ardent support to the editorial, designing and production team. Their endless efforts to recruit the best for this project, has resulted in the accomplishment of this book. They are a veteran in the field of academics and their pool of knowledge is as vast as their experience in printing. Their expertise and guidance has proved useful at every step. Their uncompromising quality standards have made this book an exceptional effort. Their encouragement from time to time has been an inspiration for everyone.

The publisher and the editorial board hope that this book will prove to be a valuable piece of knowledge for researchers, students, practitioners and scholars across the globe.

List of Contributors

Aisha Qayyum
National University of Sciences and Technology, Pakistan

Carmen Navarro-Fontestad, Carlos Fernández-Teruel and Vicente G. Casabó-Alós
Universidad de Valencia, Spain

Victor Mangas-Sanjuán, Isabel González-Álvarez and Marival Bermejo
Universidad Miguel Hernández de Elche, Spain

Alfredo García-Arieta
Agencia Española de Medicamentos y Productos Sanitarios (AEMPS), Spain

Nobuhiro Goi, Katsunori Morishita, Akihito Taniguchi and Takayuki Ishii
Mikasa Seiyaku Company Limited, Japan

Debasis Mondal, Samantha L. Gerlach, Amrita Datta, Geetika Chakravarty and Asim B. Abdel-Mageed
Tulane University School of Medicine, Department of Pharmacology, New Orleans, LA, USA

Balmukunda Regmi and Laxman Bharati
Tribhuvan University Institute of Medicine, Maharajgunj, Kathmandu, Nepal

Ghada F. Ahmed
University of Minnesota, USA

Ayman M. Noreddin
Hampton University, USA

Obiageri O. Obodozie
Department of Medicinal Chemistry and Quality Control, National Institute for Pharmaceutical Research and Development, Abuja, Nigeria

S. K. Bhavsar and A. M. Thaker
Department of Pharmacology and Toxicology, College of Veterinary Science and Animal Husbandry, Anand Agricultural University, Anand, Gujarat, India

Akos Jerzsele
Szent Istvan University-Faculty of Veterinary Science, Department of Pharmacology and Toxicology, Hungary

Jin-Oh Hahn
University of Alberta, Canada

Guy A. Dumont and J. Mark Ansermino
University of British Columbia, Canada

Hironori Takeuchi
Department of Practical Pharmacy, Tokyo University of Pharmacy and Life Sciences, Tokyo, Japan

Bundit Yuangsoi
Department of Fisheries, Faculty of Agriculture, Khon Kaen University, Khon Kaen, Thailand

Emmanuel Adelaja Bamigbola
Department of Pharmaceutics and Pharmaceutical Technology, Faculty of Pharmacy, Niger Delta University, Wilberforce Island, Amassoma, Bayelsa State, Nigeria

Malkanthi Evans, Prachi Sharma and Najla Guthrie
KGK Synergize Inc., Canada

Mohammad-Reza Rashidi and Roghiyeh Pashaei-Asl
Research Center for Pharmaceutical Nanotechnology, Tabriz University of Medical Sciences, Tabriz, Iran

Daniel Lexcen
University of Minnesota, USA

Ahmed Salem
Abbott Co Ltd., USA

Walid M. El-Khatib
Ain-Shams University, USA

Virginia Haynes
Lake Superior College, USA

Ayman Noreddin
Hampton University, USA

Qigui Li and Mark Hickman
Division of Experimental Therapeutics, Walter Reed Army Institute of Research, Silver Spring, MD, USA

Matthew Links and Peter Galettis
St. George Cancer Pharmacology and Therapeutic Group, University of New South Wales, St. George Clinical School, South Eastern Illawarrawa Area Health Service, Australia